SEVENTH EDITION

LANGE Q&A™

PHYSICIAN ASSISTANT EXAMINATION

Rachel A. Carlson, EdD, MSBS, PA-C, DFAAPA
Associate Professor & Director
Division of Physician Assistant Studies
Shenandoah University
Winchester, Virginia

Albert F. Simon, DHSc, PA-C
Professor and Chair
Department of Physician Assistant Studies
Arizona School of Health Sciences
A.T. Still University
Mesa, Arizona

Bob McMullen, EdD, PA-C
Associate Professor and Director of Assessment
Department of Physician Assistant Studies
Arizona School of Health Sciences
A.T. Still University
Mesa, Arizona

Mc
Graw
Hill
Education

New York   Chicago   San Francisco   Athens   London   Madrid   Mexico City
Milan   New Delhi   Singapore   Sydney   Toronto

Lange Q&A™: Physician Assistant Examination, 7th edition

Copyright © 2016 by McGraw-Hill Education. All rights reserved. Printed in the United States of America. Except as permitted under the United States Copyright Act of 1976, no part of this publication may be reproduced or distributed in any form or by any means, or stored in a data base or retrieval system, without the prior written permission of the publisher.

Lange Q&A™ is a trademark of McGraw-Hill Education Global Holdings, LLC.

1 2 3 4 5 6 7 8 9 0 RHR/RHR 19 18 17 16

ISBN 978-0-07-184505-2
MHID 0-07-184505-4

Notice

Medicine is an ever-changing science. As new research and clinical experience broaden our knowledge, changes in treatment and drug therapy are required. The authors and the publisher of this work have checked with sources believed to be reliable in their efforts to provide information that is complete and generally in accord with the standards accepted at the time of publication. However, in view of the possibility of human error or changes in medical sciences, neither the authors nor the publisher nor any other party who has been involved in the preparation or publication of this work warrants that the information contained herein is in every respect accurate or complete, and they disclaim all responsibility for any errors or omissions or for the results obtained from use of the information contained in this work. Readers are encouraged to confirm the information contained herein with other sources. For example and in particular, readers are advised to check the product information sheet included in the package of each drug they plan to administer to be certain that the information contained in this work is accurate and that changes have not been made in the recommended dose or in the contraindications for administration. This recommendation is of particular importance in connection with new or infrequently used drugs.

This book was set in Times LT Std by Aptara, Inc.
The editors were Catherine A. Johnson, Andrew Moyer, and Cindy Yoo.
The production supervisor was Catherine Saggese.
Project management was provided by Amit Kashyap at Aptara, Inc.
The cover designer was Dreamit, Inc.
RR Donnelley was printer and binder.

This book is printed on acid-free paper.

Library of Congress Cataloging-in-Publication Data

Names: Carlson, Rachel A., editor. | Simon, Albert F., editor. | McMullen,
   Bob (Physician assistant), editor.
Title: Lange Q & A. Physician assistant examination / [edited by] Rachel A.
   Carlson, Albert F. Simon, Bob McMullen.
Other titles: Lange Q and A. Physician assistant examination | Physician
   assistant examination
Description: Seventh edition. | New York : McGraw-Hill Education, [2016] |
   Preceded by Lange Q & A. Physician assistant / [edited by] Anthony A.
   Miller, Albert F. Simon, Rachel A. Carlson. 6th ed. c2011. | Includes
   bibliographical references and index.
Identifiers: LCCN 2015026219| ISBN 9780071845052 (pbk. : alk. paper) | ISBN
   0071845054 (pbk. : alk. paper)
Subjects: | MESH: Physician Assistants–Examination Questions.
Classification: LCC R697.P45 | NLM W 18.2 | DDC 610.73/72069076–dc23 LC record available
at http://lccn.loc.gov/2015026219

McGraw-Hill Education books are available at special quantity discounts to use as premiums and sales promotions or for use in corporate training programs. To contact a representative, please visit the Contact Us pages at www.mhprofessional.com.

This goes out to all my PA colleagues, PA students, and to my husband and children:
Nothing worth ever having was achieved without effort—Theodore Roosevelt
My best to you all.

RAC

Never say never again

AFS

To Amy, my greatest supporter
To Bert, Randy, and Richard, my mentors

BM

Contents

Contributors

Frank A. Acevedo, PA-C, MS, DFAAPA
Assistant Professor
Department of Physician Assistant Studies
New York Institute of Technology
Old Westbury, New York
Senior Surgical Critical Care Physician Assistant
Winthrop University Hospital
Mineola, New York

William Cody Black, MHS, PA-C
Assistant Professor
Director of Didactic Education
A.T. Still University
Arizona School of Health Sciences
Department of Physician Assistant Studies
Mesa, Arizona

Rachel A. Carlson, EdD, MSBS, PA-C, DFAAPA
Associate Professor & Director
Division of Physician Assistant Studies
Shenandoah University
Winchester, Virginia

James F. Cawley, MPH, PA-C, DHL (Hon)
Professor
Department of Prevention and Community Health
Milken Institute School of Public Health
Senior Research Fellow
American Academy of Physician Assistants
Professor of Physician Assistant Studies
School of Medicine and Health Sciences
The George Washington University
Washington, District of Columbia

Daniel S. Cervonka, PA-C, CAS, DHSc
Associate Professor, Health Science
Director, Physician Assistant Institute
University of Bridgeport
Bridgeport, Connecticut

Ji Hyun Chun (CJ), PA-C, MPAS, BC-ADM
Adjunct Faculty, Physician Assistant Department
A.T. Still University Arizona School of Health Sciences
OptumCare Medical Group: Endocrinology
Orange County, California

Randy D. Danielsen, PhD, PA-C, DFAAPA
Professor and Dean
Arizona School of Health Sciences
A.T. Still University
Mesa, Arizona

Erica N. Davis, MHS, PA-C
Metropolitan Nephrology Associates
Alexandria, Virginia

Aleece Fosnight, MSPAS, PA-C, CSC, CSE
President, Association of Physician Assistants
Obstetrics and Gynecology
Urology and Sexual Health
Transylvania Regional Hospital
Brevard, North Carolina

Camilla E. Hollen, MMS, PA-C
Assistant Professor
Division of Physician Assistant Studies
School of Health Professions
Shenandoah University
Winchester, Virginia

Tricia A. Howard, MHS, PA-C, DFAAPA
Associate Professor
Physician Assistant Studies
South University
Assistant Program Director
Savannah, Georgia

Scott Lightfoot, PA-C, MPAS
Adjunct Faculty
A.T. Still University
Hematology/Oncology
Ironwood Cancer and Research Centers
Glendale, Arizona

Linda S. MacConnell, PA-C, MPAS, MAEd
Assistant Professor
Department of Physician Assistant Studies
AT Still University
Mesa, Arizona

Michael A. Mastroleo, BA, BS, PA-C
Adjunct Instructor
Physician Assistant Studies, Le Moyne College
Emergency Services, Crouse Hospital
Syracuse, New York

Ariel S. McGarry, MSPAS, PA-C
Assistant Professor
School of Health Professions
Division of Physician Assistant Studies
Shenandoah University
Winchester, Virginia

Ian McLeod, MEd, MS, PA-C, ATC
Assistant Professor
Physician Assistant Studies
Director of Didactic Education
A.T. Still University
Physician Assistant
Primary Care and Sports Medicine
Dignity Health Medical Group
Phoenix, Arizona

Phil R. Merrill, PA-C, MEd
Assistant Professor
Department of Physician Assistant Studies
Arizona School of Health Sciences
A.T. Still University
Mesa, Arizona

Natalie R. Nyren, MSPAS, PA-C
Assistant Professor
Division of Physician Assistant Studies
Shenandoah University
Winchester, Virginia

Raymond J. Pavlick Jr., PhD
Associate Dean
Pre-Clinical Education
Professor of Physiology
A.T. Still University
School of Osteopathic Medicine in Arizona
Mesa, Arizona

Brenda L. Quincy, PhD, MPH, PA-C, DFAAPA
Associate Professor
College of Pharmacy and Health Sciences
Butler University
Indianapolis, Indiana

Yunius San Nicolas, MPAS, PA-C
Inpatient Medicine—Hospitalist
Scott & White Memorial Hospital
Temple, Texas

Anne E. Schempp, MPAS, PA-C
Assistant Professor
Division of Physician Assistant Studies
Shenandoah University
Winchester, Virginia

Ashlyn Smith, MMS, PA-C
Endocrinology Associates, PA
House of Delegates
American Society of Endocrine Physician Assistants
Scottsdale, Arizona

Les Swafford Jr., MPAS, PA-C
APP Partner, Emergency Professional Services
BEMC, BUMC-P
Phoenix, Arizona

Nancy Kim Zuber, MPAS, PA-C
American Academy of Nephrology Physician Assistants
Alexandria, Virginia

Preface

In this seventh edition of *Lange Q&A™: Physician Assistant Examination*, we have responded to the changing aspects of health care by including many of the new treatments and diagnostic tests from modern medical practice in extensively updated questions, while maintaining the basic format and quality our readers have grown to expect. With this edition, overall 40% of the questions are new or substantially revised. An exciting change in this edition is access to the PAEasy.com web site for additional preparation, including a practice test.

We believe that you will find this review book a helpful and useful resource as you prepare for your initial or recertification examination. Your comments and constructive criticisms are welcome and will be considered in future editions.

We would like to thank our families, friends, and coworkers for their support, encouragement, and patience during the long hours spent working on this project. We also wish to thank Andrew Moyer, Catherine Johnson, and Cindy Yoo from McGraw-Hill and Amit Kashyap from Aptara for their editorial assistance and our contributors for their hard work and dedication. Finally, we thank you, the readers, for choosing this book as one of your resources. We wish you success on the examination.

Your comments and constructive criticisms are welcome and will be considered in future editions. Please send your comments to **OnlineCustomer_Service@mheducation.com**. Note the title of the book in the subject line.

Rachel A. Carlson, EdD, PA-C
Albert F. Simon, DHSc, PA-C
Bob McMullen, EdD, PA-C

Introduction

This book has been designed as a study aid to review for the Physician Assistant National Certification and Recertification Examination. Here, in one package, is a comprehensive review resource with 1,300 questions presented in the format seen in the national examinations. Each question is answered with a referenced, paragraph length answer. The entire book has been organized by specialty area to help evaluate your areas of relative strength and weakness and to further direct your study effort with the available references.

ORGANIZATION

This book is divided into specialty chapters preceded by an Introduction and a chapter on test-taking tips and techniques. Chapter 1 provides helpful hints on how to prepare for and take certification examinations. The remaining chapters cover the different NCCPA blueprint specialties. Supplemental chapters on pharmacology, emergency medicine, surgery, preventive medicine, and basic science aid the reader in additional content areas. The introduction provides information on question types, methods for using this book, and specific information on the national certifying and recertifying examinations. The reader is also urged to consult the National Commission on Certification of Physician Assistants' web site for up-to-date information on the examination procedures and content. The web site is *www.nccpa.net*.

QUESTIONS

The National Certifying Examination is made up of "one best answer–single item" questions. In addition, some questions have illustrative materials (graphs, x-rays, and tables) that require understanding and interpretation on your part. Finally, some of the items are stated in the negative. In such instances, we have highlighted in bold or italics the negative word (e.g., "All of the following are correct EXCEPT"; "Which of the following choices is NOT correct"; and "Which of the following is LEAST correct"). These items are discouraged, and now there are very few. Many examinees will not encounter a negative question when they take the certifying examinations.

One Best Answer–Single Item Question

This type of question presents a problem or asks a question and is followed by four to five choices, only one of which is entirely correct. The directions preceding this type of question will generally appear as below:

DIRECTIONS: Each of the numbered items or incomplete statements in this section is followed by answers or by completion of the statement. Select the ONE-lettered answer or completion that is BEST in each case.

An example for this item type follows:

1. An obese 21-year-old woman complains of increased growth of coarse hair on her lip, chin, chest, and abdomen. She also notes menstrual irregularity with periods of amenorrhea. Which of the following is the most likely cause?

   (A) polycystic ovary disease
   (B) an ovarian tumor
   (C) an adrenal tumor
   (D) Cushing disease
   (E) familial hirsutism

In this type of question, choices other than the correct answer may be partially correct, but there can be only one best answer. In the question above, the key word is "most." Although ovarian tumors, adrenal tumors, and Cushing disease are causes of hirsutism (described in the stem of the question), polycystic ovary disease is a much more common cause. Familial hirsutism is not associated with the menstrual irregularities mentioned. Thus, the most likely cause of the manifestations described can only be "(A) polycystic ovary disease."

Answers, Explanations, and References

In each of the sections of this book, the question sections are followed by a section containing the answers, explanations, and references for the questions. This section (1) tells you the answer to each question; (2) gives you an explanation, reviews the reason the answer is correct, and supplies background information on the subject matter (and in most cases, the reason the other answers are incorrect); and (3) tells you where you can find more in-depth information on the subject matter in other books and journals. We encourage you to use this section as a basis for further study and understanding. If you choose the correct answer to a question, you can read the explanation for reinforcement and to add to your knowledge of the subject matter. If you choose the wrong answer to a question, you can read the explanation for an instructional review of the material in the question. Furthermore, you can note the reference cited, look up the complete source in the references at the end of the chapter (e.g., McPhee SJ, Papadakis MA. *Current Medical Diagnosis and Treatment, 2009*, 48th ed. New York, NY: McGraw-Hill; 2009), and refer to the pages or chapter cited for a more in-depth discussion. With this edition, we have provided more detailed citations that include the chapter author in edited books in order to make it easier to find the references.

Practice Test

On the basis of user feedback, we no longer provide a chapter with a typewritten practice test. Instead, the users are provided access to the online question bank at PAeasy.com. This question bank and program aid the user in preparing for online test-taking to simulate the PANCE and PANRE.

HOW TO USE THIS BOOK

There are two logical ways to get the most value from this book. We will call them Plan A and Plan B.

In Plan A, you go straight to paeasy.com and take the comprehensive test and complete it according to the instructions provided. This will be a good indicator of your initial knowledge of the subject and will help to identify specific areas for preparation and review. You can then use the earlier chapters of the book to help you improve your relative weak points.

In Plan B, you go through each section checking off your answers and then comparing your choices with the answers and discussions in the book. It is best to complete a series of questions prior to checking off your answers and reading the explanations, as some of the explanations provide answers to following questions and therefore would not provide you with an accurate representation of your knowledge base. Once you have completed this process, you can take the Test on PAeasy.com and see how well prepared you are. If you still have a major weakness, it should be apparent in time for you to take remedial action.

In Plan A, by taking the Practice Test first, you get quick feedback regarding your initial areas of strength and weakness. You may find that you have a good command of the material, indicating that perhaps only a cursory review of each section is necessary. This, of course, would be good to know early in your examination preparation. On the other hand, you may find that you have many areas of weakness. In this case, you could then focus on these areas in your review—not just with this book but also with appropriate textbooks. (It is, however, unlikely that you will not study before taking the national boards, especially because you have this book.) Therefore, it may be more realistic to take the Practice Test after you have reviewed the chapters (as in Plan B). This is likely to provide you with a more realistic type of testing situation, as very few of us merely sit down to a test without studying. In this case, you will have done some reviewing (from superficial to in-depth) and your Practice Test will reflect this study time. If, after reviewing the question chapters and taking the Practice Test, you still have some weaknesses, you can then go back to the ends of the chapters and supplement your review with the reference texts.

We hope that through careful use of this book, whether through Plan A or Plan B, you find this text a useful and beneficial study guide.

SPECIFIC INFORMATION ON THE EXAMINATIONS

The official source for all information on the certification or recertification process is the National Commission on Certification of Physician Assistants, Inc. (NCCPA), Suite 100, 12000 Findley Road, Johns Creek, Georgia 30097. This organization comprises representatives from the major organizations of medicine, including the American Academy of Physician Assistants and the Physician Assistant Education Association. Their function is to formulate and administer the annual certification examination and to provide the means for recertification. Eligibility requires completion of a Physician Assistant program that is accredited by the Accreditation Review Commission on Education for the Physician Assistant (ARC-PA). Details regarding registration are available from the NCCPA. The entry-level examination (PANCE) consists of 300 questions addressing all aspects of physician assistant education, including basic science concepts, history taking, physical examination, laboratory and radiographic interpretation, as well as treatment modalities. Tips for improving your score on the examination are provided in Chapter 1. Currently, the recertification (PANRE) examination consists of 240 questions constructed in a similar format as the entry-level examination. For the PANRE, candidates may choose alternate forms for the examination. Sixty percent of the examination will be a generalist focus. Examination candidates may select primary care, adult medicine, or surgery for the remaining 40%. More details on this option are found through the NCCPA web site: www.nccpa.net.

CHAPTER 1

Test-Taking Skills: Tips and Techniques

Rachel A. Carlson, EdD, MSBS, PA-C, DFAAPA

To become certified and maintain their recertification status, physician assistants (PAs) are required to successfully respond to multiple-choice questions that appear on Board exams. Passing these exams requires not only medical knowledge but also test-taking skills. By providing examples, helpful explanations, and opportunities for experience and practice, this chapter and the subsequent chapters will help the PA student, or graduate, prepare for the Board exams and use effective test-taking strategies for answering the types of questions found on these standardized tests.

For initial certification, new graduates are required to complete and pass the Physician Assistant National Certifying Examination (PANCE). This 300-item multiple-choice exam covers primary care medical knowledge. For recertification, graduates are required to complete, in addition to a prescribed number of continuing medical education credits, one of the recertification exams, the Physician Assistant National Recertifying Examination (PANRE), which contains 240 multiple-choice questions. Sixty percent of the content will be generalist in nature, and the candidate can select remaining 40% to be focused in adult medicine, surgery, or primary care.

These exams are designed by the National Commission on Certification of Physician Assistants (NCCPA). The PANCE and PANRE are timed, multiple-choice tests that are presented and answered on a computer screen in local commercial testing centers. Information about exam development and scoring is available at the NCCPA Web site (http://www.nccpa.net). Examination candidates are encouraged to review the content blueprint to better understand the types of practices, tasks, and diseases covered by the Board examinations.

Three conditions are generally necessary for successfully passing multiple-choice examinations: (1) knowing about or recognizing the medical information contained in the questions; (2) using appropriate test-taking skills and strategies; and (3) avoiding situations that are likely to cause mistakes or impede performance. Test anxiety is an example; any standardized exam can produce anxiety that leads to error. However, remembering that clinicians like yourself who aim to be fair created most test questions can help you keep the exam's purpose in perspective. Multiple-choice questions are limited in what they can evaluate; they generally assess only fundamental cognitive knowledge (*Ballantyne, 2002*; *Burton & Miller, 1999*) and test-wise individuals use strategies that enable them to respond correctly to these types of questions.

The fact is, written tests—even at their psychometric "best"—are crude evaluation devices (*Ballantyne, 2002*; *Burton & Miller, 1999*). Multiple-choice questions cannot reflect a clinician's total fund of clinical skills. For example, patient rapport and the mechanics of examining patients are not accurately measured through multiple-choice questions. These questions can, however, successfully measure certain cognitive or knowledge skills. Computer-administered and scored exams have limited assessment capabilities. Test taking is a discrete skill that is different from clinical skills, and expert clinicians are not necessarily expert test takers.

Clinicians who must pass standardized tests should master the skill of test taking the same way they have mastered clinical skills. This may be accomplished by practicing the methods suggested in this chapter and answering the questions in the chapters. Reading and answering questions directly on a computer screen may be unfamiliar to some PAs, and learning to become accustomed and at ease with this format are skills well worth mastering prior to test time.

This chapter is organized into four sections: (1) what to do when preparing for the exam; (2) what to do during the exam; (3) illustrative questions; and (4) "dos" and "don'ts" that bring together the strategies explained in the previous three sections.

OBJECTIVES

In this chapter, the student or graduate PA will:

1. Identify proven techniques from the psychology of learning and educational measurement that will enhance test performance.
2. Identify information from testing theory that will help avoid "careless" errors.
3. Practice using clues to help identify correct and incorrect responses to exam questions.

WHAT TO DO WHEN PREPARING FOR THE EXAM

Getting into Practice

To develop test-taking skills, you must *actively* practice what you will be doing on the test, that is, answering multiple-choice questions. Reading and reviewing without active practice are rarely sufficient. To become proficient in suturing wounds, you need to not only *read* about suturing but also *practice* suturing. Some PAs have not taken a written exam in weeks, months, or years. Do not attempt to sit for Board exams without practicing answering multiple-choice questions any sooner than you would suture a facial laceration without having sutured skin in weeks, months, or years. You have the opportunity to practice responding to questions presented on a computer screen by going to the website paeasy.com.

Areas to Emphasize

Although you may enjoy studying the areas related directly to your own practice specialty, the task at hand is to pass the Boards. This is best accomplished by achieving a fundamental knowledge of all the medical disciplines represented on the exam. Therefore, it is suggested that you direct your studying to the primary care areas with which you are *least* familiar.

The certification and recertification exams are divided into two general dimensions: (1) organ systems, and the disorders and assessments PAs encounter; and (2) the knowledge and skills PAs should exhibit (*NCCPA Connect, 2015*). Up-to-date knowledge and skill content areas by percentages, additional testing categories, and a sampling of the diseases and disorders that are included in the content blueprint are available on the NCCPA Web site (www.nccpa.net).

As you prepare, you are strongly encouraged to write several of your own test questions. Those who do so frequently comment that their questions were surprisingly similar to those on the Boards. This occurs because only a limited amount of knowledge is amenable to the written exam format. In addition to identifying clinical information that is likely to be tested, you will gain valuable insight into the logic of test-item construction, which, in turn, helps you to select the intended correct answers from among the foils.

Scheduling Preparation Time

Using a planner, schedule specific periods for test preparation, setting aside specific times for actively reviewing and answering multiple-choice questions. Regular preparation over several months is preferred to cramming; studying just before the exam is usually nonproductive.

For the recertification exam, the amount of preparation needed depends largely on your practice. If your knowledge in primary care family medicine is current, you will need less preparation time than a PA practicing a subspecialty. Primary care knowledge will enhance test performance because in designing the Boards it is assumed that all PAs should have fundamental and broad knowledge in primary care medicine regardless of specialty.

The usual learning aids, such as the use of mnemonics, are highly recommended. The reader is referred to appropriate references for general information about study skills (*Academic Skills Center, 2015*; *Kelman & Straker, 2000*; *Study Skills Information, 2015*). The remainder of this chapter addresses specific information about the Board examinations.

WHAT TO DO DURING THE EXAM

Meeting Your Physical Needs

Your anticipated physical and environmental needs during the testing period should be considered when sitting for the PANCE or PANRE. Arriving early may allow you to select a computer terminal in an optimal location. If permitted, choose one that has few or no distractions, avoiding places near doorways and thoroughfares. Repeated interference can hinder your test performance.

Observe the lighting conditions. Extremely bright fore- and overhead lights or glare on computer screens have been reported. Examine the conditions when you arrive and, if possible, request a terminal that meets your needs.

Temperature extremes may be possible. Therefore, dress in layers that will allow you to be comfortable if the temperature is too low or too high. The room situation and your own thermoregulatory mechanisms may change over the course of the day, so be prepared and avoid conditions that may prevent your best performance. In addition, you may wish to consider bringing ear plugs if you are easily distracted by environmental noises; most testing centers provide headphones.

The exam is divided into several blocks of questions, approximately 60 questions per block for both the PANRE and PANCE. Even though the time frame within each block is conveniently provided on the computer screen, you are responsible for the amount of time taken between blocks and completing all blocks within the designated time frame. (See "Time Allowance.") Therefore, you should take a watch (nondigital) in case a clock is not easily visible. However, a timer is generally embedded in the examination and can be accessed via a keystroke.

You are entitled to a comfortable and quiet environment. However, be alert for potential distractions and make reasonable requests that may be honored by the testing center.

Consider Your Nutritional Needs

Consider nutritional and other personal needs. It is recommended that a heavy meal not be eaten within 2 hours prior to the exam, but a complex carbohydrate snack approximately 30 minutes before test time and between blocks of questions may be beneficial. You may also wish to bring with you packaged drinks and other supplies, such as tissues and cough drops. Although these items are not allowed in the testing room, keep snacks, food for lunch, and drinks handy for breaks taken between blocks of questions.

Get Proper Rest

Your exam performance should reflect your knowledge fund rather than mental and physical endurance. You are encouraged to experience the energy required for answering hundreds of multiple-choice questions by using the online testing available on paeasy.com.

Research has demonstrated that lack of sleep may result in deterioration of normal cognitive and psychomotor functioning similar to that seen with alcohol intoxication (*Williamson & Feyer, 2000*). No one could be expected to perform optimally on an exam while intoxicated! Lacking even 1 hour of sleep can be expected to impede your test performance. Try to get adequate sleep and rest

before the exam by practicing the same sleep hygiene advice given to patients.

Time Allowance

You are allowed a specified number of hours to complete the test on exam day. The amount of time you spend on breaks for rest, bathroom breaks, and meals between blocks of questions is up to you, but you must complete the entire exam within the designated time frame. You may check the number of questions per block and the number of blocks for the entire exam on the NCCPA Web site.

Before beginning each block of questions, calculate the average amount of time you can spend on each question. Typically, you have approximately 1 minute per question. Never go over the calculated time limit on your first attempt at each question. If you do not know an answer, you can mark it by clicking on the appropriate icon and return to it at the end of the block. Always allow for a few extra minutes at the end for returning to marked items and checking your answers. Your subconscious processes items you have previously encountered while you work on other questions. Also, clues often appear in other items. (See "Test Mechanics.") Candidates with learning disabilities who require extended time for examinations should contact the NCCPA significantly before the anticipated test date to schedule accommodations and provide necessary documentation.

Maintain a Positive Attitude

Set yourself up for success by maintaining a positive, confident attitude. Remind yourself that you prepared as best you could. Practice other self-coaching suggestions presented here and use others that have been successful for you in the past.

Do not become discouraged by questions you cannot answer. Test questions with a predetermined discrimination level are retained for use in future exams. If too many test takers answer a particular test item correctly, it is not used again. Therefore, many of the items you will be answering are those that other test takers have failed to answer. So keep in mind that there will be a number of questions you are not expected to answer correctly.

Also, be aware that some pre-test questions appear on standardized exams. Pre-test questions are those being field-tested, and they are not counted in your score. Because you do not know which items these are, assume that any absurd or very difficult question is experimental. Try not to become irate or unnecessarily concerned about any question.

Self-coaching and imaging or visualization techniques are helpful for all test takers (*Davis et al., 2000*; *Rossman, 2000*). Stress management methods may be especially useful for anxious test takers (*Davis et al., 2000*). Resources are also available to assess your own level of test anxiety (*Kelman & Straker, 2000*). Most professional athletes and stage performers master and routinely use these techniques to manage their stress and avoid situations likely to interfere with optimal performance.

Techniques should be learned and practiced several weeks before the exam and used the day of the exam. These techniques will not bring to mind medical information you have never studied, but they help you retrieve learned information and avoid exam errors due to extreme stress. Effectively managing stress generally results in improved concentration and the ability to reason logically. The suggested techniques may be learned through special courses and by consulting appropriate references (*Davis et al., 2000*; *Rossman, 2000*). Certain brief imaging procedures and breathing techniques described by Davis et al. (2000) and Paul et al. (2007) may be used for relaxing and improving concentration during the exam.

Keeping Your Concentration

During the exam, think of nothing except the questions in front of you. When working in the operating room, you concentrate on the operative field. Similarly, give the exam your full, serious, and undivided attention. Problems at work or home should be left at the exam room doorstep knowing you will later have the opportunity to return to them. Your one and only task during the exam period is to answer questions to the best of your ability.

Test Mechanics

The mechanics of navigating through the computer-administered Board exams may be unfamiliar to most. However, the instructions are explained in detail and practice opportunities are provided on the NCCPA Web site. To conserve your mental focus and energy on the exam day, and to maximize the time allotted for rest between blocks, it is helpful to thoroughly master the test instructions well before exam day on a computer without any time constraints. Never find yourself confused because you arrived at the testing center uninformed. In addition, always read the instructions as you begin each section of the exam.

Once you are into the exam, if you do not know the answer to a question, mark it on the computer screen. You will be able to return to it at the end of the block. Unanswered questions are counted incorrect, so it is

beneficial to answer the questions you plan to return to, just in case you run out of time at the end. Continue answering the questions you know. Frequently, you will find clues in other questions. In addition, your subconscious will have processed the questions you marked. It has been found that a great deal of information is successfully stored in your memory, but information *retrieval* is often the problem during exam time. Retrieval is enhanced by getting proper rest before the exam, using well-practiced stress management skills, and varying mental tasks during the exam to help keep your mind fresh and alert.

Should You Change Your Answer?

Contrary to some popular misconceptions, if you doubt an answer selection and want to change it, it is suggested that you do so. In numerous studies across disciplines examining thousands of changed responses, answers were changed approximately twice as often from incorrect responses to correct ones (*Bauer et al., 2007*; *Fischer et al., 2005*). It might not seem this way because we tend to remember mistakes when we have changed answers from right to wrong, but pay no attention to the times we changed answers correctly. On the other hand, if you really have no idea which response is correct and you find yourself purely guessing, perhaps your first instinct will have been accurate. However, if you do have a reason to change your answer, you will probably change from an *incorrect* to a *correct* response.

Answering by Elimination

Answering multiple-choice questions resembles the process of elimination used when arriving at a diagnosis from a differential diagnosis list. Selecting an answer on the exam by the process of elimination increases the probability of choosing the correct response. Using the stem of the question, form a sentence with each choice provided. After reading the stem, it may be helpful to think out the answer before examining the foils. However, be cautioned against selecting the first answer you think is correct; consider *all* possibilities before making a final selection.

Most test questions have in common the following anatomic features: (1) one choice is easily recognized as an outlier and incorrect; (2) two choices appear plausible as either slightly off the topic or the opposite of the correct answer (e.g., artery vs. arteriole, left vs. right hemithorax); and (3) two choices are correct, but one is better than the other.

The test taker's job is to first (1) eliminate the outlier; next (2) identify the two plausible choices and reject them after weighing them against the two that are more likely to be correct; and finally (3) select the better answer of the remaining two. As with a differential diagnosis, this job is most effectively accomplished through the process of elimination.

By using the process of elimination, almost anyone can eliminate the outlier. By doing so, the probability of selecting the wrong answer by guessing alone is now decreased by 20%. If the two plausible but incorrect choices are identified, you now have two remaining items, and the more correct choice should be selected. At this point, even a pure guess will have a 50–50 chance of being correct. When in doubt, play the odds to your advantage.

Always Triage First

Some exam questions involve dangerous, invasive, expensive, or potentially harmful choices. On the exam, as in real life, you must be alert for such errors. Screen each and every question for potentially harmful or invasive choices. Just as patients are triaged, you should similarly triage each test item encountered. There are three question categories that should be identified.

The first is the "friendly" question—the one that assesses your medical knowledge simply by asking for information. The second category includes those questions designed to trap. Unlike the "friendly" question, the item designed to trap has a preconceived attractor or distracter that may catch the test taker off guard. The third type of question is the one containing a potentially harmful choice. It may refer to a treatment, procedure, finding, or diagnosis.

The third category might not be necessarily tricky, but the test-item writer had in mind a possible pitfall that must *not* be selected. Examples of each question type are presented and discussed in the section "Illustrative Questions."

Some General Hints

Certain "hints" of test taking apply to most multiple-choice questions. These hints are not, however, as likely to work on standardized exams as on other tests, because standardized examinations are subject to many reviews and statistical analyses; but they may be useful as a last resort instead of guessing randomly.

The choices "all of the above" or "none of the above" have an increased probability of being correct. If a single-answer multiple-choice question contains two alternatives that mean exactly the same thing, they probably are both incorrect.

Finally, if you must make a pure guess, (C) is most likely the correct choice. The next most likely choice is (B).

Board exam test writers try to guard against these probabilities, but the odds might prove useful to you if all else fails.

ILLUSTRATIVE QUESTIONS

You may encounter the following types of questions on Board exams. Each example presented illustrates a strategy to help identify correct choices. As always, first triage each question and identify its category as (1) friendly, (2) designed to identify a harmful choice, or (3) designed to trap.

The Oversimplification

Some questions appear tricky because you think, "No question could be this simple!" If you really know the answer to a question, answer it without belaboring or looking for booby traps that are not there. The following is an example.

A 22-year-old woman presents with abdominal pain and fever of 2 days' duration. During the digital pelvic examination, she experiences exquisite pain when the cervix is moved. This suggests a diagnosis of

(A) Uterine fibroids
(B) Vaginitis
(C) Peritonitis
(D) Cystitis
(E) Cervical carcinoma

The item least likely to cause pain, (E), is eliminated. Any of the remaining four are possibilities, but peritonitis of any etiology is usually a safe diagnostic consideration. Do not get bogged down considering the unlikely diagnostic possibilities when an obvious choice is present. The oversimplification in this case is the correct answer, (C).

The Oversimplification that is Dangerous by Omission

As always, triage questions for traps. In the following question, the correct choice is an oversimplification that is dangerous by omission.

A painless testicular mass is found in an otherwise normal 29-year-old. Which of the following diagnoses should be pursued?

(A) Varicocele
(B) Carcinoma
(C) Furuncle
(D) Torsion
(E) Strangulation

Choices (C), (D), and (E) are ruled out because they usually are painful. (A) and (B), however, usually are painless. Because of its prognosis if left untreated, a testicular mass should be considered cancer until proven otherwise. Not to do so would be considered a life-threatening omission. The correct choice is (B).

Always screen questions for dangerous or critical choices whether harmful by omission or commission. A potentially harmful choice may present itself as an oversimplification.

Clues from Logic

Sometimes a logical (and correct) answer is contained in the stem, as shown in the following example.

The diagnosis of congenital hip dislocation is made

(A) In utero
(B) At birth
(C) At 6 weeks of age
(D) At 6 months of age
(E) Fluoroscopically

The term *congenital* means "present at birth." This is when the diagnosis of congenital hip dislocation is made. The correct choice is (B).

Clues from Related Areas

Similar to clues from logic, knowledge about related disciplines can provide additional hints.

An obese 45-year-old woman presents with acute genital pain. Upon examination, a 2- to 3-cm soft mass is found in the right labia majora. This is most likely

(A) Marked lymphadenopathy
(B) An inguinal hernia
(C) A femoral hernia
(D) A femoral aneurysm
(E) Neurofibroma

If the mass were located in the scrotum of an obese man, you would probably not miss the common diagnosis of inguinal hernia. Remembering from developmental anatomy that the labia majora and scrotum are corresponding tissues, (B) would be selected as the correct response, even if the test taker had minimal knowledge about surgical emergencies.

The "Odd" Choice

This test-taking clue is demonstrated by way of two examples. The first example comes from psychiatry.

Which of the following is NOT a sign of transsexualism?

(A) Rejecting one's anatomic sex
(B) Sex identity problems during childhood
(C) Dressing in clothing of the opposite sex
(D) Aversion toward one's own genitalia
(E) Sex identity problems during adolescence

Transsexualism is considered pathological because the patient considers a serious and invasive procedure preferable to living as his/her designated gender. Each choice except (C) implies pathology—rejecting one's own anatomy, sex identity problems, and aversion. The odd choice, (C), has, however, no associated pathology and is the correct response.

The second example follows:

A 65-year-old man complains of burning pain in the distal extremities especially upon exposure to heat. Upon examination, the hands and feet are warm and erythematous. The findings are most consistent with

(A) Diabetes mellitus
(B) Arteriosclerosis
(C) Raynaud phenomenon
(D) Thromboembolism
(E) Erythromelalgia

With the limited amount of information provided in the stem, it is unlikely that you can differentiate precisely among the choices provided. Your only clue is the odd choice. Even if you are unfamiliar with the infrequently seen problem of erythromelalgia, notice that choices (A) through (D) are associated with problems causing impaired circulation and cold extremities. "Erythro" or "red" implies *increased* circulation and warmth. (E), the odd choice among the options provided, is the correct answer.

Qualifying Words

Test-item stems containing qualifying words, such as *most, more, usually, often, less, seldom,* and *few,* will sometimes lead you to the correct answer.

A 32-year-old man presents with suspected alcohol withdrawal. The most likely finding would be

(A) Visual hallucinations
(B) Auditory hallucinations
(C) Fine motor tremors
(D) Major motor seizures
(E) Autonomic hyperactivity

Any of the above may be seen with alcohol withdrawal. However, fine motor tremors are the most common by far. The stem contains a qualifying word suggesting (C) as the correct choice.

If a qualifying word appears among the choices presented, it deserves special attention. Words such as *best*, *entirely*, *completely*, *always*, and *all* imply that something is always true; words such as *worst*, *never*, *no*, and *none* imply that something is never true. In clinical practice, *always* and *never* are rarely correct.

The Overqualified Choice

To make an answer acceptable, test-item writers sometimes must qualify a choice to the point at which the savvy test taker recognizes the ploy. The following example illustrates an overqualified choice.

In a 66-year-old emphysematous man with a 100-pack-per-year smoking history, clubbing is most appropriately described as

(A) Discoloration
(B) A flattened angle between the dorsal surface of the distal phalanx and the proximal nail
(C) An abnormal inwardly curved nail
(D) A measurably increased eponychium

The overqualified (lengthy) choice, (B), is likely to be correct, as in this example.

However, remember the "odd choice" described earlier! Sometimes, the very short "odd choice" is correct. You will recognize this variation because it will be attractively precise and succinct. Having at least some knowledge about the item, you will identify it as accurate.

Strange Terms

Choices containing completely unfamiliar words are likely to be distracters. Do not assume that you somehow missed an important chapter of Harrison's or that there is a gap in your education. If the choice appears completely bizarre, the test-item writer was probably scraping the barrel for a distracter.

On a routine peripheral blood smear from a 13-year-old boy there is a nucleated cell that is filled with bright red granules and is approximately three times the diameter of a typical red blood cell. This should be recognized as a(an)

(A) Franz–Kulig cell
(B) Myelocyte
(C) Eosinophil
(D) Olson cell
(E) Kupffer cell

Choices (A), (D), and (E) are fictitious. The test-item writer obviously did not lack imagination. (B) is familiar—remember basic anatomy or hematology? However, identifying a myelocyte on the peripheral smear is not basic primary care that the Board exam covers. PAs should recognize the morphology and significance of an eosinophil; thus, the correct response is (C).

"Apple Pie" Choices

There are some responses to which no one would object. Consider the following test question.

When evaluating a 23-year-old woman with vaginal bleeding, the most important clinical information is gained from the

(A) Prothrombin time
(B) Partial thromboplastin time
(C) CBC and iron studies
(D) Physical examination
(E) Detailed history

A patient's history provides a clinician's best information and is almost never incorrect. (E) is an "apple pie" choice.

The "apple pie" choice, however, can also be used by test-item writers to set traps.

The most important physical examination component(s) in the emergency evaluation of an unconscious patient is(are)

(A) Body symmetry
(B) A carefully performed and prompt neurological examination
(C) The cardiopulmonary examination
(D) Vital signs
(E) Blood gases

The initial triage of this question would identify it as a "trap" question because of the critical nature of the scenario combined with an incorrect "apple pie" choice. Blood gases are promptly dismissed because they are not physical examination components, for which the stem asks. (B) appears attractive because of its "apple pie" component. Nevertheless, remember your ABCs of emergency care! The correct response is (D).

Hints from Inconsistencies in Terminology

Grammar inconsistencies between the stem and a choice (e.g., tense, number, gender) are usually recognized by expert educational evaluators who screen Board exam test questions. You will, therefore, seldom encounter this type of "hint" on Board exams, although it will be found more frequently in classroom situations. Hints due to inconsistencies in terminology are more frequent than other types and you may benefit from being alert for this inconsistency.

A 19-year-old unconscious motorcycle accident victim with suspected multiple trauma is brought to the emergency department. The most significant physical findings usually will result from

(A) Undressing the patient
(B) A prompt neurological examination
(C) Interviewing the family
(D) Interviewing a witness to the accident
(E) All the above

Choices (C) and (D) can be excluded because they refer to historical, not physical, findings. This also excludes foil (E). Although indicated, at this point of presentation, the neurological examination is too focused. A more general, overall assessment provides the best clinical information. Therefore, critical, life-saving information across organ systems may be gained from observing the patient. Choice (A) is correct. Similarly, choice (E), blood gases, in the previous example was eliminated because it was inconsistent with the information asked for in the stem.

Rank Orders

When given a list of numbers or other rank orders, the correct response most often occurs somewhere between the extremes, as shown in these examples.

A 17-year-old woman presents with a history of pelvic discomfort during menses. She states that the amount of blood lost during each cycle is normal. The amount of her blood loss would be approximately

(A) 25 mL
(B) 35 mL
(C) 70 mL
(D) 100 mL
(E) 125 mL

Here is the second example:

A 45-year-old patient presents for follow-up on his diagnosis of chronic schizophrenia. To be termed *chronic*, this disorder should have been present for at least

(A) 3 months
(B) 1 year
(C) 2 years
(D) 3 years
(E) 4 years

Most test-item writers try to bury the correct answer somewhere in the middle. (C) is the correct answer in each example.

As with hints from inconsistencies in terminology, this clue does not work as often on Board exams as it does on classroom tests. Educational evaluators try to randomize the position of correct responses as much as possible. However, when in doubt, it is better to avoid the extremes when presented with rank-ordered options.

DOS AND DON'TS

The following dos and don'ts summarize some of the important points made earlier in this chapter.

DO practice what you will be doing during the exam, that is, answering multiple-choice questions on a computer. Answering these questions is a skill different from knowing clinical information. Get into practice for answering Board questions by actually answering similar questions. This is imperative for the clinician who has not taken a written or computer-based exam recently.

DO direct your studying to the primary care areas with which you are *least* familiar. Passing the Boards is best accomplished by achieving a fundamental knowledge level in each medical discipline assessed on the exam. This is especially important for PANRE candidates who have worked in a narrow subspecialty.

DO write your own multiple-choice questions. Not only will you gain insights into the mechanics of test-item writing and correctly answering questions, but also it is likely that many of your items will resemble actual Board exam questions.

DO get adequate sleep and rest before the exam. Some individuals elect to stay at a hotel located near the testing center in order to help get a good night's sleep and to avoid being late due to traffic conditions.

DO dress comfortably in layers that prepare you for temperature extremes, hot or cold. Coats or jackets may not be allowed.

DO arrive alert, calm, and well-rested.

DO bring beverages, food for lunch, and between-question block snacks. They are not allowed in the exam room but may be checked outside and accessed during breaks.

DO reread instructions provided by the testing agency the night before to ensure you arrive on time, at the right place, and with the right supplies. Recheck directions to the test center.

DO review in detail the information on the PANCE or PANRE content, instructions, and format found at www. nccpa.net

DO remember to bring admissions materials (such as your permit and government-issued identification).

DO examine the computer station you are assigned. Be alert for glare or other lighting problems, and potential traffic flow as others arrive and leave throughout the day.

DO consider that the proctor is there to support you. Ask for any reasonable support or change of computer location that will help you do your best.

DO pace yourself, allowing a calculated amount of time per question. In your time allocation, allow for some extra minutes at the end for returning to items you have marked as unsure.

DO avoid situations that might put you in an unfavorable mindset before the exam. For example, if you anticipate heavy highway traffic, arrive at the exam site a day early. If disturbances bother you during an exam, come early and request a computer in a far corner of the testing room. Let nothing interfere with your best possible performance on the day of the exam.

DO relate test questions to your own practice and experience. Test-item writers are people who have derived many of the test questions from their own clinical experience. What would *you* expect a primary care PA to know? Use this mindset to understand the goal of a question and to keep a positive attitude throughout the exam.

DO practice effective stress management techniques daily several weeks before the exam. During the exam, slow breathing always induces a parasympathetic response that will calm the mind and increase your concentration and focus. If you have any tendency for test anxiety, participate in programs designed to help you do your best.

DO change your answer if you have a good reason to do so. You are twice as likely to change from an incorrect response to a correct one. However, if you are only playing a hunch with no information about the topic at all, your first "gut" reaction might be correct.

DO triage each and every question before selecting your answer. Evaluate it as a question designed: (1) to test knowledge in a "friendly" way; (2) to trap by including common pitfalls; or (3) to evaluate your knowledge about potentially dangerous choices. In the first case, the apparent oversimplification is probably the correct choice. In questions designed to trap, beware of the "apple pie" choice—by omission or commission.

DO use the process of elimination. Your job is to find the single-best answer. As with a patient's differential diagnosis, this usually is done by *elimination*. Avoid choosing an answer until after you have considered all of the choices.

DO read the question stem and combine it with each foil to form a sentence. After doing this, use the process of elimination to arrive at the final answer.

DO mark items if you are not sure of the answer. Return to these items when you finish the question block.

DO make *educated* guesses, if you must guess. Use the information provided in this chapter to help in your decision. By also using your medical knowledge and judgment, your chances will be much improved.

DO be alert for qualifying words such as *most*, *more*, *usually*, *often*, *less*, *seldom*, and *few*, which will sometimes lead you to the correct answer.

DO eliminate choices containing completely unfamiliar words as distracters. If the choice appears completely unfamiliar, it is probably incorrect.

DO consider "apple pie" choices as probably correct. However, beware that they may also be used to trap.

DO consider choices that are different from the others—the "odd choice." This may involve the choice having the "odd" meaning or the "odd" length—long or short. The overqualified choice often is correct.

DO select item (C) when purely guessing. It is most frequently the correct response on many one-choice-only multiple-choice questions. If you eliminate (C) as a possibility, (B) is the next most likely choice. This is a "last-ditch" strategy that works more often on classroom tests than on Board exams.

DO select "all the above" or "none of the above" as a last-ditch strategy. When appearing as choices, they are more likely to be correct.

DO consider taking the exam as a positive experience. Keep your motivation high through self-coaching and imaging techniques. Use recommended stress management methods, especially if you are anxious when taking tests.

DO plan to reward yourself for a good performance after the exam. This facilitates a positive attitude.

DON'T cram at the last minute. This kind of preparation will not be adequate for an exam that covers mostly primary care breadth rather than depth.

DON'T eat a large meal within 2 hours of the beginning of the exam. Be well nourished, but not full.

DON'T leave any item blank at the end of the exam. Unanswered items will be counted wrong.

DON'T discuss the exam during the administration, during breaks, or after the exam; this adds to anxiety and may result in disqualification or revocation of your certification.

DON'T become irate over seemingly absurd or difficult questions. Answer them to the best of your ability, realizing that they probably are experimental questions that will not affect your score. Other test takers probably will also consider them absurd.

DON'T guess randomly. Even if you are completely unsure of the answer to a question, use the hints suggested in this chapter to increase the probability of guessing the correct response. Make educated, not random, guesses.

DON'T think of anything except the exam in front of you. Think of it as your "operative field." Concentrate on giving your best possible performance.

DON'T engage in any behavior that could be interpreted by the proctor as cheating or unprofessional conduct. All examination administration irregularities are reported to the NCCPA and could result in severe sanctions.

REFERENCES

Academic Skills Center. *Study Skills Library*. California Polytechnic State University; 2015. http://sas.calpoly.edu/asc/ssl.html. Accessed April 15, 2015.

Ballantyne C. *Multiple Choice Tests*. Perth, Western Australia: The Teaching and Learning Centre of Murdoch University; 2002.

Bauer D, Kopp V, Fischer MR. Answer changing in multiple choice assessment change that answer when in doubt – and spread the word! *BMC Med Educ* 2007;7:28.

Burton RF, Miller DJ. Statistical modelling of multiple-choice and true/false tests. *Assess Eval High Educ* 1999;24:399–411.

Davis M, Eshelman ER, McKay M. *The Relaxation and Stress Reduction Workbook*. Oakland, CA: New Harbinger Publications; 2000.

Fischer MR, Herrmann S, Kopp V. Answering multiple-choice questions in high-stakes medical examinations. *Med Educ* 2005;39:890–894.

Kelman EG, Straker KC. *Study Without Stress*. Thousand Oaks, CA: Sage Publications; 2000.

NCCPA Connect. *National Commission on Certification of Physician Assistants*. 2015. http://www.nccpa.net. Accessed April 15, 2015.

Paul G, Elam B, Verhulst SJ. A longitudinal study of students' perceptions of using deep breathing meditation to reduce testing stresses. *Teac Learn Med* 2007;19:287–292.

Rossman ML. *Guided Imagery for Self-Healing*. Tiburon, CA: H.J. Kramer, Inc; 2000.

Study Skills Information. *Cook Counseling Center, Virginia Polytechnic Institute and State University*. http://www.ucc.vt.edu/academic_support_students/study_skills_information/. Accessed April 15, 2015.

Williamson AM, Feyer AM. Moderate sleep deprivation produces impairments in cognitive and motor performance equivalent to legally prescribed levels of alcohol intoxication. *Occup Environ Med* 2000;57:649–655.

CHAPTER 2

Cardiology

Yunius San Nicolas, MPAS, PA-C

DIRECTIONS: Each of the numbered questions or incomplete statements is followed by possible answers or completions of the statement. Select the ONE-lettered answer or completion that is BEST in each case.

1. In which of the following situations would coronary artery bypass grafting (CABG) be preferred over percutaneous coronary intervention (PCI)?

    (A) Uncomplicated distal LAD of 85% stenosis in 2 areas
    (B) RCA lesion with 95% occlusion in someone with diabetes
    (C) Left main stenosis of 65%
    (D) LAD and RCA with 60% stenosis

2. A 62-year-old woman comes into the office complaining of substernal chest pain and diaphoresis. Her electrocardiograph (ECG) indicates ST elevation in leads I, aVL, V5, and V6. What is the next step of care for this patient?

    (A) Obtain a stat chest radiograph
    (B) Start a verapamil drip
    (C) Have the patient chew an aspirin
    (D) Repeat the ECG

3. Anticoagulation therapy for a mechanical heart valve should target what international normalized ratio (INR) range?

    (A) 1.0 to 2.0
    (B) 2.1 to 3.0
    (C) 2.5 to 3.5
    (D) 3.5 to 4.5

4. Indications for abdominal aortic aneurysm (AAA) repair include:

    (A) 4-cm aneurysm with tenderness to palpation
    (B) 5-cm aneurysm in a patient with coronary artery disease
    (C) 4.5-cm aneurysm that has grown 0.5 cm over the last 6 years
    (D) 5-cm aneurysm in a patient with a recent cerebrovascular accident

5. Definitive treatment for ascending aortic dissections (Stanford Type A) is:

    (A) Serial CT scans to follow changes
    (B) Emergent surgical intervention
    (C) Admit to the intensive care unit and manage the hypertension with intravenous (IV) labetalol
    (D) Admit to a step down unit for observation

6. A 71-year-old female with long history of heavy tobacco use and COPD presents with increasing dyspnea on exertion, abdominal fullness, and lower extremity edema. The physical examination reveals elevated jugular venous pressure, a right ventricular heave, S3 gallop, holosystolic murmur at the lower LSB, RUQ tenderness with hepatomegaly, and bilateral peripheral edema. ECG demonstrates right axis deviation, right ventricular hypertrophy without significant ST-T abnormalities, and peaked P waves. What is her likely diagnosis?

    (A) Heart failure
    (B) Pulmonary embolus
    (C) Acute coronary syndrome
    (D) Cor pulmonale

7. A 33-year-old woman presents for a routine physical examination and was noted to have hypertension 175/93 mm Hg. She is asymptomatic but is noted to have an abdominal bruit on examination. Which of the following is her most likely diagnosis?

(A) Primary hyperaldosteronism
(B) Renovascular hypertension
(C) Isolated systolic hypertension
(D) Primary essential hypertension

8. A 27-year-old male with remote history of endocarditis secondary to intravenous drug use presents with complaints of abdominal fullness and edema. On examination, he has jugular venous distention, hepatic congestion, and peripheral edema. A blowing holosystolic murmur is heard along the lower left sternal border than is intensified with inspiration. What is this murmur?

(A) Tricuspid regurgitation
(B) Mitral regurgitation
(C) Aortic stenosis
(D) Mitral stenosis

9. A 43-year-old man presents to the clinic with left-sided chest pain with shortness of breath that started 1 hour ago. An ECG was performed and shows ST elevation in II, III, and AVF at 2 mm. Where is the location of his myocardial infarction?

(A) Anterior
(B) Posterior
(C) Inferior
(D) Lateral

10. A 63-year-old morbidly obese female presents to the clinic with complaints of progressive bilateral lower extremity edema with itching. On physical examination, patient is found to have symmetric peripheral edema in the calves with brown pigmentation of the skin. The skin is taught over the pretibial and ankle regions, and a shallow ulcer is seen just above the right medial malleolus. What is the most likely diagnosis?

(A) Peripheral neuropathy
(B) Lymphedema
(C) Peripheral neuropathy
(D) Venous insufficiency

11. A 32-year-old male with a 10-pack-year history of smoking presents to the clinic with an ulceration to the top of the right great toe for the last 3 days. Prior to the ulceration, the patient had noticed intermittent episodes of severe pain and cyanosis to his right foot with pallor over the last 3 months. What is the most likely diagnosis?

(A) Atherosclerotic peripheral vascular disease
(B) Thromboangiitis obliterans
(C) Acute arterial thrombosis
(D) Raynaud phenomenon

12. Patients with systemic lupus erythematosus (SLE) have an increased predilection to which cardiovascular abnormality?

(A) Congestive heart failure
(B) Acute myocardial infarction
(C) Abdominal aortic dissection
(D) Pericarditis

13. A 68-year-old man presents to the emergency department with fatigue, dyspnea, and generalized weakness that has been getting worse over the past month or so. He has faint heart sounds with weak pulses and bradycardia on physical examination. His ECG demonstrates sinus bradycardia with low-voltage QRS and T wave flattening. His chest x-ray demonstrates enlarged cardiac silhouette with a globular appearance and pleural effusions. What is his most likely underlying diagnosis?

(A) Pulmonary embolism
(B) Hypothyroidism
(C) Hyperthyroidism
(D) Pheochromocytoma

14. What ECG change may be noted when a patient has a potassium level of 6.4 mEq/L?

(A) Prolongation of the ST segment
(B) Peaked T waves
(C) Loss of P waves
(D) Prominent U waves

15. The differential diagnosis of a patient with an ECG demonstrating prominent U waves includes:

(A) Digitalis toxicity
(B) Hypothermia
(C) Hypokalemia
(D) Hypermagnesemia

16. A 37-year-old female with history of hypertension and hyperlipidemia presents to the emergency department with acute, nonradiating, left-sided chest pain that she reports is 9/10. ECG reveals sinus tachycardia with nonspecific ST-T abnormalities. Which of the following labs is most sensitive for the diagnosis of a myocardial infarction?

(A) Arterial blood gases
(B) CPK enzymes
(C) Troponin levels
(D) AST and ALT

17. A 52-year-old male with a remote history of ionizing radiation to the chest wall presents to the ED with progressive dyspnea, fatigue, and edema. Physical examination reveals tachycardia, positive jugular venous distention (JVD) with a rise in inspiration, and mild to moderate peripheral edema of the extremities. ECG shows atrial fibrillation with low-voltage QRS complexes. Chest x-ray is unremarkable. What test should be ordered next in this patient to confirm diastolic heart failure?

(A) Holter monitor
(B) Echocardiogram
(C) Cardiac catheterization
(D) Stress test

18. A febrile patient with petechiae and a new-onset murmur of aortic regurgitation should have which of the following diagnostic tests to confirm the clinical suspicion?

(A) Holter monitor
(B) Transthoracic echocardiogram
(C) Cardiac catheterization
(D) Transesophageal echocardiogram

19. What is the modality of choice to demonstrate the anatomy and size of a thoracic aortic aneurysm?

(A) Chest x-ray
(B) Cardiac catheterization
(C) Echocardiogram
(D) CT scan of the chest and abdomen

20. A 29-year-old female with history of Marfan's syndrome presents to the clinic for an annual follow-up. On physical examination, a mid-systolic click is heard that occurs in a delayed fashion with squatting. What is the most likely diagnosis?

(A) Aortic stenosis
(B) Mitral valve stenosis
(C) Aortic regurgitation
(D) Mitral valve prolapse

21. A 3-year-old female presents for a well-child visit and was found to have a rough, continuous murmur heard over the left pulmonary area. What is this murmur?

(A) Aortic stenosis
(B) Patent ductus arteriosus
(C) Mitral regurgitation
(D) Pulmonic stenosis

22. A 21-year-old woman presents to the clinic with complaints of palpitations and a headache. On physical examination, the patient is anxious and diaphoretic with a blood pressure of 175/105 mm Hg and heart rate of 122 bpm. ECG demonstrates sinus tachycardia. Based on this presentation, what is a likely diagnosis?

(A) Supraventricular tachycardia
(B) Acute coronary syndrome
(C) Aortic dissection
(D) Pheochromocytoma

23. Which of the following radiographic findings is associated with tetralogy of Fallot (TOF)?

(A) Decrease in right ventricular size
(B) Rib notching
(C) Increased pulmonary vascular markings
(D) Boot-shaped heart

24. What is the cardiac auscultatory hallmark of an atrial septal defect?

    (A) Paradoxical split S2
    (B) Wide, fixed split S2
    (C) Systolic ejection murmur second right intercostal space
    (D) Holosystolic murmur heard at apex that radiates to axilla

25. A 53-year-old man with history of tobacco presents to the emergency department complaining of severe, ripping, substernal chest pain that radiates to his back. His blood pressure is 175/92 mm Hg. Chest x-ray reveals a widened mediastinum. What is his most likely diagnosis?

    (A) Acute coronary syndrome
    (B) Pneumothorax
    (C) Aortic dissection
    (D) Mitral stenosis

26. An 81-year-old woman with a 10-year history of well-controlled atrial fibrillation complains of a 6-day history of fatigue, dyspnea, and a 10-lb weight gain. She denies angina or diaphoresis. Based on this history what is the most likely diagnosis?

    (A) Acute coronary syndrome
    (B) Heart failure
    (C) Sinus tachycardia
    (D) Cardiac tamponade

27. A 67-year-old male with history of coronary artery disease with prior myocardial infarction and stable, chronic heart failure returns to the clinic for follow-up. Which of the following medication regimens is most appropriate for him?

    (A) Aspirin, metoprolol, valsartan, clopidogrel, morphine, diuretic
    (B) Heparin, atenolol, atorvastatin, clonidine, nitroglycerin
    (C) Amlodipine, lisinopril, aspirin, valsartan, atorvastatin, diuretic, metoprolol
    (D) Aspirin, metoprolol, lisinopril, atorvastatin, diuretic, nitroglycerin

28. A 37-year-old diabetic patient with history of paroxysmal atrial fibrillation and hypertension presents with a sudden onset of severe pain in his left arm. On physical examination, the left arm is cool and pale with nonpalpable radial and ulnar pulses. What is the most likely cause for his pain?

    (A) Atherosclerotic peripheral vascular disease
    (B) Venous stasis disease
    (C) Raynaud syndrome
    (D) Arterial embolization

29. Which of the following is the most likely cause of paradoxical splitting of S2?

    (A) Pulmonic stenosis
    (B) Left bundle branch block
    (C) Atrial septal defect
    (D) Right ventricular failure

30. Orthostatic hypotension is defined as a drop in systolic blood pressure of at least ___ or a drop of diastolic blood pressure of at least ___ within 3 minutes of standing from the sitting position.

    (A) 5 mm Hg; 10 mm Hg
    (B) 10 mm Hg; 20 mm Hg
    (C) 10 mm Hg; 5 mm Hg
    (D) 20 mm Hg; 10 mm Hg

31. A 47-year-old male presents with shortness of breath. On physical examination, the patient is sitting upright with moderately labored breathing, marked jugular venous distention (JVD), bilateral pulmonary rales, and a S3 gallop. Blood pressure is 120/90 and heart rate is 110 bpm. Chest x-ray shows pulmonary congestion. ECG demonstrates sinus tachycardia with low-voltage QRS. Which class of medication should be given to this patient immediately to improve symptoms?

    (A) Ace inhibitors
    (B) Beta blockers
    (C) Calcium channel blockers
    (D) Diuretics

32. Which of the following medications is used to control the ventricular rate during an acute event of rapid atrial fibrillation?

(A) Beta blocker

(B) Digoxin

(C) Warfarin

(D) Nitroglycerin

33. Which of the following is a contraindication for an exercise treadmill stress test?

(A) Mild aortic stenosis

(B) Unstable angina

(C) Previous myocardial infarction

(D) Nonspecific ECG changes

34. Which of the following antiarrhythmic drugs most potently blocks sodium channel current in the myocardium?

(A) Flecainide

(B) Procainamide

(C) Amiodarone

(D) Lidocaine

35. According to the American Diabetes Association, risk reduction for cardiovascular events in patients with diabetes can be achieved by the use of:

(A) Beta blockers

(B) Statins

(C) Cholesterol absorption inhibitors

(D) Aldosterone

36. A 58-year-old female with history of type 2 diabetes mellitus presents for a routine follow-up. Which of the following would have the LEAST impact on prevention of her risk of developing macrovascular complications from diabetes?

(A) Strict control of blood glucose levels

(B) HMG-CoA reductase inhibitor therapy

(C) Estrogen/progestin combination therapy

(D) ACE inhibitors to control her hypertension

37. Secondary prevention of an ST-elevation myocardial infarction should include which of the following measures?

(A) Estrogen therapy

(B) ACE inhibitors

(C) Folate or Vitamin B6

(D) Calcium channel blockers

38. An increase in which of the following factors is most likely to increase the preload?

(A) Arterial vascular tone

(B) Stroke volume

(C) Heart rate

(D) Intravascular volume

39. What is the mechanism by which cardiac tamponade impedes cardiac output?

(A) Decreased inflow of blood to the ventricles

(B) Decreased pressure in pericardium

(C) Increased pressure decreases sinus rhythm

(D) Increase in end-diastolic volume

40. Which of the following is used to describe diastolic dysfunction?

(A) Increased afterload

(B) Decreased preload

(C) Decreased stroke volume

(D) Decreased ventricular myocardial compliance

41. A 37-year-old woman with a history of hypertension presents to the emergency department with complaints of shortness of breath. She was placed on a telemetry monitor. What is your diagnosis?

(A) Normal sinus rhythm

(B) Atrial fibrillation

(C) Sinus tachycardia

(D) Nodal rhythm

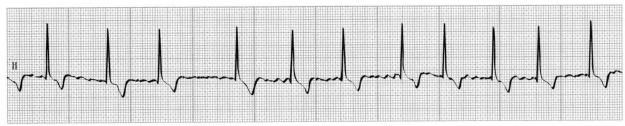

Figure 2-1.

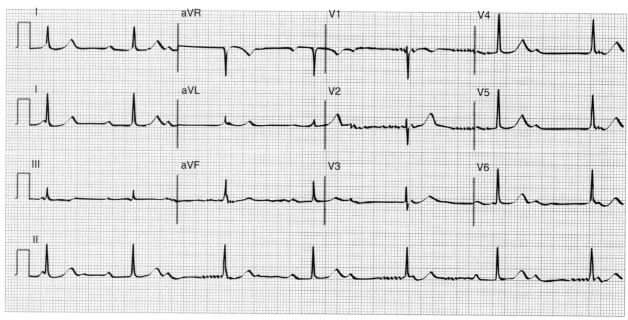

Figure 2-2. Reproduced with permission from Kasper D, Fauci A, Hauser S, et al. *Harrison's Principles of Internal Medicine.* 19th ed. New York: McGraw-Hill Education; 2015. Figure 278E-6.

42. A 29-year-old man presents with extreme fatigue and shortness of breath. What is the abnormality noted in this ECG?

    (A) Complete AV block
    (B) Type II second-degree AV block
    (C) Junctional rhythm
    (D) Atrial fibrillation

43. You have started your patient who has giant cell arteritis on her glucocorticoid therapy. Which of the following laboratory studies would be used to monitor her response to this therapy?

    (A) Cardiac enzymes
    (B) Sedimentation rate
    (C) Rheumatoid factor
    (D) Complete blood cell count

44. A 50-year-old woman presents to the office with a 1-week history of substernal chest pain. The symptoms occur with climbing the stairs in her home and with moderate-paced walking. The pain is relieved with rest. She denies any current chest pain. Her physical examination and ECG are normal. What is the next test you would order?

    (A) Exercise treadmill stress test
    (B) Cardiac enzymes

    (C) Radionuclide stress myocardial perfusion imaging
    (D) Echocardiogram

45. A 19-year-old woman presents for a physical examination. Physical examination is unremarkable except for an irregular heartbeat. An ECG was ordered and demonstrates normal sinus rhythm with premature atrial contractions (PACs). She denies any symptoms. What is the most appropriate treatment plan for this patient?

    (A) Catheter ablation
    (B) Observation only
    (C) Metoprolol
    (D) Class Ic antiarrhythmics

46. A 47-year-old man who is 1-week status-post coronary artery bypass grafting (CABG) presents to the emergency department with complaints of dizziness. Vital signs include blood pressure of 82/60 and heart rate of 122. Physical examination reveals a mildly anxious and diaphoretic patient with positive jugular venous distention and distant heart sounds. ECG shows sinus tachycardia with low-voltage QRS. Chest x-ray demonstrates a markedly enlarged cardiac silhouette. What is the most appropriate treatment?

(A) Cardiac catheterization

(B) Redo coronary artery bypass grafting

(C) Echocardiograph-guided pericardiocentesis

(D) Limited thoracotomy with pericardial window

47. The causative agent of Chagas' disease is

(A) *Brucella*

(B) *Trypanosoma cruzi*

(C) Coxsackie B virus

(D) *Francisella tularensis*

48. Which of the following is *not* considered a key feature of tetralogy of Fallot?

(A) Ventricular septal defect

(B) Overriding aorta

(C) Right ventricular hypertrophy

(D) Left ventricular outflow obstruction

49. A 69-year-old patient with a history of mitral stenosis and heart failure presents to the clinic complaining of a 2-week history of fatigue and dyspnea when taking her morning shower. Her symptoms resolve after resting for 10 minutes. What is the functional classification based on the New York Heart Association classification?

(A) Class I

(B) Class II

(C) Class III

(D) Class IV

50. A 50-year-old male with history of coronary artery disease has a 10-second run of monomorphic ventricular tachycardia (VT) without a history of prolonged QT. What is the first-line pharmacologic treatment for this patient?

(A) Propafenone

(B) Adenosine

(C) Verapamil

(D) Amiodarone

51. What is the most serious toxic effect of amiodarone?

(A) Corneal deposits

(B) Photodermatitis

(C) Peripheral neuropathy

(D) Pulmonary toxicity

52. A 61-year-old healthy man presents with an episode of presyncope and a 3-week history of palpitations. Physical examination reveals vital signs that are stable except tachycardia with an irregularly irregular rhythm. The remainder of his examination is normal. A 12-lead ECG reveals an irregular rhythm with no P waves appreciated. He is admitted for anticoagulation therapy and cardioversion is planned for a later date. What is the minimum target INR and the length of anticoagulation recommended before proceeding with elective electrocardioversion?

(A) 1.5

(B) 1.8

(C) 2.5

(D) 3.0

53. A 90-year-old female with a history of tachycardia–bradycardia syndrome (sinoatrial node dysfunction) with subsequent pacemaker insertion presents to the emergency department with complaints of a 4-day history of increasing fatigue, dyspnea on exertion, and palpitations. Physical examination is remarkable for marked bradycardia with an irregular heart rate, marked jugular pulsations, and canon A waves. What is the next most appropriate step to manage this patient?

(A) 12-lead ECG

(B) Chest x-ray

(C) Diuretics

(D) Dobutamine

54. What ECG finding is suggestive of type II second-degree AV block?

(A) PR interval greater than 0.2 seconds that remains fixed

(B) Progressive lengthening of the PR interval with a dropped beat

(C) An occasional dropped beat with fixed PR intervals

(D) Complete dissociation between P waves and QRS complexes

55. An 83-year-old woman with a history of hypertension is admitted to the hospital for asymptomatic bradycardia. On the telemetry monitor, she is in sinus bradycardia of 38 bpm and is noted to be taking a beta blocker. While the patient is on the telemetry floor, the nurse calls to inform you that the patient's heart rate is 130 bpm and her monitor tracing lacks P waves. The nurse states the patient is asymptomatic and her vitals are stable. Given this patient's history, what is her likely diagnosis?

(A) AV node re-entrant tachycardia

(B) Multifocal atrial tachycardia

(C) Premature atrial contractions

(D) Sinoatrial (SA) node dysfunction

56. A 20-year-old healthy, active male comes to the office for his annual evaluation. He denies any symptoms or previous medical illness. He is noted to have a grade I mid-systolic murmur at the left sternal border. What is the next step in his work-up?

(A) Echocardiogram

(B) Electrocardiogram

(C) Coronary arteriogram

(D) No further evaluation needed

57. A patient who has just had a minimally invasive coronary artery bypass grafting (CABG) is in the intensive care unit and has a decrease in his cardiac output. Vital signs are stable. Hemodynamic monitoring suggests hypovolemia. Blood count is stable. What is the most appropriate way to improve his cardiac output pharmacologically?

(A) Dobutamine

(B) Epinephrine

(C) Intravenous fluids

(D) Intra-aortic balloon pump

58. Metabolic syndrome is a cluster of risk factors. Which of the following is one of the diagnostic criterion for metabolic syndrome?

(A) HDL less than 50 mg/dL in a male

(B) Blood pressure greater than 130/85 mm Hg

(C) Fasting blood sugar greater than 96 mg/dL

(D) Male abdominal girth greater than 35 in

59. The goal of treatment for pulmonary arterial hypertension is to decrease pulmonary artery pressures in an effort to unload the right ventricle. Which drug should be tried in a patient who had a marked reduction in pulmonary artery pressures with vasodilators during the cardiac catheterization?

(A) Epoprostenol

(B) Bosentan

(C) Sildenafil

(D) Iloprost

60. A 28-year-old woman is admitted to the hospital for further evaluation of her syncopal episodes after a Holter monitor reveals three runs of sustained ventricular tachycardia that lasted between 20 and 30 seconds. While in the hospital, her monitor tracings reveal multifocal premature ventricular contractions. She has no symptoms, and a 12-lead ECG is without evidence of ST-segment elevation or depression. What study would you recommend to evaluate her ventricular excitability?

(A) Loop recorder

(B) Electrophysiology study

(C) Exercise treadmill stress test

(D) Transesophageal echocardiogram

61. Pharmacologic management of peripheral arterial disease includes:

(A) Elastic compression stockings

(B) Calcium channel blockers

(C) Cilostazol

(D) Warfarin

62. A 33-year-old male with diabetes mellitus type I and end-stage renal disease presents to the difficulty breathing. He has missed his last two hemodialysis (HD) treatments. On examination, he has bilateral inspiratory crackles and peripheral edema. ECG demonstrates bradycardia with peaking of the T waves, a widened QRS, and flattening of the P waves. What would be the most likely etiology for these ECG changes?

(A) Hypercalcemia

(B) Hypomagnesemia

(C) Digitalis effect

(D) Hyperkalemia

63. Which of the following symptoms is most specific for cardiac disease?

(A) Shortness of breath

(B) Paroxysmal nocturnal dyspnea

(C) Pedal edema

(D) Orthopnea

64. Outpatient Holter monitoring is *not* indicated in which of the following scenarios?

(A) Incidental discovery of premature atrial contractions

(B) Suspected tachycardia-induced cardiomyopathy

(C) Patients with a reduced left ventricular systolic function after myocardial infarction

(D) Asymptomatic atrial fibrillation

65. A 71-year-old man presents to the emergency department with complaints of chest pain and shortness of breath. Vital signs include blood pressure 86/40 and heart rate 139 bpm. Physical examination is remarkable for an anxious male with diaphoresis and an irregularly, irregular rhythm with tachycardia. ECG demonstrates tachycardia with heart rate of 155 bpm, an irregularly irregular rhythm with no discernible T waves, and ST-segment depressions V5, V6, I, and aVL. What is the next appropriate treatment for this patient?

(A) Beta blocker

(B) Adenosine

(C) Amiodarone

(D) Electrocardioversion

66. Which of the following medications has a positive inotropic effect on the heart?

(A) Digoxin

(B) Metoprolol

(C) Lisinopril

(D) Furosemide

67. A 47-year-old female presents with weakness, fatigue, and shortness of breath. Vital signs reveal a blood pressure 80/50 mm Hg and heart rate is 40 and irregular. ECG shows bradycardia with fixed PR intervals and dropped QRS beats in a 3:1

pattern. What is the most appropriate treatment for this patient?

(A) Atropine

(B) Adenosine

(C) Transvenous pacemaker

(D) Observation only

68. A 57-year-old male with history of hypertension presents to the emergency department with crushing, left-sided chest pain, and shortness of breath starting 30 minutes prior. The pain is severe and not alleviated with nitroglycerin. Vital signs are stable. Physical examination demonstrates an S4 gallop. What are the most appropriate next steps in management in this patient?

(A) Discharge patient, outpatient stress test, aspirin, follow-up in 1 week

(B) Thrombolytic therapy, emergent heart catheterization, oxygen

(C) Cardiac enzymes, aspirin, oxygen, morphine, metoprolol, ECG

(D) ECG, cardiac enzymes, enoxaparin, aspirin, metoprolol, oxygen

69. Diastolic heart failure is commonly seen in which of the following conditions?

(A) Alcohol-related cardiomyopathy

(B) Hypovolemia

(C) Left ventricular hypertrophy

(D) Chagas' disease

70. A 37-year-old female presents with chest pain, shortness of breath, and fatigue upon mild exertion. Last week she was diagnosed with iron deficiency anemia secondary to menorrhagia. She denies any other previous medical history. ECG today is unremarkable. What is the next appropriate step in management of this patient's cardiac type symptoms?

(A) Admit patient for unstable angina

(B) Patient should have a prompt exercise stress test

(C) Treat anemia first and re-evaluate patient if symptoms persist

(D) Cardiac catheterization

71. A 37-year-old male with history of insulin resistance, hypertension, and hyperlipidemia presents to the emergency department with chest pain and shortness of breath while mowing the grass today. He has had episodes of chest pain that occur with exertion and is relieved by rest over the last 2 weeks. An exercise treadmill stress test was performed with 2-mm ST-segment depressions laterally with chest pain symptoms. Subsequently, a cardiac catheterization was performed and was found to have normal coronary arteries. What is his most likely diagnosis?

(A) Prinzmetal angina

(B) Atypical angina

(C) Cardiac syndrome X

(D) Obstructive coronary artery disease

72. A 43-year-old male with history of an anterior myocardial infarction with LAD stent placed 9 days ago presents to the clinic with chest pain. The pain is worsened when he is supine and improves with sitting up. His temperature is 100.9°F. On physical examination, you hear a high-frequency, scratching sound that is increased with inspiration. ECG shows sinus tachycardia with diffuse J-point elevation. What is this patient's diagnosis?

(A) Acute myocardial infarction

(B) Dressler syndrome

(C) Acute viral pericarditis

(D) Stable angina

73. A patient with history of systolic heart failure is taking digoxin. Which of the following situations would predispose this patient to an increased risk of digoxin toxicity?

(A) Hypernatremia

(B) Hyperkalemia

(C) Hypocalcemia

(D) Hypomagnesemia

74. A 59-year-old male presents with chest pain, dyspnea, and presyncope. The symptoms occurred after climbing a flight of stairs. He has a late systolic-ejection murmur (SEM) heard in the second intercostal space (ICS) at the right sternal border with radiation to the carotids and the apex. The murmur is decreased with Valsalva maneuver. What is this murmur?

(A) Aortic stenosis

(B) Hypertrophic obstructive cardiomyopathy

(C) Ventricular septal defect

(D) Pulmonary stenosis

75. A 57-year-old male has had an acute inferior wall myocardial infarction. He had stent placed to his RCA and found to have a preserved left ventricular function. However, the patient received an intra-aortic balloon pump for hypotension in the cath lab. The patient remains hypotensive with cool, cyanotic extremities and has low urine output. What is the most appropriate initial pharmacologic management in this patient?

(A) Dopamine, intravenous fluids

(B) Beta blocker, low-dose diuretic, intravenous fluids

(C) Dopamine, dobutamine, diuretic

(D) Dobutamine, beta blocker, ace inhibitor, diuretic

76. An 18-year-old male presents with an episode of palpitations followed by a brief loss of consciousness. ECG shows delta waves and a short PR interval. Which of the following is the preferred long-term treatment for this patient's diagnosis?

(A) Digoxin

(B) Verapamil

(C) Radiofrequency catheter ablation

(D) Percutaneous coronary intervention

77. An 18-year-old patient comes to the office for a well-visit. The patient has a history of a completely repaired ventricular septal defect with no residual side effects. Which of the following procedures does the American Heart Association recommend for endocarditis prophylaxis in this type of patient?

(A) Routine dental cleaning

(B) Esophageal stricture dilation

(C) Bronchoscopy with biopsy

(D) Patient does not require routine endocarditis prophylaxis

78. A 37-year-old female with a 10-year history of amyloidosis complains of progressive weakness, fatigue, abdominal fullness, and pedal edema progressive over the last month. She denies any recent illness. On physical examination, the patient has positive jugular venous distention, pitting edema of bilateral lower extremities, and hepatomegaly with mild tenderness to palpation. On auscultation a holosystolic murmur is heard at the left sternal border that increases with inspiration. What is the most likely diagnosis?

(A) Cor pulmonale
(B) Cardiac tamponade
(C) Restrictive cardiomyopathy
(D) Infectious myocarditis

79. A 39-year-old previously health female presents to the emergency department for chest pain episodes. She reports substernal chest pain that occurs at rest and usually in the morning. She is chest pain free on initial arrival to the emergency department; however, toward the end of her physical examination she has return of her chest pain with ST-segment elevation seen on telemetry. The ST-segment elevation lasts less than 1 minute. She was taken to the cath lab and cardiac angiogram demonstrates transient right coronary artery vasospasm with ST-segment elevation but otherwise has normal coronaries. What is the appropriate treatment in this patient?

(A) Betablocker
(B) ACE-inhibitor
(C) Aldosterone antagonist
(D) Calcium channel blocker

80. Which of the following refers to conduction velocity of the atrioventricular node?

(A) Chronotropy
(B) Dromotropy
(C) Inotropy
(D) Lusitropy

81. A 12-year-old boy was diagnosed with an atrial septal defect (ASD). What would you expect to see on his ECG?

(A) Left ventricular hypertrophy (LVH)
(B) Right ventricular hypertrophy (RVH)
(C) Right bundle branch block (RBBB)
(D) Left bundle branch block (LBBB)

82. Which of the following conditions can lead to high-output heart failure?

(A) Leukocytosis
(B) Hyperthyroidism
(C) Restrictive cardiomyopathy
(D) Aortic stenosis

83. A 20-year-old female complains of palpitations. Vitals signs are stable. Physical examination is normal except for tachycardia. ECG shows a narrow-complex tachycardia with heart rate 180 bpm with a regular rhythm. What is the most appropriate initial treatment for this patient?

(A) Electrocardioversion
(B) Amiodarone
(C) Adenosine
(D) Carotid massage

84. A 62-year-old male with a history of mild mitral stenosis complains of fatigue and palpitations. Physical examination is unremarkable except an irregularly, irregular rhythm with mild tachycardia. ECG shows atrial fibrillation with heart rate of 119 bpm and no evidence of ischemia. What is the recommended initial therapy for this patient?

(A) Rivaroxaban
(B) Dabigatran
(C) Heparin
(D) Clopidogrel

85. A 23-year-old female comes to the emergency department for a syncopal episode. Just prior to the syncopal episode, the patient experienced painful menstrual cramping. She experienced a cold sweat and palpitations with the cramping. The patient describes similar episodes to her menstrual cramps in the past. Her vital signs and physical examination are normal. ECG is unremarkable. What is the likely diagnosis for her syncope?

(A) Vasovagal syndrome
(B) AV-nodal re-entrant tachycardia
(C) Long QT syndrome
(D) Hypertrophic obstructive cardiomyopathy

86. Which of the following are signs/symptoms consistent with digoxin toxicity?

(A) Anorexia

(B) Constipation

(C) Sinus tachycardia

(D) Scooped ST segments

87. What is the pathophysiologic basis for a widened pulse pressure commonly seen in the elderly?

(A) Dehydration

(B) Diastolic dysfunction

(C) Decreased arterial compliance

(D) Increased heart rate

88. A 79-year-old female presents with an acute, systolic heart failure exacerbation. Which of the following medications is contraindicated?

(A) Diuretic

(B) Beta blocker

(C) ACE inhibitor

(D) Nitroglycerin

89. A 20-year-old male is found to have bicuspid aortic valve stenosis. Which of the following is true concerning bicuspid aortic valve stenosis?

(A) Antimicrobial endocarditis is recommended

(B) Offspring of these patients have 75% risk of the disease

(C) Decreased risk for thoracic aortic aneurysms

(D) Higher likelihood of aortic valve replacement in adulthood

90. A 69-year-old female with history of severe COPD is found to have atrial fibrillation. Which of the following medications is preferred in this patient for rate control?

(A) Cardizem

(B) Nebivolol

(C) Sotalol

(D) Adenosine

91. A 7-year-old patient is diagnosed with congenital long QT syndrome. Which of the following situations could cause the patient to experience sudden cardiac death due to torsades de pointes?

(A) Sleeping

(B) Eating

(C) Exercising

(D) Resting

92. Which of the following is a hallmark of unstable angina?

(A) Pain that occurs at rest

(B) Pain without radiation

(C) Pain precipitated by stress and relieved with rest

(D) Pain lasting for 4 days

93. You are taking the history of a patient who is scheduled to have an internal cardiac defibrillator placed when the patient becomes unresponsive without a pulse. The nurse attaches a cardiac monitor and a chaotic rhythm with no discernible pattern is seen. What is the most likely diagnosis?

(A) Atrial flutter

(B) Ventricular tachycardia

(C) Asystole

(D) Ventricular fibrillation

94. A 2-week-old infant is found to have a harsh, continuous, machine-like murmur heard over the upper left sternal border. What treatment is initially used in an effort to close this type of murmur?

(A) Aspirin

(B) Indomethacin

(C) Open heart surgery

(D) Cardiac catheterization with stent

95. Torsades de pointes should be suspected in which of the following descriptions?

(A) A narrow-complex tachycardia that is regular

(B) Irregular P waves every other beat

(C) Polymorphic, wide-complexed tachycardia

(D) Prolonged PR interval with tachycardia

96. A 43-year-old male comes into the office with atrial fibrillation of unknown duration. He is asymptomatic. He has history of paroxysmal atrial fibrillation in the past. He has no other medical history. Vital signs are blood pressure 120/64 mm Hg and heart rate is 68 bpm. What is the most appropriate medication to start on this patient?

(A) Aspirin

(B) Warfarin

(C) Digoxin

(D) Metoprolol and warfarin

97. A 6-year-old female comes into the office for an annual visit. The child has a grade II murmur over the bilateral upper sternal borders that disappears when jugular vein is compressed. What is the best next step in treatment for this murmur?

(A) Echocardiogram

(B) Referral to cardiology

(C) Angiogram of neck

(D) No intervention is needed

98. A 60-year-old male presents with shortness of breath and orthopnea. The patient was found to have an S3 gallop and an apical holosystolic murmur that radiates to the axilla. What is this murmur?

(A) Tricuspid regurgitation (TR)

(B) Mitral regurgitation (MR)

(C) Aortic stenosis (AS)

(D) Ventricular septal defect (VSD)

99. A 47-year-old female with newly diagnosed atrial fibrillation of unknown duration presents with increasing symptoms of dizziness and fatigue due to episodes of rapid ventricular response despite maximal medical management. What diagnostic study should be performed before elective cardioversion?

(A) Transthoracic echocardiogram

(B) Chest x-ray

(C) Transesophageal echocardiogram

(D) CT scan of chest with angiogram

100. A 37-year-old male was recently diagnosed with systolic heart failure secondary to alcohol use. He admits to drinking 12 beers nightly for the last 8 years. Which of the following is the most appropriate counseling for this patient to slow the progression of his condition?

(A) Sodium-restricted diet

(B) Discontinue alcohol use

(C) Vigorous exercise regimen

(D) Fluid restrictive diet

101. A 49-year-old female presents to the emergency department with acute, substernal chest pain. She lost her husband recently in an automobile accident. The ECG shows anterior ST-segment elevation consistent with anterior myocardial infarction. She undergoes emergent cardiac catheterization which demonstrates normal coronaries; however, her ejection fraction is depressed and has left apical ballooning. Which of the following is true regarding this patient's diagnosis?

(A) Prognosis is extremely poor

(B) Most patients with this diagnosis have no symptoms

(C) Majority of patients with this diagnosis will need heart transplant

(D) Discharge medications are similar to those who have had myocardial infarction with obstructive coronary artery disease

102. A 51-year-old female with history of diabetes mellitus type 2 presents for blood pressure management. At her last two visits her blood pressure was 145/91 and 155/97 mm Hg. Today, her blood pressure is 141/99. Recent lab work shows basic metabolic panel normal. Which of the following is the best treatment in this patient?

(A) Lisinopril

(B) Hydrochlorothiazide

(C) Metoprolol

(D) No treatment is recommended

103. A 45-year-old male with 20-year history of diabetes mellitus type I develops pain with walking that radiates from the right thigh to calf. Pain is worsened with walking and is relieved by rest. Patient denies edema. Which of the following is the most appropriate test to order?

(A) Venogram

(B) Ankle-brachial index with Dopplers

(C) X-ray of the right hip and lumbar-sacral spine

(D) Venous Doppler with ultrasound

104. A 67-year-old male with history of hypertension and tobacco use presents with tearing chest pain. Blood pressure is 130/80 and heart rate is 68. Chest x-ray demonstrates a widened mediastinum. ECG shows no significant abnormalities. What is the most appropriate first step in treating this patient while awaiting a CT scan?

(A) Repeat ECG

(B) Order MRA of thoracic aorta

(C) Prepare for cardiac catheterization and stent placement

(D) Administer intravenous labetalol

105. Coarctation of the aorta is associated with which finding on chest x-ray?

(A) Rib notching

(B) Pulmonary vascular congestion

(C) Dextrocardia situs inversus

(D) Enlarged cardiac silhouette

106. A 37-year-old female who is a tobacco smoker and on oral contraceptive pills comes in for left calf pain. On physical examination, she has positive Homan's sign and left lower extremity edema. Which of the following diagnostic tests is most appropriate?

(A) Arterial ultrasound with ankle-brachial index

(B) Venous ultrasound

(C) Arteriogram

(D) CT scan with angiography

Answers and Explanations

1. **(C)** The 2011 ACCF/AHA Guideline for Coronary Artery Bypass Graft Surgery states CABG is recommended (Class Ib) for patients with significant left main stenosis (≥50% diameter). Uncomplicated distal left anterior descending (LAD) stenosis and right coronary artery (RCA) lesions are both significant but suitable for percutaneous coronary intervention (PCI). LAD and RCA stenosis of 60% does not meet criteria for PCI (≥70% deemed significant). *(Bashore et al., 2016, p. 361, Hillis & Anderson, 2011, pp. 16–26)*

2. **(C)** Patient is having a lateral ST-elevation myocardial infarction (STEMI). Aspirin doses 162 to 325 mg should be administered acutely in the prehospital and/or emergency department setting as it has been shown to be effective in the initial management of patients with suspected STEMI. It should be chewed to allow more rapid absorption buccally. *(Mega & Morrow, 2015)*

3. **(C)** The international normalized ratio (INR) range recommended for patients with a mechanical heart valve replacement is 2.5 to 3.5. Patients with mechanical aortic valve replacement have a target INR of 2.0 to 3.0. Patients with an INR greater than 3.5 are at a high risk of developing warfarin-associated bleeding. *(Bashore et al., 2016, pp. 349—351)*

4. **(A)** Repair of abdominal aortic aneurysm is recommended for those aneurysms that are associated with symptoms despite size, larger than 5.5 cm in diameter, expansion of greater than 0.5 cm in 6 months. *(Collins, 2013; Owens et al., 2016, pp. 476–468)*

5. **(B)** Acute ascending aortic dissection (Stanford type A) is a surgical emergency. Patients with descending aortic dissections (Stanford type B) and hemodynamically stable may be treated with conservative therapy and should be followed every 6 months with serial CT scans. In addition, both patients with type A and type B dissections benefit from intravenous beta-blockade as well as intravenous nitroprusside. *(Manning, 2013)*

6. **(D)** Given the patient's long history of tobacco use with prior diagnosis of COPD who presents with pulmonary artery hypertension and right ventricular overload findings, the best answer is cor pulmonale. Acute pulmonary embolus can present similarly but hepatomegaly from bilateral peripheral edema, and peaked P waves leads to cor pulmonale as the most likely diagnosis. Acute coronary syndrome may have ECG changes will include ST-segment changes and will not usually present with acute tricuspid regurgitation. Patients who have severe heart failure will have similar symptoms but also have pulsus alternans and pulmonary rales. *(Klings, 2014; Thompson & Hales, 2014)*

7. **(B)** This patient likely has renovascular disease given her abdominal bruit and hypertension. Essential hypertension is diagnosed in those in whom secondary hypertension has not been implicated. Primary hyperaldosteronism is a differential diagnosis; however, the presence of an abdominal bruit makes renovascular hypertension more likely. Isolated systolic hypertension is defined as a systolic blood pressure of greater than 140 mm Hg but a diastolic blood pressure of less than 90 mm Hg. *(Sutters, 2016, pp. 438–439)*

8. **(A)** Tricuspid regurgitation is associated with a holosystolic murmur heard best at the left sternal border and the intensity may increase with inspiration. The patient most likely had endocarditis of his

tricuspid valve in the past due to intravenous drug abuse. Aortic stenosis is a systolic ejection murmur with a crescendo–decrescendo quality that is heard at the aortic area and can radiate to carotids and/or the apex of the heart. The murmur of mitral regurgitation is heard best at the apex and radiates to the axilla in severe cases. Mitral stenosis is described as a low-pitched rumbling diastolic murmur. *(Bashore et al., 2016, pp. 347–348)*

9. **(C)** ST-elevation myocardial infarction (STEMI) is defined as new ST-segment elevation in ≥2 contiguous leads and ≥1 mm high. Reciprocal changes of ST-segment depression can often be found. Inferior STEMI involves leads II, II, and AVF. Anterior STEMI involves V2–V4. Acute posterior STEMI is usually associated with ST depressions in V1–V3 with relative early R-wave progression in leads V1–V3. Lateral wall STEMI involves ST elevation in leads V5, V6, I, and aVL. *(Goldberger, 2014)*

10. **(D)** Patients with chronic venous insufficiency classically present with pitting edema, itching, discomfort worsened with standing, and brawny skin pigmentation. Ulcerations of venous insufficiency are usually low on the medial ankle or anterior aspect of leg. Patients with arterial insufficiency normally have symptoms of claudication and they are found to have decreased pulses, distal hair loss, thick nails, and pallor. Peripheral neuropathy tends to present with paresthesias, numbness, or burning pains and the ulcer is most commonly at areas of increased pressure at sites of bony prominences. Lymphedema presents normally with pitting edema but without brawny pigmentation changes or ulcerations. *(Alguire & Mathes, 2015; Owens et al., 2016, pp. 485–487)*

11. **(B)** Thromboangiitis obliterans or Buerger's disease is a nonatherosclerotic, inflammatory disease that occurs segmentally in small- to medium-sized arteries and veins of the extremities. Patients are usually <40 years of age and it is strongly associated with smoking cigarettes. Acute arterial thrombosis will present as an acute complaint of ischemia and pain with pulselessness. Raynaud phenomenon is most commonly seen in young women, occurs bilaterally, and is precipitated by emotional stress or cold environment and relieved with warmth. *(Hellman & Imboden, 2016, p. 476; Mohler & Olin, 2013; Owens et al., 2016, p. 476)*

12. **(D)** The heart is frequently involved in SLE with the pericardium affected in the majority of cases. *(Hellmann & Imboden, 2016, pp. 825–828)*

13. **(B)** Patients with hypothyroidism will complain of fatigue and dyspnea when pleural effusions are present. Many variations can be seen in a patient with hypothyroidism but bradyarrhythmias are seen predominantly. Diabetic patients may have ST changes and evidence of silent ischemia on their ECG. Sinus bradycardia does not usually occur in these patients. Pheochromocytoma, hyperthyroidism, and pulmonary embolism are associated with tachycardia. *(Fitzgerald, 2016, pp. 1099–1104)*

14. **(B)** Peaked T waves are the first electrocardiographic changes seen in mild hyperkalemia. Late changes are associated with higher morbidity and mortality. Potassium levels higher than 7.0 mEq/L include prolonged PR interval and QRS duration, atrioventricular conduction delays, and loss of the P wave. Prominent U waves are associated with hypokalemia and antiarrhythmic medication toxicity. *(Goldberger, 2015)*

15. **(C)** The most distinct features of hypokalemia is ST-segment depressions with T wave flattening and prominent U waves. Hypothermia is associated with J waves sometimes called Osborn waves. Hypermagnesemia does not have any distinct ECG features but with severe elevations can lead to prolonged QRS and PR intervals. *(Goldberger, 2015)*

16. **(C)** Troponin levels have a high sensitivity and specificity in the diagnosis of MI and have become almost universally used. It detects small quantities of necrotic myocardial tissue and is more specific to cardiac tissue compared to CPK, AST, and ALT enzymes. *(Bashore et al., 2016, pp. 368–369)*

17. **(B)** This patient presents with a constrictive pericarditis secondary to history of ionizing radiation to chest wall. Echocardiogram should be ordered to determine left ventricular ejection fraction. Cardiac catheterization can be used but echocardiogram is noninvasive, readily available, and is performed prior to catheterization. Holter monitor should be used to aid in the diagnosis of arrhythmias but is not a diagnostic tool used for the diagnosis of diastolic heart failure. Electrocardiographic stress tests are

used to screen for cardiac ischemia in an ambulatory patient who is complaining of chest discomfort. *(Bashore et al., 2016, p. 425)*

18. **(D)** The most probable diagnosis is infective endocarditis. Transesophageal echocardiogram is sensitive for detecting valvular vegetations more so than transthoracic echocardiogram. Holter monitors and cardiac catheterization do not detect vegetations on valves. *(Schwartz, 2016, pp. 1433–1438)*

19. **(D)** CT scan is the modality of choice to evaluate the size and anatomy of a thoracic aortic aneurysm (TAA). Cardiac catheterization and an echocardiogram can be used to determine the approximate size of a TAA but is better used to evaluate the relationship of the coronary arteries to the aneurysm. CT scan gives a more precise location, measurement, and will indicate if there is an associated dissection. Chest x-ray cannot clearly define size and anatomy of the aneurysm. *(Owens et al., 2016, pp. 479–480)*

20. **(D)** Mitral valve prolapse is characterized as a mid- to late-systolic click that may or may not be associated with a murmur. It is a frequent finding in patients with connective tissue disorders, such as Marfan's syndrome. The murmur associated with aortic stenosis is a systolic-ejection murmur. Aortic regurgitation is characterized by a high-pitched decrescendo murmur in early diastole. Mitral valve stenosis is associated with a low-pitched, mid-diastolic murmur that may be associated with an opening snap. *(O'Gara & Loscalzo, 2015)*

21. **(B)** Patent ductus arteriosus is a continuous murmur heard at the pulmonic area. Aortic stenosis is a systolic-ejection murmur. Mitral regurgitation is a blowing, systolic murmur heard at apex and may radiate to axilla. Pulmonic stenosis is a systolic murmur. *(Bashore et al., 2016, p. 329; O'Gara & Loscalzo, 2015)*

22. **(D)** Pheochromocytoma is related to an increase in catecholamine release with symptoms of palpitations, anxiety, sweating, and headache. Supraventricular tachycardia can present with anxiety and palpitations but is normally not associated with severe hypertension. This patient is not complaining of chest pain and is a young adult, so it is unlikely that the patient has acute coronary syndrome (ACS). The patient is not complaining of chest pain and

does not list a history of trauma or connective tissue disease, so it is less likely she has aortic dissection. *(Fitzgerald, 2016, pp. 1158–1163; Kotchen, 2015)*

23. **(D)** Radiographic finding associated with tetralogy of Fallot (TOF) is a normal-sized, boot-shaped heart with diminished pulmonary vascular markings. Rib notching is associated with coarctation of the aorta. *(Webb et al., 2015)*

24. **(B)** A wide, fixed split S2 is the auscultatory hallmark of an ASD. A systolic murmur is best heard at the upper left sternal border. A pansystolic murmur at left sternal border can be heard if right ventricular failure with tricuspid regurgitation is present. *(Webb et al., 2015)*

25. **(C)** The patient's symptoms of a ripping pain that radiates to the back and a chest x-ray that reveals a widened mediastinum are classic findings for thoracic aortic dissection and not typical for acute coronary syndrome. On the other hand, a normal chest x-ray cannot rule out an aortic dissection. Pneumothorax would most likely demonstrate a visceral pleural line and present with chest pain and dyspnea. *(Creager & Loscalzo, 2015a)*

26. **(B)** The typical symptoms of heart failure are fatigue and shortness of breath. Weight gain is secondary to fluid retention from humoral and neurohumoral mechanisms that promote water reabsorption. Sinus tachycardia is unlikely because this patient has had long-standing atrial fibrillation. Cardiac tamponade classically presents as tachypnea and tachycardia with a narrowed pulse pressure. *(Bashore et al., 2016, pp. 401–411; Mann & Chakinala, 2015)*

27. **(D)** For a patient with coronary artery disease (CAD) and stable, chronic heart failure the following medications are recommended: aspirin, beta blocker, statin, ACE inhibitor, diuretic, nitroglycerin. Heparin and morphine are not recommended normally as an outpatient for long-term use for heart failure (HF). Calcium channel blockers are not recommended in CAD or HF. *(Bashore et al., 2016, pp. 408–409; Mann & Chakinala, 2015)*

28. **(D)** The pain associated with arterial occlusion occurs as a sudden onset of severe pain and associated with pallor, poikilothermia, and nonpalpable pulses. He is

at risk given the history of paroxysmal atrial fibrillation. Atherosclerotic peripheral vascular disease has symptoms of claudication and develops as more of a chronic arterial insufficiency picture and not typically with acute findings. Raynaud syndrome has cycles of vasoconstrictions that have similar symptoms but are often triggered by exposure to stress or cold environments. *(Owens et al., 2016, pp. 472–473; Hellmann & Omboden, 2016, pp. 829–831)*

29. **(B)** Paradoxical splitting of S2 occurs on expiration and disappears on inspiration: the opposite of physiologic splitting. The most common cause is left bundle branch block. Atrial septal defect and right ventricular failure are associated with fixed splitting. Pulmonic stenosis is associated with a wide split. *(Bickley & Szilagyi, 2013, p. 396)*

30. **(D)** Orthostasis is defined as a drop of greater than 20 mm Hg in the systolic pressure or a drop of greater than 10 mm Hg in the diastolic pressure within 3 minutes of posture change. When the drop in pressure is related to neurogenic causes, the compensatory change in the pulse rate is not seen. *(Bickley & Szilagyi, 2013, pp. 124, 945)*

31. **(D)** This is an acute event of heart failure, and intravenous (IV) diuretic therapy is indicated. IV diuretic therapy should be initiated even if the patient did not have a previous episode of fluid retention. Beta blockers should be used with extreme caution in uncompensated heart failure as it may aggravate the acute uncompensated state. ACE inhibitors should be considered a part of the recommended treatment but does not relieve the volume overload. Calcium channel blockers are not indicated for the treatment of acute heart failure. *(Bashore et al., 2016, pp. 410–411; Colucci, 2014)*

32. **(A)** Beta blockers should be used to control the ventricular rate in rapid atrial fibrillation. While digoxin will slow the ventricular rate, it is no longer the drug of choice. Warfarin is used for anticoagulation and the prevention of clot formation that is a risk with the occurrence of atrial fibrillation. There is not a clear need for nitroglycerin at the time because there is no mention of angina. *(Ganz, 2014)*

33. **(B)** Unstable angina is a contraindication for exercise treadmill stress test. Mild aortic stenosis is not

a contraindication. Severe aortic stenosis is a contraindication. Previous myocardial infarction is not a contraindication and neither is nonspecific ECG changes. New LBBB would be a contraindication. *(Balady & Morise, 2015)*

34. **(A)** Flecainide is a Class Ic antiarrhythmic whose mechanism of action blocks sodium channels more potently than Class Ia (Procainamide) of Ib (Lidocaine). Class Ic medications are indicated for life-threatening ventricular tachycardia or fibrillation. They may also be used in refractory supraventricular tachycardia. *(Kumar & Zimetbaum, 2014)*

35. **(B)** Patients with diabetes have an increased risk for atherosclerosis due to diabetes and other risk factors. Statins, aspirin, and ACE inhibitors are recommended for those deemed high risk for cardiovascular events. *(McCulloch, 2014)*

36. **(C)** Aggressively modifying risk factors lower the development of macrovascular complications of diabetes. Smoking cessation, management of hypertension with an ACE inhibitor, cholesterol lowering with statins, and the use of aspirin is of benefit for those diabetics with high cardiovascular disease risk. The Women's Health Initiative study concludes that there was no reduction in coronary events with the use of estrogen/progestin tablets. *(Libby, 2015; McCulloch, 2014)*

37. **(B)** Beta blockers, ACE inhibitors, and aspirin have been shown to improve the morbidity and mortality rates in patients who have had a myocardial infarction and are Class I and IIa recommendations. Calcium channel blockers are recommended in those that beta blockers are contraindicated. Estrogen therapy is not recommended for use with the intention of improving cardiovascular outcomes. Folate or vitamin B6 to treat elevated homocysteine levels is not recommended for the purpose of improving cardiac outcomes. *(Mega & Morrow, 2015)*

38. **(D)** Preload is defined as the ventricular end-diastolic volume. Factors that increase the ventricular end-diastolic volume include an increase in the intravascular volume. Arterial vascular tone increases the blood pressure, which may decrease the venous return to the heart. Increases in the stroke volume occur when the ventricle is more efficient, thus

increasing the cardiac output; increases in the stroke volume have little to no effect on the end-diastolic volume. The heart rate does not increase the ventricular end-diastolic volume. In fact, if the heart rate increases, it provides less time for ventricular filling so that it may decrease the ventricular end-diastolic volume. *(Loscalzo et al., 2015)*

39. **(A)** Cardiac tamponade is the result of accumulation of fluid in the pericardial space with increased pressure in the pericardium, in amounts sufficient to compress the vena cava and decrease inflow of blood to the ventricles. The increase in pressure in the pericardium is decrease in blood flow into the ventricles demonstrating a decrease in preload. *(Braunwald, 2015)*

40. **(D)** Diastolic dysfunction occurs when the ventricle has a decreased ability to draw the blood from the left atrium because of a decrease in ventricular myocardial compliance. Diastolic dysfunction can lead to decreased stroke volume and increase in preload, but that is not the defining factor. *(Zile & Little, 2015)*

41. **(B)** This patient has atrial fibrillation. Atrial fibrillation is characterized by an irregularly irregular rhythm with the absence of P waves. Sinus tachycardia exists when the heart rate is greater than 100 bpm with discernible P waves. Nodal (or junctional) rhythm is characterized by heart rates in the 40s and the lack of (or inverted) P waves in lead II. *(Bashore et al., 2016, p. 387)*

42. **(A)** Complete AV block results from failure of conduction of any impulse from the atrium so the ventricles will beat independently of each other. Type II second-degree AV block is characterized by dropped QRS beats without changes in the preceding PR or RR intervals. A junctional rhythm will have flat or inverted P waves in lead II and a narrow QRS complex with heart rate of 40 to 60 bpm. Atrial fibrillation is normally an irregularly, irregular rhythm with disorganized and irregular atrial activation. *(Bashore et al., 2016, pp. 398–399)*

43. **(B)** Patients with giant cell arteritis present with an elevated erythrocyte sedimentation rate (ESR). ESR is used to monitor the inflammatory disease process and is a useful indicator when judging the glucocorticoid tapering dosing. These patients do present

with anemia but it is not a useful indicator for response therapy. Patients may also have a positive rheumatoid factor, but this is not an indicator for successful therapy. *(Langford & Fauci, 2015)*

44. **(A)** This patient has typical symptoms for angina pectoris and is an intermediate category based on symptoms and age. The 2012 ACC/AHA guidelines give this type of patient a Class I indication to perform exercise treadmill stress testing without radionuclide imaging. Cardiac enzymes are indicated for EKG changes consistent with ischemia or infarct. Echocardiogram should be performed if the patient has a positive exercise stress test result. *(Fihn et al., 2012, p. 2574; Garber & Hlatky, 2013)*

45. **(B)** This patient is asymptomatic; therefore, no intervention is needed at this time. If a patient requires intervention, beta-blockade should be initiated as a first-line therapy. *(Bashore et al., 2016, p. 383)*

46. **(C)** This patient presents with the three clinical indicators (Beck's triad: hypotension, soft heart sounds, JVD) for cardiac tamponade and should be treated with emergent pericardiocentesis. Pericardial window is used for recurrent pericardial effusions. There is no indication for cardiac catheterization or redo coronary bypass grafting at this time. *(Braunwald, 2015)*

47. **(B)** Chagas' disease is the most common cause of cardiomyopathy in the world. It is caused by the protozoan parasite *Trypanosoma cruzi* which is found most commonly in patients from Central and South America. *Brucella* is transmitted through infected milk and meat of farm animals. Coxsackie B virus is an RNA enterovirus virus which is associated with acute myocarditis and pericarditis. *Francisella tularensis* is a zoonotic infection of wild rodents and rabbits. *(Rosenthal, 2016, pp. 1484–1485; Schwartz, 2016, pp. 1484–1485)*

48. **(D)** Five features are characteristic findings of tetralogy of Fallot: ventricular septal defect, right ventricular hypertrophy, overriding aorta, right ventricular outflow tract obstruction, and a right-sided aortic arch (25% of cases). *(Bashore et al., 2016, pp. 327–329)*

49. **(C)** This patient has Class III symptoms characterized by marked limitations with less than ordinary

activities. Class I demonstrates no limitations of physical activity. Class II symptoms are noted in patients who have mild symptoms with ordinary exertion. Class IV patients have symptoms even at rest. *(Mann & Chakinala, 2015)*

50. **(D)** Amiodarone and sotalol are indicated to prevent recurrent, monomorphic ventricular tachycardia (VT) in a patient with cardiac disease without evidence of prolonged QT. Propafenone is not indicated for use in patients with coronary artery disease and VT. Most VT does not respond to adenosine. Verapamil has a higher propensity to cause cardiovascular collapse in patients with heart disease and VT. *(Bashore et al., 2016, pp. 394–396; Hume & Grant, 2015)*

51. **(D)** Amiodarone's most serious adverse effect is a dose-related pulmonary toxicity that can cause fatal pulmonary fibrosis, even at low doses. Corneal deposits, photodermatitis, and peripheral neuropathies associated with amiodarone use are generally not life threatening. *(Hume & Grant, 2015)*

52. **(B)** An INR of >1.8 for 3 weeks on at least two separate occasions is recommended before cardioversion. INRs between 2.0 and 3.0 are recommended for patients with persistent and long-standing atrial fibrillation in which cardioversion has failed. *(Bashore et al., 2016, pp. 386–392)*

53. **(A)** This patient presents with symptoms of pacemaker syndrome. This condition is the result of interruption or failure to capture atrial and ventricular synchrony. The best initial test to diagnose this condition is the ECG as it can be quickly obtained. Pacemaker interrogation would be indicated as well. Pacemaker exchange is indicated. Chest x-ray and other laboratory data will not help you to diagnose this condition. *(Spragg & Tomaselli, 2015)*

54. **(C)** Type II second-degree block has a fixed PR interval with occasional dropped beats. Wenckebach (type I second-degree AV block) is characterized by a progressive lengthening of the PR interval. First-degree heart block is characterized by a PR interval that is longer than 0.2 seconds, while complete dissociation between the electrical activity of the atrium and the ventricle is noted in third-degree AV block. *(Spragg & Tomaselli, 2015)*

55. **(D)** This patient has a short history of both profound bradycardia and tachycardia consistent with SA node dysfunction (also called tachy–brady syndrome). Premature atrial contractions have P waves before the QRS complex and AV-node re-entrant tachycardia usually generates a faster rhythm. Multifocal atrial tachycardias have P waves from differing ectopic sources before the QRS complexes. *(Spragg & Tomaselli, 2015)*

56. **(D)** In an active and young adult without symptoms, a grade I–II mid-systolic murmur at the left sternal border is unlikely to cause harm and is usually a benign finding. No further evaluation is recommended. Echocardiogram should be performed in patients who are symptomatic, with diastolic or continuous murmurs, and in patients with a systolic murmur that is greater than grade II. Coronary arteriogram is used to evaluate patients suspicious for coronary ischemia. *(O'Gara & Loscalzo, 2015)*

57. **(C)** Cardiac output is impacted by the heart rate and the stroke volume. Stroke volume is impacted by volume status (preload), myocardial contractility, and systemic vascular resistance (afterload). The patient is hypovolemic with a stable blood count. Intravenous fluids would increase the preload and is most appropriate. Dobutamine would be indicated for reduced ejection fraction with reduced cardiac output. Intra-aortic balloon pump and epinephrine are not indicated for a patient with stable blood pressure. *(Owens et al., 2016, pp. 492–493)*

58. **(B)** A person must have three or more of the five diagnostic criteria for metabolic syndrome. The criteria include a blood pressure greater than 130/85 mm Hg, waist circumference greater than 40 inches in male, HDL less than 40 mg/dL in male, fasting blood sugar greater than 100 mg/dL, and triglycerides greater than 150 mg/dL. *(Bickley & Szilagyi, 2013, p. 358)*

59. **(C)** Sildenafil is recommended in this patient as the vasodilator challenge demonstrated pulmonary artery responsiveness. Bosentan (an endothelial receptor antagonist), iloprost, and epoprostenol (both prostacyclin analogs) all are indicated when the pulmonary arterial hypertension is not responsive to the vasodilator challenge. *(Bashore et al., 2016, pp. 425–426)*

60. **(B)** Electrophysiology studies are used to evaluate the excitability of the myocardium and to reproduce the ventricular tachycardia (VT). Catheter ablation can cure VT in 90% of cases in those without structural heart disease. Repeating the ECG when she has no symptoms and documented Holter monitor demonstrates the likely etiology of the syncope. Exercise treadmill test is not indicated as she has had multiple sustained ventricular tachycardia episodes. Transesophageal echocardiography is used most commonly to evaluate the aorta for evidence of dissection, to elucidate evidence of atrial clots, and to assess for evidence of valvular vegetations. *(Bashore et al., 2016, p. 395)*

61. **(C)** Cilostazol (a phosphodiesterase inhibitor) increases claudication distance by 40% to 60% in patients with peripheral arterial disease. Elastic compression stockings should be avoided as it can decrease arterial circulation to the skin. Calcium channel blockers have not proven to be beneficial. Warfarin may prevent more cardiovascular events but causes more major bleeding and has not been shown to improve outcomes in those with chronic PAD. *(Creager & Loscalzo, 2015b).*

62. **(D)** Moderate hyperkalemia will present with flattening/absence of the P wave, bradycardia, widened QRS pattern, and peaked T waves. The patient is high risk given his end-stage renal disease and having missed his HD appointments. The QT shortens in hypercalcemia. The QT shortens with digitalis effect but the ST-segment scoops downward. Hypomagnesemia is not associated with specific findings but a nonspecific QT prolongation but not with tenting of the T waves. *(Goldberger, 2014)*

63. **(B)** Paroxysmal nocturnal dyspnea is most specific for cardiac disease. Orthopnea and shortness of breath is a common symptom for heart failure, pulmonary disease, and obesity. Pedal edema is a cardinal manifestation of heart failure but is nonspecific and can present in a number of disorders such as nephrotic syndrome, venous insufficiency, etc. *(Mann & Chakinala, 2015)*

64. **(A)** Asymptomatic premature atrial contractions are not an indication for Holter monitoring. Holter monitor is indicated for suspected tachycardia-induced cardiomyopathy, patients with reduced left

ventricular systolic function after myocardial infarction to determine risk of sudden cardiac death, and asymptomatic atrial fibrillation to determine need for anticoagulation. Holter monitor is also indicated for non–life-threatening arrhythmias or palpitations if it is accompanied with daily symptom, intermittent symptoms with a prolonged duration, and/or severe symptoms. *(Bashore et al., 2016, p. 383)*

65. **(D)** Electrocardioversion is indicated based on clinical parameters of angina and ischemia and hemodynamic compromise with a low blood pressure with diaphoresis. Amiodarone has less success at terminating atrial fibrillation and it takes longer to administer compared to electrocardioversion. Beta blocker is contraindicated given his hypotension. Adenosine is not indicated. *(Bashore et al., 2016, p. 387)*

66. **(A)** Inotropy is a term used for cardiac contractility. Digoxin is a positive inotropic drug, increasing contractility. Lisinopril and furosemide have no effect on inotropy. Metoprolol can have a negative inotropic effect and therefore is not recommended for use in acute heart failure. *(Katzung, 2015)*

67. **(A)** The bradycardia algorithm in the AHA ACLS manual describes the preferred treatment of symptomatic bradycardia is atropine. If it is ineffective then transcutaneous pacing, dopamine, or epinephrine are recommended. Transvenous pacing should be considered but requires more invasive measures and the above measures can be done in a more rapid fashion. *(Sinz et al., 2011, p. 84)*

68. **(D)** This patient is having an acute coronary syndrome. ECG will be needed to evaluate for ST-elevation myocardial infarction (STEMI) and/or ischemia. Cardiac enzymes will evaluate for positive myocardial infarction. Aspirin, beta blocker, and enoxaparin demonstrate morbidity and mortality benefits. Thrombolytics are not considered unless you have an STEMI diagnosed and there is not a cardiac cath lab readily available. *(Bashore et al., 2016, pp. 363–378)*

69. **(C)** Diastolic heart failure is defined as heart failure in the presence of a normal or near-normal left ventricular ejection fraction due to increased stiffness in the left ventricular muscle. Diastolic heart failure is most commonly associated with left ventricular hypertrophy. Diastolic heart failure can also be seen in infiltrative diseases such as amyloidosis. Alcohol-related cardiomyopathy and Chagas' disease normally present with systolic heart failure. *(Mann & Chinkala, 2015)*

70. **(C)** Patient has a low risk of myocardial infarction given no previous medical history. Her symptoms are most likely as the result of decreased oxygen carrying capacity due to anemia. Treating anemia should improve her symptoms. If it does not, then further testing is warranted. *(Nadler& Gonzalez, 2016, pp. 26–29)*

71. **(C)** Cardiac syndrome X is described by the presence of a classical angina pattern, treadmill test with cardiac ischemia, and normal coronaries on cardiac catheterization. Patients with atypical angina have chest pain at rest. Prinzmetal angina is caused by a focal spasm of a major coronary artery with ST-segment elevation than can be seen on cardiac catheterization. *(Bashore et al., 2016, p. 363; Pinto, 2014)*

72. **(B)** Dressler syndrome is an autoimmune pericarditis that can occur days to months post myocardial infarction (MI). It normally presents with low-grade fever, malaise, and chest pain, lessened by sitting up. Repolarization changes can be seen on ECG. Acute MI does not typically have diffuse J-point elevation with no reciprocal changes present and the pain is atypical to that of an acute MI. Although viral pericarditis is the most common cause of acute pericarditis, it is less likely given the patient's recent MI. This is not stable angina as the symptoms are not exertional but are positional and at rest. *(Bashore et al., 2016, p. 377; Braunwald, 2015)*

73. **(D)** Hypomagnesemia, hypokalemia, and hypercalcemia increase the risk of potential digoxin toxicity. *(Katzung, 2015)*

74. **(A)** Severe aortic stenosis may present with a classic triad of exertional symptoms: chest pain, dyspnea, and syncope/presyncope. Hypertrophic cardiomyopathy does not radiate to the carotids and the murmur intensity is increased with Valsalva maneuver. Ventricular septal defects cause a harsh, holosystolic murmur heard at lower left sternal border. Pulmonary stenosis is heard at the mid left sternal border. *(Bashore et al., 2016, pp. 339–344)*

75. **(A)** This patient has had an acute inferior infarct and now develops right-sided heart failure and cardiogenic shock. They had stent placed and intra-aortic balloon pump and remains in cardiogenic shock. The patient's left ventricular ejection fraction (LVEF) is normal so does not have systolic heart failure. The treatment of choice is IV fluids and dopamine. Dobutamine would not likely help as the patient has normal left ventricular function. Avoid diuretics as this could cause cardiovascular collapse by lowering preload and blood pressure. Avoid beta blockers and ACE inhibitors as patient is hypotensive at the present time. *(Bashore et al., 2016, p. 376)*

76. **(C)** Patient has symptomatic Wolff–Parkinson–White syndrome with a short PR interval and delta wave. Radiofrequency catheter ablation is the treatment of choice for those with symptomatic WPW syndrome. Verapamil and digoxin should be avoided in patients with WPW syndrome as these drugs can increase ventricular rates. Percutaneous coronary intervention is not indicated. *(Bashore et al., 2016, p. 385; Biase, 2014)*

77. **(D)** This patient does not require endocarditis prophylaxis. He has a completely repaired congenital heart defect that is greater than 6 months after surgery. *(Sexton, 2012)*

78. **(C)** The patient has amyloidosis which is the most common cause of restrictive cardiomyopathy. She presents with right heart failure and tricuspid regurgitation as a result of probable pulmonary hypertension. Right heart failure predominates over left heart failure in restrictive cardiomyopathy and cor pulmonale, but given the patient's history of amyloidosis and no history of pulmonary illness in the past, the more likely diagnosis is restrictive cardiomyopathy. The patient does not present with tachycardia, hypotension, or distant heart sounds that is seen in cardiac tamponade. *(Bashore et al., 2016, pp. 419–420; Mann & Chakinala, 2015)*

79. **(D)** This patient has variant (Prinzmetal) angina given the chest pain with coronary vasospasm seen with transient ST elevation during cardiac catheterization. Calcium channel blockers with or without nitrates is recommended for variant angina with no significant coronary artery disease. *(Bashore et al., 2016, p. 363; Giugliano et al., 2015)*

80. **(B)** By definition, dromotropy is conduction velocity of the atrioventricular node. Chronotropy refers to heart rate. Inotropy is a term used for cardiac contractility. Lusitropy affects the rate of relaxation. *(Katzung, 2015)*

81. **(C)** Almost all patients with an atrial septal defect will have an RBBB on their ECG. Left ventricular hypertrophy (LVH) can be seen on conditions such as a ventriculoseptal defect. Right ventricular hypertrophy and right axis deviation can be seen with tetralogy of Fallot. Left bundle branch block in pediatric patients can be seen in LVH, left ventricular noncompaction, and Wolff–Parkinson–White syndrome. *(Bashore et al., 2016, pp. 323–325)*

82. **(B)** Hyperthyroidism is a cause for high-output heart failure. Restrictive cardiomyopathy and aortic stenosis are structural and underlying causes for heart failure. *(Givertz & Haghighat, 2012)*

83. **(D)** Carotid massage or vagal maneuvers is the most appropriate treatment for this patient and are usually used as the first step to terminate the supraventricular tachycardia. If this fails to work, adenosine can be used. Adenosine is preferred over other antiarrhythmics initially as it has a rapid onset of action. If adenosine fails, a calcium channel blocker or beta blocker or an antiarrhythmic can be used. Electrocardioversion is used for those patients that are hemodynamically compromised. *(Miller & Zipes, 2015)*

84. **(C)** Those patients with atrial fibrillation and mitral stenosis have a high risk for thromboembolism. Even with return to sinus rhythm, atrial fibrillation often recurs and 20% to 30% of these patients may have systemic embolization if not anticoagulated appropriately. Heparin is recommended initially. Dabigatran and rivaroxaban are for the indication of nonvalvular atrial fibrillation. Clopidogrel is not recommended as this patient is high risk for thromboembolism. *(Ganz, 2014)*

85. **(A)** Vasovagal syncope (also known as neurocardiogenic or neutrally mediated syncope) is characterized by an abrupt onset of hypotension followed by a syncopal episode. Bradycardia may or may not accompany the hypotension. The reason has been hypothesized due to a paradoxical reflex when ventricular preload is decreased by venous pooling causing decreased cardiac output temporarily. This leads to a cascade of events with the end result increase in vagal tone which causes vasodilation and bradycardia and then syncope. Vasovagal episodes can occur due to a trigger from orthostatic stress, emotional stress, temperature changes, and pain. *(Calkins et al., 2015)*

86. **(A)** Critical digoxin toxicity usually presents with cardiac signs of frequent PVCs, life-threatening arrhythmias (ventricular tachycardia/fibrillation, complete heart block), and symptomatic bradycardia. Gastrointestinal symptoms include anorexia, nausea, weight loss, diarrhea, and vomiting. Neurologic symptoms of digoxin toxicity include drowsiness, lethargy, fatigue, dizziness, confusion, changes in visual acuity, and paresthesias. *(Levine & O'Connor, 2013)*

87. **(C)** Pulse pressure is the difference between systolic and diastolic blood pressure. Increase in pulse pressure is commonly seen in the elderly. In the elderly an increase in the systolic and decrease in the diastolic components of the pulse pressure usually as the result of stiffness in the large arteries. *(Townsend, 2014)*

88. **(B)** Beta blockers are not recommended for acute heart failure as they can cause a decrease in cardiac contractility (negative inotropy). Diuretics and ACE inhibitors are indicated. Nitroglycerin can achieve early symptomatic improvement of acute heart failure. *(Felker & Teerlink, 2015)*

89. **(D)** Congenitally abnormal bicuspid aortic valve may have symptoms in adolescents but normally emerges at ages 50 to 65 years old. These patients have higher risk of thoracic aortic aneurysms. Endocarditis prophylaxis is no longer recommended for these individuals. Up to 30% of the offspring of these patients have risk of bicuspid aortic valve. *(Bashore et al., 2016, pp. 339–344)*

90. **(A)** Calcium channel blocker is recommended for rate control in this type of patient as beta blockers are contraindicated and could cause severe respiratory distress. Sotalol is not first-line and should not be used in this patient for this reason and can cause respiratory distress in a COPD patient. Adenosine is not indicated. *(Bashore et al., 2016, pp. 387–392)*

91. **(C)** Patients with congenital long QT syndrome have increased risk of sudden cardiac death (SCD).

Generally speaking, SCD risk is highest during times of sympathetic nervous system activation as in exercise and emotional distress. *(Zimetbaum et al., 2012)*

92. **(A)** Unstable angina is characterized by at least one of three descriptions: (1) occurs at rest or minimal exertion, (2) severe and/or new onset, (3) increase in pain frequency and/or severity. *(Bashore et al., 2016, pp. 363–368)*

93. **(D)** Ventricular fibrillation is a chaotic electrical rhythm that is described as an erratic ventricular rhythm without identifiable waves. Asystole is characterized by flat line description. Ventricular tachycardia is very rapid ventricular activity with wide QRS pattern seen. Atrial flutter is rapid firing atrial complexes that resemble a saw tooth like pattern followed by a QRS complex. *(Dubin, 2000, p. 338)*

94. **(B)** Probably due to patent ductus arteriosus, indomethacin or ibuprofen is used initially in effort to close this type of murmur in the first 2 weeks of life. *(Bashore et al., 2016, p. 329)*

95. **(C)** Torsades de pointes is described as a polymorphic, wide-complex tachycardia that looks similar to a twisting ribbon. *(Dubin, 2000, p. 158)*

96. **(A)** This patient's CHADS2 score is 0. The recommendation is either aspirin or nothing. Warfarin is indicated for CHADS2 score of 1 and above. The patient does not appear to need heart rate control at the present time and digoxin and metoprolol are not indicated. *(Bashore et al., 2016, pp. 386–388; Miller & Zipes, 2015)*

97. **(D)** This is a venous hum. Venous hums are benign and do not need intervention. *(Bickley & Szilagyi, 2013, p. 844)*

98. **(B)** Mitral regurgitation presents as an apical holosystolic murmur and when severe, radiates to the axilla. Heart failure signs of fatigue, shortness of breath, and orthopnea are present with severe MR. Aortic stenosis would present with a systolic ejection murmur that is heard right upper sternal border and may radiate to carotids and apex. Tricuspid regurgitation is a holosystolic murmur best heard at left sternal border. Ventricular septal defects are described as a harsh, holosystolic murmur heard at lower left sternal border and may radiate across sternal area. *(Bashore et al., 2016, pp. 336–338)*

99. **(C)** Transesophageal echocardiogram (TEE) is recommended prior to elective cardioversion, more so for those in low risk of thromboembolism group. Cardioversion can be performed with low risk of thromboembolic event. Transthoracic echocardiogram does not visualize the left appendage area as clearly as a TEE. Chest x-ray and CT scan of the chest with angiogram does not evaluate for thrombus of the left atrial appendage. *(Bashore et al., 2016, pp. 386–392; Miller & Zipes, 2015)*

100. **(B)** This patient likely has a dilated cardiomyopathy with left ventricular dysfunction secondary to alcohol. Alcohol use should be discontinued if there is any chance of recovery of cardiac function. Sodium intake and fluid restriction would also be appropriate but alcohol cessation is the most important to slow the progression of left ventricular dysfunction. A vigorous exercise regimen is not appropriate. *(Bashore et al., 2016, pp. 413–415; Mehra, 2015)*

101. **(D)** This is an example of Takotsubo cardiomyopathy. This is an acute cardiomyopathy that is provoked from a stressful or emotional situation. It presents like an acute myocardial infarction but with the absence of coronary stenosis. Apical ballooning is seen on ventriculogram. Most cases are fully reversible with time and supportive care. Treatment is similar to treatment to those who have an ST-elevation myocardial infarction. *(Bashore et al., 2016, p. 416; Falk & Hershberger, 2015)*

102. **(A)** ACE inhibitors should be part of the initial treatment of hypertension in diabetic patients because of the beneficial benefits in delaying diabetic nephropathy. ACE inhibitors are the most appropriate initial medication in this patient. *(Bashore et al., 2016, p. 462)*

103. **(B)** The patient has a long-standing history of diabetes mellitus and has signs of intermittent claudication. This patient is at high risk for peripheral arterial disease. Evaluation of ankle-brachial index is the initial tool of choice. Venous Doppler with ultrasound and venogram are not indicated as they do not evaluate arterial perfusion. *(Owens et al., 2016, pp. 468–469; Creager & Loscalzo, 2015b)*

104. (D) Aggressive measures should be initiated to lower blood pressure even before you confirm diagnosis. Intravenous beta blockers are the drug of choice until patient can go for surgery. The patient does not have time to wait for an MRA of the thoracic aorta as it takes time to complete the test. *(Owens et al., 2016, pp. 481–482; Creager & Loscalzo, 2015a)*

105. (A) Rib notching is associated with coarctation of the aorta. Pulmonary vascular congestion with enlarged cardiac silhouette can be seen in dilated cardiomyopathy with heart failure. *(Bashore et al., 2016, pp. 322–323; Creager & Loscalzo, 2015a)*

106. (B) Venous ultrasound is the technique of choice to detect venous thrombosis of the leg. *(Goldhaber, 2015)*

REFERENCES

Alguire PC, Mathes BM. Clinical manifestations of lower extremity chronic venous disease. In: Eidt JF, Mills JL, eds. *UpToDate.* Waltham, MA: UpToDate; 2015. Accessed November 16, 2015.

Balady GJ, Morise AP. Chapter 13: Exercise testing. In: Mann DL, Zipes DP, Libby P, Bonow RO, eds. *Braunwald's Heart Disease: A Textbook of Cardiovascular Medicine.* 10th ed. Philadelphia, PA: Saunders; 2015. Accessed November 16, 2015.

Bashore TM, Granger CB, Jackson KP, Patel MR. Chapter 10: Heart disease. In: Papadakis MA, McPhee SJ, Rabow MW, eds. *CURRENT Medical Diagnosis & Treatment 2016.* New York, NY: McGraw-Hill; 2016.

Bickley LS, Szilagyi PG. *Bates' Guide to Physical Examination and History Taking.* 11th ed. Philadelphia, PA: Lippincott Williams & Wilkins; 2013.

Braunwald E. Chapter 288: Pericardial disease. In: Kasper DL, Fauci AS, Hauser SL, Longo DL, Jameson J, Loscalzo J, eds. *Harrison's Principles of Internal Medicine.* 19th ed. New York, NY: McGraw-Hill; 2015. Accessed November 16, 2015.

Calkins HG, Zipes DP. Chapter 40: Hypotension and syncope. In: Mann DL, Zipes DP, Libby P, Bonow RO, eds. *Braunwald's Heart Disease: A Textbook of Cardiovascular Medicine.* 10th ed. Philadelphia, PA: Saunders; 2015. Accessed November 16, 2015.

Collins, KA. Overview of abdominal aortic aneurysm. In: Eidt JF, Mills JL, eds. *UpToDate* . Waltham, MA: UpToDate; 2013. Accessed June 30, 2014.

Colucci WS. Treatment of acute decompensated heart failure: components of therapy. In: Gottlieb SS, Hoekstra J, Yeon SB, eds. *UpToDate.* Waltham, MA: UpToDate; 2014. Accessed June 30, 2014.

Creager MA, Loscalzo J. Chapter 301: Diseases of the aorta. In: Kasper DL, Fauci AS, Hauser SL, Longo DL, Jameson J, Loscalzo J, eds. *Harrison's Principles of Internal Medicine.* 19th ed. New York, NY: McGraw-Hill; 2015a. Accessed November 16, 2015.

Creager MA, Loscalzo J. Chapter 302: Arterial diseases of the extremities. In: Kasper DL, Fauci AS, Hauser SL, Longo DL, Jameson J, Loscalzo J, eds. *Harrison's Principles of Internal Medicine.* 19th ed. New York, NY: McGraw-Hill; 2015b. Accessed November 16, 2015.

Dubin D. *Rapid Interpretation of EKG's.* 6th ed. Fort Myers, FL: Cover; 2000. Accessed November 16, 2015.

Falk RH, Hershberger RE. Chapter 65: The dilated, restrictive, and infiltrative cardiomyopathies. In: Mann DL, Zipes DP, Libby P, Bonow RO, eds. *Braunwald's Heart Disease: A Textbook of Cardiovascular Medicine.* 10th ed. Philadelphia, PA: Saunders; 2015. Accessed November 16, 2015.

Felker GM, Teerlink JR. Diagnosis and management of acute heart failure. In: Mann DL, Zipes DP, Libby P, Bonow RO, eds. *Braunwald's Heart Disease: A Textbook of Cardiovascular Medicine.* 10th ed. Philadelphia, PA: Saunders; 2015. Accessed November 16, 2015.

Fihn SD, Gardin JM, Abrams J, et al. 2012 ACCF/AHA/ACP/AATS/PCNA/SCAI/STS Guideline for the diagnosis and management of patients with stable ischemic heart disease: A Report of the American College of Cardiology Foundation/American Heart Association task force on practice guidelines, and the American College of Physicians, American Association for thoracic surgery, preventive cardiovascular Nurses Association, Society for Cardiovascular Angiography and Interventions, and Society of Thoracic Surgeons. *J Am Coll Cardiol.* 2012;60:2564–2603. http://dx.doi.org/10.1016/j.jacc.2012.07.012. Accessed November 16, 2015.

Fitzgerald PA. Chapter 26: Endocrine disorders. In: Papadakis MA, McPhee SJ, Rabow MW, eds. *CURRENT Medical Diagnosis & Treatment 2016.* New York, NY: McGraw-Hill; 2016.

Ganz LI. Control of ventricular rate in atrial fibrillation. In: Knight BP, eds. *UpToDate.* Waltham, MA: UpToDate; 2014. Accessed June 30, 2014.

Garber AM, Hlatky MA. Stress testing for the diagnosis of coronary heart disease. In: Kaski JC, Pellikka PA, Downey BC, eds. *UpToDate*. Waltham, MA: UpToDate; 2013. Accessed June 30, 2014.

Giugliano RP, Cannon CP, Braunwald E. Chapter 53: Non-ST elevation acute coronary syndrome. In: Mann DL, Zipes DP, Libby P, Bonow RO, eds. *Braunwald's Heart Disease: A Textbook of Cardiovascular Medicine*. 10th ed. Philadelphia, PA: Saunders; 2015. Accessed November 16, 2015.

Givertz MM, Haghighat A. High-output heart failure. In: Gottlieb SS, Yeon SB, eds. *UpToDate*. Waltham, MA: UpToDate; 2012. Accessed June 30, 2014.

Goldberger AL. Electrocardiogram in the diagnosis of myocardial ischemia and infarction. In: Verheugt F, Mirvis DM, eds. *UpToDate*. Waltham, MA: UpToDate; 2014. Accessed June 30, 2014.

Goldberger AL. Chapter 268: Electrocardiography. In: Kasper DL, Fauci AS, Hauser SL, Longo DL, Jameson J, Loscalzo J, eds. *Harrison's Principles of Internal Medicine*. 19th ed. New York, NY: McGraw-Hill; 2015. Accessed November 16, 2015.

Goldhaber SZ. Chapter 300: Deep venous thrombosis and pulmonary thromboembolism. In: Kasper DL, Fauci AS, Hauser SL, Longo DL, Jameson J, Loscalzo J, eds. *Harrison's Principles of Internal Medicine*. 19th ed. New York, NY: McGraw-Hill; 2015. Accessed November 16, 2015.

Hellmann DB, Imboden JB Jr. Chapter 20: Rheumatologic & immunologic disorders. In: Papadakis MA, McPhee SJ, Rabow MW, eds. *CURRENT Medical Diagnosis & Treatment 2016*. New York, NY: McGraw-Hill; 2016.

Hillis LD, Smith PK, Anderson JL, et al. 2011 ACCF/AHA Guideline for Coronary Artery Bypass Graft Surgery: a report of the American College of Cardiology Foundation/ American Heart Association Task Force on practice guidelines. *Circulation*. 2011;124:e652–e735. Accessed November 16, 2015.

Hume JR, Grant AO. Chapter 14: Agents used in cardiac arrhythmias. In: Katzung BG, Trevor AJ, eds. *Basic & Clinical Pharmacology*. 13th ed. New York, NY: McGraw- Hill; 2015. Accessed November 16, 2015.

Katzung BG. Chapter 13: Drugs used in heart failure. In: Katzung BG, Trevor AJ, eds. *Basic & Clinical Pharmacology*. 13th ed. New York, NY: McGraw-Hill; 2015. Accessed November 16, 2015.

Klings ES. Cor pulmonale. In: Mandel J, ed. *UpToDate*. Waltham, MA: UpToDate; 2014. Accessed June 30, 2014.

Kotchen TA. Chapter 247: Hypertensive vascular disease. In: Kasper DL, Fauci AS, Hauser SL, Longo DL, Jameson J, Loscalzo J, eds. *Harrison's Principles of Internal Medicine*. 19th ed. New York, NY: McGraw-Hill; 2015. Accessed November 16, 2015.

Kumar K, Zimetbaum PJ. Antiarrhythmic drugs to maintain sinus rhythm in patients with atrial fibrillation: clinical trials. In: Knight B, Saperia G, eds. *UpToDate*. Waltham, MA: UptoDate; 2014. Accessed June 30, 2014.

Langford CA, Fauci AS. Chapter 385: The vasculitis syndromes. In: Kasper DL, Fauci AS, Hauser SL, Longo DL, Jameson J,

Loscalzo J, eds. *Harrison's Principles of Internal Medicine*. 19th ed. New York, NY: McGraw-Hill; 2015. Accessed November 16, 2015.

Levine M, O'Connor A. Digitalis (cardiac glycoside) poisoning. In: Traub SJ, Burns MM, Grayzel J, eds. *UpToDate*. Waltham, MA; UpToDate; 2013. Accessed June 30, 2014.

Libby P. Chapter 291e: The pathogenesis, prevention, and treatment of atherosclerosis. In: Kasper DL, Fauci AS, Hauser SL, Longo DL, Jameson J, Loscalzo J, eds. *Harrison's Principles of Internal Medicine*. 19th ed. New York, NY: McGraw-Hill; 2015. Accessed November 16, 2015.

Loscalzo J, Libby P, Epstein J. Chapter 265e: Basic biology of the cardiovascular system. In: Kasper DL, Fauci AS, Hauser SL, Longo DL, Jameson J, Loscalzo J, eds. *Harrison's Principles of Internal Medicine*. 19th ed. New York, NY: McGraw-Hill; 2015. Accessed November 16, 2015.

Mann DL, Chakinala M. Chapter 279: Heart failure: pathophysiology and diagnosis. In: Kasper DL, Fauci AS, Hauser SL, Longo DL, Jameson J, Loscalzo J, eds. *Harrison's Principles of Internal Medicine*. 19th ed. New York, NY: McGraw-Hill; 2015. Accessed November 16, 2015.

Manning WJ. Management of aortic dissection. In: Mohler ER, Eidt JF, Mills JL, eds. *UpToDate*. Waltham, MA: UpToDate; 2013. Accessed June 30, 2014.

McCulloch DK. Overview of medical care in adults with diabetes mellitus. In: Nathan DM, Mulder JE, eds. *UptoDate*. Waltham, MA: UptoDate; 2014. Accessed June 30, 2014.

Mega ML, Morrow DA. Chapter 52: ST-elevation myocardial infarction : management. In: Mann DL, Zipes DP, Libby P, Bonow RO, eds. *Braunwald's Heart Disease: A Textbook of Cardiovascular Medicine*. 10th ed. Philadelphia, PA: Saunders; 2015. Accessed November 16, 2015.

Mehra MR. Chapter 280: Heart failure: management. In: Kasper DL, Fauci AS, Hauser SL, Longo DL, Jameson J, Loscalzo J, eds. *Harrison's Principles of Internal Medicine*. 19th ed. New York, NY: McGraw-Hill; 2015. Accessed November 16, 2015.

Miller JM, Zipes DP. Chapter 35: Therapy for cardiac arrhythmias. In: Mann DL, Zipes DP, Libby P, Bonow RO, eds. *Braunwald's Heart Disease: A Textbook of Cardiovascular Medicine*. 10th ed. Philadelphia, PA: Saunders; 2015. Accessed November 16, 2015.

Mohler ER, Olin JW. Thromboangiitis obliterans (Buerger's disease). In: Hunder GG, Eidt JF, Mills JL, eds. *UpToDate*. Waltham, MA; UpToDate; 2013. Accessed June 30, 2014.

Nadler PL, Gonzalez R. Chapter 2: Common symptoms. In: Papadakis MA, McPhee SJ, Rabow MW, eds. *CURRENT Medical Diagnosis & Treatment 2016*. New York, NY: McGraw-Hill; 2016.

O'Gara P, Loscalzo J. Chapter 286: Multiple and mixed valvular heart disease. In: Kasper DL, Fauci AS, Hauser SL, Longo DL, Jameson J, Loscalzo J, eds. *Harrison's Principles of*

Internal Medicine. 19th ed. New York, NY: McGraw-Hill; 2015. Accessed November 16, 2015.

Owens CD, Gasper J, Johnson MD. Chapter 12: Blood vessel & lymphatic disorders. In: Papadakis MA, McPhee SJ, Rabow MW, eds. *CURRENT Medical Diagnosis & Treatment 2016.* New York, NY: McGraw-Hill; 2016.

Pinto DS, Beltrame JF, Crea F. Variant angina. In: Kaski JC, Saperia GM, eds. *UpToDate.* Waltham, MA: UpToDate; 2014. Accessed June 30, 2014.

Rosenthal PJ. Chapter 35: Protozoal & helminthic infections. In: Papadakis MA, McPhee SJ, Rabow MW, eds. *CURRENT Medical Diagnosis & Treatment 2016.* New York, NY: McGraw-Hill; 2016.

Schwartz BS. Chapter 33: Bacterial and chlamydial infections. In: Papadakis MA, McPhee SJ, Rabow MW, eds. *CURRENT Medical Diagnosis & Treatment 2016.* New York, NY: McGraw-Hill; 2016.

Sexton DJ. Antimicrobial prophylaxis for bacterial endocarditis. In: Otto CM, Baron EL, Yeon SB, eds. *UpToDate.* Waltham, MA: UptoDate; 2012. Accessed June 30, 2014.

Sinz E, Navarro E, Soderberg ES. *Advanced Cardiovascular Life Support Provider Manual.* American Heart Association. First American Heart Association Printing; 2011.

Spragg DD, Tomaselli GF. Chapter 274: The bradyarrhythmias. In: Kasper DL, Fauci AS, Hauser SL, Longo DL, Jameson J, Loscalzo J, eds. *Harrison's Principles of Internal Medicine.*

19th ed. New York, NY: McGraw-Hill; 2015. Accessed November 16, 2015.

Sutters M. Chapter 11: Systemic hypertension. In: Papadakis MA, McPhee SJ, Rabow MW, eds. *CURRENT Medical Diagnosis & Treatment 2016.* New York, NY: McGraw-Hill; 2016.

Thompson, BT, Hales CA. Overview of acute pulmonary embolism. In: Mandel J, ed. *UpToDate.* Waltham, MA: UpToDate; 2014. Accessed June 30, 2014.

Townsend RR. Increased pulse pressure. In: . Bakris GL, Forman JP, eds. *UpToDate.* Waltham, MA: UpToDate; 2014. Accessed June 30, 2014.

Webb GD, Smallhorn JF, Therrien J, Redington AN. Chapter 62: Congenital heart disease. In: Mann DL, Zipes DP, Libby P, Bonow RO, eds. *Braunwald's Heart Disease: A Textbook of Cardiovascular Medicine.* 10th ed. Philadelphia, PA: Saunders; 2015. Accessed November 16, 2015.

Zile MR, Little WC. Chapter 27: Heart failure with a preserved ejection fraction. In: Mann DL, Zipes DP, Libby P, Bonow RO, eds. *Braunwald's Heart Disease: A Textbook of Cardiovascular Medicine.* 10th ed. Philadelphia, PA: Saunders; 2015. Accessed November 16, 2015.

Zimetbaum PJ, Seslar SP, Berul CI, Josephson ME. Prognosis and management of congenital long QT syndrome. In: Triedman JK, Asirvatham S, Downey BC, eds. *UpToDate.* Waltham, MA: UpToDate; 2012. Accessed June 30, 2014.

CHAPTER 3

Dermatology
Natalie R. Nyren, MSPAS, PA-C

DIRECTIONS: Each of the numbered questions or incomplete statements is followed by possible answers or completions of the statement. Select the ONE-lettered answer or completion that is BEST in each case.

1. Erythema with yellowish scale-forming plaques on the eyebrows, nasolabial folds, glabella, and presternal area best describes which of the following dermatologic disorders?

    (A) Allergic contact dermatitis
    (B) Bacterial folliculitis
    (C) Rosacea
    (D) Seborrheic dermatitis

2. A 36-year-old patient reporting sudden hair loss is found to have a round, well-circumscribed, 3-cm area of alopecia on the parietal scalp area with exclamation point hair. Which of the following is the most likely diagnosis?

    (A) Alopecia areata
    (B) Anagen effluvium
    (C) Androgenetic alopecia
    (D) Tinea capitis

3. An acute eruption of violaceous, pruritic, polygonal, shiny, flat-topped papules involving the flexor surfaces is suggestive of which of the following?

    (A) Lichen planus
    (B) Pityriasis rosea
    (C) Psoriasis
    (D) Seborrheic dermatitis

4. Bites that typically reveal a central blue color of impending necrosis with a surrounding white area of vasospasm and a peripheral red halo of inflammation are associated with which of the following conditions?

    (A) Black widow spiders
    (B) Brown recluse spiders
    (C) Deer ticks
    (D) Scabies

5. A 41-year-old male presents with a pruritic rash that appeared after a recent hiking trip. Physical examination reveals linear vesicles with underlying erythema on the hands, arms, and legs. Which of the following is the most likely diagnosis?

    (A) Herpes simplex virus
    (B) Impetigo
    (C) Toxicodendron dermatitis
    (D) Varicella zoster virus

6. A 25-year-old obese female presents for a screening employment physical. Her skin examination reveals velvety, hyperpigmented, papillomatous lesions of the neck and axillae. The remainder of the examination is unremarkable. Which of the following diagnostic tests should be ordered in the initial work-up of this patient?

    (A) Chest x-ray
    (B) Fasting blood sugar
    (C) KOH (potassium hydroxide) test of skin scrapings
    (D) Mineral oil skin scraping

7. A patient with a past medical history of allergic rhinitis and asthma presents with chronic pruritic inflammatory lesions of the flexor surfaces, wrists, and dorsal areas of the feet. The lesions are excoriated and lichenified with crusted patches and plaques. Which of the following is the most likely diagnosis?

   (A) Atopic dermatitis
   (B) Dermatitis nummular eczema
   (C) Psoriasis
   (D) Seborrheic dermatitis

8. A 65-year-old patient presents with a 4-week history of dark red pruritic urticarial plaques on the flexor surfaces, which now have begun developing tense bullae on the surface of the plaques. Which of the following conditions is this clinical presentation most suggestive of?

   (A) Bullous impetigo
   (B) Bullous pemphigoid
   (C) Dermatitis herpetiformis
   (D) Pemphigus vulgaris

9. Mupirocin (Bactroban) ointment is indicated for the treatment of the mild to moderate form of which of the following conditions?

   (A) Cellulitis
   (B) Impetigo
   (C) Rosacea
   (D) Tinea pedis

10. A 73-year-old white male with a history of organ transplantation presents with a 6 mm, red irregularly shaped, sharply demarcated, eroded lesion on his forehead. Which of the following is the most likely diagnosis for this patient?

   (A) Basal cell carcinoma
   (B) Bullous pemphigoid
   (C) Erythema multiforme
   (D) Squamous cell carcinoma

11. A 12-year-old girl presents with complaints of pruritus of the scalp for 2 weeks that started at the occiput and postauricular areas but has now spread. Microscopic examination of the hair shows the following (see Fig. 3-1). Based on the findings, which of the following is the most likely diagnosis?

   (A) Pediculosis capitis
   (B) Scabies
   (C) Seborrheic dermatitis
   (D) Tinea capitis

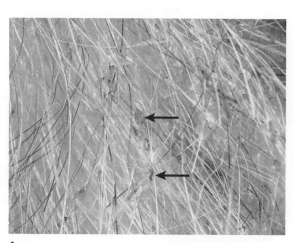

A

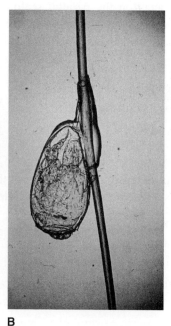

B

Figure 3-1. Reproduced with permission from Fitzpatrick, Johnson, Wolff, et al. *Dermatology in General Medicine.* 4th ed. New York, NY: McGraw-Hill, 1993. (See also Color Insert).

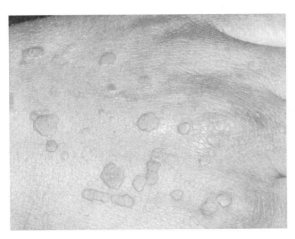

Figure 3-2. Reproduced, with permission, from Goldsmith LA, Katz SI, Gilchrest BA, et al. *Fitzpatrick's Dermatology in General Medicine.* 8th ed. New York, NY: McGraw-Hill Education, 2012. Figure 196–8. (See also Color Insert).

12. A 11-year-old patient presents with multiple, flat, round, light brown lesions measuring 1 to 5 mm in diameter on the dorsum of the left hand as seen in Figure 3-2. Several are noted to form a linear pattern. Which of the following is the most likely diagnosis?

(A) Lichen planus

(B) Seborrheic keratoses

(C) Syringomas

(D) Verruca plana

13. A 19-year-old male presents with the minimally pruritic rash seen in Figure 3-3. The lesion on the

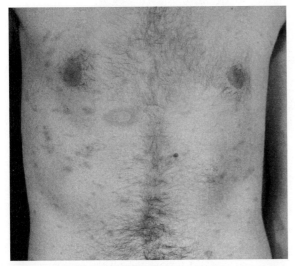

Figure 3-3. Reproduced, with permission, from Wolff K, Johnson RA, Suurmond D. *Fitzpatrick's Color Atlas & Synopsis of Clinical Dermatology.* 5th ed. New York, NY: McGraw-Hill Education, 2005:119. (See also Color Insert).

right chest was the first to appear, followed a week later by the remaining lesions. He states he had cold-like symptoms about a week before the eruption, but feels fine now. Which of the following is the most likely diagnosis?

(A) Guttate psoriasis

(B) Pityriasis rosea

(C) Scabies

(D) Tinea corporis

14. A 17-year-old white female presents with a recurrent rash to her upper chest and back, which seems to worsen during the summer months. She has become increasingly self-conscious of the lesions and is requesting treatment. On physical examination the patient's skin appears tan with discrete, hypopigmented lesions present on her chest and upper back. Which of the following is the treatment of choice for this patient?

(A) Selenium sulfide shampoo

(B) Topical glucocorticoid

(C) Topical 4% hydroquinone

(D) Topical salicylic acid

15. A 45-year-old African-American woman presents with an indurated, reddish orange lesion on her cheek and indurated painful nodules on the shins bilaterally. Which of the following is the initial best test to order in the management of this patient?

(A) Antinuclear antibody

(B) Chest x-ray

(C) KOH Prep

(D) Thyroid stimulating hormone

16. Which of the following is the best management plan for a 4-mm macular lesion that is asymmetrical, black and red, located on the left forearm, and has progressed rapidly over the past 6 months?

(A) Completely excise the lesion as soon as possible

(B) Have the patient document changes to the lesion in a journal for 4 months

(C) Remove the lesion with a vascular laser

(D) Schedule visits with a provider every 6 months to photograph changes

17. A patient with recurrent erythema multiforme minor lesions approximately every month should be treated prophylactically with which of the following oral medications?

(A) Acyclovir (Zovirax)

(B) Dapsone

(C) Prednisone

(D) Terbinafine (Lamisil)

18. Painful, erythematous, indurated nodules on the lower extremities of a woman on an oral contraceptive pill are most likely due to which of the following conditions?

(A) Erythema annulare centrifugum

(B) Erythema chronica migrans

(C) Erythema multiforme

(D) Erythema nodosum

19. Which of the following disease states is associated with the nail findings in the following image (Fig. 3-4)?

(A) Endocarditis

(B) Liver disease

(C) Psoriasis

(D) Tinea unguium

20. A patient presents with multiple 1- to 2-mm, flesh-colored, dome-shaped, umbilicated, waxy papules. Which of the following is the most likely cause for the patient's symptoms?

(A) Chronic UV light exposure

(B) Pox virus

(C) *Staphylococcus aureus*

(D) Varicella zoster virus

21. Folliculitis under occlusion of a bathing suit is most likely secondary to which of the following organisms?

(A) *Candida albicans*

(B) Group A β-hemolytic streptococcus

(C) *Pseudomonas aeruginosa*

(D) *Staphylococcus aureus*

22. Which of the following conditions can be described as pink lesions on the distal extremities and face that rapidly depigment?

(A) Contact dermatitis

(B) Guttate psoriasis

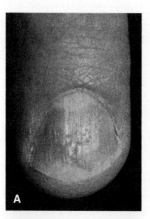
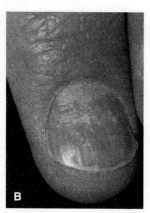
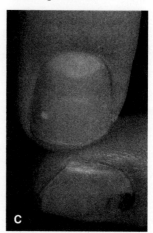
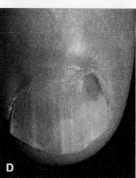

Figure 3-4. Reproduced, with permission, from Wolff K, Johnson RA, Saavedra AP. Fitzpatrick's Color Atlas and Synopsis of Clinical Dermatology. 7th ed. New York: McGraw-Hill Education, 2013. Figure 32-8.

(C) Pityriasis alba

(D) Vitiligo

23. Which of the following is the best treatment option for a 2-cm plaque of Bowen's disease on the lower leg of a young woman with concerns about her cosmetic outcome?

(A) Intralesional glucocorticoid

(B) Topical clobetasol (Temovate)

(C) Topical imiquimod (Aldara)

(D) Surgical excision

24. A 67-year-old male presents with a 1-cm pearly papule with central ulceration and telangiectasias on the left temple. Which of the following is the most likely diagnosis?

(A) Basal cell carcinoma

(B) Ecthyma

(C) Rosacea

(D) Sebaceous gland hyperplasia

25. Which of the following medications best treats comedonal acne?

(A) Benzoyl peroxide

(B) Oral antibiotics

(C) Topical antibiotics

(D) Topical retinoids

26. A 64-year-old man with a history of Hodgkin lymphoma presents with a 6-month history of a fish-like scale most prominent on the lower extremities that is getting progressively worse. He has no history of atopy and is currently on no medications. Which of the following is the most likely diagnosis?

(A) Acquired ichthyosis

(B) Eczema craquelé

(C) Ichthyosis vulgaris

(D) Lichen simplex chronicus

27. A 46-year-old white woman presents with facial flushing that she notes is worse when she has her morning coffee and when she is stressed at work. Physical examination reveals the presence of localized facial erythema, telangiectasias as well as several scattered papules and pustules on her cheeks. Which of the following is the most likely diagnosis?

(A) Acne vulgaris

(B) Folliculitis

(C) Impetigo

(D) Rosacea

28. A 16-year-old female with type 1 diabetes mellitus presents with a lesion on the finger pad of the fourth digit of the left hand. She states it came up rapidly and bleeds easily if she bumps it. On physical examination, there is a vascular, sessile, dome-shaped lesion. What is the most likely diagnosis?

(A) Cherry angioma

(B) Nodular melanoma

(C) Pyoderma gangrenosum

(D) Pyogenic granuloma

29. A 47-year-old man presents with complaints of blisters that form on sun-exposed areas of skin, leaving behind scars. He admits to being an alcoholic but has been sober for the past 6 months. On physical examination there are atrophic scars and milia on the dorsum of the hands. He has a tense bulla noted on his fifth digit of the right hand. He is also noted to have hypertrichosis of the face. Which of the following disorders would you test for?

(A) Human immunodeficiency virus

(B) Hepatitis C virus

(C) Herpes simplex virus

(D) Herpes zoster

30. A 32-year-old patient presents with grouped vesicles that are intensely pruritic noted on the elbows, knees, sacral area, and buttocks. The patient also notes a history of chronic diarrhea. Immunofluorescence of a skin biopsy shows IgA deposits. Which of the following is the treatment of choice for this patient?

(A) Acyclovir

(B) A gluten-free diet

(C) Dapsone

(D) Topical glucocorticoids

31. Which of the following forms of alopecia occurs because of sensitivity to dihydrotestosterone (DHT)?

(A) Alopecia areata

(B) Anagen effluvium

(C) Androgenetic alopecia

(D) Telogen effluvium

32. A 44-year-old male with a history of obesity and newly diagnosed type 2 diabetes presents with 2-week history of redness, pruritus, and white discharge to the head of his penis. Patient denies history of STDs and is in a monogamous relationship with his wife. Based on the most likely diagnosis, which of the following is the best treatment for this patient?

(A) Oral acyclovir (Zovirax)

(B) Oral azithromycin (Zithromax)

(C) Topical clotrimazole (Mycelex)

(D) Topical tolnaftate (Tinactin)

33. A 35-year-old female complains of worsening hyperpigmentation to her face, particularly her cheeks. Physical examination of the face reveals diffuse light-to-dark brown macules to bilateral upper cheeks. Based on the most likely diagnosis, which of the following should be asked regarding this patient's history?

(A) History of breast cancer

(B) Oral contraceptive use

(C) Tobacco abuse

(D) Recent antibiotic use

34. A mother brings in her 2-year-old child with complaints of increased fussiness, decreased appetite, and multiple lesions to the child's face and mouth. Physical examination reveals several ulcers to the hard palate and gingiva as well as several reddened lesions to the right vermilion border. Right submandibular lymphadenopathy is present on palpation. Which of the following is the most likely cause of the patient's lesions?

(A) Aphthous ulceration

(B) Candida species

(C) Coxsackievirus A16

(D) Herpes simplex

35. A mother brings in her 9-month-old child with a several day history of high fever and clear rhinorrhea. This morning she reports the appearance of the following rash (see Fig. 3-5). Mother denies any change in the child's physical activity or appetite or any other associated symptoms. Which of the following is the most likely diagnosis?

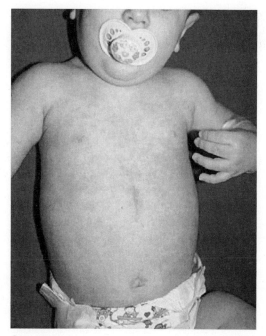
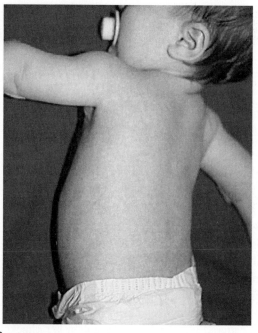

A   B

Figure 3-5. Reproduced, with permission, from Goldsmith LA, Katz SI, Gilchrest BA, et al. *Fitzpatrick's Dermatology in General Medicine.* 8th ed. New York, NY: McGraw-Hill Education, 2012. Figure 192–14.

(A) Fifth disease

(B) Roseola

(C) Rubella

(D) Rubeola

36. Which of the following patients is at the highest risk for acquiring a methicillin-resistant *Staphylococcus aureus* (MRSA) infection?

(A) 3-year-old in day care

(B) 27-year-old inmate with no significant past medical history

(C) 31-year-old female healthcare worker

(D) 50-year-old male with a 40 pack-year smoking history

37. A 4-year-old child presents with low-grade fever, malaise, irritability followed by the vesicular rash which now has developed into multiple hole–punched lesions around the child's mouth and nose. The patient's past medical history is significant for eczema. Which of the following is the most likely diagnosis?

(A) Eczema herpeticum

(B) Impetigo

(C) Perioral dermatitis

(D) Varicella

38. A 13-year-old female athlete presents with the following pruritic rash to her neck (see Fig. 3-6), which she first noticed approximately 1 week ago. Which of the following is the treatment of choice for this patient?

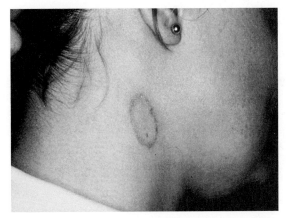

Figure 3-6. Reproduced with permission from Longo DL, Fauci AS, Kasper DL, et al. *Harrison's Principles of Internal Medicine.* 18th ed. New York, NY: McGraw-Hill Education, 2012. Figure E16–49.

(A) Clotrimazole/betamethasone (Lotrisone)

(B) Mupirocin (Bactroban)

(C) Terbinafine 1% (Lamisil)

(D) Triamcinolone 0.1%

39. Which of the following accurately describes Mohs micrographic surgery?

(A) Surgical technique to excise skin cancer under microscopic control

(B) Surgical technique using an elliptical incision extending into the subcutaneous fat

(C) Surgical technique involving a cylindrical excision extending into the subcutaneous tissue

(D) Surgical technique involving a tangential excision of a lesion

40. *Haemophilus influenzae* type B (Hib) vaccination may help to prevent which of the following skin disorders in children?

(A) Atopic dermatitis

(B) Cellulitis

(C) Toxic shock syndrome

(D) Varicella

41. A 4-month-old child is brought in by his mother for a rash to his neck fold that began approximately 1 week ago (see Fig. 3-7). Although the temperature is warm outside she admits to keeping the child bundled up lately due to having a "cold." She states she has been applying topical OTC hydrocortisone cream with no relief. Which of the following is the most likely diagnosis for this patient?

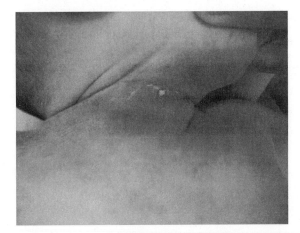

Figure 3-7. (Courtesy of K Zipperstein.) Source: McPhee SJ, Papadakis MA. Chapter 6. Dermatologic disorders. *Current Medical Diagnosis and Treatment 2011.* 50th ed. http://www.accessmedicine.com

(A)   Allergic contact dermatitis

(B)   Atopic dermatitis

(C)   Impetigo

(D)   Intertrigo

42.   Hidradenitis suppurativa is a disorder associated with which of the following glands?

(A)   Apocrine

(B)   Eccrine

(C)   Lacrimal

(D)   Sebaceous

43.   Which of the following best describes the clinical findings associated with lichen simplex chronicus?

(A)   Poorly defined erythematous patches, papules, and plaques with or without scale

(B)   Severe pruritus leading to a thickened scaly plaque with excoriations

(C)   Severe pruritus associated with firm to hard nodules with excoriations

(D)   Well-demarcated plaques that form from coalescing papules and papulovesicles with oozing crust and scale

44.   Which of the following presentations is most consistent with signs of physical abuse?

(A)   2-year-old with burns to both hands

(B)   4-year-old with a 2-cm facial laceration

(C)   8-year old with a black eye

(D)   12-year-old with diffuse lower extremity palpable purpura

45.   A 34-year-old female presents with severe pruritus, redness to her face, and scalp starting shortly after applying a new hair treatment 1 day ago. Patient states that she experienced a similar episode a year ago, however it was not as severe and resolved on its own. Which of the following is the best next step in the management of this patient?

(A)   Administer patch testing

(B)   Check erythrocyte sedimentation rate

(C)   Check lymphocyte transformation test

(D)   Perform punch biopsy

46.   An 80-year-old nursing home resident is noted to have non-blanchable erythema to her sacrum while being bathed. Her skin is intact. Which of the following stages of pressure ulcers best fits the description of this patient's symptoms?

(A)   Stage I

(B)   Stage II

(C)   Stage III

(D)   Stage IV

47.   A 45-year-old patient presents to the ER with sudden onset of facial edema, tongue swelling, and now difficulty breathing shortly after beginning a new blood pressure medication. Which of the following medications is most likely to cause the patient's symptoms?

(A)   Amlodipine (Norvasc)

(B)   Hydrochlorothiazide (Microzide)

(C)   Metoprolol (Lopressor)

(D)   Quinapril (Accupril)

48.   A 31-year-old male presents with newly acquired milk-white patches with a uniform color distribution to the left chin and neck. He denies trauma, pain or pruritus to the lesions, or any other associated symptoms. Given the most likely diagnosis, which of the following diagnostic tests should be included in the work-up of this patient?

(A)   Lipid panel

(B)   Punch biopsy

(C)   Thyroid stimulating hormone

(D)   Vitamin D level

49.   Which of the following lesions, if left untreated, may progress to squamous cell carcinoma?

(A)   Actinic keratosis

(B)   Bowen disease lesion

(C)   Seborrheic keratosis

(D)   Verrucae

50. A 25-year-old female presents with 1-week history of persistent redness to her cheeks, which began after spending a day at an amusement park (see Fig. 3-8). She denies taking any medications and has NKDA. PMH is significant only for occasional arthralgias. Physical examination is unremarkable. Laboratory results reveal normal CBC and complete metabolic panel (CMP) and an anti-nuclear antigen (ANA) titer of >1:320. Based on the information, which of the following is the most likely diagnosis?

(A) Acne rosacea

(B) Atopic dermatitis

(C) Dermatomyositis

(D) Systemic lupus erythematosus

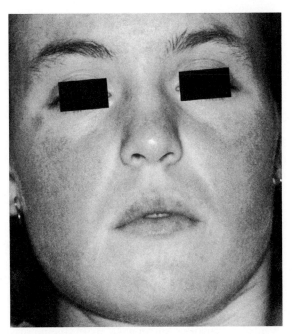

Figure 3-8. Reproduced, with permission, from Goldsmith LA, Katz, SI, Gilchrest BA, et al. *Fitzpatrick's Dermatology in General Medicine.* 8th ed. New York, NY: McGraw-Hill Education, 2012. Figure 155–1.

Answers and Explanations

1. **(D)** This is a classic distribution pattern for seborrheic dermatitis, a common, chronic inflammatory condition that affects the sebum-producing areas of the body, associated with the yeast *Malassezia* as well as genetic and environmental factors. Bacterial folliculitis is characterized by the formation of papules or pustules surrounded by erythema arising from hair follicles. Allergic contact dermatitis is characterized by the presence of vesicles, edema, erythema, and pruritus. Rosacea often presents with erythema, pustules, and papules with the absence of scales. *(Castanedo-Tardan & Zug, 2012, pp. 152–164; Collins & Hivnor, 2012, pp. 259–266; Wolff et al., 2013, pp. 8–9, 785–789)*

2. **(A)** Alopecia areata (AA) is an autoimmune process presenting with well-circumscribed round or oval areas of hair loss, without visible evidence of inflammation, most commonly on the scalp. The hallmarks of AA are "black dots," resulting from hair that breaks before reaching the skin and exclamation point hair (hair pushed out from the black dots). Anagen effluvium is diffuse hair loss involving the entire scalp and is commonly caused by drugs or chemotherapy. Androgenetic alopecia is progressive balding secondary to genetic predisposition and the influence of androgen and typically spares the parietal region. Tinea capitis is caused by dermatophyte infection, and is a common cause of hair loss in children. Hair breaks off at the surface of the skin causing the presence of "black dots" on physical examination as well as minimal scaling and inflammation. *(Otberg & Shapiro, 2012, pp. 981–1008)*

3. **(A)** Lichen planus is an idiopathic inflammatory disorder affecting the skin and mucous membranes, with lesions characterized by the four P's: papule, purple, polygonal, and pruritic. Pityriasis rosea is typically confined to the trunk, beginning with a single red oval plaque (Herald patch) that is followed by a number of similar smaller plaques with spontaneous resolution in 6 to 12 weeks. Psoriasis has red well-demarcated plaques covered by silvery scales commonly presenting as scaly plaques involving the elbows, knees, and scalp. Seborrheic dermatitis is a common, chronic inflammatory disease commonly seen on the scalp and scalp margins, eyebrows, nasolabial folds, and presternal areas. *(Wolff et al., 2013, pp. 49–52, 65–67, 320–324)*

4. **(B)** Brown recluse (*Loxoscelidae recluses*) spider bites can vary from mild local reaction to severe ulcerative necrosis. The hallmark "red, white and blue" sign is characterized by a central violaceous area surrounded by a rim of blanched skin, which is further surrounded by erythema. Scabies (*Sarcoptes scabiei*) lesions are often vesicular, pustular, or excoriated with linear, curved, or S-shaped burrows. Black widow (*Latrodectus mactans*) bites are often painful, associated with localized erythema, piloerection, and sweating around the wound. Deer tick (*Ixodes dammini*) lesions can present as an erythematous macule or papule, which can expand with a distinct red border (erythema migrans), a solitary bluish-red nodule can also be seen (borrelial lymphocytoma). *(Schwartz & Steen, 2012, pp. 2599–2610; Wolff et al., 2013, pp. 585–589)*

5. **(C)** Allergic phytocontact dermatitis due to the toxicodendrons occurs most commonly on areas at risk of contact (hands, arms, and legs) with the plants of poison ivy, poison sumac, or poison oak. They form linear pruritic vesicles caused by the resin of the plant being dragged by scratching. Impetigo presents with superficial vesicles, bullae, pustules, and

honey-colored crusts commonly involving the face. Varicella causes a pruritic vesicular rash that begins prominently on the face, scalp and trunk, later involving the extremities. Herpes simplex virus usually presents with grouped vesicles or discrete erosions. *(Wolff et al., 2013, pp. 28–30, 525–530, 660–662, 673–674)*

6. **(B)** Acanthosis nigricans is commonly associated with obesity, insulin resistance, and diabetes mellitus. A fasting blood sugar is a first step in screening patients for insulin resistance. Potassium hydroxide (KOH) of skin scrapings is used to look for hyphae and spores indicating a fungal infection or tinea versicolor. While tinea versicolor is velvety and can be hyperpigmented, it is not papillomatous. Mineral oil skin scrapings are used to look for the mites of scabies. Scabies can occur in the axillae but appear as erythematous papules or nodules. A chest x-ray would be used to look for pulmonary changes associated with cutaneous findings, such as sarcoidosis. Acanthosis nigricans is not associated with pulmonary changes. *(Masharani, 2015, pp. 1186–1187)*

7. **(A)** Atopic dermatitis is commonly known as the "itch that rashes." Patients have dry skin and pruritus; consequent rubbing leads to increased inflammation and lichenification, which add to further itching–scratching. Psoriasis is a papulosquamous disease commonly presenting as scaly plaques involving the elbows, knees, and scalp. Nummular eczema is a chronic, extremely pruritic, inflammatory dermatitis with coin-shaped plaques with small papules and vesicles on an erythematous base, typically seen on the extremities of atopic individuals in winter months. Seborrheic dermatitis presents as erythema with yellowish scale-forming plaques on the eyebrows, nasolabial folds, glabella, and presternal area of the chest. *(Wolff et al., 2013, pp. 31–38, 43, 49–52)*

8. **(B)** Bullous pemphigoid is an autoimmune blistering disease of older adults. A hallmark is the presence of tense bullae overlying erythematous plaques. Direct immunofluorescence is positive for IgG and C3 deposition at the dermal–epidermal junction. Bullous impetigo is a superficial skin infection caused by streptococci and/or staphylococci, with flaccid vesicles typically distributed on the face and distal extremities in children and adolescents. Pemphigus vulgaris is a rare autoimmune disorder that is characterized by painful flaccid bulla and erosions that may be present on the skin or mucous membranes. It is associated with a high morbidity and mortality. Dermatitis herpetiformis is a gluten-sensitive enteropathy presenting with severe pruritus and clustered herpetiform grouped vesicles on the extensor surfaces and trunk. It is not a viral infection or related to the herpes viruses. *(Culton et al., 2012, pp. 608–616; Payne & Stanley, 2012, pp. 586–599; Ronaghy et al., 2012, 642–648; Wolff et al., 2013, pp. 525–530)*

9. **(B)** Mupirocin is the first topical antibiotic approved for the treatment of impetigo. The topical treatment of choice for rosacea is metronidazole. Tinea pedis is a dermatophyte infection treated with antifungals. Cellulitis typically requires treatment with oral or parenteral antibiotics. *(Berger, 2015, pp. 94–97, 137–138; Schieke & Garg, 2012, pp. 2277–2297; Wolff et al., 2013, pp. 8–9)*

10. **(D)** Immunosuppressive agents required following organ transplant greatly increase the risk (65-fold) for developing squamous cell carcinoma. Erythema multiforme, a reaction pattern of idiopathic, drug, and infectious origin, is unrelated to organ transplant immunosuppression, as is bullous pemphigoid, an autoimmune subepidermal blistering disease. Pseudomonas folliculitis is an acute skin infection that follows exposure to contaminated water and is also known as "hot tub folliculitis." *(Culton et al., 2012, pp. 608–616; Grossman & David, 2012, pp. 1283–1294; Wolff et al., 2013, pp. 314–316, 785–789)*

11. **(A)** Pediculosis capitis (head lice) begins most commonly at the occiput and postauricular area where grayish white, oval-shaped nits are seen adhered to the hair shaft. Scabies is caused by a superficial epidermal infestation of the mite *S. scabiei*, which causes intense pruritus where it burrows, however rarely affects the head and neck areas. Seborrheic dermatitis presents with diffuse erythema with a greasy yellow scale throughout the scalp. Tinea capitis appears as an area of alopecia with scale and broken off hair or "black dots." *(Collins & Hivnor, 2012, pp. 259–266; Wolff et al., 2013, pp. 704–705, 710–712)*

12. **(D)** Flat warts or verruca plana are light brown- or flesh-colored papules ranging from 1 to 5 mm in diameter. Because the virus spreads with scratching

or shaving, a linear pattern forms. Lichen planus lesions are pruritic, planar (flat), polyangular/polygonal, purple papules, generally seen on the volar aspects of the wrist and forearm as opposed to the dorsum. Seborrheic keratoses are round to oval hyperpigmented plaques with a "stuck-on" appearance; some may present with horn cysts. Syringomas are small soft skin-colored to brown papules that occur on the lower eyelids, face, neck, and trunk. *(Srivastava & Taylor, 2012, pp. 1337–1343; Thomas et al., 2012, pp. 1319–1323; Wolff et al., 2013, pp. 320–324, 641)*

13. **(B)** Pityriasis rosea first presents with the herald patch (in 80% of cases) followed 1 to 2 weeks later by a secondary eruption of small oval-shaped fine scaly papules and patches in a typical Christmas tree pattern that is confined to the trunk and proximal extremities. The rash is self-limiting resolving in 6 to 12 weeks. Tinea corporis affects glabrous skin excluding the soles, palms, and groin. It commonly presents as an annular lesion with scaling and an erythematous border. A KOH will help confirm the diagnosis. Scabies presents with burrows at the edge of vesicles or papules and excoriations in the interdigital web spaces, axillae, groin, breasts, buttocks, wrist, and waist-band area. Guttate psoriasis presents as a sudden eruption of small, 2- to 10-mm, scattered, discrete, erythematous plaques that present with or without a scale that tend to coalesce, appearing after group A streptococcal pharyngitis. *(Schieke & Garg, 2012, pp. 2277–2297; Wolff et al., 2013, pp. 49–52, 65–67, 710–712)*

14. **(A)** Tinea versicolor comes and goes but tends to flare in hot and humid weather. Treatment options include selenium sulfide shampoo daily in the warm months and 2 to 3 times per week in the cooler months. Alternatively, patients can be treated with ketoconazole 400 mg orally once followed by vigorous exercise (to induce sweating) or with topical ketoconazole shampoo. Topical glucocorticoids will exacerbate the condition. Topical hydroquinone (4%) is a bleaching agent that could even out skin pigment but will not affect the tinea versicolor. Cryotherapy is not indicated as a therapy option and could leave permanent hypopigmentation of the skin. *(Berger, 2015, p. 113)*

15. **(A)** Sarcoidosis most commonly affects Caucasians in Denmark, Sweden, and African Americans. In the United States, disease onset has its highest peak in the third decade and is slightly more common in women. The most common cutaneous lesions seen are the papular form, which presents as 2 to 5 mm, translucent, yellow-brown lesions, most commonly seen on the face and neck. Erythema nodosum is the most common nonspecific cutaneous lesion seen with sarcoidosis. There is no diagnostic test that can confirm the diagnosis, therefore the diagnosis must be made based on the entire clinical picture. Sarcoidosis affects many organs but most commonly the lungs, eyes, and liver. The chest radiograph is abnormal in 90% of patients with sarcoidosis. Other recommended examinations include pulmonary function tests, peripheral blood counts, serum chemistries, electrocardiogram, routine ophthalmologic examination, and tuberculin skin testing. *(Marchell et al., 2012, pp. 1869–1880)*

16. **(A)** Based on the ABCDE criteria, this lesion falls into four categories: asymmetrical, irregular borders, two colors particularly black and red, which are ominous, and rapid enlargement or elevation. It is less than 6 mm in diameter. However, this lesion is highly suspicious for a melanoma and should be excised as soon as possible for diagnosis. *(Wolff et al., 2013, pp. 261, 282–283)*

17. **(A)** Recurrent erythema multiforme is most commonly due to recurrent herpes simplex virus outbreaks. Prophylactic treatment with acyclovir or related compound should suppress future herpes simplex virus outbreaks, and therefore, future erythema multiforme recurrences. *(Wolff et al., 2013, pp. 314–316)*

18. **(D)** Erythema nodosum presents with painful nodules generally on the lower extremities. The most common causes are oral contraceptive use, sarcoidosis, and Behçet's. Erythema multiforme is usually due to herpes simplex virus infection or a drug reaction, but the lesions are targetoid in appearance. Erythema annulare centrifugum (EAC) is a chronic idiopathic condition that presents as one or more urticarial-type papules that enlarge to form indurated ringed lesions. EAC lesions are further classified as either superficial or deep with most deep lesions being lupus tumidus. Erythema chronica migrans is the classic rash associated with Lyme disease and is usually a solitary ringed lesion at the

site of the tick bite. *(Aronson et al., 2012, pp. 734–736; Burgdorf, 2012, pp. 463–466; Wolff et al., 2013, pp. 314–316)*

19. **(C)** Nail findings in psoriasis include pitting, onycholysis (detachment of the nail plate from the nail bed), subungual hyperkeratosis, and yellowish-brown discolorations under the nail plate, known as oil spots. Endocarditis can present with red or black longitudinal lines under the nail bed, known as splinter hemorrhages. Liver disease can present with Terry nails where the nail bed is white with a normal distal band (cirrhosis) or in the case of Wilson disease, azure (blue) lunulae. Tinea unguium presents as thickened, yellow, crumbly nails. *(Tosti & Piraccini, 2012, pp. 1009–1029)*

20. **(B)** Molluscum contagiosum is described as 1- to 2-mm, dome-shaped, umbilicated waxy papules. Varicella starts as erythematous papules that progress to vesicles, then pustules that umbilicate and crust in crops. Basal cell carcinoma can have central ulceration but are not waxy lesions and generally are larger than 1 to 2 mm. In addition, they usually have telangiectasias on the lesion that are not seen in molluscum. Impetigo begins as vesicles or bulla that umbilicate and then rapidly becomes a honey-colored crust. *(Carucci et al., 2012, pp. 1294–1303; Wolff et al., 2013, pp. 525–530, 629–633, 673–674)*

21. **(C)** Hot tub folliculitis occurs under areas of occlusion of the bathing suit and is usually due to improperly cleaned hot tubs caused by *Pseudomonas aeruginosa*. *Staphylococcus aureus* tends to occur in areas of trauma, such as shaving with a predilection of the beard area in men and the legs in women. Group A b-hemolytic streptococcus does not generally cause a folliculitis. It tends to cause impetiginization of open skin areas. *Candida albicans* folliculitis is seen in febrile bedridden patients generally on the back due to occlusion. *(Wolff et al., 2013, pp. 525–530, 785–789)*

22. **(D)** Vitiligo presents as pink lesions that depigment on the extremities and central face (periorbital and perioral areas). Pityriasis alba is hypopigmentation secondary to an inflammatory rash of eczema. Guttate psoriasis are pink–red teardrop lesions of psoriasis but do not depigment. Contact dermatitis presents as erythematous areas that on resolution

can leave postinflammatory hypopigmentation but not depigmentation. *(Birlea et al., 2012, pp. 792–803; Castanedo-Tardan & Zug, 2012, pp. 152–164; Wolff et al., 2013, pp. 49–52, 297–300)*

23. **(C)** Intralesional steroids are of no benefit in the treatment of squamous cell carcinoma in situ (Bowen disease). Topical clobetasol, a glucocorticoid, will also have no effect on squamous cell carcinoma. Of the other two modalities, imiquimod topically and surgical excision will both lead to resolution of Bowen disease or squamous cell carcinoma in situ. However, because the plaque is 2 cm in size, the use of imiquimod will lead to resolution without scarring, so it is the better choice in this scenario. *(Grossman & David, 2012, pp. 1283–1294)*

24. **(A)** Basal cell carcinoma is most commonly found on the sun-exposed areas of the head and neck. Common features include translucency, ulceration, telangiectasias, and a rolled border and they generally appear in the elderly, however it is appearing more frequently in patients younger than 50 years of age. Rosacea is adult acne characterized by papules, pustules, a notable absence of comedones, and flushing that can lead to permanent telangiectasia formation on the central face. Ecthyma is caused by group A b-hemolytic streptococcus and seen most commonly in diabetic patients, the elderly, and alcoholic patients and is usually found on the lower extremities. Sebaceous gland hyperplasia are enlarged oil glands, approximately 3 mm, yellowish-white, with telangiectasias and generally more than one are noted on the central face, but rarely, if ever, get as large as 1 cm. *(Carucci et al., 2012, pp. 1294–1303; Craft, 2012, pp. 2128–2147; Srivastava & Taylor, 2012, pp. 1337–1343; Wolff et al., 2013, pp. 8–9)*

25. **(D)** The four treatment areas for acne are decrease sebum production, normalize abnormal desquamation of follicular epithelium, inhibit *Propionibacterium acnes* proliferation and colonization, and reduce the inflammatory response. Topical retinoids normalize follicular desquamation, which is the key factor in comedonal production. They also reduce the inflammatory response preventing the development of papules and pustules. Benzoyl peroxide and topical and oral antibiotics have a weak effect on comedones and follicular desquamation, but all three work to

inhibit *P. acnes* proliferation and colonization as well as reduce the inflammatory response. *(Berger, 2015, pp. 125–128)*

26. **(A)** HIV infection, lymphoma, sarcoidosis, and thyroid disease are all associated with the development of acquired ichthyosis, a sudden appearance of fish-like scales, usually on the lower extremities, but possibly throughout the entire body. Ichthyosis vulgaris is an inheritable form of ichthyosis that presents with the triad of atopic dermatitis, keratosis pilaris, and ichthyosis is generally on the lower extremities. Eczema craquelé is also referred to as asteatotic eczema or winter itch and occurs in high temperature/low humidity environments (heated homes and desert climates). It is more common in older patients and presents as dry, cracked skin with pruritus. Lichen simplex chronicus is the name for lichenification that occurs secondary to scratching. *(Berger, 2015, pp. 104–105; Wolff et al., 2013, pp. 48, 72–74, 84)*

27. **(C)** Impetigo presents with vesicles that rapidly become honey-colored crusts around the nose and mouth predominantly. Folliculitis and acne vulgaris both have pustules that arise from hair follicles. Neither will have associated flushing and telangiectasia. Rosacea presents with erythematous papules and pustules, a noted absence of comedones, and flushing that is exacerbated by caffeine, alcohol, stress, extremes of temperature, and certain foods. *(Wolff et al., 2013, pp. 8–9, 125–128, 525–545, 785–789)*

28. **(D)** Pyogenic granulomas occur frequently after trauma and can occur anywhere on the body. They arise rapidly and are sessile and friable. Nodular melanoma should be kept in the differential and a biopsy considered. However, based on the history and the fact that nodular melanomas in this age group are quite rare, it is less likely to be the diagnosis. Cherry angiomas are generally not sessile, but rather small, red papules that predominantly occur on the trunk. They are hereditary and do not arise from trauma. Pyoderma gangrenosum lesions begin as a painful hemorrhagic pustule surrounded by an erythematous halo that eventually breaks down to form an ulcer with perforations that drain pus. It is associated most commonly with inflammatory bowel disease and rheumatoid arthritis. *(Wolff et al., 2013, pp. 116–119, 159, 166, 272–272)*

29. **(B)** The patient has symptoms that would indicate a diagnosis of porphyria cutanea tarda (PCT). This can be an acquired or inherited defect in hepatic uroporphyrinogen decarboxylase. PCT can manifest in the presence of iron overload, ethanol abuse, hepatitis C, and estrogen use, although most patients in the United States have concomitant hepatitis C. Therefore, all patients with PCT should be screened for hepatitis C. The other diseases do not impact the formation or course of PCT. *(Berger, 2015, pp. 121–122)*

30. **(B)** Dermatitis herpetiformis (DH) is associated with gluten-sensitive enteropathy and granular IgA deposits in normal skin are considered diagnostic for the condition. Presentation includes intense suppress, grouped papules and vesicles on the extensor surfaces of the elbows, knees, buttocks, and back. Dapsone is the first-line therapy for DH. Sulfapyridine is a second-line option. A gluten-free diet may help suppress the disease or allow for lower dosage of dapsone, however this is variable among patients and requires strict adherence to a gluten-free diet. *(Ronaghy et al., 2012, pp. 643–648)*

31. **(C)** In androgenetic alopecia in men, 5-α reductase activity and DHT are increased as opposed to non-balding scalp skin. Therefore, finasteride (Propecia), a 5-α reductase inhibitor, can halt or slow further hair loss in men. Alopecia areata is due to an autoimmune disorder in which antibodies to the hair follicles are produced leading to alopecia. Telogen effluvium occurs after trauma and physical and emotional stressors, which leads to an increase in diffuse shedding. Anagen effluvium occurs generally after chemotherapy or radiation therapy. *(Otberg & Shapiro, 2012, pp. 981–1008)*

32. **(C)** First-line treatment for candida balanitis includes topical azoles, such as topical clotrimazole or oral fluconazole. Topical tolnaftate is used to treat tinea infections, including corporis, cruris, and pedis. It is not effective against candida. Oral azithromycin is used to treat sexually transmitted infections such as chlamydia. Oral acyclovir is indicated for the treatment of herpes simplex infection, which is associated with outbreaks of vesicular lesions without white discharge. *(Schwartz, 2015, Ch. 33; Vashi-Kundu & Garg, 2012, pp. 2301–2306; Wolff et al., 2013, Section 27)*

33. **(B)** Hormonal birth control is a common trigger for melasma, as well as pregnancy, family history, and sun exposure. Other factors that may contribute are certain cosmetic products, estrogen replacement therapy and certain antiepileptic drugs. *(Lapeere et al., 2012, p. 819)*

34. **(D)** Gingivostomatitis, caused by primary oral herpes simplex begins as vesicular lesions, which quickly ulcerate. It is commonly associated with systemic manifestations such as malaise and fever. Coxsackievirus A16 causes hand-foot-mouth disease, which causes painful ulcers in the mouth including the tongue, buccal mucosa, and hard palate. Aphthous ulcers are painful small round ulcerations with yellow-gray centers and red halos, involving the buccal and labial mucosa and rarely the tongue, gums, and palate. *(Belazarian et al., 2012, pp. 2360–2362, Vashi-Kundu & Garg, 2012, pp. 2298–2300; Wolff et al., 2013, pp. 660–662, 824–826)*

35. **(B)** Roseola infantum is caused by human herpes virus-6 (HHV-6). It is commonly seen in younger children (6 months–4 years), associated with a fever that lasts 3 to 7 days and can be followed by rose red macules or papules surrounded by a white halo mainly seen on the neck and trunk. Rubella, German measles, has a short prodrome followed by a rash that lasts 2 to 3 days, it commonly presents with lymphadenopathy. Fifth disease, caused by parvovirus B-19, has a similar prodrome to roseola; the rash typically begins with "slapped cheeks" followed by erythematous lacy eruption on the trunk and extremities and may be pruritic. Rubeola is associated with high fever, cough, coryza, Koplik spots, followed by erythematous, non-pruritic macules and papules that start on the face followed by neck and trunk. *(Belazarian et al., 2012, pp. 2337–2345, 2356–2357)*

36. **(B)** Methicillin-resistant *Staphylococcus aureus* (MRSA) is present in more than 50% of cases of cellulitis in which a pathogen has been isolated. Although MRSA can affect healthy people, patients who are immunocompromised, those with chronic illnesses (such as end-stage renal disease and diabetes), inmates and athletes are affected at higher rates than the general population. *(Lipworth et al., 2012, pp. 2160–2162)*

37. **(A)** Eczema herpeticum, caused by HSV, infects broken epidermis and can be transmitted from parental herpes labialis to child with atopic dermatitis. Along with cutaneous lesions, which progress into "punched-out" erosions, patients can present with fever, malaise, and irritability. As opposed to lesions of the herpes simplex virus, eczema herpeticum lesions are not grouped, but dispersed. Impetigo is most often caused by *Staphylococcus aureus* and presents with honey-crusted lesions typically without systemic symptoms. Perioral dermatitis is associated with erythematous papules, vesicles, and pustules, vermillion border sparing and is not associated with systemic symptoms. Varicella begins as vesicles, which evolve into pustules, crusts and sometimes scars; lesions typically begin on the head and spread inferiorly. *(Wolff et al., 2013, pp. 12–13, 525–530, 668–669)*

38. **(C)** Although all topical antifungals may be effective against tinea corporis, evidence shows a greater effectiveness of allylamines (terbinafine) over azoles. Topicals are also preferred to oral agents for smaller lesions such as this patient's. Lotrisone and corticosteroids alone are not recommended for tinea corporis and may make symptoms worse. Mupirocin is a topical antibiotic used first line for the treatment of impetigo. *(Berger, 2015, pp. 94–97)*

39. **(A)** Mohs micrographic surgery is a precise method of treating skin cancer that results in the highest cure rate with maximum tissue conservation and most desirable cosmetic outcome. The other scenarios describe surgical excision, punch biopsy, and shave biopsy procedures. *(Alcalay & Alkalay, 2012, pp. 2950–2956; Duncan et al., 2012, p. 1268; Sheehan et al., 2012, pp. 2921–2949)*

40. **(B)** *Haemophilus influenzae* causes cellulitis typically involving the face, neck, and upper extremities. Most cases occur in young children (6–24 months), however due to immunization with *H. influenzae* conjugate vaccine cases have nearly disappeared in westernized countries. It continues to be a problem in developing nations. Varicella and atopic dermatitis have no connection to the *H. influenzae* vaccine. Toxic shock syndrome is associated with many staphylococcal and streptococcal species rather than *H influenzae*. *(Cohen et al., 2012, pp. 2188–2190; Travers & Mousdicas, 2012, pp. 2154–2156)*

41. **(D)** Intertrigo, caused by *C. albicans*, has a predilection for colonizing in skin folds and is provoked by warm, moist environments. Presentation includes pruritic red macerated patches. Atopic dermatitis is most commonly seen on flexor surfaces associated with dry erythematous skin and pruritus. Impetigo is commonly seen on the face and is associated with vesicular and honey-crusted lesions. In the acute phase of allergic contact dermatitis symptoms include erythema, papules, and nonumbilicated vesicles, which progress to erosions and crusts. In the chronic phase symptoms include papules, which progress to scaling and lichenification. *(Vashi-Kundu & Garg, 2012, pp. 2301–2302; Wolff et al., 2013, pp. 24–28, 31–38, 525–530)*

42. **(A)** Hidradenitis suppurativa is a disease caused by the occlusion of the apocrine gland, part of the terminal hair follicle, which leads to eventual follicular rupture perifollicular inflammation and possible secondary infection. Disorders of the eccrine sweat gland most commonly include hyperhidrosis and anhidrosis. The disorders of the sebaceous gland play a large role in the cause of acne. Lacrimal gland disorders are most commonly associated with Sjögren's syndrome. *(Illei & Danielides, 2012, pp. 1976–1985; Wolff et al., 2013, pp. 14–17)*

43. **(B)** Lichen simplex chronicus is a disorder associated with highly sensitive skin, which elicits an itch response, causing a pleasurable response when scratched that would not occur in normal skin. Symptoms include severe pruritus and a solid plaque of lichenification arising from the confluence of small papules with excoriations. The nuchal area in females is commonly involved, as well as the scalp, ankles, lower legs, upper thighs, forearms, and genital area. The other descriptions describe nummular eczema, prurigo nodularis, and atopic dermatitis. *(Burgin, 2012, pp. 182–187)*

44. **(A)** Signs of abuse can include bruising to soft padded areas of the body in multiple stages of healing and burns that are uniform and bilateral in appearance. Some medical conditions can mimic abusive bruising, such as palpable purpura of vasculitis. Facial lacerations and black eyes in children are not considered suspicious for child abuse. *(Pride, 2012, pp. 1177–1183)*

45. **(A)** Patch testing is the current diagnostic test of choice for allergic contact dermatitis and it includes applying numerous suspected allergens to the patient's back covered with an occlusive dressing and then examining the area after 48 hours. Lymphocyte transformation test is used mostly for suspected metal allergies but has a low specificity and sensitivity. A punch biopsy is used to excise a piece of full-thickness skin and is useful in the diagnosis of many lesions that extend into the deeper dermis such as sarcoidosis, psoriasis, pemphigus, and benign tumors. The erythrocyte sedimentation rate is a nonspecific highly sensitive test for inflammation. *(Castanedo-Tardan & Zug, 2012, pp. 152–164; Zuber, 2012, p. 462)*

46. **(A)** Nonblanchable erythema and intact skin are the clinical findings for stage I pressure ulcers. Stage II includes partial-thickness skin loss involving the epidermis, dermis, or both. Stage III includes full-thickness skin loss extending down to the underlying fascia. Finally, stage IV includes full-thickness wounds that extend into the muscle and bone. *(Powers et al., 2012, pp. 1121–1129)*

47. **(D)** ACE inhibitors, such as quinapril, rarely have the potential to cause anaphylaxis associated with laryngeal or tongue or pharyngeal edema which can be life threatening. It is believed this reaction is due to the inhibition of kinin metabolism of ACE. Metoprolol, hydrochlorothiazide, and amlodipine are not associated with angioedema as an adverse reaction. *(Kaplan, 2012, pp. 414–430; Skidgel et al., 2011, Ch. 32)*

48. **(C)** Vitiligo is a diagnosis commonly made clinically and is often associated with other autoimmune conditions particularly hypothyroidism (Hashimoto's thyroiditis) or hyperthyroidism (Grave's disease). Lipid panel and vitamin D levels are not needed unless indicated for other reasons unrelated to vitiligo. Rarely a skin biopsy is needed to confirm the diagnosis, however histology will show the epidermis devoid of melanocytes. *(Birlea et al., 2012, pp. 792–803)*

49. **(A)** Actinic keratoses are rough scaly lesions that are the precursors to squamous cell carcinoma, caused by excessive UV exposure. Bowen disease is squamous cell carcinoma in situ. Seborrheic

keratoses are hyperpigmented lesions with a "stuck on" appearance and are not precancerous. Verrucae (warts) are caused by the Human papillomaviruses, more commonly seen in younger patients and mostly resolve spontaneously. *(Duncan et al., 2012, pp. 1261–1269; Wolff et al., 2013, pp. 176–178, 641)*

50. **(D)** Systemic lupus erythematosus is characterized by the development of a malar rash, commonly after UV exposure lasting days to weeks. It can include a wide variety of other cutaneous and systemic manifestations based on the sub-type. A high titer antinuclear antibody (ANA) and double-stranded (ds) DNA are highly specific for diagnosis. Dermatomyositis is an autoimmune disorder that presents with muscle weakness as well as painful and pruritic cutaneous lesions in 60% of cases. The Gottron sign and Gottron papules are pathognomonic for dermatomyositis. Acne rosacea, associated with facial erythema and flushing, and atopic dermatitis, associated pruritic erythematous facial skin lesions with scaling and crusting, are not associated with an elevated ANA. *(Costner & Sontheimer, 2012, pp. 1909–1926; Sontheimer et al., 2012, pp. 1926–1942)*

REFERENCES

Alcalay J, Alkalay R. Chapter 244: Mohs micrographic surgery. In: Goldsmith LA, Katz SI, Gilchrest BA, Paller AS, Leffell DJ, Wolff K, eds. *Fitzpatrick's Dermatology in General Medicine.* 8th ed. New York, NY: McGraw-Hill; 2012.

Aronson IK, Fishman PM, Worobec SM. Chapter 70: Panniculitis. In: Goldsmith LA, Katz SI, Gilchrest BA, Paller AS, Leffell DJ, Wolff K, eds. *Fitzpatrick's Dermatology in General Medicine.* 8th ed. New York, NY: McGraw-Hill; 2012.

Belazarian LT, Lorenzo ME, Pearson AL, Sweeney SM, Wiss K. Chapter 192: Exanthematous viral diseases. In: Goldsmith LA, Katz SI, Gilchrest BA, Paller AS, Leffell DJ, Wolff K, eds. *Fitzpatrick's Dermatology in General Medicine.* 8th ed. New York, NY: McGraw-Hill; 2012.

Berger TG. Chapter 6: Dermatologic disorders. In: Papadakis MA, McPhee SJ, Rabow MW, eds. *Current Medical Diagnosis & Treatment 2015.* New York, NY: McGraw-Hill; 2015.

Birlea SA, Spritz RA, Norris DA. Chapter 74: Vitiligo. In: Goldsmith LA, Katz SI, Gilchrest BA, Paller AS, Leffell DJ, Wolff K, eds. *Fitzpatrick's Dermatology in General Medicine.* 8th ed New York, NY: McGraw-Hill; 2012.

Burgdorf WC. Chapter 43: Erythema annulare centrifugum and other figurate erythemas. In: Goldsmith LA, Katz SI, Gilchrest BA, Paller AS, Leffell DJ, Wolff K, eds. *Fitzpatrick's Dermatology in General Medicine.* 8th ed. New York, NY: McGraw-Hill; 2012.

Burgin S. Chapter 15: Nummular eczema, lichen simplex chronicus, and prurigo nodularis. In: Goldsmith LA, Katz SI, Gilchrest BA, Paller AS, Leffell DJ, Wolff K, eds. *Fitzpatrick's Dermatology in General Medicine.* 8th ed. New York, NY: McGraw-Hill; 2012.

Carucci JA, Leffell DJ, Pettersen JS. Chapter 115: Basal cell carcinoma. In: Goldsmith LA, Katz SI, Gilchrest BA, Paller AS, Leffell DJ, Wolff K, eds. *Fitzpatrick's Dermatology in General Medicine.* 8th ed. New York, NY: McGraw-Hill; 2012.

Castanedo-Tardan M, Zug KA. Chapter 13: Allergic contact dermatitis. In: Goldsmith LA, Katz SI, Gilchrest BA, Paller AS, Leffell DJ, Wolff K, eds. *Fitzpatrick's Dermatology in General Medicine.* 8th ed. New York, NY: McGraw-Hill; 2012.

Cohen MS, Rutala WA, Weber DJ. Chapter 180: Gram-negative coccal and bacillary infections. In: Goldsmith LA, Katz SI, Gilchrest BA, Paller AS, Leffell DJ, Wolff K, eds. *Fitzpatrick's Dermatology in General Medicine.* 8th ed. New York, NY: McGraw-Hill; 2012.

Collins CD, Hivnor C. Chapter 22: Seborrheic dermatitis. In: Goldsmith LA, Katz SI, Gilchrest BA, Paller AS, Leffell DJ, Wolff K, eds. *Fitzpatrick's Dermatology in General Medicine.* 8th ed. New York, NY: McGraw-Hill; 2012.

Costner MI, Sontheimer RD. Chapter 155: Lupus erythematosus. In: Goldsmith LA, Katz SI, Gilchrest BA, Paller AS, Leffell DJ, Wolff K, eds. *Fitzpatrick's Dermatology in General Medicine.* 8th ed. New York, NY: McGraw-Hill; 2012.

Craft N. Chapter 176: Superficial cutaneous infections and pyodermas. In: Goldsmith LA, Katz SI, Gilchrest BA, Paller AS, Leffell DJ, Wolff K, eds. *Fitzpatrick's Dermatology in General Medicine.* 8th ed. New York, NY: McGraw-Hill; 2012.

Culton DA, Liu Z, Diaz LA. Chapter 56: Bullous pemphigoid. In: Goldsmith LA, Katz SI, Gilchrest BA, Paller AS, Leffell DJ, Wolff K, eds. *Fitzpatrick's Dermatology in General Medicine.* 8th ed. New York, NY: McGraw-Hill; 2012.

Duncan KO, Geisse JK, Leffell DJ. Chapter 113: Epithelial precancerous lesions. In: Goldsmith LA, Katz SI, Gilchrest BA, Paller AS, Leffell DJ, Wolff K, eds. *Fitzpatrick's Dermatology in General Medicine.* 8th ed. New York, NY: McGraw-Hill; 2012.

Grossman D, David JL. Chapter 114: Squamous cell carcinoma. In: Goldsmith LA, Katz SI, Gilchrest BA, Paller AS, Leffell DJ, Wolff K, eds. *Fitzpatrick's Dermatology in General Medicine*. 8th ed. New York, NY: McGraw-Hill; 2012.

Illei G, Danielides S. Chapter 161: Sjögren's syndrome. In: Goldsmith LA, Katz SI, Gilchrest BA, Paller AS, Leffell DJ, Wolff K, eds. *Fitzpatrick's Dermatology in General Medicine*. 8th ed. New York, NY: McGraw-Hill; 2012.

Kaplan AP. Chapter 38: Urticaria and angioedema. In: Goldsmith LA, Katz SI, Gilchrest BA, Paller AS, Leffell DJ, Wolff K, eds. *Fitzpatrick's Dermatology in General Medicine*. 8th ed. New York, NY: McGraw-Hill; 2012.

Lapeere H, Boone B, De Schepper S, et al. Chapter 75: Hypomelanoses and hypermelanoses. In: Goldsmith LA, Katz SI, Gilchrest BA, Paller AS, Leffell DJ, Wolff K, eds. *Fitzpatrick's Dermatology in General Medicine*. 8th ed. New York, NY: McGraw-Hill; 2012.

Lipworth AD, Saavedra AP, Weinberg AN, Johnson R. Chapter 178: Non-necrotizing infections of the dermis and subcutaneous fat: cellulitis and erysipelas. In: Goldsmith LA, Katz SI, Gilchrest BA, Paller AS, Leffell DJ, Wolff K, eds. *Fitzpatrick's Dermatology in General Medicine*. 8th ed. New York, NY: McGraw-Hill; 2012.

Marchell RM, Thiers B, Judson MA. Chapter 152: Sarcoidosis. In: Goldsmith LA, Katz SI, Gilchrest BA, Paller AS, Leffell DJ, Wolff K, eds. *Fitzpatrick's Dermatology in General Medicine*. 8th ed. New York, NY: McGraw-Hill; 2012.

Masharani U. Chapter 27: Diabetes mellitus & hypoglycemia. In: Papadakis MA, McPhee SJ, Rabow MW, eds. *Current Medical Diagnosis & Treatment 2015*. New York, NY: McGraw-Hill; 2015.

Otberg N, Shapiro J. Chapter 88: Hair growth disorders. In: Goldsmith LA, Katz SI, Gilchrest BA, Paller AS, Leffell DJ, Wolff K, eds. *Fitzpatrick's Dermatology in General Medicine*. 8th ed. New York, NY: McGraw-Hill; 2012.

Payne AS, Stanley JR. Chapter 54: Pemphigus. In: Goldsmith LA, Katz SI, Gilchrest BA, Paller AS, Leffell DJ, Wolff K, eds. *Fitzpatrick's Dermatology in General Medicine*. 8th ed. New York, NY: McGraw-Hill; 2012.

Powers JG, Odo L, Phillips TJ. Chapter 100: Decubitus (Pressure) ulcers. In: Goldsmith LA, Katz SI, Gilchrest BA, Paller AS, Leffell DJ, Wolff K, eds. *Fitzpatrick's Dermatology in General Medicine*. 8th ed. New York, NY: McGraw-Hill; 2012.

Pride HB. Chapter 106: Skin signs of physical abuse. In: Goldsmith LA, Katz SI, Gilchrest BA, Paller AS, Leffell DJ, Wolff K, eds. *Fitzpatrick's Dermatology in General Medicine*. 8th ed. New York, NY: McGraw-Hill; 2012.

Ronaghy A, Katz SI, Hall RP. Chapter 61: Dermatitis herpetiformis. In: Goldsmith LA, Katz SI, Gilchrest BA, Paller AS, Leffell DJ, Wolff K, eds. *Fitzpatrick's Dermatology in General Medicine*. 8th ed. New York, NY: McGraw-Hill; 2012.

Schieke SM, Garg A. Chapter 188: Superficial fungal infection. In: Goldsmith LA, Katz SI, Gilchrest BA, Paller AS, Leffell DJ, Wolff K, eds. *Fitzpatrick's Dermatology in General Medicine*. 8th ed. New York, NY: McGraw-Hill; 2012.

Schwartz BS. Bacterial & chlamydial infections. In: Papadakis MA, McPhee SJ, Rabow MW, eds. *Current Medical Diagnosis & Treatment 2015*. New York, NY: McGraw-Hill; 2014. http://accessmedicine.com. Accessed March 23, 2015.

Schwartz RA, Steen CJ. Chapter 210: Arthropod bites and stings. In: Goldsmith LA, Katz SI, Gilchrest BA, Paller AS, Leffell DJ, Wolff K, eds. *Fitzpatrick's Dermatology in General Medicine*. 8th ed. New York, NY: McGraw-Hill; 2012.

Sheehan JM, Kingsley M, Rohrer TE. Chapter 243: Excisional surgery and repair, flaps, and grafts. In: Goldsmith LA, Katz SI, Gilchrest BA, Paller AS, Leffell DJ, Wolff K, eds. *Fitzpatrick's Dermatology in General Medicine*. 8th ed. New York, NY: McGraw-Hill; 2012.

Skidgel RA, Kaplan AP, Erdös EG. Chapter 32: Histamine, bradykinin, and their antagonists. In: Brunton LL, Chabner BA, Knollmann BC, eds. *Goodman & Gilman's The Pharmacological Basis of Therapeutics*. 12th ed. New York, NY: McGraw-Hill; 2011. Available on AccessMedicine.

Sontheimer RD, Hansen CB, Costner MI. Chapter 156: Dermatomyositis. In: Goldsmith LA, Katz SI, Gilchrest BA, Paller AS, Leffell DJ, Wolff K, eds. *Fitzpatrick's Dermatology in General Medicine*. 8th ed. New York, NY: McGraw-Hill; 2012.

Srivastava D, Taylor R. Chapter 119: Appendage tumors and hamartomas of the skin. In: Goldsmith LA, Katz SI, Gilchrest BA, Paller AS, Leffell DJ, Wolff K, eds. *Fitzpatrick's Dermatology in General Medicine*. 8th ed. New York, NY: McGraw-Hill; 2012.

Thomas VD, Snavely NR, Lee KK, Swanson NA. Chapter 118: Benign epithelial tumors, hamartomas, and hyperplasias. In: Goldsmith LA, Katz SI, Gilchrest BA, Paller AS, Leffell DJ, Wolff K, eds. *Fitzpatrick's Dermatology in General Medicine*. 8th ed. New York, NY: McGraw-Hill; 2012.

Tosti A, Piraccini B. Chapter 89: Biology of nails and nail disorders. In: Goldsmith LA, Katz SI, Gilchrest BA, Paller AS, Leffell DJ, Wolff K, eds. *Fitzpatrick's Dermatology in General Medicine*. 8th ed. New York, NY: McGraw-Hill; 2012.

Travers JB, Mousdicas N. Chapter 177: Gram-positive infections associated with toxin production. In: Goldsmith LA, Katz SI, Gilchrest BA, Paller AS, Leffell DJ, Wolff K, eds. *Fitzpatrick's Dermatology in General Medicine*. 8th ed. New York, NY: McGraw-Hill; 2012.

Vashi-Kundu R, Garg A. Chapter 189: Yeast infections: candidiasis, tinea (Pityriasis) versicolor, and malassezia (pityrosporum) folliculitis. In: Goldsmith LA, Katz SI, Gilchrest BA, Paller AS, Leffell DJ, Wolff K, eds. *Fitzpatrick's Dermatology in General Medicine*. 8th ed. New York, NY: McGraw-Hill; 2012.

Wolff K, Johnson R, Saavedra AP. *Fitzpatrick's Color Atlas and Synopsis of Clinical Dermatology*. 8th ed. New York, NY: McGraw-Hill; 2013.

Zuber T. Skin biopsy techniques: when and how to perform Punch Biopsy. Consultant360. June 2012.

CHAPTER 4

Endocrinology

Ji Hyun Chun (CJ), PA-C, MPAS, BC-ADM
Ashlyn Smith, MMS, PA-C

DIRECTIONS: Each of the numbered questions or incomplete statements is followed by possible answers or completions of the statement. Select the ONE-lettered answer or completion that is BEST in each case.

1. A patient was incidentally found to have a thyroid nodule on carotid ultrasound and formal thyroid US shows a calcified nodule with irregular borders and increased blood flow. The patient had a biopsy done which proved thyroid cancer and underwent total thyroidectomy. She forgot the type of cancer but was told that it is the most common type of thyroid cancer. She is on levothyroxine (LT4) therapy and is feeling well. Aside from ultrasound of the neck, what serum testing should be used to assess thyroid cancer recurrence?

   (A) Thyroid stimulating hormone (TSH)
   (B) Free T4
   (C) Thyroglobulin
   (D) Thyroid peroxidase antibody (TPOab)
   (E) Calcitonin

2. A 12-year-old boy is being seen for concerns of development of breast tissue. Upon physical examination, he is noted to have a firm, slightly tender mass under the left areola. What is the most appropriate action at this time?

   (A) Referral to pediatric surgery for resection
   (B) Measurement of serum hCG
   (C) Measurement of testosterone and estrogen levels
   (D) Reassurance and observation
   (E) Prescribe aromatase inhibitor

3. A 22-year-old man is being evaluated for extremity enlargement unlike anyone in his family. Over the past 2 years, he has noticed that his rings no longer fit and his feet are so wide that he cannot find shoes to fit. He has always been tall for his age, greater than the 95th percentile throughout his teenage years. He has very coarse facial features, macroglossia, and a very deep voice. What is the most likely cause of this patient's condition?

   (A) Adrenal neoplasm
   (B) Multinodular goiter
   (C) Pituitary macroadenoma
   (D) Rathke cleft cyst
   (E) Testicular neoplasm

4. A 23-year-old woman presents with joint pain, anorexia, amenorrhea, and fatigue. On further questioning, she says that she has been craving salty foods and gets dizzy easily when she stands. Upon physical examination, she is found to have darkened skin over her palms and extensor surfaces and postural hypotension. An 8 AM plasma cortisol level is low. What test is the gold standard to diagnose her condition?

   (A) Abdominal CT scan
   (B) Rapid ACTH stimulation test
   (C) Thyroid stimulating antibody
   (D) Urine catecholamines
   (E) GH stimulation test

5. A 25-year-old male presents for consultation of hyperparathyroidism. He asks what parathyroid hormone does. What is the most accurate explanation?

   (A) Indirectly decreases bone resorption
   (B) Enhances the activation of vitamin D
   (C) Decreases serum calcium levels
   (D) Stimulated by a rise in serum vitamin D levels

6. A 41-year-old Caucasian man presents to the office following a health fair screening of his cholesterol because he was told that it is high. He watches his diet, plays tennis, exercises three to five times a week, and appears in good physical condition. He is a nonsmoker, and has no family history of cardiovascular disease. His blood pressure today is 106/72 mm Hg. His lipid profile is total cholesterol 202 mg/dL, HDL 65 mg/dL, LDL 128 mg/dL, and triglycerides 145 mg/dL. His 10-year atherosclerotic cardiovascular event risk is 0.6%. According to the 2013 ACC/AHA cholesterol guideline, what is the most appropriate recommendation for the following patient?

(A) Prescribe gemfibrozil

(B) Prescribe HMG-CoA reductase inhibitor

(C) Prescribe low-dose niacin and slowly increase to achieve 3 g daily

(D) Prescribe omega-3 fatty acid 4 g daily

(E) Give diet education and continued exercise program

7. A 28-year-old female was diagnosed with hypothyroidism 15 years ago. Her thyroid function has been stable for the past 4 years on levothyroxine (LT4). She noticed palpitations, nervousness, heat intolerance, and irregular periods. Her thyroid function test reveals low TSH and high free T4. What could explain this sudden change in her thyroid hormone levels?

(A) Stopping birth control pill

(B) Taking calcium supplements with LT4

(C) Taking iron supplements with LT4

(D) Missing LT4 one to two times a week

(E) Eating high fiber diet close to LT4

8. A 55-year-old man presents with tachycardia and heart palpitations. Physical examination shows a multinodular goiter. He does not have obstructive symptoms. He has low TSH and elevated T3 and T4, and a thyroid scan shows multiple functioning nodules. What is the treatment of choice for this patient?

(A) Propylthiouracil

(B) Beta-blockers

(C) ^{131}I ablation

(D) Surgical resection

(E) Methimazole

9. Which of the following is true concerning insulin?

(A) Triggers translocation of GLUT4 transporters to fat cell membrane

(B) Produced by pancreatic alpha cells

(C) Suppressed by glucagon-like peptide-1

(D) Stimulated by low serum glucose levels

10. A 23-year-old patient with type 1 diabetes mellitus (DM) has been having difficulty sleeping at night. Usually around 3 am the patient will wake up feeling sweaty, nauseated, and tachycardic. He has recorded the following blood glucose levels:

| At 10 PM, glucose = 90 mg/dL |
| At 3 AM, glucose = 40 mg/dL |
| At 7 AM, glucose = 200 mg/dL |

What advice is the best for this patient?

(A) Stop eating a bedtime snack

(B) Increase the evening regular dosage

(C) Decrease the evening basal insulin dosage

(D) Exercise before going to bed at night

(E) Add sulfonylurea at bed time

11. A 35-year-old male with known pituitary macroadenoma develops sudden onset of excruciating headache and blurry vision. He was rushed to the hospital due after syncopal episode. He was subsequently diagnosed with pituitary apoplexy with multihormonal deficiency. After stabilizing the patient, which hormone has to be instituted first?

(A) Thyroid hormone

(B) Growth hormone

(C) Testosterone

(D) Glucocorticoids

(E) Mineralocorticoids

12. Which of the following is major risk to fetus of poorly controlled diabetic mother during gestation?

(A) Diabetic retinopathy

(B) Diabetic nephropathy

(C) Diabetic gastroenteropathy

(D) Neonatal hyperglycemia

(E) Macrosomia

13. A 43-year-old obese man presents for a health maintenance visit. On physical examination, it is noted that his waist circumference is 106 cm and blood pressure is 148/92 mm Hg. Which of the following fasting laboratory levels would suggest a diagnosis of metabolic syndrome (syndrome X) in this patient?

    (A) HDL of 45 mg/dL
    (B) LDL of 180 mg/dL
    (C) Triglyceride of 190 mg/dL
    (D) Random glucose of 100 mg/dL
    (E) Total cholesterol of 250 mg/dL

14. An obese patient with type 2 diabetes mellitus is started on initial therapy to improve glycemic control. Which of the following would be a contraindication for treatment with metformin?

    (A) Renal failure
    (B) History of ketoacidosis
    (C) Inflammatory bowel disease
    (D) Anemia
    (E) History of pancreatitis

15. A 25-year-old man presents to the clinic complaining of nocturnal enuresis, weight loss, and blurred vision. On further questioning, he relates that he has increased appetite and thirst. His fasting blood glucose level is 225 mg/dL. Which of the following would also be indicative of type 1 versus type 2 diabetes mellitus?

    (A) Increased triglycerides
    (B) Presence of glutamic acid decarboxylase
    (C) Presence of C-peptide
    (D) Decreased urine catecholamines
    (E) Increased proteinuria

16. A 41-year-old female had a total thyroidectomy due to compressive symptoms (dysphagia, dyspnea but no dysphonia). Her dysphagia and dyspnea resolved right after surgery but now she has noticed dysphonia. It was thought to be from tracheal intubation and was expected to resolve with time. However, her dysphonia did not improve after 6 months and endoscopy revealed paralyzed vocal cord. Which nerve is most likely injured from the surgery?

    (A) Trigeminal nerve—Ophthalmic division
    (B) Trigeminal nerve—Maxillary division
    (C) Trigeminal nerve—Mandibular division
    (D) Recurrent laryngeal nerve
    (E) Facial nerve

17. The adrenal medulla is responsible for synthesizing:

    (A) Catecholamines
    (B) Cortisol
    (C) Aldosterone
    (D) Dehydroepiandrosterone
    (E) Androstenedione

18. How often should urine be obtained to screen for microalbuminuria in the management of a type 2 diabetic patient?

    (A) Every month
    (B) Every 6 months
    (C) Annually
    (D) Every 2 years
    (E) Every 5 years

19. Which of the following oral agents used to treat type 2 diabetes mellitus is effective in lowering fasting blood glucose levels without causing hypoglycemia?

    (A) Glyburide
    (B) Metformin
    (C) Repaglinide
    (D) Glyburide
    (E) Insulin glargine

20. A 17-year-old female was brought in by her parents to check her cholesterol due to family history of hypertriglyceridemia. Her dad and paternal aunt have history of pancreatitis. Family history is negative for premature arteriosclerotic cardiovascular disease. Her cholesterol panel is as following:

    > Total cholesterol 188 mg/dL (<200), triglyceride 851 mg/dL (<150), HDL 15 mg/dL (>50), LDL 102 mg/dL (<130).

    Based on her results, which pharmacologic intervention would you recommend first line?

    (A) Fibric acid derivatives (fenofibrates)
    (B) HMG-CoA reductase inhibitor (statins)
    (C) Bile acid sequestrants (colesevelam)
    (D) Cholesterol absorption inhibitor (ezetimibe)
    (E) Proprotein convertase subtilisin/kexin type 9 (PCSK9)

21. A 35-year-old male presents with incidentally found thyroid nodule that was found on CT scan of his head. Patient's paternal grandmother, dad, and sister were all diagnosed with thyroid cancer as well that was surgically treated followed by radioactive iodine therapy. Thyroid ultrasound was ordered which shows 2.5-cm solid nodule in left lobe. Nodule has irregular borders, microcalcification, and increased vascular supply. Eight enlarged lymph nodes are seen near the thyroid nodule. Thyroid function test reveals normal TSH and free T4. What is the most appropriate next step for this patient?

(A) Thyroid nodule is very common with predominantly benign lesions. No further work up is needed as long as patient has no symptoms

(B) Reassure patient and recheck thyroid ultrasound in 6 months

(C) Order ultrasound guided fine needle aspiration (FNA)

(D) Order 24-hour uptake and scan

(E) Take levothyroxine 100 µg and recheck thyroid ultrasound in 1 year

22. An 11-year-old boy is being seen in the clinic for well-child care. His father inquires whether his son is starting to show physical signs of puberty. Which of the following is the first sign of puberty in males?

(A) Change of voice

(B) Scrotal and testicular enlargement

(C) Gynecomastia

(D) Pubic hair development

(E) Prognathia

23. You are considering the addition of glipizide therapy to the treatment regimen for a patient with type 2 diabetes mellitus. Which of the following would be a contraindication if present in this patient?

(A) Hypertension

(B) Diabetic retinopathy

(C) Liver impairment

(D) Age less than 85 years

(E) Osteoporosis

24. A 30-year-old patient presents 2 months post thyroidectomy. The patient has had symptoms of increased irritability, muscle spasms, and hair loss for the past month. On physical examination, a positive Chvostek sign is noted. Which of the following is the most likely diagnosis?

(A) Hypothyroidism

(B) Hypopituitarism

(C) Hypoparathyroidism

(D) Hypogonadism

(E) Vocal cord paralysis

25. A 39-year-old male presents with complaints of excessive weight gain, low libido, and mood changes. Patient has "buffalo hump" (dorsocervical fat pad), moon face, truncal obesity with relatively atrophied extremities, and purple striae on his abdomen (see Fig. 4-1). His blood pressure is 161/102 mm Hg. Which of the following is the most common etiology for this condition?

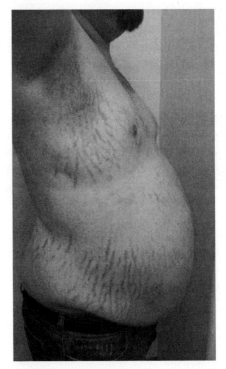

Figure 4-1. Reproduced, with permission, from Ji Hyun Chun, PA-C.

(A) Pituitary adenoma (Cushing's disease)

(B) Adrenal neoplasm

(C) Bronchogenic carcinoma

(D) Familial adrenal dysplasia (Carney's syndrome)

(E) Exogenous glucocorticoids usage (iatrogenic)

26. You are treating a 60-year-old man with a history of angina. He has been on the therapeutic lifestyle change (TLC) diet for 12 weeks (with solid effort). This patient has no other medical conditions and takes nitroglycerin as needed and daily enteric-coated aspirin. His fasting lipid panel from last week demonstrates the following:

> total cholesterol (TC): 295 mg/dL
> low-density lipoproteins (LDL): 145 mg/dL
> high-density lipoproteins (HDL): 48 mg/dL

What is the most appropriate treatment at this time?

(A) Prescribe colestipol

(B) Prescribe ezetimibe

(C) Prescribe atorvastatin

(D) Prescribe niacin

(E) No pharmacologic treatment

27. Which of the following antidiabetic medication has the highest potential risk of hypoglycemia?

(A) Metformin

(B) Glyburide

(C) Rosiglitazone (Actos)

(D) Sitagliptin (Januvia)

(E) Canagliflozin (Invokana)

28. A 30-year-old woman presents to the office with polyuria, fatigue, and a chronic white vaginal discharge with vaginal pruritus. She has been having the discharge off and on for the past 6 months with recurrent treatment failures. Which of the following is the most likely diagnosis?

(A) Type 2 diabetes mellitus

(B) Hyperthyroidism

(C) Hypothyroidism

(D) Diabetes insipidus

(E) Familial glucosuria

29. A 38-year-old man presents to the emergency department experiencing a severe headache and heart palpitations. He appears to be anxious and perspiring heavily. On examination, he is found to be tachycardic and his blood pressure is 158/102 mm Hg. His urine catecholamines are increased. If imaging were performed, what is the most likely location where a lesion would be found?

(A) Pituitary gland

(B) Liver

(C) Adrenal gland

(D) Testicle

(E) Kidney

30. A 37-year-old female complains of constant fatigue, weight gain, cold intolerance, depression, and irregular menses with menorrhagia. Laboratory result shows elevated TSH, low free T4, and positive TPO antibodies. What is the treatment of choice for her?

(A) Iodine supplement

(B) Levothyroxine (Synthroid)

(C) Liothyronine (Cytomel)

(D) Methimazole (Tapazole)

(E) Propylthiouracil (PTU)

31. A 54-year-old woman is taking glyburide, a second-generation sulfonylurea, to control her type 2 diabetes mellitus. Which of the following is the most likely mechanism of the therapeutic effect of glyburide on this patient's disease?

(A) Increase pancreatic insulin secretion, in part by acting on potassium channels

(B) Delay postprandial carbohydrate and glucose absorption

(C) Reduce hepatic glucose production by suppressing gluconeogenesis

(D) Inhibit cholesterol synthesis and carbohydrate uptake

(E) Increase glucagon-like peptide 1 by inhibiting dipeptidyl peptidase-4

32. A 45-year-old man with a history of neck irradiation for Hodgkin lymphoma at the age of 15 is found to have a 1.5-cm, nontender, firm thyroid nodule. Upon laboratory evaluation, the patient is found to be euthyroid, and fine needle biopsy reveals malignancy. What histologic type is most likely?

(A) Anaplastic

(B) Follicular

(C) Medullary

(D) Papillary

(E) Hürthle cell

33. A 41-year-old male came to urgent care due to development of excessive urination and frequent thirst. Symptoms started suddenly 10 days ago where he noticed urinating every 40 to 50 minutes even overnight. He is feeling very tired as he is not sleeping well. He is drinking lots of fluid but thinks this is in response to polyuria rather than the cause of polyuria. He denies polyphagia or weight loss. He did suffer car accident about 2 weeks ago and had concussion. He was cleared from the emergency room the day of accident.

Laboratory results show sodium 166 mmol/L, potassium 4.2 mmol/L, chloride 123 mmol/L, and bicarbonate 27 mmol/L. His fasting serum glucose is 80 mg/dL and creatinine 1.2 mg/dL. His serum osmolality is 343 mOsm/kg.

What is the treatment of choice for this patient?

(A) Caffeinated beverage
(B) Sports drinks to balance his electrolytes
(C) IV insulin
(D) Transsphenoidal pituitary surgery
(E) Desmopressin (DDAVP)

34. A 63-year-old woman presents with shortness of breath, cough, and proximal muscle weakness of 1-month duration. On clinical examination, she is noted to have a blood pressure of 156/102 mm Hg, facial flushing, mild hirsutism, truncal obesity, marked proximal muscle weakness of both the upper and lower extremity, and hyperpigmentation over the palms and back of the neck. Laboratory examination reveals hypercortisolism and increased ACTH. Which of the following would be the most likely primary diagnosis in this patient?

(A) Lymphoma
(B) Ovarian cancer
(C) Renal cell carcinoma
(D) Cushing's disease
(E) Hyperfunctioning adrenal adenoma

35. A 31-year-old woman is being evaluated for irregular, infrequent menstrual periods. On further questioning, she complains of headaches, fatigue, and breast discharge. She takes ibuprofen only occasionally. Which of the following labs would most likely be elevated in this patient?

(A) BUN and creatinine
(B) Luteinizing hormone (LH) and follicle-stimulating hormone (FSH)
(C) Oxytocin
(D) Prolactin
(E) TSH

36. A 24-year-old female who is 30-week gestation complains of constant nervousness, increased appetite, weight loss, heat intolerance, and irregular heartbeat. Her thyroid function test showed suppressed TSH with elevated T4, T3, and positive thyroid-stimulating immunoglobulin (TSI). She denies prior thyroid disorder. She was placed on methimazole (Tapazole) and was advised to return in 3 weeks for reassessment. She returns sooner than expected due to rash preceded by pruritus. She also noticed frequent nose bleeding, easy bruising, and bleeding gums when brushing her teeth. She has some sore neck as well. Which of the following is the most appropriate action to take?

(A) Continue with methimazole and add propranolol
(B) Stop methimazole and check a STAT CBC
(C) Stop methimazole and add propylthiouracil
(D) Stop methimazole and do urgent radioactive iodine treatment
(E) Reassure patient as these are common harmless side effect/adverse effect of methimazole

37. A 36-year-old female with history of parathyroid adenoma status postsurgical resection. He returns due to recurrent hypercalcemia/hyperparathyroidism. She also notes amenorrhea for the past 10 months and breast discharge for the past 6 months. She has been having poor sleep mainly due to nightmares, night sweats, feeling very jittery and sweaty in the middle of the night that improves with orange juice. High parathyroid runs in her family extensively. Her dad and paternal uncle have tumor in pituitary gland. Her sister was diagnosed with severe acid reflux when she was 15 years old. Which syndrome is most suspicious in this patient?

(A) Familial hyperparathyroidism syndrome
(B) MEN 1 syndrome
(C) MEN 2A syndrome

(D) MEN 2B syndrome

(E) Familial medullary thyroid cancer syndrome

38. A 53-year-old Caucasian female presents to the ER with epigastric pain. Past medical history is significant for breast cancer for which she takes tamoxifen, antiestrogen therapy. She is otherwise healthy and previously felt well. She denies a previous history of abdominal pain prior to this episode. She is subsequently diagnosed with pancreatitis on abdominal CT. Subsequent abdominal ultrasound is unremarkable. What is the most likely cause of this patient's pancreatitis?

(A) Hypertriglyceridemia secondary to estrogen blockade

(B) Alcohol consumption secondary to underlying substance abuse and depression

(C) Undiagnosed type 2 diabetes mellitus

(D) Breast cancer recurrence

(E) Cholelithiasis

39. A 57-year-old male with a history of metabolic syndrome, obesity, sleep apnea, chronic back pain, presents to clinic with decreased libido, erectile dysfunction and depression which have been going on for about 6 to 12 months. He has two biological children and reports no prior infertility and went through puberty normally. He is on chronic narcotic medications for his back pain. His sleep apnea is not currently treated as he doesn't like to use machines while sleeping. Which laboratory findings would be characteristics of secondary hypogonadism?

(A) Normal gonadotropins (LH/FSH) and normal testosterone

(B) High gonadotropins and low testosterone

(C) High gonadotropins and high testosterone

(D) Low gonadotropins and low testosterone

(E) Low gonadotropins and high testosterone

40. A previously healthy, 28-year-old pregnant woman undergoes a routine prenatal glucose tolerance test. She is found to have increased serum glucose levels at 1 and 3 hours following a glucose challenge. What is the most likely consequence of gestational diabetes?

(A) Future onset of type 2 diabetes

(B) Macrosomic baby

(C) Diabetic ketoacidosis

(D) Nephropathy

(E) Postpartum thyroiditis

41. Which of the following is the most likely cause of hypercalcemia in an ambulatory patient?

(A) Parathyroid adenoma

(B) Renal insufficiency

(C) Malabsorption

(D) Multiple myeloma

(E) Lithium

42. Which of the following drugs can cause syndrome of inappropriate antidiuretic hormone (SIADH)?

(A) Carbamazepine

(B) Glyburide

(C) Lithium carbonate

(D) Metoprolol

(E) Furosemide

43. A patient seen at the prenatal clinic develops Graves' disease at 9 weeks' gestation. Which of the following is the most appropriate treatment?

(A) PTU 100 mg po tid

(B) Methimazole 10 to 30 mg po qd

(C) Propranolol 80 mg po qid

(D) Radioactive iodine therapy (RAI, ^{131}I)

(E) Levothyroxine 0.1 mg po qd

44. An 8-year-old boy presents with parental concerns that he is the "shortest boy in his class." His growth chart indicates decreased growth velocity falling below the fifth percentile. Laboratory studies show subnormal growth hormone secretion. What additional finding would you expect to see in this child?

(A) Inadequate weight gain

(B) Delayed skeletal maturation

(C) Precocious puberty

(D) Normal facies

(E) Hypoglycemia

45. A 65-year-old woman presents to the office with decreased hearing, and pain over her sternum, pelvis, and her right tibial tubercle. On x-ray, the involved bones are noted to be expanded and denser than normal. Her serum calcium and phosphorus levels are normal, but serum alkaline phosphatase level is markedly elevated. Which of the following would be the appropriate initial treatment for this patient?

(A) Ibuprofen 600 mg po every 6 hours

(B) Indomethacin 25 mg po tid

(C) Meclizine 25 mg po tid

(D) Methotrexate 7.5 mg po qd

(E) Tiludronate 400 mg po qd

46. A 63-year-old diabetic male presents today for recent onset of fatigue, weight gain, lower extremity swelling, and shortness of breath with only 10 to 20 steps. Physical examination reveals 3+ pitting edema on both shin and fine, crepitant rales are heard in lower lungs upon auscultation. He has been on insulin (unsure of type) once a day for the past 5 years and was placed on an oral diabetic medication 2 months ago which he doesn't remember the name of. Which antidiabetic agent is most likely to explain his signs and symptoms?

(A) Metformin

(B) Glimepiride

(C) Pioglitazone

(D) Sitagliptin

(E) Liraglutide

47. A 68-year-old woman complains of loss of appetite, weakness, fatigue, constipation, and impaired memory. She has a history of two episodes of nephrolithiasis. Laboratory evaluation reveals calcium levels and PTH are high. Which one of the following is a common manifestation of this disease?

(A) Anxiety

(B) Osteoporosis

(C) Heart failure

(D) Hirsutism

(E) Proximal muscle weakness

48. A 57-year-old female complains of increasing head size, her rings not fitting anymore and her shoe size getting bigger as well. She has read about gigantism and acromegaly and would like to be tested. Which of the following is the most appropriate initial testing?

(A) Growth hormone (GH)

(B) Insulin-like growth hormone factor 1 (IGF-1)

(C) Growth hormone releasing hormone (GHrH)

(D) Oral glucose tolerance test

(E) Insulin tolerance test

49. The mechanism of action of a cardioembolic event secondary to hyperlipidemia is:

(A) Progressive atherosclerosis

(B) Diminished blood flow secondary to plaque accumulation

(C) Concomitant tobacco use

(D) HDL deficiency

(E) Rupture from an unstable plaque

50. A 26-year-old woman presents to the clinic with a 3-month history of galactorrhea and amenorrhea. Her serum HCG is negative and her serum prolactin is elevated at 220. You suspect a pituitary adenoma. Which of the following physical examination findings is most likely to suggest a macroadenoma versus a microadenoma?

(A) Visual field defects

(B) Significant weight loss

(C) Bilateral nipple discharge

(D) Elevated blood pressure

(E) Amenorrhea

Answers and Explanations

1. **(C)** The most common thyroid malignancy is papillary carcinoma (80–90%) and the treatment of choice is total thyroidectomy followed by radioactive iodine ablation in selected cases. Monitoring for thyroid cancer recurrence should be performed with neck ultrasound, whole-body scan, and serum thyroglobulin. *(Fitzgerald, 2014, pp. 1085–1092)*

2. **(D)** Type 1 idiopathic gynecomastia in adolescent men presents with a firm mass under the areola ("breast bud") typically during sexual maturation stages (SMR), stages II to III. This is a result of normal estrogen and androgen activity at the breast tissue level. Appropriate action is observation and to reassure the patient that the condition will likely resolve in 1 to 2 years. *(Kaplan & Sass, 2012, p. 134)*

3. **(C)** This patient's signs and symptoms are consistent with acromegaly, which is caused by an increased secretion of GH. These are almost always caused by pituitary macroadenomas. The tumors may be locally invasive into the cavernous sinus but are typically not malignant. *(Fitzgerald, 2014, pp. 1059–1062)*

4. **(B)** Adrenal crisis may present with a history of fatigue, anorexia, weight loss, oligomenorrhea, or amenorrhea, joint or back pain, and darkening of the skin. Patients may have postural dizziness, food cravings, hyponatremia, hypoglycemia, hyperkalemia, and prerenal azotemia. The 8 am plasma cortisol levels may serve as a screening tool for adrenal insufficiency. The gold standard test to diagnose this is an ACTH stimulation test. This test will also differentiate between primary and secondary adrenal insufficiency. *(Fitzgerald, 2014, pp. 1112–1113)*

5. **(B)** Parathyroid hormone directly increases bone resorption and indirectly increases calcium absorption. This hormone also enhances the activation of vitamin D, and increases serum calcium levels. Vitamin D deficiency is a cause of hyperparathyroidism. *(Guyton & Hall, 2006, pp. 985–988)*

6. **(E)** The patient does not fit any of the four criteria who would benefit by pharmacologic intervention. Four criteria: clinical atherosclerotic cardiovascular disease (ASCVD), LDL-C >190, type 1 or 2 diabetes mellitus age between 40 and 75, and 10-year estimated risk >7.5%. *(Stone, 2013, pp. 13–20)*

7. **(A)** Estrogen therapy raises serum-binding protein. Free thyroid hormones will bind to those binding globulins and patient may become hypothyroid. Conversely, stopping estrogen can lower binding globulins and previously bound thyroid hormones will now become free and patient can become thyrotoxic. Concurrent administration of calcium, iron, and high-fiber diet can interfere with LT4 absorption and decrease the available thyroid hormone levels. *(Anderson et al., 2011, p. 171)*

8. **(C)** The treatment of choice for multinodular goiter is ^{131}I ablation. In patients with very large thyroid glands with obstructive symptoms, surgical resection may be the best option. *(Fitzgerald, 2014, pp. 1081–1085)*

9. **(A)** Insulin is produced by pancreatic beta cells in response to elevated serum to stimulate translocation of GLUT4 transporters in fat, muscle, and liver cells. Glucagon-like peptide-1 stimulates further insulin secretion from pancreas in response to oral glucose. *(Guyton & Hall, 2006, pp. 961–971)*

10. **(C)** The patient has described the Somogyi effect. This effect occurs because the patient is receiving

too much intermediate insulin at dinnertime. This occurs when nocturnal hypoglycemia results in counter-regulatory hormones producing hyperglycemia. Either the intermediate insulin dosage can be shifted to a lower dosage at bedtime or the patient can eat a larger snack at bedtime. *(Masharami, 2014, p. 1177)*

11. **(D)** Adrenal hormones (glucocorticoids and mineralocorticoids) are essential for life. In multihormonal deficiency, it is critical to replace adrenal hormones first before others. Starting thyroid replacement with low adrenal reserve will induce adrenal crisis as it will enhance the clearance of adrenal hormones that are deficient to begin with. Unmanaged adrenal insufficiency remains important contraindication for thyroid hormone medications. Mineralocorticoids are not affected in secondary adrenal insufficiency and do not need to be replaced in this case (only in primary adrenal insufficiency such as Addison's disease). *(Anderson et al., 2011, pp. 97–99)*

12. **(E)** Due to free transport of glucose through placenta, maternal hyperglycemia would lead to fetal hyperglycemia/hyperinsulinemia which causes fetal macrosomia. Neonatal hypoglycemia is common postdelivery due to chronic hyperinsulinemia and lack of glucose perfusion once placenta is detached. Worsening of underlying diabetic retinopathy/nephropathy/gastroenteropathy can happen to diabetic mother during pregnancy. *(Anderson et al., 2011, pp. 646–648)*

13. **(C)** Metabolic syndrome is found in approximately 25% of Americans. It is defined as three or more of the following findings: waist circumference of greater than 102 cm in men or greater than 88 cm in women; serum triglyceride level of at least 150 mg/dL, HDL level of less than 40 mg/dL in men or less than 50 mg/dL in women; blood pressure of at least 130/85 mm Hg; and fasting serum glucose level of ≥100 mg/dL or specific medication or previously diagnosed type 2 diabetes. *(Masharami, 2014, pp. 1154–1155)*

14. **(A)** Metformin should not be used in patients with renal insufficiency due to its ability to produce lactic acidosis. Other contraindications include liver disease, severe congestive heart failure, metabolic

acidosis, or history of alcohol abuse. *(Masharami, 2014, pp. 1166–1167)*

15. **(B)** Type 1 diabetes mellitus (DM) is an autoimmune disease. New-onset type 1 diabetic patients have islet cell antibodies. A variety of beta-cell antibodies including insulin and glutamic acid decarboxylase may exist. GAD 65 is present in 70% to 90% of patients with new-onset type 1 DM. *(Masharami, 2014, pp. 1150–1152)*

16. **(D)** Recurrent laryngeal nerves traverse the lateral borders of the thyroid gland and must be identified during thyroid surgery to avoid vocal cord paralysis. *(Fitzgerald, 2014, p. 1088)*

17. **(A)** Catecholamines are synthesized in the adrenal medulla. Cortisol, aldosterone, DHEA, and androstenedione are synthesized in the adrenal cortex. *(Guyton & Hall, 2006, pp. 944–947)*

18. **(B)** Screening for proteinuria should be done annually in type 2 diabetic patients starting at the time of diagnosis and yearly in type 1 diabetic patients beginning after 5 years of disease. Approximately 20% to 30% of diabetic patients develop nephropathy. *(Masharami, 2014, p. 1182)*

19. **(B)** Metformin is considered a "euglycemic" or "antihyperglycemic" drug because it does not cause a hypoglycemic reaction at therapeutic levels. Insulin glargine primarily works on lowering fasting glucose but has risk of hypoglycemia. *(Masharami, 2014, pp. 1163–1171)*

20. **(A)** The patient has familial hypertriglyceridemia which shows high triglyceride and low HDL with normal LDL. Fibrate drugs or fish oils (omega-2 fatty acids) are reasonable first-line approach and niacin can also be considered. Bile acid sequestrants can further raise triglycerides and should not be prescribed. *(Baron, 2014, pp. 1210–1211)*

21. **(C)** This patient has multiple risk factors for thyroid malignancy (family history, suspicious ultrasound characteristics, lymphadenopathy) and FNA is warranted to differentiate benign versus malignant nodule. Monitoring is appropriate for benign looking nodule (purely cystic, lack of calcification,

vascularity, or lymphadenopathy). *(Anderson et al., 2011, pp. 215–216)*

22. **(B)** Scrotal and testicular enlargement is the first sign of puberty in boys. This typically occurs at the average age of 10 to 12 years. *(Kaplan & Sass, 2012, p. 123)*

23. **(C)** At least 90% of glipizide is metabolized in the liver to inactive products, and 10% is excreted unchanged in the urine. Because of the short half-life, it is preferable to use glyburide in elderly patients because of lessened risk of hypoglycemia. *(Masharami, 2014, pp. 1165–1166)*

24. **(C)** Hypoparathyroidism commonly presents following thyroidectomy surgery. This patient has classic signs and symptoms of a low calcium level and hypoparathyroidism. Chvoestek sign is a physical examination finding that is positive after tapping in front of the ear in the facial nerve region, the muscle contracts. When the calcium level is low, this occurs. Hypothyroidism can occur following a thyroidectomy but the symptoms are not the same. *(Fitzgerald, 2014, pp. 1094–1097)*

25. **(E)** Patient has Cushing's syndrome. Most common cause for Cushing's syndrome is iatrogenic (long-term exogenous glucocorticoids usage for various conditions). Most common cause for endogenous Cushing's syndrome is Cushing's disease (pituitary–hypothalamic dysfunction). *(Fitzgerald, 2014, pp. 1117–1120)*

26. **(C)** The history of ASCVD warrants high-potency statin which is either atorvastatin 40 to 80 mg or rosuvastatin 20 to 40 mg. *(Stone, 2013)*

27. **(B)** Sulfonylureas such as glyburide, glipizide, and glimepiride stimulate insulin secretion by interacting with the ATP-sensitive potassium channel on the beta cell. These are not glucose dependant and may cause hypoglycemia if meals are delayed, unexpected physical activities and alcohol intake. Other agents have low risk of hypoglycemia unless used with other insulin secretagogues and/or insulin. *(Masharami, 2014, pp. 1163–1171)*

28. **(A)** Polyuria, polydipsia, and fatigue are all findings that can be consistent with both type 1 and type 2 diabetes. Any woman who presents with a chronic vaginal discharge or chronic vaginal pruritus should be screened for type 2 diabetes. *(Masharami, 2014, p. 1185)*

29. **(C)** Pheochromocytomas produce, store, and secrete catecholamines. They are usually derived from the adrenal medulla, although they may be found in other locations. *(Fitzgerald, 2014, pp. 1125–1130)*

30. **(B)** Patient has hypothyroidism due to Hashimoto's thyroiditis. The treatment of choice is levothyroxine. Iodine supplements are not used for hypothyroid treatment unless hypothyroid is due to iodine deficiency. Liothyronine is not standard therapy for hypothyroidism. Methimazole and propylthiouracil are medications for hyperthyroidism. *(Fitzgerald, 2014, pp. 1079–1081)*

31. **(A)** Sulfonylureas have a principal action of the stimulation of endogenous insulin secretion from pancreatic beta cells. The drug acts to close adenosine triphosphate-dependent potassium channels. *(Masharami, 2014, pp. 1163–1165)*

32. **(D)** Thyroid carcinoma often presents as an asymptomatic thyroid nodule. The most common histologic form is papillary carcinoma, representing more than 80% of cases. *(Fitzgerald, 2014, pp. 1085–1092)*

33. **(E)** Patient most likely developed diabetes insipidus (DI) posttraumatic brain injury. Treatment for choice for DI is desmopressin. *(Fitzgerald, 2014, pp. 1058–1059)*

34. **(D)** Tumor cells may secrete hormones that have the same biologic actions as the normal hormone. This patient's symptoms are consistent with secondary adrenocorticoid hyperfunction (due to elevated ACTH level). Primary disease would have suppressed ACTH. *(Fitzgerald, 2014, pp. 1117–1120)*

35. **(D)** This patient's symptoms are consistent with a pituitary adenoma. Prolactinomas account for about half of all functioning pituitary tumors and may secrete PRL, GH, and ACTH. *(Fitzgerald, 2014, p. 1062)*

36. **(A)** This patient might be having rare but serious side effect of antithyroid medication, agranulocytosis (<1%). Once suspected, stop the antithyroid

medication and get a STAT CBC. Once confirmed, one should not restart antithyroid agent. More common side effects of antithyroid drugs are rash, urticaria, fever, and arthralgia (1–5%). These may resolve spontaneously or after substituting an alternative antithyroid drug. Pregnancy and breast feeding are absolute contraindication for RAI treatment. (*Fitzgerald, 2014, p. 1074*)

37. **(B)** MEN 1 syndrome is the so-called "P disease" which consists of pituitary, parathyroid, and enteropancreatic disorders. MEN 2 can be subdivided into A and B. Both A and B have medullary thyroid cancer and pheochromocytoma. MEN 2A also includes parathyroid disorder and MEN 2B also includes mucosal and GI neuromas and marfanoid features. (*Fitzgerald, 2014, pp. 1146–1148*)

38. **(A)** Antiestrogen therapy tamoxifen has the side effect of hypertriglyceridemia. While alcohol abuse is a common cause of pancreatitis, there is no indication of underlying depressive disorder or substance abuse. Breast cancer recurrence is not associated with pancreatitis. There is no evidence of diabetic symptoms in her history. A normal abdominal US rules out cholelithiasis. (*Baron, 2014, pp. 1210–1211*)

39. **(D)** Low testosterone with uncompensated (low) gonadotropins would suggest secondary hypogonadism (pituitary and/or hypothalamus dysfunction). Low testosterone with elevated gonadotropins would suggest primary hypogonadism (testicular dysfunction). (*Fitzgerald, 2014, pp. 1131–1135*)

40. **(B)** Gestational diabetes is the presence of glucose intolerance developing during pregnancy. This usually returns to normal following delivery. Screening is routinely performed at 24 and 28 weeks' gestation. The most common complication of gestational diabetes is the delivery of a large for gestational age baby. (*Rogers & Worley, 2014, pp. 778–779*)

41. **(A)** The most common cause of hypercalcemia in an ambulatory patient is a primary hyperparathyroid condition. These include parathyroid adenomas and parathyroid malignancies. Both of these account for 90% of the causes of hypercalcemia. Renal insufficiency, malabsorption, and multiple myeloma are all causes of elevated calcium level but they are all secondary causes. (*Fitzgerald, 2014, pp. 1097–1099*)

42. **(A)** Many medications can enhance the release or potentiate the effects of ADH. Carbamazepine may increase ADH release. (*Cho, 2014, p. 840*)

43. **(A)** In nonpregnant patients, PTU and methimazole are the drugs of choice for the management of Graves' disease. During first trimester of pregnancy, PTU has a lower incidence of crossing the placental barrier than methimazole. It also is excreted into breast milk to a lesser degree than is methimazole. Propranolol will help with the symptoms of Graves' but not treat it. It can also cause low birth rate in the infant. RAI is contraindicated in pregnancy. Levothyroxine will worsen a Graves' patient's hyperthyroidism. (*Anderson et al., 2011, p. 203*)

44. **(B)** Children with growth failure due to growth hormone deficiency have delayed skeletal maturation. This is assessed by left hand/wrist radiographs. These children also often have distinctive facial appearances and truncal obesity. (*Zeitler et al., 2009, pp. 1013–1019*)

45. **(E)** This patient's signs and symptoms are consistent with Paget disease of bone. Bisphosphates have become the treatment of choice for this disease. Tiludronate, taken orally for 3 months, is very effective in treatment of this disease. (*Fitzgerald, 2014, pp. 1110–1112*)

46. **(C)** Thiazolidinediones (TZD) such as rosiglitazone (Avandia) and pioglitazone (Actos) have a risk of onset of or worsening congestive heart failure due to increased plasma volume, especially patients who are on insulin. (*Masharami, 2014, pp. 1167–1168*)

47. **(B)** This patient has hyperparathyroidism. The most common clinical manifestation of disease is nephrolithiasis due to elevated levels of PTH. There is a high rate of bone resorption due to increased PTH and thereby developing osteopenia or osteoporosis. (*Fitzgerald, 2014, pp. 1097–1103*)

48. **(B)** IGF-1 has longer half-life and provides a useful laboratory screening measure. GH, on the other hand, is pulsatile and single random GH value does not diagnose or rule out the disease. Once high IGF-1 is documented, oral glucose tolerance has to be done which is GH suppression test. Insulin

tolerance test is used to stimulate GH to diagnose GH deficiency. *(Anderson et al., 2011, p. 39)*

49. **(E)** The outdated theory of progressive plaque accumulation impeding blood flow has been disproven. The current theory involves inflammation from an unstable plaque that causes clotting and resulting embolism. Tobacco use and atherosclerosis contribute to overall vascular disease but do not cause embolism. HDL is cardioprotective. Therefore HDL deficiency indirectly increases cardiovascular

disease by allowing proliferation of plaques. However, HDL does not play a role in embolism. *(Baron, 2014, pp. 1210–1211)*

50. **(A)** Mass effects of an enlarging pituitary tumor are often related to the location of the optic chiasm related to the sella turcica. Expansion of a macroadenoma places pressure on the optic chiasm. Bitemporal hemianopia is the most common visual field abnormality. *(Fitzgerald, 2014, pp. 1062–1065)*

REFERENCES

Anderson M, Aron DC, Badell ML, et al. *Greenspan's Basic & Clinical Endocrinology*. 9th ed. New York, NY: The McGraw-Hill Companies, Inc.; 2011.

Baron RB. Lipid disorders. In: McPhee SJ, Papadakis MA, eds. *Current Medical Diagnosis and Treatment*. 53rd ed. New York, NY: McGraw-Hill; 2014.

Cho KC. Electrolyte & acid-base disorders. In: McPhee SJ, Papadakis MA, eds. *Current Medical Diagnosis and Treatment*. 53rd ed. New York, NY: McGraw-Hill; 2014.

Fitzgerald PA. Endocrine diseases. In: McPhee SJ, Papadakis MA, eds. *Current Medical Diagnosis and Treatment*. 53rd ed. New York, NY: McGraw-Hill; 2014.

Guyton AC, Hall JE. *Textbook of Medical Physiology*. 11th ed. Philadelphia, PA: Elsevier Saunders; 2006.

Kaplan DW, Sass AE. Adolescence. In: Hay WW, Levin MJ, Sondheimer JM, et al., eds. *Current Pediatric Diagnosis and Treatment*. 21st ed. New York, NY: McGraw-Hill; 2012.

Masharami U. Diabetes mellitus and hypoglycemia. In: McPhee SJ, Papadakis MA, eds. *Current Medical Diagnosis and Treatment*. 53rd ed. New York, NY: McGraw-Hill; 2014.

Rogers VL, Worley KC. Obstetrics and obstetric disorders. In: McPhee SJ, Papadakis MA, eds. *Current Medical Diagnosis and Treatment*. 53rd ed. New York, NY: McGraw-Hill; 2014.

Stone NJ, Robinson J, Lichtenstein AH, et al. 2013 ACC/AHA Blood Cholesterol Guideline. *Circulation*. 2013.

Zeitler PS, Travers SH, Hoe F, et al. Endocrine disorders. In: Hay WW, Levin MJ, Sondheimer JM, et al., eds. *Current Pediatric Diagnosis and Treatment*. 21st ed. New York, NY: McGraw-Hill; 2012.

CHAPTER 5

GI/Nutrition

Phil R. Merrill, PA-C, MEd

DIRECTIONS: Each of the numbered questions or incomplete statements is followed by possible answers or completions of the statement. Select the ONE-lettered answer or completion that is BEST in each case.

1. Chronic gastroesophageal reflux disease can put patients at risk for which of the following diseases?

    (A) Achalasia
    (B) Barrett esophagus
    (C) Esophageal varices
    (D) Candidal esophagitis
    (E) Zenker's diverticulum

2. Chronic hepatitis B carries a more serious short-term prognosis when coinfected with which of the following viruses?

    (A) Hepatitis A
    (B) Hepatitis C
    (C) Hepatitis D
    (D) Hepatitis E
    (E) Hepatitis G

3. Which of the following is a risk factor for an increased incidence of duodenal and gastric ulcers, as well as a decrease in rate of healing?

    (A) Age greater than fifty
    (B) Dietary factors
    (C) Cigarette smoking
    (D) Stress
    (E) Alcohol use

4. In a patient with chronic hepatitis C infection, which of the following comorbidities would be considered a contraindication to using interferon A as a treatment?

    (A) Hypertension
    (B) Hyperlipidemia
    (C) Diabetes
    (D) Migraine headaches
    (E) Systemic lupus erythematosus

5. A 50-year-old female presents to the office with elevated alkaline phosphatase levels. She denies abdominal pain. The history is negative for medications of any kind, and she denies alcohol use. Surgical history is negative. Which of the following is the most likely diagnosis?

    (A) Primary biliary cirrhosis
    (B) Pancreatitis
    (C) Cholecystitis
    (D) Fatty liver
    (E) Primary sclerosing cholangitis

6. A 25-year-old patient presents with an acute onset of mid abdominal pain, nausea, vomiting, and voluminous diarrhea. The patient denies blood in the stool, or fever. Which of the following organisms is the most likely cause?

    (A) *Clostridium difficile*
    (B) Enterotoxic *Escherichia coli*
    (C) *Salmonella typhi*
    (D) *Shigella flexneri*
    (E) *Campylobacter jejuni*

7. A 25-year-old male presents to you complaining of 6 to 8 weeks of chronic diarrhea. Stool cultures were collected and the laboratory reported cultures positive for *Cryptosporidium*. What would be an important follow-up?

   (A) Test the patient for HIV
   (B) Check family members for the organism
   (C) Perform a colonoscopy
   (D) Perform blood cultures
   (E) Isolate the patient

8. A patient is hepatitis C positive. What should be included in educating them and their family about this disease?

   (A) The incubation period for hepatitis C is 5 to 7 days
   (B) Hepatitis C and D infections must be acquired simultaneously
   (C) Hepatitis C is less likely than hepatitis B to cause chronic hepatitis
   (D) Hepatitis C is a DNA virus with similarities to rotavirus
   (E) The risk of maternal–neonatal transmission is low with hepatitis C

9. A patient presents with an acute onset of left lower quadrant abdominal pain with fever. Laboratory testing shows a white blood cell count of 15,000. If the primary concern is that the patient has diverticulitis, which of the following is most likely to be confirmatory on the CT scan?

   (A) Toxic megacolon
   (B) Air–fluid levels
   (C) Soft tissue inflammation of the pericolic fat
   (D) Thinning of the colon wall
   (E) Paucity of bowel gas in the colon

10. A young mother is positive for HBsAg. She just delivered a child. The proper treatment of this child includes:

   (A) Observation of the child, and HBV testing at 18 months
   (B) HBIG, followed by cautious observation
   (C) HBV vaccination series, followed by cautious observation

   (D) HBIG, followed by HBV vaccination series
   (E) No observation needed, the child will be OK

11. An African-American male patient was just diagnosed with a malignant tumor of the esophagus. What type of tumor is more common in this population?

   (A) Adenocarcinoma
   (B) Leiomyoma
   (C) Small cell carcinoma
   (D) Squamous cell carcinoma
   (E) Granular cell carcinoma

12. In a patient with colorectal cancer, what area of the body would you most likely expect to find evidence of metastasis?

   (A) Thyroid
   (B) Spleen
   (C) Brain
   (D) Stomach
   (E) Liver

13. Hepatocellular carcinoma has a higher incidence of occurrence when associated with which of the listed disorders?

   (A) Hepatitis A
   (B) Acute alcoholic hepatitis
   (C) Long-term use of oral contraceptives
   (D) The use of statins in diabetes
   (E) Cirrhosis

14. When a patient is seen for drug-induced acute liver failure, what is the drug most commonly found to be the cause?

   (A) Estradiol
   (B) Ketoconazole
   (C) Lisinopril
   (D) Acetaminophen
   (E) Methotrexate

15. Your patient has positive serology testing for celiac sprue. To confirm the diagnosis, you need to perform which of the following tests?

   (A) Stool for fecal fat
   (B) Barium enema

(C) Intestinal biopsy

(D) Antimitochondrial antibodies

(E) Food challenge

16. Mrs. Jones was referred for screening colonoscopy at the age of 50. She has no personal or family history of colorectal cancer. No polyps or lesions were found during the examination. She should be advised that a colonoscopy should be repeated in how many years?

(A) 1 year

(B) 2 years

(C) 3 years

(D) 5 years

(E) 10 years

17. A patient describes multiple episodes of forceful vomiting with hematemesis. After evaluation, the report comes back as a nonpenetrating mucosal tear at the gastroesophageal junction. What is this finding called?

(A) Boerhaave syndrome

(B) Plummer–Vinson syndrome

(C) Peutz–Jeghers syndrome

(D) Mallory–Weiss syndrome

(E) Zollinger–Ellison syndrome

18. The laboratory reports *Giardia lamblia* on a stool specimen submitted for a work-up on diarrhea. What is the treatment of choice for this infection?

(A) Erythromycin

(B) Tetracycline

(C) Quinolones

(D) Metronidazole

(E) Ampicillin

19. A patient with suspected acute appendicitis complains of abdominal pain in the right lower quadrant region when he walks and strikes his heel to the ground. What diagnostic sign is he demonstrating?

(A) Grey Turner sign

(B) Rebound tenderness

(C) Jar sign

(D) Psoas sign

(E) Kernig sign

20. A 50-year-old alcoholic presents with dark scaling skin lesions on the sun-exposed areas of his skin. He also has signs of confusion, hallucinations, and psychosis. He complains of chronic severe diarrhea. What nutrient is he lacking?

(A) Thiamine

(B) Vitamin K

(C) Riboflavin

(D) Niacin

(E) Pyridoxine

21. An elderly patient is brought into the emergency department complaining of incontinence of liquid stool. He also reports rectal pressure and lower abdominal pain. The pain is cramping in quality and the patient's abdomen is "bloated." Digital rectal examination reveals a large amount of stool in the rectum. Which of the following should be selected as the initial treatment for this patient?

(A) Passing a nasogastric tube

(B) Milk of magnesia

(C) Opiate analgesics for pain

(D) Oral sodium phosphate

(E) Manual disimpaction

22. The initial diagnosis of cholelithiasis is best made with which of the following imaging techniques?

(A) CT scan of the abdomen

(B) Ultrasound of the abdomen

(C) Oral cholecystogram

(D) Abdominal plain film

(E) MRI of the abdomen

23. Cullen sign (periumbilical ecchymosis) is associated with which disorder?

(A) Diastasis recti

(B) Ventral hernia

(C) Musculoskeletal injury

(D) Umbilical hernia

(E) Retroperitoneal bleeding

24. Which of the following vitamins help increase the absorption of calcium in the GI tract?

    (A) Vitamin A
    (B) Vitamin B
    (C) Vitamin C
    (D) Vitamin D
    (E) Vitamin E

25. The presence of which of the following risk factors are an important clue in the diagnosis of colitis due to *C. difficile*?

    (A) Advanced age
    (B) Non–insulin-dependent diabetes mellitus
    (C) Travel to an underdeveloped country
    (D) Recent hospital stay
    (E) Attending a daycare or preschool center

26. A 30-year-old woman presents for evaluation of chronic diarrhea. Physical examination reveals a papulovesicular rash on the extensor surfaces of her arms, legs, trunk, and neck. The patient reports this to be pruritic. The most likely diagnosis is dermatitis herpetiformis. Which of the following disorders is the most likely cause of her diarrhea?

    (A) Crohn disease
    (B) Celiac disease
    (C) Pancreatitis
    (D) Diverticulitis
    (E) Chronic hepatitis

27. Which of the clinical profiles is consistent with a diagnosis of Whipple disease?

    (A) Forty-year-old female with right upper quadrant pain and vomiting related to fatty food ingestion
    (B) Seventy-year-old woman with left lower quadrant pain with a mass and fever
    (C) Fifty-year-old man with fever, arthritis, and malabsorption
    (D) Twenty-year-old man with abdominal cramps, frequent bloody diarrhea, and anemia

28. Which of the following is more likely to be associated with Crohn disease versus ulcerative colitis?

    (A) Anemia
    (B) Large bowel involvement
    (C) Anal fissure
    (D) Bloody diarrhea
    (E) Arthritis

29. Which of the following medications is a significant risk factor for the development of erosive gastropathy?

    (A) Acetaminophen (Tylenol)
    (B) Fluoxetine (Prozac)
    (C) Isoniazid (INH)
    (D) Ibuprofen (Advil)
    (E) Trazodone (Desyrel)

30. A patient's esophageal biopsy was positive for Barrett esophagus. Of the following, which is a complication of this disease?

    (A) Achalasia
    (B) Adenocarcinoma
    (C) Diffuse spasm
    (D) Varices
    (E) Stricture

31. After hospitalization for pneumonia, your patient has developed moderate greenish, foul-smelling watery diarrhea 5 to 15 times per day with lower abdominal cramps. You suspect antibiotic-associated colitis. What antibiotic is most appropriate for treatment?

    (A) Oral ciprofloxacin (Cipro)
    (B) Intravenous vancomycin (Vancocin)
    (C) Oral sulfasalazine (Azulfidine)
    (D) Intravenous penicillin
    (E) Oral metronidazole (Flagyl)

32. A 2-year-old baby girl is brought to the emergency department with a history of abdominal pain and diarrhea. Mother states that the child was playing normally and then doubled over with what appears to be abdominal pain. The abdomen appears slightly distended and is tender to palpation. While in the emergency department the child has a loose bloody

bowel movement. Which of the following is the most likely diagnosis?

(A) Pyloric stenosis

(B) Mesenteric ischemia

(C) Crohn disease

(D) Intussusception

(E) Hirschsprung disease

33. Among different ethnic groups, cholesterol cholelithiasis is unusually common in which group?

(A) African Americans

(B) Native Americans

(C) Northern Europeans

(D) Chinese

(E) Dutch

34. A 50-year-old woman reports a 3-month history of fatigue, constipation, and crampy abdominal pain. Over this same time she has lost 15 lb. She is undergoing a divorce and feels stressed. On physical examination you note mild tenderness without masses in the left lower quadrant during palpation of the abdomen. Rectal examination was benign, but the fecal occult blood test was positive. Which of the following is the most appropriate next step to evaluate her symptoms?

(A) Keep a food diary for the next 2 weeks

(B) Flexible sigmoidoscopy

(C) Increase dietary fiber and daily water intake

(D) Refer for psychologic evaluation to help with stress

(E) Colonoscopy and upper endoscopy

35. A patient is ill looking and reports a sudden onset of severe, diffuse abdominal pain. Physical examination demonstrates a ridged abdomen with rebound tenderness. Perforated peptic ulcer is suspected. What would be the best initial diagnostic study for this condition?

(A) Abdominal ultrasound

(B) Upper GI barium swallow

(C) Esophagogastroduodenoscopy

(D) Upright/decubitus abdominal plain film

(E) Colonoscopy

36. A patient is having recurrent episodes of pancreatitis and there is a concern about the development of malignant cysts or tumors. If endoscopic cholangiopancreatography was not available, what other methods could be used to evaluate and treat these problems?

(A) Multiphasic CT scan

(B) Abdominal MRI

(C) Endoscopic ultrasound

(D) Percutaneous cholangiography

(E) Push enteroscopy

37. A 23-year-old man presents with the complaint of rectal pain and bleeding. The pain is described as "tearing and intense" and occurs only during bowel movements. He notices bright red blood on the toilet paper after defecation but at no other time. Rectal examination is very painful but otherwise negative. His vital signs are within normal limits. Which of the following is the most likely diagnosis?

(A) Anal fissure

(B) Colon cancer

(C) Proctalgia fugax

(D) Internal hemorrhoids

(E) Anorectal abscess

38. A patient is diagnosed with mild to moderate ulcerative colitis. Of the following medications, which is commonly used as a first-line treatment for this disorder?

(A) Cimetidine (Tagamet)

(B) Metronidazole (Flagyl)

(C) Sulfasalazine (Azulfidine)

(D) Infliximab (Remicade)

(E) Dexamethasone (Decadron)

39. A patient who presents with hematemesis is most likely having problems with which of the following disorders?

(A) Meckel diverticulum

(B) Diverticulitis

(C) Mesenteric ischemia

(D) Peptic ulcer

(E) Hiatal hernia

40. An ICU patient with sepsis who is being mechanically ventilated due to respiratory failure is at significantly increased risk for which of the following?

(A) Esophageal varices

(B) Stress ulcer

(C) Gastroparesis

(D) Mallory–Weiss tear

(E) Volvulus

41. A 50-year-old female is complaining of sporadic midepigastric pain and episodes of increased flatus with meals. She has been on a strict diet and exercise program for the last 2 weeks for weight loss. She does not use tobacco or alcohol.

> Vitals: blood pressure 130/89, height 64 in, weight 190 lb, BMI 32.6. History: married with three children.

From this information, you are concerned about her developing which disorder?

(A) Gallstones

(B) Gastritis

(C) Pancreatitis

(D) Colitis

(E) Peptic ulcer

42. A diet high in nitrates or salt and low in vitamin C is a significant risk factor for cancer of which of the following?

(A) Oropharynx

(B) Esophagus

(C) Stomach

(D) Pancreas

(E) Liver

43. A 5-week-old male infant presents with a 1-week history of forceful vomiting which occurs shortly after feeding. The vomitus is occasionally blood streaked. The infant has not had diarrhea. Physical examination shows evidence of slight dehydration. Weight loss from the check-up 2 weeks ago is documented. Which of the following is the most likely diagnosis?

(A) Peptic ulcer disease

(B) Viral gastroenteritis

(C) Hirschsprung disease

(D) Pyloric stenosis

(E) Intussusception

44. A 14-year-old boy presents for evaluation of diarrhea, bloating, flatulence, nausea, and anorexia for the past 2 weeks. He has four to five loosely formed stools per day. He thinks that his symptoms may have started after returning from a camping trip about 1 month ago. He denies fever, or blood in the stools. Which of the following tests should be ordered to confirm the diagnosis?

(A) Stool assay for rotavirus

(B) Stool assay for *C. difficile*

(C) Stool for ova and parasites

(D) Stool for fecal leukocytes

(E) Stool cultures

45. An elderly man with a history of cirrhosis is admitted to the hospital with an upper GI bleed. He is also showing signs of increasing confusion and lethargy, which cause you to be concerned for the development of hepatic encephalopathy. What test should be ordered to determine if this is the case?

(A) Blood alcohol

(B) Serum sodium

(C) Alkaline phosphatase

(D) Creatinine

(E) Serum ammonia

46. An anxious 60-year-old man presents to the emergency department with an acute onset of left upper quadrant and midepigastric pain radiating to the left scapula. The pain is severe, constant, and worsening over the last 2 hours. He has vomited once. There is no rebound or masses noted. Vitals: temperature 100.8 F, BP 90/40 mm Hg, Pulse 120 bpm, respirations 26/min. What is the most likely diagnosis?

(A) Cholecystitis

(B) Pancreatitis

(C) Diverticulitis

(D) Appendicitis

(E) Gastroenteritis

47. A patient's laboratory results show an indirect (unconjugated) bilirubin of 1.0 (normal: 0.2–0.7 mg/dL). Of the following, which condition is most likely to cause this finding?

    (A) Cholelithiasis
    (B) Sclerosing cholangitis
    (C) Primary biliary cirrhosis
    (D) Gilbert syndrome
    (E) Cholangiocarcinoma

48. Which of the following hernias is most common in women and will typically be palpated below the inguinal ligament?

    (A) Obturator
    (B) Indirect inguinal
    (C) Direct inguinal
    (D) Femoral
    (E) Ventral

49. The majority of cases of thiamine deficiency in the United States are due to which of the following underlying conditions?

    (A) Alcoholism
    (B) Pernicious anemia
    (C) Celiac disease
    (D) Bulimia
    (E) Cholestatic liver disease

50. Which symptom would not be a typical finding and be considered a red flag finding in a patient who has irritable bowel syndrome?

    (A) Passage of mucus in the stool
    (B) Hematochezia
    (C) Constipation
    (D) Abdominal cramping
    (E) Watery stools

51. Your patient reports a 12-month history of episodic right upper quadrant and midepigastric pain that occurs after eating greasy foods. He denies fever. He has not been seen for this before. An abdominal ultrasound is done on your patient showing evidence of gallbladder irritation with thickening of the walls and inflammation. The report also shows multiple stones in the gallbladder. The radiologist says that the patient has a "strawberry gallbladder." Complete metabolic panel is normal. What is your diagnosis?

    (A) Chronic cholecystitis
    (B) Choledocholithiasis
    (C) Cholangitis
    (D) Sclerosing cholangitis
    (E) Biliary dyskinesia

52. During a new patient work-up your patient reports a past history of malaise, fatigue, nausea, anorexia, arthralgia's, and low-grade fever with jaundice, and dark urine. You run laboratories that show IgG Anti-HAV. What does this finding demonstrate?

    (A) Lifelong immunity to hepatitis A
    (B) Chronic active hepatitis A
    (C) Super infection with hepatitis D
    (D) Reinfection with hepatitis A
    (E) Coinfection with hepatitis G

53. What does a positive surface antibody for hepatitis B (anti-HBs) indicate?

    (A) Reinfection
    (B) Acute infection
    (C) Chronic infection
    (D) Carrier state
    (E) Previous immunization

54. A 70-year-old male presents to your clinic complaining of an acute onset of severe periumbilical pain with nausea and vomiting. Past medical history is remarkable for coronary artery disease with atrial fibrillation. Physical examination is remarkable for minimal abdominal distension and guaiac positive stool. The suspected diagnosis is acute mesenteric ischemia. Which is the gold standard diagnostic imaging study to confirm the suspected diagnosis?

    (A) Doppler ultrasound
    (B) Angiography
    (C) Computed tomography
    (D) Plain radiography
    (E) Colonoscopy

55. A patient has cancer in the ascending (right side) colon. What findings are typically found in this situation?

(A) Patients often report "pencil-thin" stools

(B) Constipation and intestinal obstruction frequently occurs

(C) Bright red blood coating the surface of the stool is often present

(D) Iron deficiency anemia from chronic blood loss frequently occurs

(E) Patients develop jaundice

56. Born in 1955, a patient is being seen for the first time for a physical examination. He has never had a physical examination or any type of laboratory work before. He has no complaints. Family history is negative. What special laboratory test should be ordered on this patient?

(A) EGD

(B) MRCP

(C) Hepatitis panel

(D) HIDA scan

(E) Antinuclear antibody

57. A patient who was reporting "just a little blood when I wipe" has multiple perianal fistulas found on rectal examination. On further questioning, there is also a chronic history of episodic diarrhea, mid and lower abdominal pain/cramping, fatigue, and weight loss. Which of the following is the most likely diagnosis?

(A) Hemorrhoids

(B) Crohn disease

(C) Irritable bowel syndrome

(D) Ischemic bowel disease

(E) Diverticulosis

58. A volunteer travels to Haiti on a medical mission. After drinking water from a river, she experiences an abrupt onset of voluminous watery diarrhea which appeared pale with flecks of mucus. She denies fever, abdominal pain, or blood in the diarrhea. Which is the most likely causative organism?

(A) *S. typhi*

(B) *Entamoeba histolytica*

(C) *S. sonnei* (Shigellosis)

(D) *Vibrio cholerae*

(E) Enteroinvasive *E. coli*

59. On physical examination, a patient has jaundice with a tender distended abdomen, dilated abdominal veins, spider nevi, and gynecomastia. What is the most likely diagnosis?

(A) Cirrhosis

(B) Acute hepatitis B

(C) Cholecystitis

(D) Heterozygous hemochromatosis

(E) Cholangitis

60. A patient presents with splenomegaly, Coombs-negative hemolytic anemia, portal hypertension, neurologic/psychiatric abnormalities, and moderately elevated AST and ALT liver enzymes. During the HEENT portion of the physical examination, Kayser–Fleischer rings are present. What laboratory finding is expected if the patient has Wilson's disease?

(A) Decreased ceruloplasmin levels

(B) Elevated CA19–9 levels

(C) Positive antimitochondrial antibodies

(D) Decreased Alpha-1 antitrypsin levels

(E) Elevated glucose levels

61. A patient has a history of abdominal discomfort with gas and bloating, which seems to get worse whenever they eat bread or other wheat products. They also have a problem maintaining a normal weight; having been underweight most of their life. Of the following studies, which will best help establish a diagnosis?

(A) Urinary D-xylose test

(B) Small bowel biopsy

(C) Small bowel Barium contrast x-ray

(D) Schilling test

(E) Abdominal CT scan

62. A patient has Crohn disease and you are advising them on lifestyle changes to improve their symptoms. What advice will you give them?

(A) Increase fiber in their diet

(B) Go on a low cholesterol diet

(C) Lose weight

(D) Avoid gluten

(E) Discontinue smoking cigarettes

63. A patient presents to the office for a yearly check up. He reports no current problems or concerns. His social history is benign, and he leads a healthy life-style. His family history is negative. His physical examination is unremarkable. He asks you when he should be screened for colon cancer. According to the U.S. Preventive Services Task Force, when should colon cancer screening be performed in a Caucasian with average risk?

(A) Screening is not necessary in an asymptomatic patient

(B) Beginning at age 40 and repeated every 5 years

(C) Beginning at age 65 and repeated every 3 to 5 years

(D) Beginning at age 50 and repeated every 10 years

(E) Beginning at the age of the oldest family member minus 5 years

64. A patient has developed a carrier state of salmonel-losis which is not responding to chemotherapy, which is the most likely site of colonization?

(A) Liver

(B) Spleen

(C) Gallbladder

(D) Bone marrow

(E) Colon

65. A patient with cirrhosis develops acute hepatic encephalopathy. Initial pharmacologic treatment of this disorder consists of which of the following?

(A) Lactulose (Enulose)

(B) Omega-3–10-fatty acids

(C) Neomycin (Neo-Fradin)

(D) Mannitol (Osmitrol)

(E) Amoxicillin

66. A 45-year-old female presents with a 10-lb weight loss and recurrent greasy stools mixed with diar-rhea. The patient notes that these symptoms are worse when she eats pastas and breads. Which of the following laboratory tests should be ordered for the initial work-up of celiac sprue?

(A) Antiendomysial antibodies

(B) Antimitochondrial antibodies

(C) Antiglomerular basement membrane antibodies

(D) Antiphospholipid antibodies

(E) Antismooth muscle antibodies

67. Which of the following subtypes of viral hepatitis requires the presence of the hepatitis B virus for replication?

(A) Hepatitis G

(B) Hepatitis C

(C) Hepatitis D

(D) Hepatitis E

(E) Hepatitis A

68. A patient has hepatitis that was obtained by eating contaminated food. He was told that he should get over the infection. What is the most commonly seen form of hepatitis that can be transmitted via the oral route and does not typically become a chronic problem?

(A) Hepatitis A

(B) Hepatitis B

(C) Hepatitis C

(D) Hepatitis D

(E) Hepatitis E

69. An individual's gallbladder releases stored bile after a meal to perform what action?

(A) Digestion of proteins

(B) Digestion of fats

(C) Digestion of carbohydrates

(D) Activation of enzymes

(E) Conversion of iron

70. Your patient has an acute onset of left lower quad-rant pain without fever or other complicating find-ings, and you suspect that she has mild diverticulitis. You decide to treat her on an outpatient basis with oral antibiotics while you do further studies. Which of the following antibiotics offers the best treatment when combined with metronidazole?

(A) Ciprofloxacin

(B) Erythromycin

(C) Penicillin

(D) Doxycycline

(E) Keflex

Answers and Explanations

1. **(B)** Barrett esophagus is a condition in which the squamous epithelium of the esophagus is replaced by metaplastic columnar epithelium containing goblet and columnar cells (specialized intestinal metaplasia), which is believed to carry an increased risk of neoplasia. It is present in up to 10% of patients with chronic reflux.

   Candidal esophagitis is found in patients who are immunosuppressed, with uncontrolled diabetes, or are taking systemic steroids or antibiotics. Zenker's diverticulum is a protrusion of the pharyngeal mucosa that develops at the pharyngoesophageal junction, and is not a complication of GERD. Esophageal varices are associated with cirrhosis and portal hypertension, and may result in serious UGI bleeding. *(McQuaid, 2014, pp. 576–577)*

2. **(C)** In chronic hepatitis B, superinfection by HDV appears to carry a worse short-term prognosis, often resulting in fulminant hepatitis or severe chronic hepatitis that progress rapidly to cirrhosis. *(Friedman, 2014, p. 651)*

3. **(C)** Cigarette smoking is known to retard ulcer healing. Alcohol, dietary factors, and stress do not appear to cause or exacerbate ulcer disease. Ulcers occur more frequently in the age range of 30 to 55, but age is not implicated in nonhealing. *(McQuaid, 2014, pp. 592, 596)*

4. **(E)** Peginterferon alfa is contraindicated in pregnant or breast-feeding patients and those with decompensated cirrhosis, profound cytopenias, severe psychiatric disorders, autoimmune diseases, or an inability to self-administer treatment. *(Friedman, 2014, p. 657; Sanjiv C, Sanjeev A, UpToDate)*

5. **(A)** Primary biliary cirrhosis is a chronic disease of the liver characterized by autoimmune destruction of small intrahepatic bile ducts and cholestasis. It is insidious in onset, occurs usually in women aged 40 to 60 years, and is often detected by the chance finding of elevated alkaline phosphatase levels. It presents often without pain, which is more common with cholecystitis or pancreatitis. Primary sclerosing cholangitis is more likely to occur in a patient with known inflammatory bowel disease. *(Friedman, 2014, pp. 671–673)*

6. **(B)** Watery, nonbloody diarrhea associated with periumbilical cramps, bloating, nausea, or vomiting suggests a small bowel source caused by either a toxin-producing bacterium (enterotoxigenic *E. coli* [ETEC], *Staphylococcus aureus*, *Bacillus cereus*, *Clostridium perfringens*) or other agents (viruses, *Giardia*). The diarrhea (which originates in the small intestine) can be voluminous. The presence of fever and bloody diarrhea (dysentery) indicates colonic tissue damage caused by invasion (shigellosis, salmonellosis, *Campylobacter* or *Yersinia* infection, amebiasis) or a toxin (*C. difficile*, Shiga-toxin–producing *E. coli* [STEC; also known as enterohemorrhagic *E. coli*]). Because these organisms involve predominantly the colon, the diarrhea is small in volume. *(McQuaid, 2014, p. 558)*

7. **(A)** Chronic diarrhea from *cryptosporidiosis* may be indicative of underlying immunodeficiency. Patients with a positive culture should be checked for HIV. Rarely do patients with intact immune systems have problems with this organism, so checking family members would not be useful. Isolation also is not indicated. Blood cultures and colonoscopy study would not offer increased information with

this diagnosis. *(Rosenthal, 2014, pp. 1457, 1458; Zolopa, Katz, 2014, p. 1283)*

8. **(E)** The maternal–neonatal transmission with hepatitis C is low. Hepatitis C is an RNA virus that is similar to flaviviruses. The incubation period averages 6 to 8 weeks, and is more likely to become chronic than hepatitis B. Coinfection with hepatitis D occurs with hepatitis B, not hepatitis C. *(Friedman, 2014, pp. 649–650)*

9. **(C)** CT scan of the abdomen can be obtained to look for evidence of diverticulitis and determine its severity, and to exclude other disorders that may cause lower abdominal pain. The presence of colonic diverticula and wall thickening, pericolic fat infiltration, abscess formation, or extraluminal air or contrast suggest diverticulitis. *(McQuaid, 2014, p. 631)*

10. **(D)** All pregnant women should be screened for HBsAg. Transmission of the virus to the baby after delivery is likely if both surface antigen and e-antigen are positive. Vertical transmission can be blocked by the immediate postdelivery administration to the newborn of hepatitis B immunoglobulin and hepatitis B vaccine intramuscularly. The vaccine dose is repeated at 1 and 6 months of age. *(Rogers, Worley, 2014, pp. 783, 784)*

11. **(D)** Esophageal cancer usually develops in persons between 50 and 70 years of age. The overall ratio of men to women is 3:1. There are two histologic types: squamous cell carcinoma and adenocarcinoma. In the United States, squamous cell cancer is much more common in blacks than in whites. Chronic alcohol and tobacco use are strongly associated with an increased risk of squamous cell carcinoma. Adenocarcinoma is more common in whites. The majority of adenocarcinomas develop as a complication of Barrett metaplasia due to chronic gastroesophageal reflux. Benign tumors such as leiomyomas are rare. *(Kelly & McQuaid, 2014, p. 1558)*

12. **(E)** Approximately 20% of patients in the United States have distant metastatic disease at the time of presentation. CRC can spread by lymphatic and hematogenous dissemination, as well as by contiguous and transperitoneal routes. The most common metastatic sites are the regional lymph nodes, liver, lungs, and peritoneum. *(Cornett & Dea, 2014, p. 1569; Fletcher, UpToDate)*

13. **(E)** Hepatocellular carcinomas are associated with cirrhosis in 80% of cases. Evidence for an association with long-term use of oral contraceptives is inconclusive. In diabetic patients, the use of statins, metformin, and thiazolidinediones appear to be protective. Acute (not chronic) alcoholic hepatitis without cirrhosis is not a factor. *(Cornett & Dea, 2014, p. 1549)*

14. **(D)** An estimated 1,600 cases of acute liver failure occur each year in the United States. Acetaminophen toxicity is the most common cause, accounting for at least 45% of cases. Suicide attempts account for 44% of cases of acetaminophen-induced hepatic failure. All the drugs listed can cause acute liver failure. *(Friedman, 2014, p. 651–652; Goldberg, Chopra, UpToDate)*

15. **(C)** Endoscopic mucosal biopsy of the proximal duodenum (bulb) and distal duodenum is the standard method for confirmation of the diagnosis in patients with a positive serologic test (IgA endomysial antibody) for celiac disease. "Classic" symptoms of malabsorption more commonly present in infants (<2 years). Older children and adults are less likely to manifest signs of serious malabsorption. Stool for fecal fat is a nonspecific finding. Antimitochondrial antibodies are positive in primary biliary cirrhosis. *(Kelly, UpToDate; McQuaid, 2014, pp. 602–603)*

16. **(E)** In average risk individuals aged 50 or greater, screening colonoscopy should be repeated every 10 years following and initial normal examination. If the individual has a first-degree relative with a history of adenomas or colorectal cancer, screening should begin earlier, generally at age 40 or 10 years younger than the age at diagnosis of the youngest affected relative. *(Cornett & Dea, 2014, pp. 1571–1572)*

17. **(D)** Mallory–Weiss syndrome is characterized by a nonpenetrating mucosal tear at the gastroesophageal junction that is hypothesized to arise from events that suddenly raise transabdominal pressure, such as lifting, retching, or vomiting. Alcoholism is

a strong predisposing factor. Plummer–Vinson is a congenital syndrome associated with anemia and webbing of the esophagus. Boerhaave syndrome is a rare life-threatening problem characterized by a full-thickness tear of the esophageal wall. Zollinger–Ellison syndrome is caused by gastrin-secreting neuroendocrine tumors resulting in acid hypersecretion. *(Guelrud, UpToDate; McQuaid, 2014, pp. 551, 581–582, 600)*

18. **(D)** The treatments of choice for giardiasis are metronidazole (250 mg orally three times daily for 5 to 7 days) or tinidazole (2 g orally once). Erythromycin can be used to treat Campylobacter. Doxycycline or tetracycline can be used to treat cholera. Fluoroquinolones can also be used to treat cholera and shigellosis. *(Rosenthal, 2014, pp. 1460–1461)*

19. **(C)** Jar sign is also known as Markle sign and it may prove to be superior to rebound tenderness as a localizing sign of peritoneal irritation, especially in the pelvis. It is done by quickly dropping down on the heels and noting the location of the patient's abdominal pain. Rebound tenderness is elicited by pressing the fingers gently into the abdomen, then suddenly withdrawing them. Psoas sign is performed by flexing the thigh against resistance to elicit muscle irritation from an inflamed appendix. Kernig sign is a test for spinal cord irritation. *(Bickley, 2009, p. 468; LeBlond, 2009, p. 481; McQuaid, 2014, p. 610)*

20. **(D)** Niacin deficiency is known as pellagra. It is rare in the United States and is most often a compilation of alcoholism or malabsorption syndrome. Clinical signs of pellagra are known as the 3 Ds—dermatitis, diarrhea, and dementia. *(Baron, 2014, p. 1219; Sassan, Clifford, David, UpToDate)*

21. **(E)** Mechanical bowel obstruction in the rectum does not usually respond to oral laxatives, and they may cause complications. A nasogastric tube would not be used for an obstruction in the distal colon/rectum. One would avoid opiates in fecal impactions and other constipation problems because they tend to be more constipating. This patient needs to be disimpacted. *(McQuaid, 2014, p. 555; Rao, UpToDate)*

22. **(B)** Ultrasound has replaced oral cholecystograms as the test of choice for diagnosing cholelithiasis.

CT is useful in the evaluation of the acute abdomen, but the sensitivity for viewing the gallstones is poor. KUB is also not a sensitive study for cholelithiases. MRI is expensive and not recommended as an initial screening examination for gallstones but can be used if ultrasound is equivocal. *(Friedman, 2014, pp. 681–684)*

23. **(E)** A faint blue coloration, or bruising may occur as a result of retroperitoneal bleeding. This is known as Cullen sign. Diastasis recti occurs when the rectus muscles lack a normal fibrous band that attaches at midline. An umbilical/ventral hernia will occur when a weakness occurs in the abdominal wall. *(Kendall, Moreira, UpToDate; Leblond, 2009, p. 478)*

24. **(D)** Vitamin D increases the absorption of calcium and phosphorus in the GI tract and induces osteoclast activity, which causes an overall increase in serum calcium levels. *(Fitzgerald, 2014, p. 1107; Hutton, 2005, p. 32)*

25. **(D)** Antibiotic-associated colitis is a significant clinical problem almost always caused by *C. difficile* infection. Hospitalized patients are most susceptible. *C. difficile* colitis is the major cause of diarrhea in patients hospitalized for more than 3 days, affecting 22 patients of every 1,000. *(Kelly, Lamont, UpToDate; McQuaid, 2014, p. 616)*

26. **(B)** Dermatitis herpetiformis is regarded as a cutaneous variant of celiac disease. It is a characteristic skin rash consisting of pruritic papulovesicles over the extensor surfaces of the extremities and over the trunk, scalp, and neck. Dermatitis herpetiformis occurs in <10% of patients with celiac disease; however, almost all patients who present with dermatitis herpetiformis have evidence of celiac disease on intestinal mucosal biopsy, though it may not be clinically evident. *(Hull, UpToDate; McQuaid, 2014, p. 602)*

27. **(C)** Whipple disease is a rare multisystemic illness caused by infection with the bacillus *Tropheryma whippelii*. It may occur at any age but most commonly affects white men in the fourth to sixth decades. The most common findings are arthralgias, diarrhea, abdominal pain, and weight loss. Other symptoms include abdominal pain, diarrhea, and some degree of malabsorption with distention,

flatulence, and steatorrhea. Weight loss is the most common presenting symptom—seen in almost all patients. *(McQuaid, 2014, p. 604)*

28. **(C)** One-third of cases of Crohn disease involve the small bowel only, most commonly the terminal ileum (ileitis). Half of all cases involve the small bowel and colon, most often the terminal ileum and adjacent proximal ascending colon (ileocolitis). In 20% of cases, the colon alone is affected. One-third of patients have associated perianal disease (fistulas, fissures, abscesses). Ulcerative colitis is an idiopathic inflammatory condition that involves the mucosal surface of the colon, resulting in diffuse friability and erosions with bleeding. Extra intestinal manifestations such as arthritis, arthralgias, and skin rash may occur with both conditions. Both conditions may have bloody diarrhea although it is more common in ulcerative colitis. *(McQuaid, 2014, pp. 621, 626)*

29. **(D)** The most common causes of erosive gastropathy are medications (especially NSAIDs), alcohol, stress due to severe medical or surgical illness, and portal hypertension ("portal gastropathy"). Major risk factors for stress gastritis include mechanical ventilation, coagulopathy, trauma, burns, shock, sepsis, central nervous system injury, liver failure, kidney disease, and multiorgan failure. *(McQuaid, 2014, p. 588)*

30. **(B)** Barrett esophagus is a condition in which the squamous epithelium of the esophagus is replaced by metaplastic columnar epithelium containing goblet and columnar cells (specialized intestinal metaplasia). The most serious complication of Barrett esophagus is esophageal adenocarcinoma. It is believed that most adenocarcinomas of the esophagus and many such tumors of the gastric cardia arise from dysplastic epithelium in Barrett esophagus. *(McQuaid, 2014, pp. 576, 577)*

31. **(E)** Antibiotic-associated colitis is a significant clinical problem almost always caused by *C. difficile* infection. Hospitalized patients are most susceptible. Although almost all antibiotics have been implicated, colitis most commonly develops after use of ampicillin, clindamycin, third-generation cephalosporins, and fluoroquinolones. *C. difficile* colitis will develop in approximately one-third of infected patients If possible, antibiotic therapy

should be discontinued and therapy with metronidazole, vancomycin, or fidaxomicin (a poorly absorbable macrolide antibiotic) should be initiated. Vancomycin and fidaxomicin are significantly more expensive than metronidazole. Therefore, metronidazole remains the preferred first-line therapy in patients with mild disease, except in patients who are intolerant of metronidazole, pregnant women, and children. *(McQuaid, 2014, p. 616)*

32. **(D)** Patients with intussusception typically develop the sudden onset of intermittent, severe, crampy, progressive abdominal pain, accompanied by inconsolable crying and drawing up of the legs toward the abdomen. In up to 70% of cases, the stool contains gross or occult blood. It is the most frequent cause of obstruction in the first 2 years. Pyloric stenosis typically presents prior to the age of 6 months with vomiting, but not with diarrhea. Hirschsprung disease is an absence of ganglion cells in the colon with failure to pass meconium, followed by vomiting and abdominal distention. Crohn disease and mesenteric ischemia occur later in life. *(Kitagawa, Migdady, UpToDate; Sondgeimer, 2007, pp. 607–608, 612, 617, 634)*

33. **(B)** Gallstones are more common in women than in men and increase in incidence in both sexes and all races with age. In the United States, the prevalence of gallstones is 8.6% in women and 5.5% in men, with the highest rates in persons over age 60 and higher rates in Mexican-Americans than in non-Hispanic whites and African Americans. Although cholesterol gallstones are less common in black people, cholelithiasis attributable to hemolysis occurs in over a third of individuals with sickle cell disease. Native Americans of both the Northern and Southern Hemispheres have a high rate of cholesterol cholelithiasis, probably because of a predisposition resulting from "thrifty" *(LITH)* genes. *(Friedman, 2014, pp. 681, 682)*

34. **(E)** Asymptomatic adults with positive fecal occult blood test or fecal immunochemical test that are performed for routine colorectal cancer screening should undergo colonoscopy. All symptomatic adults with positive FOBTs or FITs or iron deficiency anemia should undergo evaluation of the upper and lower gastrointestinal tract with colonoscopy and upper endoscopy, unless the anemia can be

definitively ascribed to a nongastrointestinal source. The chief disadvantage of screening with flexible sigmoidoscopy is that is does not examine the proximal colon. The prevalence of proximal versus distal neoplasia is higher in people over 65 years of age, African Americans, and women. *(Cornett & Dea, 2014, pp. 1572, 1573; McQuaid, 2014, p. 569)*

35. **(D)** Ulcer perforation should be suspected in patients who suddenly develop severe, diffuse abdominal pain. If imaging is required, plain x-rays are typically obtained first. Careful interpretation of upright chest and abdominal films can detect diagnostic free air in many cases of perforated gastric and duodenal ulcers. If there is no free air on the plain film, computed tomography or ultrasound can be useful to detect small amounts of free air or fluid. Barium studies are contraindicated in patients with a possible perforation. *(McQuaid, 2014, p. 599; Soll, Vakil, UpToDate)*

36. **(C)** Endoscopic ultrasound was developed as a diagnostic modality but rapidly gained a role for a variety of therapeutic applications. EUS has been used increasingly for drainage of pancreatic pseudocysts, treatment of cystic lesions of the pancreas, EUS-guided cholangiopancreatography, localized therapy for pancreatic tumors, and treatment of subepithelial lesions and gastric varices. Endoscopic ultrasonography (with pancreatic tissue sampling) is a less invasive alternative to ERCP. CT and MRI can offer images, but cannot provide diagnostic tests. Percutaneous cholangiography evaluates the biliary tract, and push enteroscopy evaluates the small bowel. *(Fasanella & Sanders, UpToDate; Friedman, 2014, pp. 691, 692, 695)*

37. **(A)** Anal fissure is thought to be due to trauma to the anal canal during defecation. Patients will complain of severe pain during defecation with occasional blood noted on the surface of the stool or on the toilet paper. Proctalgia fugax presents with acute, severe rectal pain but without bleeding. Internal hemorrhoids may have bleeding but are typically painless. Colorectal cancer more typically presents with a change in bowel habits or obstructive symptoms. Anorectal abscess typically manifests as continuous, throbbing perianal pain. *(Cornett & Dea, 2014, p. 1569; McQuaid, 2014, pp. 637, 639, 640)*

38. **(C)** Disease extending above the sigmoid colon is best treated with oral 5-ASA agents (mesalamine, balsalazide, or sulfasalazine), which result in symptomatic improvement in 50% to 75% of patients. Oral sulfasalazine is comparable in efficacy to mesalamine and because of its low cost it is still commonly used as a first-line agent by many providers. Patients with disease confined to the rectum or rectosigmoid region generally have mild to moderate but distressing symptoms. They may be treated with topical mesalamine, topical corticosteroids, or oral aminosalicylates (5-ASA). The anti-TNF agents infliximab and adalimumab are approved in the United States for the treatment of patients with moderate to severe ulcerative colitis who have had an inadequate response to conventional therapies. *(McQuaid, 2014, p. 627)*

39. **(D)** Peptic ulcers account for half of major upper gastrointestinal bleeding with an overall mortality rate of 6%. Meckel diverticulum, diverticular disease, and mesenteric ischemia may present with lower GI bleeding. Hiatal hernias usually cause no symptoms. *(McQuaid, 2014, p. 563)*

40. **(B)** The most common causes of erosive gastropathy are medications (especially NSAIDs), alcohol, stress due to severe medical or surgical illness, and portal hypertension ("portal gastropathy"). Major risk factors for stress gastritis include mechanical ventilation, coagulopathy, trauma, burns, shock, sepsis, central nervous system injury, liver failure, kidney disease, and multiorgan failure. Mallory–Weiss tears follow a prolonged period of retching/vomiting. Volvulus is most frequently due to adhesions or redundant colon. Gastroparesis is a slowing of the transit of stomach contents, and does not typically cause ulcers. *(McQuaid, 2014, pp. 588, 589)*

41. **(A)** Obesity is a risk factor for gallstones, especially in women. Rapid weight loss, as occurs after bariatric surgery, also increases the risk of symptomatic gallstone formation. Diabetes mellitus, glucose intolerance, and insulin resistance are risk factors for gallstones, and a high intake of carbohydrate and high dietary glycemic load increase the risk of cholecystectomy in women. *(Friedman, 2014, p. 681, 682)*

42. **(C)** Chronic *H. pylori* gastritis is a strong risk factor for gastric carcinoma. Other risk factors for

intestinal-type gastric cancer include pernicious anemia, a history of partial gastric resection more than 15 years previously, smoking, and diets that are high in nitrates or salt and low in vitamin C. *(Cornett & Dea, 2014, p. 1561)*

43. (D) The classic presentation of infantile hypertrophic pyloric stenosis is the 3- to 6-week-old infant who develops immediate postprandial vomiting that is nonbilious and forceful. The majority (83%) were boys, and 31% were firstborn. Patients were classically described as being emaciated and dehydrated. Peptic ulcer is commonly found at an older age. Intussusception presents with colicky abdominal pain, vomiting, and bloody diarrhea. *(Olivé, Endom, UpToDate)*

44. (C) Giardiasis is a protozoal infection of the upper small intestine caused by the flagellate *G. lamblia*. The parasite occurs worldwide, most abundantly in areas with poor sanitation. In developing countries, young children are very commonly infected. Groups at special risk include travelers to *Giardia*-endemic areas, those who swallow contaminated water during recreation or wilderness travel, men who have sex with men, and persons with impaired immunity. *(Rosenthal, 2014, p. 1460)*

45. (E) Hepatic encephalopathy is a state of disordered central nervous system function resulting from failure of the liver to detoxify noxious agents of gut origin because of hepatocellular dysfunction and portosystemic shunting. The clinical spectrum ranges from day-night reversal and mild intellectual impairment to coma. Ammonia is the most readily identified and measurable toxin but is not solely responsible for the disturbed mental status. Bleeding into the intestinal tract may significantly increase the amount of protein in the bowel and precipitate encephalopathy. Hyponatremia can cause confusion, but this would not be specific to hepatic encephalopathy. *(Friedman, 2014, p. 669)*

46. (B) Acute pancreatitis typically presents with epigastric abdominal pain, generally abrupt in onset, is steady, boring, and severe. The pain usually radiates into the back but may radiate to the right or left. Nausea and vomiting are usually present. Weakness, sweating, and anxiety are noted in severe attacks. There may be a history of alcohol intake or a heavy meal immediately preceding the attack. Fever of 38.4–39°C, tachycardia, hypotension (even shock), pallor, and cool clammy skin are often present. Older age and obesity increase the risk of a severe course. Cholecystitis, diverticulitis, and appendicitis are located in different quadrants. Gastroenteritis typically presents without pain or hypovolemia. *(Bickley, Szilagy, Bates, pp. 472, 473; Friedman, 2014, p. 690)*

47. (D) Unconjugated hyperbilirubinemia (predominant indirect-reacting bilirubin). Increased bilirubin production, or impaired bilirubin uptake and storage (e.g., posthepatitis hyperbilirubinemia, Gilbert syndrome, Crigler–Najjar syndrome, drug reactions). Conjugated hyperbilirubinemia (predominant direct-reacting bilirubin). Faulty excretion of bilirubin conjugates (e.g., Dubin–Johnson syndrome, Rotor syndrome). Or, obstruction of the bile ducts (e.g., cholelithiasis, sclerosing cholangitis, and cancer of the bile ducts). *(Friedman, 2014, pp. 641, 642, 643)*

48. (D) A hernia may bulge through the femoral canal, which is medial to the femoral vein and inferior to the inguinal ligament. Direct and indirect inguinal hernias are typically palpated above the inguinal ligament. Obturator hernias are rare and typically occur in elderly women. *(Bickley, Szilagyi, pp. 521, 538)*

49. (A) Most thiamine deficiency in the United States is due to alcoholism. Patients with chronic alcoholism may have poor dietary intakes of thiamine and impaired thiamine absorption, metabolism, and storage. Thiamine deficiency is also associated with malabsorption, dialysis, and other causes of chronic protein–calorie undernutrition. Early manifestations of thiamine deficiency include anorexia, muscle cramps, paresthesias, and irritability. Advanced deficiency primarily affects the cardiovascular system. *(Baron, 2014, p. 1218)*

50. (B) Consensus definition of irritable bowel syndrome is abdominal discomfort or pain that has two of the following three features: (1) relieved with defecation, (2) onset associated with a change in frequency of stool, or (3) onset associated with a change in form (appearance) of stool. Other symptoms supporting the diagnosis include abnormal stool frequency; abnormal stool form (lumpy or hard; loose or watery); abnormal stool passage (straining, urgency, or feeling of incomplete evacuation); passage of mucus; and bloating or a feeling of abdominal distention. The patient should be asked about "alarm symptoms" that suggest a diagnosis other than irritable bowel syndrome and warrant further investigation. The acute onset of symptoms raises the likelihood of organic disease, especially in patients aged >40 to 50 years. Nocturnal diarrhea, severe constipation or diarrhea, hematochezia, weight loss, and fever are incompatible with a diagnosis of irritable bowel syndrome. *(McQuaid, 2014, pp. 612, 613)*

51. **(A)** Chronic cholecystitis results from repeated episodes of acute cholecystitis or chronic irritation of the gallbladder wall by stones and is characterized pathologically by varying degrees of chronic inflammation of the gallbladder. Calculi are usually present. In about 4% to 5% of cases, the villi of the gallbladder undergo polypoid enlargement due to deposition of cholesterol that may be visible to the naked eye ("strawberry gallbladder," cholesterolosis). Choledocholithiasis is stones in the bile duct. Cholangitis involves pain, fever, and jaundice. Sclerosing cholangitis is associated with colitis. Biliary dyskinesia involves spasm of the biliary tract. *(Friedman, 2014, p. 684)*

52. **(A)** Titers of IgG anti-HAV rise after 1 month of the disease and may persist for years. IgG anti-HAV (in the absence of IgM anti-HAV) indicates previous exposure to HAV, noninfectivity, and immunity. *(Friedman, 2014, p. 645)*

53. **(E)** Specific antibody to HBsAg (anti-HBs) appears in most individuals after clearance of HBsAg and after successful vaccination against hepatitis B. Disappearance of HBsAg and the appearance of anti-HBs signals recovery from HBV infection, noninfectivity, and immunity. *(Friedman, 2014, p. 647)*

54. **(B)** In patients with acute or chronic intestinal ischemia, a CTA or MRA can demonstrate narrowing of the proximal visceral vessels. In acute intestinal ischemia from a nonocclusive low flow state, angiography is needed to display the typical "pruned tree" appearance of the distal visceral vascular bed. *(Rapp, Owens, Johnson, p. 454)*

55. **(D)** Symptoms depend on the location of the carcinoma. Chronic blood loss from right-sided colonic cancers may cause iron deficiency anemia, manifested by fatigue and weakness. Obstruction, however, is uncommon because of the large diameter of the right colon and the liquid consistency of the fecal material. Lesions of the left colon often involve the bowel circumferentially. Because the left colon has a smaller diameter and the fecal matter is solid, obstructive symptoms may develop with colicky abdominal pain and a change in bowel habits. *(Cornett & Dea, 2014, p. 1569)*

56. **(C)** Birth cohort screening of persons born between 1945 and 1965 ("baby boomers") for HCV infection has been recommended by the CDC. *(Friedman, 2014, p. 650)*

57. **(B)** In chronic inflammatory disease patients report malaise, weight loss, and loss of energy. In patients with ileitis or ileocolitis, there may be diarrhea, which is usually nonbloody and often intermittent. In patients with colitis involving the rectum or left colon, there may be bloody diarrhea and fecal urgency, which may mimic the symptoms of ulcerative colitis. Cramping or steady right lower quadrant or periumbilical pain is common. Physical examination reveals focal tenderness, usually in the right lower quadrant. *(McQuaid, 2014, p. 621)*

58. **(D)** Cholera is an acute diarrheal illness caused by certain serotypes of *V. cholerae* producing hypersecretion of water and chloride ion and a massive diarrhea of up to 15 L/day. Cholera occurs in epidemics under conditions of crowding, war, and famine (e.g., in refugee camps) and where sanitation is inadequate. The liquid stool is gray; turbid; and without fecal odor, blood, or pus ("rice water stool"). Enteroinvasive *E. coli* invade cells, causing bloody diarrhea. *Shigella* dysentery is a common disease with diarrheal stool often mixed with blood and mucus. *S. typhi* symptoms consist of fever (often with chills), nausea and vomiting, cramping abdominal pain, and diarrhea, which may be grossly bloody. *Entamoeba* causes diarrhea, but not as much, and frequently has abdominal pain. *(Schwartz, 2014, pp. 1398–1400)*

59. **(A)** In cirrhosis, abdominal pain may be present and is related either to hepatic enlargement and stretching

of Glisson capsule or to the presence of ascites. Skin manifestations consist of spider angiomas. Jaundice is a late finding. The superficial veins of the abdomen and thorax are dilated, and gynecomastia in men may occur. The other choices typically do not have signs of chronic liver disease. *(Friedman, 2014, p. 665)*

60. **(A)** Wilson disease (hepatolenticular degeneration) is a rare autosomal recessive disorder that usually occurs in persons under age 40. The major physiologic aberration in Wilson disease is excessive absorption of copper from the small intestine and decreased excretion of copper by the liver, resulting in increased tissue deposition, especially in the liver, brain, cornea, and kidney. The diagnosis can be challenging, even with the use of scoring systems, and is generally based on demonstration of increased urinary copper excretion or low serum ceruloplasmin levels. *(Friedman, 2014, pp. 675, 676)*

61. **(B)** Celiac disease (also called sprue, celiac sprue, and gluten enteropathy) is a permanent dietary disorder caused by an immunologic response to gluten, a storage protein found in certain grains, resulting in diffuse damage to the proximal small intestinal mucosa with malabsorption of nutrients. Endoscopic mucosal biopsy of the proximal duodenum (bulb) and distal duodenum is the standard method for confirmation of the diagnosis in patients with a positive serologic test for celiac disease. *(McQuaid, 2014, pp. 601–603)*

62. **(E)** Cigarette smoking is strongly associated with the development of Crohn disease, resistance to medical therapy, and early disease relapse. *(McQuaid, 2014, p. 621)*

63. **(D)** Colonoscopy has also been advocated as a screening examination. It is more accurate than flexible sigmoidoscopy for detecting cancer and polyps. Screening is recommended for all men and women aged 50 through 75 years of age who are at average risk for cancer. Some guidelines recommend screening for African Americans beginning at age 45. *(Cornett & Dea, 2014, pp. 1571,1572; Fletcher, UpToDate)*

64. **(C)** Frequently, aggressive antibiotic therapy, combined with cholecystectomy is required to eradicate

a carrier state of salmonellosis. *(Hohmann, UpToDate; Schwartz, 2014, p. 1399)*

65. **(A)** For the treatment of hepatic encephalopathy, initiate measures to lower blood ammonia concentrations with medications such as lactulose. Lactulose should be administered in a dosage of 30 mL orally every 1 to 2 hours until evacuation occurs then reduced to 15 to 45 mL/h every 8 to 12 hours as needed to promote two or three bowel movements daily. *(Ferenci, UpToDate; McQuaid, 2014, p. 584)*

66. **(A)** Serologic tests should be performed in all patients in whom there is a suspicion of celiac disease. The two tests with the highest diagnostic accuracy are the IgA endomysial antibody and IgA tissue transglutaminase antibody tests, both of which have a ≥90% sensitivity and ≥95% specificity for the diagnosis of celiac disease. *(McQuaid, 2014, p. 603)*

67. **(C)** HDV is a defective RNA virus that causes hepatitis only in association with HBV infection and specifically only in the presence of HBsAg; it is cleared when the latter is cleared. *(Friedman, 2014, p. 651)*

68. **(A)** Hepatitis A is transmitted by the fecal–oral route, and its spread is favored by crowding and poor sanitation. Common source outbreaks may still result from contaminated water or food, including inadequately cooked shellfish. The mortality rate for hepatitis A is low, and fulminant hepatitis A is uncommon except for rare instances in which it occurs in a patient with concomitant chronic hepatitis C. There is no chronic carrier state. *(Friedman, 2014, pp. 644, 645)*

69. **(B)** Central to the mechanism of fat absorption is the problem of solubilizing lipids in an aqueous environment. Emulsification begins in the upper gastrointestinal tract through mastication and gastric mixing. Fat droplets released by these mechanical means are coated with phospholipids to form a stable emulsion. Additional phospholipid from bile is added once the emulsion reaches the duodenum. Bile salts further enhance fat solubilization, producing an emulsion of microscopic micelles. *(Mason, UpToDate)*

70. **(A)** Based upon retrospective studies and expert opinion, patients with acute uncomplicated diverticulitis are generally treated with antibiotics for 10 to 14 days, depending upon resolution of symptoms. The choice of antibiotics should be based upon the usual bacteria, which are principally Gram-negative rods and anaerobes (particularly *E. coli* and *B. fragilis*). Reasonable choices include a quinolone with metronidazole, amoxicillin–clavulanate, or trimethoprim–sulfamethoxazole with metronidazole. *(McQuaid, 2014, p. 631; Young-Fadok, Pemberton, UpToDate)*

REFERENCES

Baron RB. Nutritional Disorders. In: Papadakis MA, McPhee SJ, Rabow MW, eds. *Current Medical Diagnosis & Treatment*. 53rd ed. New York, NY: McGraw-Hill; 2014.

Bickley LS, Szilagyi PG, Bates B. *Bates' Guide to Physical Examination and History Taking*. 10th ed. Philadelphia, PA: Wolters Kluwer Health/Lippincott Williams & Wilkins; 2009.

Cornett PA, Dea TO. Cancer. In: Papadakis MA, McPhee SJ, Rabow MW, eds. *Current Medical Diagnosis & Treatment 2014*. New York, NY: McGraw-Hill; 2014.

Fasanella KE, Sanders MK. Therapeutic endoscopic ultrasound. In: UpToDate, Howell DA, Travis AC, eds. UpToDate, Waltham, MA. Accessed on July 28, 2014.

Ferenci P. Hepatic encephalopathy in adults: Treatment. In: UpToDate, Runyon BA, Travis AC, eds, UpToDate, Waltham, MA. Accessed on July 28, 2014.

Fitzgerald PA. Endocrine disorders. In: Papadakis MA, McPhee SJ, Rabow MW, eds. *Current Medical Diagnosis & Treatment 2014*. New York, NY: McGraw-Hill; 2014.

Fletcher RH. Screening for colorectal cancer: Strategies in patients at average risk. In: UpToDate, Lamont JT, Sokol HN, eds. UpToDate, Waltham, MA. Accessed on July 24, 2014.

Friedman LS. Liver, Biliary Tract, and Pancreas Disorders. In: Papadakis MA, McPhee SJ, Rabow MW, eds. *Current Medical Diagnosis & Treatment*. 53rd ed. New York, NY: McGraw-Hill; 2014.

Goldberg E, Chopra S. Acute liver failure in adults: Etiology, clinical manifestations, and diagnosis. In: UpToDate, Brown RS, Travis AC, eds. UpToDate, Waltham, MA. Accessed on July 14, 2014.

Guelrud M, Mallory-Weiss syndrome. In: UpToDate, Feldman M, Travis AC, eds. UpToDate, Waltham, MA. Accessed on July 14, 2014.

Hohmann EL. Treatment and prevention of typhoid fever. In: UpToDate, Calderwood SB, Bloom A, eds. UpToDate, Waltham MA. Accessed on July 27, 2014.

Hull C. Dermatitis herpetiformis. In: UpToDate, Zone JJ, Ofori AO, eds. UpToDate, Waltham MA. Accessed on July 21, 2014.

Hutton E. Evaluation and management of hypercalcemia. *JAAPA*. 2005;18(6):30–35.

Kelly CP, Lamont JT. Clostridium difficile in adults: Treatment. In: UpToDate, Calderwood SB, Baron EL, eds. UpToDate, Waltham MA. Accessed on July 21, 2014.

Kelly RK, McQuaid KR. Esophageal cancer. In: Papadakis MA, McPhee SJ, Rabow MW, eds. *Current Medical Diagnosis & Treatment 2014*. New York, NY: McGraw-Hill; 2014.

Kendall JL, Moreira M. Evaluation of the adult with abdominal pain in the emergency department. In: UpToDate, Hockberger RS, Grayzel J, eds. UpToDate, Waltham, MA. Accessed on July 21, 2014.

Kitagawa S, Migdady M. Intussusception in children. In: UpToDate, Ferry GD, Singer JI, Hoppin AG, eds. UpToDate, Waltham, MA. Accessed on July 21, 2014.

LeBlond RF, DeGowin RL, Brown DD. *DeGowin's Diagnostic Examination*. New York, NY: McGraw-Hill; 2009.

Mason JB. Mechanisms of nutrient absorption and malabsorption. In: UpToDate, Lipman TO, Grover S, eds. UpToDate, Waltham, MA. Accessed on July 28, 2014.

McQuaid KR. Gastrointestinal disorders. In: Papadakis MA, McPhee SJ, Rabow MW, eds. *Current Medical Diagnosis & Treatment*. 53rd ed. New York, NY: McGraw-Hill; 2014.

Olivé AP, Endom EE. Infantile hypertrophic pyloric stenosis. In: UpToDate, Klish WJ, Singer JI, Hoppin AG, eds. UpToDate, Waltham, MA. Accessed on July 23, 2014.

Rao SC. Constipation in the older adult. In: UpToDate, Tally NJ, Schmader KE, Grover S, eds. UpToDate, Waltham, MA. Accessed on July 21, 2014.

Rapp JH, Owens CD, Johnson MD. Blood vessel & lymphatic disorders. In: Papadakis MA, McPhee SJ, Rabow MW, eds. *Current Medical Diagnosis & Treatment 2014*. New York, NY: McGraw-Hill; 2014.

Rogers VL, Worley KC. Obstetrics & obstetric disorders. In: Papadakis MA, McPhee SJ, Rabow MW, eds. *Current Medical Diagnosis & Treatment 2014*. New York, NY: McGraw-Hill; 2014.

Rosenthal PJ. Protozoal & helminthic infections. In: Papadakis MA, McPhee SJ, Rabow MW, eds. *Current Medical Diagnosis & Treatment 2014*. New York, NY: McGraw-Hill; 2014.

Sanjiv C, Sanjeev A. Patient evaluation and selection for antiviral therapy for chronic hepatitis C virus infection. In: UpToDate, Di Bisceglie A, ed. UpToDate, Waltham, MA. Accessed on July 8, 2014.

Sassan P, Clifford WL, David B. Overview of water-soluble vitamins. In: UpToDate, Timothy L, Alison H, eds. UpToDate, Waltham, MA. Accessed on July 21, 2014.

Schwartz BS. Bacterial & Chlamydial Infections. In: Papadakis MA, McPhee SJ, Rabow MW, eds. *Current Medical Diagnosis & Treatment 2014*. New York, NY: McGraw-Hill; 2014.

Soll AH, Vakil NB. Overview of the complications of peptic ulcer disease. In: UpToDate, Feldman M, Soybel DI, Grover S, eds. UpToDate, Waltham, MA. Accessed on July 22, 2014.

Soundgeimer JM. Gastrointestinal tract. In: Hay WW, Levin MJ, Sondheimer JM, eds. *Current Diagnosis and Treatment: Gastroenterology, Hepatology, & Endoscopy*. New York, NY: McGraw-Hill; 2009.

Young-Fadok T, Pemberton JH. Nonoperative management of acute uncomplicated diverticulitis. In: UpToDate, Weiser M, Duda RB, eds. UpToDate, Waltham, MA. Accessed on July 28, 2014.

Zolopa AR, Katz MH. HIV Infection & AIDS. In: Papadakis MA, McPhee SJ, Rabow MW, eds. *Current Medical Diagnosis & Treatment 2014*. New York, NY: McGraw-Hill; 2014.

CHAPTER 6

Hematology/Oncology

Scott Lightfoot, PA-C, MPAS

DIRECTIONS: Each of the numbered questions or incomplete statements is followed by possible answers or completions of the statement. Select the ONE-lettered answer or completion that is BEST in each case.

1. Which of the following is the most common cause of hypersegmented neutrophils on the peripheral smear?

    (A) Vitamin B-12 deficiency
    (B) Iron-deficiency anemia
    (C) Chronic myeloid leukemia
    (D) Essential thrombocytosis
    (E) History of splenectomy

2. Which of the following is the most common cause of hypercalcemia in malignancy?

    (A) Chronic renal failure leading to secondary hyperparathyroidism
    (B) Increase in calcium absorption in the renal tubules
    (C) Increased production of parathyroid hormone-related peptide
    (D) Osteoblastic lesions from bone metastasis
    (E) Granulomatous reaction to the tumor causing increased 1,25-dihydroxy vitamin D

3. A 33-year-old female presents to the emergency room with complaints of left lower extremity swelling and calf tenderness. She denies any chest pain, hemoptysis, or shortness of breath. Her past medical history is positive for three spontaneous miscarriages, all in the first trimester. On examination, her leg lower extremity is swollen and tender in the back of the calf. She denies any recent surgeries, trauma, history of prior clots, or a family history of clots. She also has a lacy erythematous rash on her upper and lower extremities, bilaterally. Which of the following is the most likely cause for her presumed diagnosis?

    (A) Livedo reticularis
    (B) Elevated factor VIII levels
    (C) Antiphospholipid antibody syndrome
    (D) Antithrombin III deficiency
    (E) Elevated protein S levels

4. A 74-year-old male comes in for a routine physical examination. He has a past medical history of hypertension, diabetes mellitus type II, and a prior history of immune thrombocytopenia purpura. His labs show an elevated white blood cell count at 28,000, a hemoglobin of 14 g/dL, a hematocrit of 45%, and a platelet count of 170,000. His peripheral smear reveals a neutrophil count of 5,000, a lymphocyte count of 22,000, and an eosinophil count of 500. He also has a basophil count of 300, and a monocyte count of 100. Which of the following is the most likely diagnosis?

    (A) Chronic myeloid leukemia
    (B) Acute lymphoblastic leukemia
    (C) A leukemoid reaction
    (D) Chronic lymphocytic leukemia
    (E) Acute myelogenous leukemia

5. Which of the following is pathognomonic for hemophilia A?

    (A) Elevated factor IX levels
    (B) Bleeding gingivae
    (C) Immediate bleeding after surgery
    (D) Petechiae on examination
    (E) Spontaneous hemarthroses

6. Which of the following is the most serious delayed toxicity that is seen with the anthracycline drug class?

(A) Cardiomyopathy
(B) Myelosuppression
(C) Pulmonary toxicity
(D) Neutropenic fever
(E) Neuropathy

7. A 68-year-old male presents for routine physical examination. He has a past medical history of hypertension which is under control with diuretics, hyperlipidemia that is diet controlled, and a 45 pack-year history of smoking. His physical examination is positive for an increase in his anterior-posterior diameter, diminished breath sounds, clubbing of his fingers, splenomegaly, and facial swelling. Physical examination did not reveal ecchymoses, hepatomegaly, ascites, lower extremity swelling, lymphadenopathy, or telangiectasias. Labs are drawn and reveal a white blood count of 13,000, a hemoglobin of 20 g/dL, a hematocrit of 59%, and a platelet count of 460,000. Which factor is the most consistent with a history of primary polycythemia?

(A) His smoking history
(B) His lack of ecchymoses
(C) His splenomegaly
(D) His history of diuretic use
(E) His lack of hepatomegaly on examination

8. A 12-year-old female presents to the office for complaints of bleeding gums and epistaxis. On examination you notice petechiae on her lower extremities. The rest of the examination is unremarkable for lymphadenopathy or hepatosplenomegaly. She admits to recovering from an upper respiratory infection 1 week prior. Her complete blood count reveals a white blood count of 8,000, a hemoglobin of 12.5, a hematocrit of 38%, and a platelet count of 12,000. Which of the following is the most appropriate therapy?

(A) Rituximab
(B) Prednisone
(C) Splenectomy
(D) Eltrombopag
(E) Platelet transfusion

9. Vitamin B-12 deficiency:

(A) Is most commonly caused by Crohn's disease
(B) Can be easily separated from folic acid deficiency by the presence of hypersegmented neutrophils
(C) If left untreated can cause irreversible neuropathy
(D) Is commonly seen in patients who have had their rectosigmoid colon removed
(E) Often seen with myeloproliferative disorders

10. A 64-year-old African-American male with a long-standing history of benign prostatic hypertrophy, comes to the office complaining of urinary dysuria and urinary frequency. Urine analysis confirms a urinary tract infection. He is given a 3-day course of antibiotics, 7 days later he presents with acute fatigue, dizziness, and exertional dyspnea. His labs reveal a hemoglobin of 8.5 g/dL, a hematocrit of 26%, and a mean corpuscle volume of 104 fenoliters. Given the presumed diagnosis, which of the following is most likely to be found?

(A) A low glucose-6-phosphate level on an acute serum draw
(B) A reticulocyte count of 2.5%
(C) The presence of Heinz bodies
(D) An elevated haptoglobin
(E) A reactive thrombocytosis

11. A 46-year-old male farmer presents to the office with complaints of fatigue, dizziness, fevers, and easy bruising for 1 week's duration. He denies any bone pain. He has no significant past medical history. On examination he is febrile with a temperature of 102°F, tachycardic, pale, and has petechiae. His complete blood count reveals a white blood cell count of 1,500, a hemoglobin of 7.2 g/dL, a hematocrit of 20%, and a platelet count of 16,000. The differential reveals a neutrophil count of 800, a lymphocyte count of 500, an eosinophil count of 200, a monocyte count of 100, and no basophils. A bone marrow biopsy is performed and reveals a hypoplastic marrow and no blasts. Which of the following is the most likely diagnosis?

(A) Aplastic anemia
(B) Acute myeloid leukemia
(C) Early evolving myelodysplastic syndrome
(D) Acute lymphoblastic leukemia
(E) Benzene toxicity

12. von Willebrand disease type I:

   (A) Is an autosomal recessive bleeding disorder

   (B) Has a predilection to affect males

   (C) Causes a prolonged prothrombin time/ international ratio (PT/INR)

   (D) Can be treated with vasopressin (DDAVP) for bleeding

   (E) Is often followed by measuring factor VII levels

13. A 75-year-old female is admitted to the hospital for chest pain. Her past medical history is positive for hypertension, diabetes mellitus type II, and smoking. Upon workup she is found to have bilateral pulmonary emboli with no upper or lower extremity deep venous thromboses. She is started on anticoagulation. After 5 days of treatment with coumadin and heparin, her platelet count starts to drop below 50,000 and she began developing thromboses at her intravenous sites. Which of the following is the most likely diagnosis?

   (A) Thrombotic thrombocytopenia purpura

   (B) Disseminated intravascular coagulation

   (C) Hemolytic uremic syndrome

   (D) ADAMTS13 deficiency

   (E) Heparin-induced thrombocytopenia

14. Hodgkin's lymphoma:

   (A) Has a bimodal age distribution

   (B) Is separated from non-Hodgkin's lymphoma by the absence of Reed–Sternberg cells

   (C) Commonly presents with persistent painful lymphadenopathy

   (D) Different histologies are not related to socioeconomic status

   (E) There is an increased risk after exposure to cytomegalovirus (CMV)

15. Lovenox:

   (A) Is best dosed 1.0 mg/kg once a day for acute deep venous thrombosis

   (B) Can be used safely in pregnancy

   (C) Does not cause heparin-induced thrombocytopenia purpura

   (D) Is not recommended as a form of anticoagulation in cancer patients with blood clots

   (E) Is best measured by following the partial thromboplastin time (PTT)

16. Myelodysplastic syndrome:

   (A) Is caused by an abnormal population of dysplastic plasma cells

   (B) Typically presents with microcytic anemia

   (C) Can progress into acute leukemia in select patients

   (D) Can be diagnosed by looking at the peripheral smear

   (E) Commonly presents in the fifth decade of life

17. A 23-year-old female with a recent history of systemic lupus for which she takes steroids, presents to the emergency room, with a complaint of shortness of breath and dizziness. When evaluated in the emergency room she is found to be pale and tachycardic. The following were obtained:

WBC: 9,500

Red blood cell count (RBC): 3.5

Hemoglobin: 7.1 g/dL

Hematocrit: 23%

Platelet count: 530,000

Mean corpuscle volume (MCV): 70 fenoliters

Red cell distribution width (RDW): 18

Retic count: 2.5%

Lactase dehydrogenase (LDH): 230

Haptoglobin: 80

Which of the following is the most useful in determining the underlying cause of her anemia?

   (A) Hemoglobin electrophoresis

   (B) Coombs; direct and indirect

   (C) Folic acid level

   (D) Bone marrow biopsy

   (E) Iron studies

18. Which of the following is true regarding blood products?

(A) Packed red cell transfusions (PRBCs) can cause temporary hypokalemia

(B) The risk of iron overload after PRBCs is increased after 15 lifetime transfusions

(C) Plasma and apheresis platelet products carry the highest risk of transfusion-related acute lung injury (TRALI) among all blood products

(D) One unit of PRBCs is expected to raise the hemoglobin 2 to 3 g

(E) Guidelines for PRBC transfusion for GI bleeds are designed to transfuse the hemoglobin when it drops below 9 g/dL

19. Which of the following findings on the peripheral smear match the disease?

(A) Target cell: Chronic myeloid leukemia

(B) Howell–Jolly bodies: Hereditary spherocytosis

(C) Heinz bodies: Thrombotic thrombocytopenia purpura

(D) Rouleaux formation: Chronic lymphocytic leukemia

(E) Poikilocytosis: Extreme iron deficiency

20. A 45-year-old female with a long-standing history of rheumatoid arthritis has been complaining of some early satiety over the last few months but denies any other symptoms. Her examination is benign except some fullness in the left upper quadrant. An ultrasound confirms no hepatomegaly, but reveals splenomegaly. What additional findings would confirm a diagnosis of Felty's syndrome?

(A) A complete blood count with a differential

(B) A sedimentation rate

(C) Flow cytometry

(D) Large granular lymphocytes in the bone marrow

(E) Anti–double-stranded DNA antibodies titers

21. A 34-year-old female is scheduled for elective cosmetic surgery. Upon her pre-op workup she is found to have a prolonged partial thromboplastin time on two separate draws; her prothrombin time is normal. A mixing study of her blood to normal serum is performed. Which of the following would cause a persistently prolonged partial thromboplastin time after a 1:1 mixing study?

(A) A circulating lupus anticoagulant

(B) Disseminated intravascular coagulation (DIC)

(C) Antithrombin III deficiency

(D) Factor VIII deficiency

(E) Dysfibrinogenemia

22. A 71-year-old African-American male presents to the emergency room. He has a past medical history of hypertension well controlled with medication, a remote history of prostate cancer treated 4 years ago by external beam radiation, a 50 pack-year history of smoking, and coronary artery disease status post coronary stent placement presents to the clinic with increasing lower back pain. He states that his pain does not get better with rest. An x-ray of his lumbar spine is taken and reveals lytic lesions throughout the lumbar spine. Blood work reveals macrocytic anemia, an elevated calcium, an elevated total serum protein level, and an increase in his globulin protein level. Urine analysis reveals Bence Jones proteins. Which of the following is the next best step to confirm the suspected diagnosis?

(A) A biopsy of the lytic lesions in the spine

(B) Serum protein electrophoresis

(C) A prostate specific antigen (PSA)

(D) Total body bone scan

(E) Bone marrow aspiration and biopsy

23. A 45-year-old male patient presents to the emergency room with complaints of bleeding gums and epistaxis. His blood work is drawn and reveals isolated thrombocytopenia with a platelet count of 18,000. The rest of the complete blood count is normal. Which of the following would be suggestive of a diagnosis of immune thrombocytopenia purpura?

(A) Absence of splenomegaly on examination

(B) Evidence of purpura on examination

(C) A prolonged prothrombin time

(D) A drastic increase in the platelet count after a platelet transfusion

(E) Evidence of schistocytes on the peripheral smear

24. Which of the following is the best choice in patients on chemotherapy to help minimize the risk of neutropenia?

   (A) Acetaminophen
   (B) Augmentin
   (C) Rituxan
   (D) Ciprofloxacin
   (E) Pegfilgrastim

25. A 32-year-old African-American asymptomatic woman presents to her gynecologist's office for a physical examination. She has no medical history. She mentions that she has recently become engaged and that she is aware that her fiancée's family has suffered from sickle cell disease, although he is "healthy." They are planning a honeymoon to the mountains. Which of the following issues would be MOST appropriate to discuss?

   (A) The risk of infertility for her husband, if he carries the sickle cell gene.
   (B) Reassure her of the low risk of illness for her children, given her and her future husband's lack of apparent sickle cell disease.
   (C) Offer to refer her for genetic counseling.
   (D) Advise against travel to high-altitude regions for her husband.
   (E) Counseling regarding the increased risk of sexually transmitted infections for those with sickle cell trait.

26. Which of the following is true of iron-deficiency anemia?

   (A) It is most commonly due to acute blood loss.
   (B) It does not frequently occur from the typical American diet.
   (C) The primary cause during pregnancy is increased red blood cells destruction.
   (D) Confirmation by bone marrow aspiration is required.
   (E) Treatment with long-term iron replacement is typically greater than 1 year.

27. Which of the following are consistent with lead poisoning?

   (A) Profound anemia
   (B) Complaints of severe fatigue and persistent muscle wasting

   (C) Acute difficulty concentrating after exposure
   (D) Basophilic stippling
   (E) Treatment with chelating agent is always required

28. A 48-year-old previously healthy, African-American man presents to his local emergency center with dyspnea on exertion while mowing the grass. He has no significant medical history. Laboratory studies reveal a white blood cell count of 6.1, a hemoglobin of 9.7, a hematocrit of 29, a mean corpuscle volume (MCV) of 78, and a platelet count of 254,000. What diagnosis is most likely causing his symptoms?

   (A) Sickle cell anemia
   (B) Thalassemia
   (C) Iron deficiency
   (D) Hemolytic anemia
   (E) TTP

29. When using tamoxifen in the treatment of malignancy, one must keep which of the following toxicities in mind?

   (A) Impotence
   (B) Peripheral neuropathy
   (C) Secondary malignancy
   (D) Pulmonary fibrosis
   (E) Osteoporosis

30. Which tumor marker may be used in the screening of patients for cancer?

   (A) Prostatic acid phosphate
   (B) Carcinoembryonic antigen
   (C) Cancer antigen 19-9
   (D) Alpha-fetoprotein
   (E) Cancer antigen 125

31. Thalassemia

   (A) is a rare cause of normocytic, normochronic anemia.
   (B) is most common in those of European descent.
   (C) may result in few problems, except during stress states.
   (D) may be diagnosed by peripheral smear.
   (E) may be an acquired or hereditary disease.

32. Common complications of external beam irradiation may include:

(A) Myelosuppresion

(B) Cancer growth

(C) Fatigue

(D) Worsening bone pain during treatment for bone metastasis

(E) Generalized hair loss

33. Choose the correct statement regarding the condition known as Christmas disease.

(A) It is a deficiency of factor XI.

(B) It is similar to factor VIII deficiency and may be treated with factor VIII concentrates.

(C) It may result in both easy bleeding and clotting.

(D) The another name for this disease is hemophilia A.

(E) It is an X-linked recessive disease, affecting primarily men.

34. A 44-year-old woman presents to the emergency department after receiving a puncture wound to the foot by a rusty nail, while working in the yard. On examination, she is found to have splenomegaly. Which of the following signs or symptoms may be helpful in identifying the underlying cause of her splenomegaly?

(A) Petechiae

(B) Spider angiomas

(C) LUQ (lower upper quadrant) fullness

(D) Reflux

(E) Early satiety

35. In which situation should you most likely consider referring a patient for genetic counseling?

(A) Personal history of breast cancer at age 52

(B) Family history of a mother with primary brain tumor at age 3

(C) Family history of maternal grandmother with breast cancer at age 62, maternal grandfather with prostate cancer diagnosed at age 78, and paternal grandfather with lung cancer diagnosed at age 64

(D) Family history of a sister with colon cancer at age 29

(E) Personal history of several skin cancers and three prior colonic polyps, now with colon cancer at age 58

36. When encountering a patient with petechiae noted on physical examination,

(A) a platelet count of 204,000 suggests evolving thrombocytopenia as the cause.

(B) a platelet count of 204,000 in a patient on clopidogrel (plavix) suggests this agent is not therapeutic in its antiplatelet effect.

(C) with a platelet count of 45,000, a bleeding time should be performed.

(D) hepatic dysfunction should be in the differential diagnosis.

(E) suspected overdose of coumadin should be considered in those on that agent.

37. A 52-year-old man presents complaining of early satiety and mild fatigue for the last 5 months. He has no other complaints and no significant medical history, other than a tonsillectomy at age 6 and well-controlled hypertension. On examination, there is no lymphadenopathy or hepatomegaly, but his spleen is palpable. A blood smear shows a hemoglobin of 13.9, a hematocrit of 42.0, a platelet count of 580,000, and a white blood cell count of 85,000 with some immature cells but only 1% blasts. A bone marrow performed the next day shows a hypercellular sample with essentially a normal differential, and again, only 1% blasts. Chromosome analysis shows presence of the Philadelphia chromosome (t(9;22)). What is the most likely diagnosis?

(A) Acute lymphocytic leukemia

(B) Acute myelogenous leukemia

(C) Chronic myelogenous leukemia

(D) Chronic lymphocytic leukemia

(E) Burkitt lymphoma

38. A 33-year-old woman presents complaining of profound fatigue for the past 6 weeks, necessitating her quitting her job. She looks pale and is tachycardic at 110 bpm, but otherwise her examination is normal. A blood smear shows a hemoglobin of 4.5, a hematocrit of 13.4, a platelet count of 19,000, and a white blood cell count of 3.1 with 21% blasts that have Auer rods. The most likely diagnosis is:

(A) Hodgkin's disease

(B) Non-Hodgkin's lymphoma

(C) Chronic myelogenous leukemia

(D) Acute myelogenous leukemia

(E) Hemolytic anemia

39. Which of the following is true regarding vitamin K deficiencies?

(A) It may result in abnormal platelet function.

(B) In the United States, it is most commonly due to inadequate intake.

(C) It should be suspected in patients with prolongation of the prothrombin time/INR.

(D) Treatment with fresh-frozen plasma is typically required.

(E) It occurs in primary biliary cirrhosis.

40. Decreased platelet production may be observed in which of the following conditions?

(A) Hypersplenism

(B) DIC

(C) Henoch–Schönlein disease

(D) Aplastic anemia

(E) Alcoholism

Answers and Explanations

1. **(A)** Of all of the following only vitamin B-12 deficiency and folic acid deficiency lead to hypersegmented neutrophils. Differentiating between the two can made on a clinical basis as well as laboratory studies. Neutrophils normally contain 3 to 4 lobes. However, in both vitamin B-12 deficiency and folic acid deficiency, the neutrophils can contain up to 5 to 6 lobes. By definition, greater than 5% of the neutrophils have to contain up to 5 or more lobes and at least one neutrophil with 6 lobes or more to be labeled as hypersegmentation. In some instances, hypersegmented neutrophils may be the only manifestation of vitamin B-12 deficiency. Hypersegmentation is a result of altered granulocyte production from impaired DNA synthesis. There have been rare reports of iron deficiency causing some hypersegmentation but it is not common. Hypersegmented neutrophils are not found in patients who had a history of a splenectomy, in patients with chronic myeloid leukemia (CML), or in patients with essential thrombocytosis. Moreover, it is common to see an elevated vitamin B-12 levels from over production of intrinsic factor in myeloproliferative neoplasms like CML. *(Hoffbrand, 2013b, pp. 94–103; Schrier, 2014)*

2. **(C)** Parathyroid hormone-related peptide or parathyroid hormone-reactive protein (PTHrP) is now recognized as the most common cause of hypercalcemia in malignancy. Hypercalcemia is encountered in approximately 20% to 30% of cancer patients (solid tumors and hematology malignancies). The most common cancers associated with hypercalcemia include lung cancer, breast cancer, and myeloma. PTHrP production accounts for up to 80% of the causes of hypercalcemia, followed by osteolytic metastasis (not osteoblastic) in up to approximately 20% of the causes; with the rest due to tumor production of 1,25 dihydroxy vitamin D. PTHrP has almost complete homology to PTH, especially the first 13 amino acids on the amino-terminal end. As a result PTHrP binds to PTH-1 receptors to drive similar pathways that are driven by PTH including osteoclast activation, renal phosphate wasting, and bone resorption. While it was recently thought PTHrP also led to an increase in renal calcium absorption, this has been found not to be the case. Hypercalcemia can be seen in chronic renal failure, however, this is not the most common cause of hypercalcemia in malignancy. *(Horwitz, 2014)*

3. **(C)** Antiphospholipid antibody syndrome, commonly abbreviated APS, is a syndrome characterized by arterial or venous thromboses with laboratory evidence of the antiphospholipid antibodies. It includes laboratory evidence as well as clinical evidence. Pregnancy morbidity is defined as: fetal loss at >10 weeks with a morphologically normal fetus; or one or more premature deliveries before 34 weeks of gestation due to eclampsia, preeclampsia, or placental insufficiency; or three or more unexplained losses at <10 weeks. This condition can be found alone or in conjunction with systemic disease such as systemic lupus erythematous. A prolonged aPTT or a slightly low platelet count in the setting of a thrombus should raise suspicion of APS. A careful history should be taken to account previous thromboses and prior fetal loss as well as systemic symptoms that could suggest underlying lupus. Testing for anticardiolipin antibodies, the lupus anticoagulant, and anti–beta-2 glycoproteins should be ordered in this setting. It is recommended to repeat these tests approximately 12 weeks apart to ensure the true presence of APS as these tests can be elevated transiently. These patients tend to be very hypercoagulable and are best treated with a

more aggressive anticoagulation regimen with a target INR between 2.5 and 3.5 on coumadin. The presence of livedo reticularis can suggest a very aggressive subtype of APS called Sneddon's syndrome which places the patient at high risk for a stroke. While antithrombin III deficiency can cause clots this history is less suggestive of that entity. Low protein S levels are associated with a hypercoagulable state whereas elevated levels are clinically irrelevant. Elevated factor VII levels also have no significance in this case. *(Bermis et al., 2014)*

4. **(D)** This history is a classic presentation of chronic lymphocytic leukemia (CLL). CLL is a B-cell lymphoproliferative disorder with an average age at diagnosis in the early seventh decade. Most cases are found incidentally on routine blood work showing a leukocytosis and lymphocytosis. Due to abnormal qualitative and potentially quantitative humoral- and cellular-mediated immune system, these patients are commonly at risk for infections and benefit from prophylactic vaccinations. Approximately one-third of patients with CLL can develop autoimmune hemolytic anemia (AIHA) and up to 5% can develop idiopathic thrombocytopenia purpura (with some cases of AIHA or ITP preceding the diagnosis of CLL), as did this patient. Chronic myeloid leukemia causes an increase in the myeloid cell line along with the presence of the Philadelphia chromosome. A leukemoid reaction by definition is the presence of a WBC >50,000 with predominantly neutrophil precursors not the lymphocytic cell line. There are no findings in this case to suggest either acute myelogenous leukemia or acute lymphoblastic leukemia due to the absence of blasts. *(Longo, 2013b)*

5. **(E)** Spontaneous hemarthroses are pathognomonic for both hemophilia A and B. The hemophilias are a group of bleeding disorders that involve defects of the secondary hemostatic pathway. These are most commonly inherited although some cases can be acquired secondary to random mutations. This is due to the fact that the gene that encodes factor VIII (the factor deficient in hemophilia A) is over 186,000 bases long making it susceptible to random mutations. Hemophilia A affects approximately 1 out of 5,000 to 10,000 males and is X-linked affecting males; females are the carriers. Hemophilia A is classified as mild, moderate, or severe depending on factor VIII levels (>5%, 1–5%, and <1%),

respectively. The sites of bleeding involve more of the muscles and joints and tend to be delayed and often times spontaneous. Primary hemostatic disorders such as von Willebrand's disease tend to present with more acute bleeding and involve superficial sites. Petechiae and bleeding gingivae are found on examination with thrombocytopenia. Elevated factor IX levels have no clinical significance. *(Hoots & Shapiro, 2014)*

6. **(A)** The anthracycline drug class is very active in lymphomas, breast cancer, ovarian cancer, leukemias, sarcomas, as well as other solid tumors. Some of the more common agents that are used include doxorubicin, idarubicin, and daunorubicin. While myelosuppression is an acute toxicity with a nadir of approximately 7 days, cardiotoxicity can be acute or chronic. Acute toxicity can cause arrhythmias, heart block, ventricular dysfunction, and pericarditis–myocarditis syndrome. Cardiomyopathy is the main chronic toxicity that can occur as soon as 3 months after exposure to years after. Before and after exposure to these agents, it is recommended to assess the left ventricular ejection fracture with a 2D echo or a MUGA scan to evaluate for pre-existing cardiomyopathy or causal cardiomyopathy. The taxane and platin drug classes are known for causing neuropathy in a stocking and glove-like pattern. Pulmonary toxicity is a known toxicity from bleomycin used in Hodgkin's lymphoma and testicular cancer. Neutropenic fever is a common side effect that occurs when patients experience myelosuppression after receiving their chemo. *(Cornet & Dea, 2013; Floyd & Morgan, 2014)*

7. **(C)** Polycythemia vera (PV) is one of the four main common types of myeloproliferative neoplasms; the others being essential thrombocytosis, chronic myeloid leukemia, and primary idiopathic myelofibrosis. True primary polycythemia vera has to be distinguished from secondary polycythemia and spurious polycythemia. Spurious PV is usually a false elevation in the hemoglobin and hematocrit caused by either dehydration, a poor sample, or the patient who is taking diuretics. Secondary polycythemia can be caused by obstructive sleep apnea, chronic obstructive pulmonary disease, or malignancies releasing exogenous erythropoietin. The presence of the JAK2 V617F mutation is found in 95 plus percent of primary PV patients but not in secondary or spurious

PV. Splenomegaly is found approximately 70% of the time on examination in true primary PV. A history of smoking is more suggestive of secondary PV. Diuretic use is more suggestive of spurious PV. Ecchymoses and hepatomegaly are not useful clinically in this patient's case. *(Tefferi, 2014)*

8. **(B)** This is a classic case of immune thrombocytopenia purpura (ITP). The first treatment of choice is still steroids. In some children treatment can be withheld and the platelet count can recover on its own. In adults it tends to be more chronic or cyclical. A platelet transfusion is seldom indicated in ITP unless the patient is bleeding or the platelet count drops below 5,000 to 10,000. Platelet transfusions can occasionally cause a flare of the ITP. Rituxan is a monoclonal antibody used for lymphomas that has gained popularity in ITP in adults. However, its use has not been established in pediatric patients. Eltrombopag is a thrombopoietin agonist approved in adults for ITP but like rituxan its use has not been established in pediatrics. Splenectomy can be offered in children or adults with ITP but this would not be first-line therapy. *(Fogarty & Minichiello, 2013, pp. 540–542)*

9. **(C)** Vitamin B-12 deficiency and folic acid deficiency are both classified as megaloblastic anemias. Vitamin B-12 is found in many meat and dairy products. The body typically has enough stores of this vitamin to last up to 3 to 4 years. The process of vitamin B-12 absorption is a complicated process that involves the separation of vitamin B-12 from R-factors that are in the saliva and gastric juices, the binding of vitamin B-12 to intrinsic factor (IF) which is produced by the parietal cells within the stomach, and ultimately absorption in the terminal ileum. The most common causes of vitamin B-12 deficiency are pernicious anemia which is an autoimmune disorder where the body produces antibodies against IF, and reduced absorption due to gastric surgery. Both folic acid and vitamin B-12 deficiency is manifested by hypersegmented neutrophils. Patients who had their ileum removed have problems with absorption, not the rectosigmoid region. Believed to be due to overproduction of IF, myeloproliferative neoplasms actually present with elevated levels of vitamin B-12. If left untreated, vitamin B-12 deficiency can cause irreversible neuropathy due to a defect in myelin formation. Stocking and glove-like paresthesias, cerebellar ataxia, spasticity, dementia, and memory loss are documented temporary or permanent effects of vitamin B-12 deficiency. *(Hoffbrand 2013b, pp. 94–104)*

10. **(C)** This case represents glucose-6-phosphate dehydrogenase deficiency (G6PD). G6PD deficiency is an X-linked disorder that afflicts approximately 200 to 400 million people worldwide. G6PD is critical to help maintain RBC integrity as it is an important catalyst in the hexose monophosphate shunt pathway. This pathway produces the RBCs only source of NADPH which is an important factor of glutathione metabolism. Glutathione in turn helps maintain RBC integrity during oxidative stressors. Certain drugs that can cause redox reactions, select viral infections, and exposure to certain foods can all lead to hemolysis. The production of methemoglobin and sulfhemoglobin leads to insoluble masses that attach to the RBC membrane. These masses are known as Heinz bodies. With hemolysis, the retic count is elevated anywhere from 4% to 9%, haptoglobin is low, lactase dehydrogenase (LDH) is high, and indirect bilirubin is commonly elevated. Reactive thrombocytosis is not seen. Measuring G6PD levels in the acute setting is not recommended since the G6PD-deficient cells have been removed during the hemolysis. Instead it is recommended to check G6PD levels approximately 3 months after the episode of hemolysis. *(Glader, 2014)*

11. **(A)** This patient is presenting with signs and symptoms similar to both acute lymphoblastic leukemia (ALL) and acute myeloid leukemia (AML) however there are no blasts found in the bone marrow and the bone marrow is hypoplastic. Aplastic anemia is caused by diminished or absent hematopoietic pluripotent stem cells in the bone marrow due to injury. Causal agents can include radiation exposure, chemical exposure to pesticides or solvents, viruses, paroxysmal nocturnal hemoglobinuria, and drugs such as gold or sulfa compounds. If the insult is severe enough, the myeloid and erythroid cell lines could be absent. In AML and ALL the bone marrow tends to be hyperplastic with blasts in the marrow and in circulation. Furthermore, they tend to present with bone pain. Benzene could be the causal agent but it is not the diagnosis. Myelodysplastic syndrome (MDS) is a bone marrow disorder that typically present with disorganized erythropoiesis and hypercellularity in the marrow. The majority of patients with myeloproliferative

disorders are diagnosed in the late sixth to eighth decade. *(Drews, 2013; Young, 2013, pp. 127–134)*

12. **(D)** von Willebrand's disease (VWD) is an inherited autosomal dominant bleeding disorder that affects men and women equally. It is the most common bleeding disorder effecting approximately 1% of the general population. VWD is caused by a qualitative or quantitative defect in von Willebrand's factor (VWF). There are three main subtypes which are classified based on clinical and laboratory findings. Type I is treated with vasopressin or DDAVP to help raise VWF levels. VWF is responsible to assist the platelets in binding to the injured vascular wall. This factor also assists in the formation of the fibrin clot by acting as a cofactor for factor VIII. VWF exists as different multimers with the high–molecular-weight multimers being the most active. The disease is assessed by measuring VWF antigen, VWF activity (ristocetin activity), and factor VIII levels. These levels can vary due to numerous physiological factors making the diagnosis sometimes difficult. If VWF levels are low enough, it can cause factor VIII levels to drop affecting the partial thromboplastin time (PTT). *(Rick, 2014)*

13. **(E)** Heparin-induced thrombocytopenia (HIT) is a serious and potentially fatal condition that results in approximately 3% to 5% of patients exposed to heparin and 0.3% of patients exposed to low–molecular-weight heparins (LMWH). This condition is caused by the formation of autoantibodies of platelet factor 4 (PF4) released by the alpha granules in the platelets to the heparin molecule forming a heparin PF4 complex. This causes the formation of antibodies to the heparin PF4 complex. The IgG subtype antibody is the one that is pathologic in this disease process that causes the thrombocytopenia and thrombosis. The thrombocytopenia is a result of the consumption of the platelets as well as the removal of the IgG-coated platelets by macrophages and the reticuloendothelial system. The thrombosis ensues from these large heparin PF4 complexes dislodging into vascular sites. This event typically occurs anywhere from 4 to 10 days after the exposure of the heparin product, and is seen more commonly in women, and in surgical patients. Thrombocytopenia is the most common finding in HIT in up to 90% of patients where the nadir of the thrombocytopenia is around 50 to 60,000. There was no evidence of

schistocytes which is seen in thrombocytopenia purpura or hemolytic uremic syndrome. In this case, the patient did not present with findings clinically consistent with disseminated intravascular coagulation. ADAMTS13 deficiency also known as Upshaw–Schulman's syndrome is a rare inherited disorder that can place patients at higher rates of TTP during their life and would not fit this clinical presentation. *(Coutre, 2014; Fogarty & Minichello, 2013; Lee & Arpally, 2104 pp. 544–545)*

14. **(A)** Hodgkin's lymphoma (HL) is a lymphoproliferative disorder that arises from the germinal center or the postgerminal center B-cells. The unique appearance of the cellular composition is described as Reed–Sternberg cells and be divided into two main categories: classic Hodgkin's lymphoma and nodular lymphocytic predominant Hodgkin's lymphoma. Classic Hodgkin's lymphoma is further subdivided into nodular sclerosis classic HL, mixed cellularity classic HL, lymphocytic rich classic HL, and lymphocytic depleted classic HL. HL accounts or approximately 10% of all lymphomas and has a bimodal age distribution affecting young adults in their 20s and 30s and older adults in their 60s. The histological subtype can vary based on geographic location and socioeconomic status. For example, in developed countries like the United States, nodular sclerosis classic HL is the most common, whereas in less developed countries there is an equal incidence of mixed cellularity classic HL and nodular sclerosis classic HL. There is a higher incidence also reported in immunocompromised patients and patients with autoimmunity. Furthermore, HL is more common in patients that have been exposed to Epstein–Barr virus (EBV). Patients afflicted with HL typically present with painless lymphadenopathy, night sweats, fatigue, and pruritus. Treatment for HL depends on the symptoms, histology, stage, and whether there is bulky disease. Therapy often includes chemotherapy with ABVD (adriamycin, bleomycin, vinblastine, and dacarbazine) often coupled with external beam radiation. *(Aster, 2014; Cozen et al., 2012)*

15. **(B)** Lovenox is a commonly used low-molecular-weight heparin (LMWH) used for the treatment of deep venous thrombosis, for anticoagulation after cardiac procedures, and for the treatment of unstable angina. Even though this product is an LMWH, there still is a slight risk of heparin-induced

thrombocytopenia of less than 1%. According to recent research, LMWHs are the preferred initial and long-term anticoagulant of choice in cancer patients. Safety data indicate that lovenox is safe for use in pregnancy. While LMWHs bind to antithrombin III and have an inhibitory effect on factor Xa, the partial thromboplastin time does not measure the efficiency. The preferred dosing of lovenox is 1 mg/kg twice a day for the treatment of venous thromboembolisms or 1.5 mg/kg once a day. *(Bhutia & Wong, 2013; Lyman et al., 2013, p. 2189)*

16. **(C)** Myelodysplastic syndrome (MDS) is a collection of malignant stem cell disorders marked by dysplastic and ineffective blood production that may have the ability to transform into acute leukemia. The exact pathogenesis of MDS has not been clearly mapped out, but it is understood to be a clonal process that arises from a single malignant clone. MDS represents a constellation of different subtypes including refractory cytopenia with unilineage dysplasia (RCUD), refractory anemia with ringed sideroblasts (RARS), MDS with 5q-, refractory cytopenia with multilineage dysplasia (RCMD), refractory anemia with excess blasts subtypes 1 and 2, and MDS unspecified based on the World Health Organization (WHO) classification system. Some disorders like chronic myelomonocytic leukemia and MDS with thrombocytosis have features of both MDS and myeloproliferative neoplasms. Evaluation of the peripheral blood work can suggest MDS but the bone marrow biopsy is diagnostic. Prognosis and treatment depends on the subtype discovered whether it's a high risk, low risk, or intermediate risk (based on the International Prognostic Scoring System taking into account, the blast count, karyotype, and the number of cytopenias). The median age at diagnosis is 65, with a slight male predominance. Patients can present with anemia that is typically macrocytic with a mean corpuscle volume between 100 and 110, thrombocytopenia, leukopenia, thrombocytosis, or bicytopenia, abnormal cell morphology is also commonly detected. *(Bejar et al., 2012, p. 3376; Damon et al., 2013, pp. 517–519)*

17. **(E)** This patient is presenting with a microcytic anemia with reactive thrombocytosis. The most common cause of microcytic anemia is iron deficiency. Reactive thrombocytosis is commonly seen with iron deficiency. Another cause of microcytic anemia is thalassemia, however in thalassemia the red blood cell count is usually normal to elevated, the platelet count and red cell distribution width are normal. Thus ordering a hemoglobin electrophoresis has no utility in this case. A bone marrow biopsy is seldom indicated unless the patient had more than one cell line affected, abnormal cells in circulation, or there was suspicion of an underlying lymphoproliferative disorder. In addition there does not appear to be any indication of hemolysis given the normal haptoglobin, retic count, and LDH. Finally, folic acid deficiency presents with macrocytic anemia. This patient likely has iron deficiency from a GI source. *(Damon et al., 2013, pp. 491–501)*

18. **(C)** Transfusion-related acute lung injury (TRALI) is a rare but potentially fatal reaction to blood product infusions that occurs during or within a 6-hour window of the infusion. The clinical presentation includes hypoxia, pulmonary infiltrates, hypotension, and cyanosis. Even though TRALI can happen after any blood product infusion, plasma blood products, apheresis platelet concentrates, and whole blood (rarely used today) confer the greatest risk of TRALI. There is evidence that female donor blood products carry a higher risk. TRALI is believed to be caused by neutrophilic sequestering, priming, and activation in the pulmonary capillary endothelium. Treatment is supportive with oxygen supplementation and possibly ventilation. The benefit of steroid use remains unclear. The risk of iron overload has been recognized after packed red blood cell transfusions of more than 20 units. PRBC transfusions are known to cause hyperkalemia from the leakage of potassium out of the RBCs. The risk is greater the longer the PRBC is stored. Potassium leakage is estimated to be at a rate of approximately 1 mEq/day. One unit of PRBCs is expected to raise the hemoglobin approximately 1 g. Previous guidelines encouraged transfusions to the keep the hemoglobin above 10 g/dL and hematocrit above 30%. In current practice, the timing for transfusions is more conservative and individualized. For patients with a GI Bleed, there were fewer reported deaths, adverse events, and less bleeding when patients were not transfused until the hemoglobin dropped below 7.0 g/dL compared to a threshold of 9.0 g/dL. *(Carson & Kleinman, 2014; Kleinman & Kor, 2014)*

19. **(E)** Target cells are RBCs that have a central area of density surrounded by a halo that looks like a target. An increased surface area to volume ratio along with a redundant cell membrane accounts for the appearance of these cells. Target cells are seen in patients who have liver disease, a hemoglobinopathy like thalassemia, and less commonly, for several weeks after splenectomy. Howell–Jolly bodies are seen in the peripheral smear in postsplenectomy or functionally asplenic patients. Howell–Jolly bodies are nuclear remnants in the RBCs that would have been removed by the spleen. Heinz bodies are aggregates of hemoglobin that was denatured and precipitated on the RBC membrane. This is seen in glucose-6 phosphate dehydrogenase deficiency patients and less commonly in thalassemia patients. Rouleaux formation is the term used for a stacked coin appearance of the RBCs that is due to elevated levels of plasma proteins most commonly seen in myeloma and less likely in polyclonal diseases. In extreme cases of iron deficiency, the RBCs not only are microcytic and hypochromic but they can have abnormal shapes; this is referred to as poikilocytosis. *(Longo, 2013a, pp. 57–68; Rosenthal, 2014)*

20. **(A)** Felty's syndrome is a rare but severe subset of seropositive rheumatoid arthritis (RA) characterized by splenomegaly and neutropenia. It can affect up to 1% of patients who have RA. Typically it does not manifest itself until the patient has had RA for at least 10 years. Despite the triad of RA, splenomegaly, and neutropenia, some experts agree that splenomegaly is not needed to make the diagnosis. The pathophysiology of the neutropenia is believed to be due to immune destruction and removal of the neutrophils and a drop in production. The neutrophil count should be below 2,000 to make the diagnosis. Splenomegaly is present in up to 90% of the patients with Felty's syndrome. While a bone marrow biopsy is commonly performed to rule out other causes such as large granular lymphocytic leukemia, the diagnosis of Felty's syndrome remains a clinical one. A sedimentation rate is expected to be elevated but will not offer any further insight to the diagnosis. Flow cytometry may assist in ruling out other causes. Anti–double-stranded DNA antibodies titers will likely be positive but are not specific for this diagnosis. *(Xio et al., 2014, pp. 713–716)*

21. **(A)** Evaluation of a prolonged partial thromboplastin time (PTT) is a common clinical dilemma both in the inpatient and outpatient setting. When confronted with a prolonged PTT, it is recommended to first repeat the test to ensure that the results are truly prolonged. Use care to take a comprehensive history searching for clues suggesting bleeding disorders and searching for medications that may be the source of the problem. The PTT is sensitive to factors XII, XI, IX, VIII, and to heparin or other inhibitors. When performing a mixing study, the patient's serum is mixed in a 1:1 ratio with a normal donor's serum. Two possibilities can occur; the first is that after the mixing, the PTT corrects; the second is the PTT stays prolonged. If the PTT corrects, then there was a deficiency of one of the factors. If it stays prolonged, then there is a presence of an inhibitor. Common inhibitors that would cause the PTT to stay prolonged after the mixing study include the lupus anticoagulant, factor VIII Inhibitors, and contamination with heparin. In DIC and with factor VIII deficiency, the PTT would correct in the mixing study. Antithrombin III deficiency and dysfibrinogenemia would not alter the PTT. *(Zehnder, 2014)*

22. **(E)** This patient's presentation and clinical findings are consistent with multiple myeloma. Myeloma is a plasma cell disorder that arises from abnormal proliferation of a malignant plasma cell clone. Myeloma is present in all races but is—two to three times more common in African Americans than in whites. The average age at diagnosis is 66 to 70 years of age. Myeloma accounts for 1% of all cancers and 10% of all hematological malignancies in the United States. The abnormal proliferation of the malignant clone can lead to multiple deleterious effects including hypercalcemia, renal failure, anemia, and lytic bone lesions (CRAB criteria). The diagnosis is made when there are more than 10% of clonal plasma cells in the bone marrow, a monoclonal spike is present in the urine, serum, or both, and the presence of organ damage (anyone of the CRAB criteria). Monoclonal proteins in the urine are commonly called Bence Jones proteins and are best assessed with a 24-hour urine collection. Serum studies include checking the immunoglobulins to ascertain which immunoglobulin is involved (e.g., IgG, IgA, or light chains), serum protein electrophoresis, immunofixation, serum total protein and globulin protein, a bone marrow biopsy, and a skeletal survey, with the bone marrow biopsy having the greatest diagnostic yield. A biopsy of a lytic lesion often times can be difficult and may not have a high yield. Obtaining a PSA would be reasonable given the patients prior history of prostate cancer, however, prostate cancer typically forms sclerotic lesions more commonly than lytic. Finally, a total body bone scan does not offer any utility in the workup myeloma as it only identifies sclerotic lesions. *(Munshi et al., 2013, pp. 214–225; Rajkumar et al., 2012, pp. 494–496)*

23. (A) Primary immune thrombocytopenia purpura, also known as immune thrombocytopenia purpura or idiopathic thrombocytopenia purpura (ITP) is an acquired thrombocytopenia that results from platelet antigen autoantibodies. These IgG autoantibodies are produced by the B-cells. ITP can be challenging to diagnose since there is no specific test to confirm its presence and there are numerous other potential etiologies for thrombocytopenia. In children ITP can be self-limiting and may not even require treatment. In adults it tends to be secondary to an underlying disorder such as lymphomas or autoimmune diseases and tends to recur. Steroids are indicated as first-line therapy. On evaluation of the patient, one would expect to see purpura or petechiae, bleeding mucous membranes, and no splenomegaly. The presence of splenomegaly suggests splenic sequestering rather than immune destruction as the cause. It is common in ITP for the platelet count not to increase at all or even get worse after platelet transfusions due to the presence of the autoantibodies. Since ITP is a primary hemostatic disorder and does not involve the coagulation cascade, the PTT and PT/INR should be normal. Evidence of schistocytes on the peripheral smear suggests the possibility of a thrombotic microangiopathic process such as thrombocytopenia purpura or hemolytic uremic syndrome rather than ITP. *(Fogarty & Minichello, 2013, pp. 540–542)*

24. (E) Neutropenic fever is commonly encountered in cancer patients undergoing chemotherapy secondary to the myelosuppressive effects that chemotherapy has on the stem cells in the bone marrow. There is an inverse relationship between the neutrophil count and risk of infection. As the absolute neutrophil count (ANC) drops, the risk of infection goes up. Neutropenia is defined as an ANC of <1,500 cells/μL. It can be subclassified as mild (ANC 1,000–1,500 cells/μL), moderate (ANC 500–1,000

cells/μL), or severe (ANC <500 cells/μL). Fever above 100.4°F (38°C) with an ANC less than 1,500 cells/μL is defined as neutropenic fever. To minimize neutropenia and thus neutropenic fever, colony-stimulating factory (CSF) support with medications like pegfilgrastim (a long-acting CSF medication) can be used and injected after chemotherapy. Other short-acting forms of CSF such as filgrastim, sargramostim, or tbo-filgrastim can be used as well. While acetaminophen and prophylactic antibiotics can be used to treat the fever and minimize the risk of infection, neither do anything to minimize the risk of neutropenia. Hydrea and rituxan have no role in minimizing the risk of neutropenia. *(Bow & Wingard, 2014)*

25. (C) Sickle cell disease (hemoglobin S disease) is an autosomal dominant hemoglobinopathy. The homozygous form (SS), sickle cell anemia, results in sickling of erythrocytes, occurring when oxygen levels decrease at the tissue level. This results in impedance of blood flow to organs. Hemolysis often accompanies these abnormal erythrocytes. Although sexual and growth maturation are often delayed, most patients with the disease are fertile. Sickle cell crises are often precipitated by infection and those with sickle cell disease are at increased risk of infections from encapsulated organisms. Given the apparent good health of this woman's fiancée, he likely does not have sickle cell disease but may carry the trait. Those heterogenous (AS) for the gene are referred to as having sickle cell trait. The risk of carrying the trait is approximately 8% to 10% for those of African decent in the United States. Approximately 2.5 million people in the United States have the trait. Therefore, those with family histories of the disease likely carry the trait and genetic testing should be offered before childbearing. Given the strong family history of this man and the woman being of African descent, testing should be offered as they both may carry the gene. Those with sickle cell trait are typically asymptomatic with mild or absent anemia. Although sickle cell crises may occur at high altitudes for those with the disease, sickle cell crises are rare in those who are only carriers. The risk of sexually transmitted diseases is not increased for those with the trait or disease. *(Vinchinsky, 2014)*

26. (B) Iron-deficiency anemia is most commonly due to chronic blood loss. In the United States, dietary

deficiency is uncommon (except during pregnancy) and should not be presumed unless potential sources of blood loss have been excluded. However, dietary deficiency often occurs in pregnancy because of increased production of erythrocytes. Supplementation during pregnancy is routinely recommended. In mild to moderate iron deficiency, the reticulocyte count is mildly elevated although the corrected reticulocyte count is usually low. Low reticulocyte counts are seen in more severe forms of the disease. Elevated TIBC and low levels of iron, ferritin, and transferrin in the setting of microcytic anemia confirm the diagnosis. Although diminished iron stores are noted on bone marrow aspiration, this is not routinely needed to confirm the diagnosis. Once the diagnosis of iron-deficiency anemia is made, the underlying cause must be found and treated. Iron replacement may be needed in moderate to severe cases and is typically accomplished within 6 to 12 months. Once iron stores have been replaced, iron supplementation should be stopped to prevent iron toxicity or mask further blood loss. *(Damon et al., 2013, pp. 490–492)*

27. **(D)** Lead poisoning usually results in a mild anemia. Patients often have vague complaints including fatigue, abdominal pain, difficulties with concentration, decreased libido, and muscle weakness. There is some evidence that genetic polymorphisms such as the presence of C282Y and H63D alleles (seen in hemochromatosis) could also lead to worse cognitive declines compared to others exposed to lead who do not have the alleles. Hypertension, cardiovascular mortality, psychiatric effects can occur due to chronic exposure. Mild anemia and the presence of basophilic stippling are often seen. Lead levels should be checked in anyone presenting with these complaints and at risk, including children and adults with an occupational/environmental exposure. Primary treatment is to remove the source of lead. Chelating agents may be needed for those who are symptomatic or with very high levels. *(Goldman & Hu, 2014)*

28. **(C)** Anemia may be the result of a wide variety of causes. Once a patient is found to be anemic, the next step is determining the underlying etiology. Anemia may be divided into microcytic, normocytic, and macrocytic on the basis of the MCV of the erythrocytes. Once this has been determined, the differential diagnosis may be narrowed and appropriate adjuvant tests can be ordered. Microcytic anemia is most commonly seen in the presence of iron deficiency. Thalassemia will also result in a microcytic anemia but is less common in the United States. Both lead poisoning and anemia of chronic illness may result in a mildly lower MCV, but a normocytosis is more commonly seen. In addition, patients with chronic illnesses often have more than one contributing factor for their anemia; and therefore, the MCV may be low, high, or normal. In a previously healthy individual with microcytic anemia, and with normal WBC and platelet counts, iron deficiency should be suspected. *(Damon et al., 2013, pp. 490–496)*

29. **(C)** Anticancer therapy often results in complications that may be mild to severe, acute, and chronic. Many chemotherapeutic agents share similar side effects including alopecia, nausea, vomiting, diarrhea, mucositis, fatigue, and myelosuppression. The frequency and severity of these common toxicities vary with each drug and dosage. Tamoxifen use has been shown to increase the risk of uterine malignancies. Although this risk remains relatively low, it must be considered and discussed with patients when considering its use in treatment and prevention of malignancy. *(Sausville & Longo, 2013, pp. 378–379)*

30. **(D)** Tumor markers are biochemical abnormalities, which are often elevated in particular malignancies. They are typically measured in the blood but may sometimes be analyzed in urine or tumor tissue. Tumor markers are often present at low levels in healthy individuals and levels may occasionally be elevated in nonmalignant conditions. Although tumor markers are often quite helpful in monitoring patients with known cancer, they are rarely sensitive enough to allow for screening of the disease. Prostate-specific antigen (PSA) is the most commonly used tumor marker for cancer screening despite recent recommendations by the United States Preventive Services Task Force discouraging PSA screening. Prostatic acid phosphate level may be elevated in prostate cancers, particularly when metastatic disease is present, but is much less sensitive than PSA and should not be used for screening. Carcinoembryonic antigen (CEA) levels may be elevated in a variety of malignancies, most commonly colon cancer, while cancer antigen 19-9 (CA 19-9) levels may be elevated in pancreatic cancer. Unfortunately, neither CEA nor CA 19-9 is sensitive

enough for cancer screening. Alpha-fetoprotein is recommended in screening for hepatocellular carcinoma in those considered at increased risk, including those with chronic hepatitis B and C and those with cirrhosis from all causes. The role of CA 125 is currently under investigation for screening of ovarian cancer but to date it is not considered standard of care. *(Croswell et al., 2013, pp. 351–357)*

31. **(C)** Thalassemia is a group of genetic disorders affecting one or more of the subunits of the hemoglobin chain resulting in a microcytic, hypochromic anemia. As a result it is not a quantitative red blood cell production problem. As a result, the red blood cell count is normal or elevated, while the mean corpuscle volume is much lower than expected than with iron deficiency. It is most common in those of African and Asian descents. Presentation may occur early or later in life, depending upon the affected subunit and number of genetic abnormalities involved. The most common form (thalassemia minor) results in only mild disease, often goes undiagnosed and requires no treatment; other forms are life-threatening. Suggestion of thalassemia can be made by calculating the Mentzer index which is calculated by dividing the mean corpuscle volume by the red blood cell count. If the result is greater than 13, iron deficiency is the more likely diagnosis. If the result is less than 13, then thalassemia is likely the diagnosis. Subsequently the diagnosis is ultimately confirmed by Hb electrophoresis, which should be ordered when the disease is suspected. *(Benz, 2014)*

32. **(C)** External beam irradiation is a common modality of anticancer therapy. In previous years, it had been used to treat benign conditions including thyroid disorders and acne. Complications may include local damage to tissues/organs, radiation enteritis, radiation esophagitis, radiation dermatitis, radiation osteonecrosis, delayed wound healing, nausea, headache, and fatigue. Myelosuppression may occur if bone marrow is involved in the radiation field. However, significant myelosuppression is not typical unless coupled with chemotherapy. Hair loss is typical over the radiation treatment field but diffuse hair loss is not seen. Radiation therapy is often used to palliate pain for patients with metastatic disease to the bone. It may produce relief of pain within a few days of initiation of treatment,

especially is radiosensitive tumors like plasmacytomas. Worsening bone pain is not expected but may signal a complication of the disease, such as a pathologic fracture. *(Dainiak, 2014; Sausville & Longo, 2013b, p. 363)*

33. **(E)** Christmas disease, also known as hemophilia B and factor IX (not factor XI) hemophilia, is a hereditary bleeding disorder. It is x-linked–like hemophilia A and the combined incidence of the hemophilias is approximately 1 in 5,000 births. Unlike hemophilia A, in hemophilia B, some have a Leyden phenotype that is a severe form of hemophilia that becomes mild after puberty. Given the deficiency of factor IX, these patients experience spontaneous bleeding in their joints, muscles, and their gastrointestinal tract. Abnormal thrombosis does not occur. It is managed with factor IX concentrates or fresh-frozen plasma. It is necessary to distinguish between hemophilia A and hemophilia B, since both diseases present similarly but require specific factor replacement. *(Hoots & Shapiro, 2014)*

34. **(B)** Splenomegaly may be associated with LUQ fullness, pain, early satiety, and reflux. Because of sequestration of platelets, petechiae are often found on examination. Splenomegaly may be caused by various illnesses including infectious, immune related, oncologic, and inflammation. Splenomegaly frequently is a result of hepatic parenchymal or veno-occlusive disease and patients presenting with unexplained splenomegaly should be examined for the presence of findings to suggest portal hypertension. Additional symptoms and signs should be sought to help in narrowing a differential diagnosis. The presence of physical findings of liver disease may be identified to include spider angiomas, caput medusa, palmar erythema, gynecomastia, and with more advanced disease, ascites, jaundice, and asterixis. Lymphadenopathy suggests possible infectious or malignant causes of splenomegaly in any patient. *(Henry & Longo, 2013, pp. 32–39)*

35. **(D)** Genetic testing has become increasingly available for various genetic mutations, although there is much work to be done in this field. Since cancer is a second leading cause of death in the United States (second to heart disease), many patients will have some family history of the disease. Personal and family histories, which may raise concern for

a possible hereditary disease, include multiple family members with malignancy and the diagnosis of malignancy at a young age (i.e., younger than expected for the particular disease). Consideration of genetic susceptibility is most important when screening tests for the disease are available and when risk reduction strategies are available. For these patients, referral to a genetics counselor should be considered. Risk factors for hereditary cancer syndromes include early age of onset, multiple family members with the same cancer, and clustering of cancers known to be caused by a single gene mutation. *(Morin 2013, pp. 300–309)*

36. **(D)** Petechiae are typically a sign of thrombocytopenia. It does not usually occur with other disorders of the coagulation cascade. It would not be expected in patients who receive excess coumadin, in the absence of a platelet abnormality. Antiplatelet medications affect platelet function but should not result in thrombocytopenia. Platelet function may be difficult to assess since bleeding times and platelet aggregations studies can be vague. Various conditions may result in thrombocytopenia, including immune, infectious, oncologic, and hepatic or splenic sequestering. *(Fogarty & Minichiello, 2013; Konkle, 2013, pp. 538–548)*

37. **(C)** The myeloproliferative disorder CML is the most likely diagnosis here. Early satiety is a common manifestation of splenomegaly; fatigue is a general complaint found in many conditions. Causes of leukemias are rarely identified, although radiation is considered a cause of some leukemias, of which CML is one. Often, splenomegaly is the only physical finding in a newly diagnosed CML patient. An elevated white blood cell count might be the only abnormality on a blood smear. If there were more blasts (20%), this would be correctly diagnosed as an acute leukemia. Bone marrow analysis is commonly done to detect the presence of the chromosomal translocation 9 (ABL) and 22 (BCR) which is referred to as the Philadelphia chromosome. This oncogene as it is referred to leads to the abnormal clonal proliferation of mature and maturing granulocytes from the stem cells. A peripheral blood test done by reverse transcriptase polymerase chain reaction or a fluorescence in situ hybridization (FISH) study used to detect the BCR/ABL gene can also be

done to make the diagnosis. CML accounts for approximately 15% to 20% of leukemias in adults. It can be separated into three phases: the chronic phase; accelerated phase, and blast phase that can transform into ALL or AML. The incidence of CML rises slowly with age until the mid-40s. After that the incidence rises more rapidly. CLL is a lymphoproliferative disorder; the Philadelphia chromosome abnormality does not occur in CLL or in Burkitt lymphoma. Typical chromosomal translocations in Burkitt lymphoma are t(8;14) and t(8;22). *(Van Etten, 2014; Wetzler et al., 2013, pp. 175–181)*

38. **(D)** Auer rods are pathognomonic for AML: This presentation is typical for AML. Lymphomas do not present with profound pancytopenias. CML could be in the differential; however, the high number of blasts rules out the chronic phase of CML. There would be no thrombocytopenia and no blasts (definitely no Auer rods) if hemolytic anemia was the cause of this woman's fatigue. Therefore, acute leukemia is the most likely diagnosis. Auer rods are eosinophilic needle-like inclusions in the cytoplasm, seen in AML. Hodgkin's and non-Hodgkin's lymphomas can present with anemia but rarely have abnormal platelet counts involved nor are Auer rods present. CML and CLL usually present with high WBC counts but no Auer rods. *(Damon et al., 2013, pp. 519–521)*

39. **(E)** Vitamin K is a fat-soluble vitamin that is stored in the liver. It is critical in the clotting cascade and deficiencies result in prolongation of the prothrombin time. It normally assists in the activity of helping the production of factors II, VII, IX, and X. With severe or prolonged deficiencies, prolongation of the prothrombin time/international ratio followed by prolongation of the partial trhomboplastin time. Deficiencies may occur from dietary deficiencies, malabsorption, and most commonly, chronic liver disease, such as cirrhosis. Treatment is with parenteral administration of vitamin K, with monthly injections in those with chronic deficiencies. FFP may be needed if patients have active hemorrhage. *(Fogarty & Minichiello, 2013, p. 553)*

40. **(D)** Various conditions may result in thrombocytopenia. Many are due to a reduction in the number of circulating platelets in the setting of adequate production. These include DIC (due to consumption of

platelets during abnormal clotting), hypersplenism resulting in sequestration of platelets, and Henoch–Schönlein purpura (a systemic vasculitis with typical manifestations of palpable purpura, abdominal pain, and hematuria). Alcoholism may result in cirrhosis, particularly in the presence of hepatitis C or other chronic liver disease. Cirrhosis results in portal hypertension, splenomegaly, and thrombocytopenia. Platelet production may be reduced in malignant conditions involving the bone marrow such as leukemia or in the setting of marrow failure with aplastic anemia. Alternatively, essential thrombocytosis is a rare myeloproliferative disorder that is identified by an elevated platelet count caused by abnormal proliferation of megakaryocytes in the bone marrow. Therefore, increased risk of thrombosis is a complication and may occur in small veins such as the mesenteric, hepatic, or portal venous system. (*Damon et al., 2013, pp. 511–516; Fogarty & Minichiello, 2013, pp. 538–542*)

REFERENCES

Aster J. Epidemiology, pathological features, and diagnosis of classic hodgkin's lymphoma. 2014. UpToDate. Available at: http://www.uptodate.com/contents/epidemiology-pathologic-features-and-diagnosis-of-classical-hodgkin-lymphoma?source=search_result&search=hodgkins+lymphoma&selectedTitle=2%7E150. Accessed August 13, 2014.

Bejar R, Stevenson KE, Caughey BA, et al. Validation of a prognostic model and the impact of mutations in patients with lower-risk myelodysplastic syndromes. *J Clin Oncol*. 2012;30:3376–3382.

Benz E. Clinical manifestations and diagnosis of thalassemias. 2014. Available at: http://www.uptodate.com/contents/clinical-manifestations-and-diagnosis-of-the-thalassemias?source=search_result&search=thalasemia&selectedTitle=1%7E150. Accessed August 31, 2014.

Bermis B, Erkan D, Schur P. Diagnosis of antiphospholipid antibody syndrome. UpToDate. 2014. Available at: http://www.uptodate.com/contents/diagnosis-of-the-antiphospholipid-syndrome?source=search_result&search=APS&selectedTitle=1%7E52. Accessed August 20, 2014.

Bhutia S, Wong PF. Once versus twice daily low molecular weight heparin for the initial treatment of venous thromboembolism. *Cohcrane Database Syst Rev*. 2013;7:CD003074.

Bow E, Wingard J. Overview of neutropenic fever syndromes. 2014. UpToDate. Available at: http://www.uptodate.com/contents/overview-of-neutropenic-fever-syndromes?source=search_result&search=neutropenia&selectedTitle=3%7E150. Accessed August 16, 2014.

Carson J, Kleinman S. Indications and hemoglobin thresholds for red blood cell transfusions in the adult. 2014. UpToDate. Available at: http://www.uptodate.com/contents/indications-and-hemoglobin-thresholds-for-red-blood-cell-transfusion-in-thadult?source=search_result&search=transfusion+medicine&selectedTitle=1%7E150. Accessed September 1, 2014.

Cornet PA, Dea TO. Cancer. In: Papadakis MA, McPhee SJ, eds. *Current Medical Diagnosis and Treatment*. New York, NY: McGraw-Hill; 2013.

Coutre S. Clinical presentation and diagnosis of heparin induced thrombocytopenia. 2014. UpToDate. Available at: http://www.uptodate.com/contents/clinical-presentation-and-diagnosis-of-heparin-induced-thrombocytopenia?source=search_result&search=HIT&selectedTitle=1%7E150. Accessed August 28, 2014.

Cozen W, Li D, Best T, et al. A genome-wide meta analysis of nodular sclerosis hodgkin's lymphoma identifies risk at loci at 6p21. 32. *Blood*. 2012;119:469–475.

Croswell JM, Brawley OW, Kramer BS. Prevention and early detection of cancer. In: Longo DO, Fauci AS, Kasper DL, et al., eds. *Harrisons Hematology and Oncology*. 2nd ed. New York, NY: McGraw-Hill; 2013.

Dainiak N. Biology and clinical features of radiation injuries in adults. 2014. UpToDate. Available at: http://www.uptodate.com/contents/biology-and-clinical-features-of-radiation-injury-in-adults?source=search_result&search=radiation+toxicity&selectedTitle=1%7E150. Accessed August 13, 2014.

Damon LE, Andrealis C, Linker CA. Blood disorders. In: Papadakis MA, McPhee SJ, eds. *Current Medical Diagnosis and Treatment*. New York, NY: McGraw-Hill; 2013.

Drews R. Hematological consequences of malignancy; anemia and bleeding. 2013. UpToDate. Available at: http://www.uptodate.com/contents/hematologic-consequences-of-malignancy-anemia-and-bleeding?source=search_result&search=anemia+in+cancer&selectedTitle=1%7E150. Accessed August 14, 2014.

Floyd J, Morgan J. Cardiotoxicity of anthracycline-like chemotherapy agents. UpToDate. 2014. Available at: http://www.uptodate.com/contents/cardiotoxicity-of-anthracycline-like-chemotherapy-agents?source=search_result&search=

adriamycin+cardiotoxicity&selectedTitle=1%7E150. Accessed August 18, 2014.

Fogarty PF, Minichiello TM. Disorders of hemostasis, thrombosis, and antithrombotic therapy. In: Papadakis MA, McPhee SJ, eds. *Current Medical Diagnosis and Treatment*. New York, NY: McGraw-Hill; 2013.

Glader B. Diagnosis and treatment of glucose-6-phosphate dehydrogenase deficiency. UpToDate. 2014. Available at: http://www.uptodate.com/contents/diagnosis-and-treatment-of-glucose-6-phosphate-dehydrogenase-deficiency?source=search_result&search=g6pd+deficiency&selectedTitle=1%7E150. Accessed August 13, 2014.

Goldman R, Hu H. *Adult Lead Poisoning*. 2014. UpToDate. Available at: http://www.uptodate.com/contents/adult-lead-poisoning?source=search_result&search=lead+poisoning&selectedTitle=1%7E107#H7. Accessed August 18, 2014.

Henry PH, Longo DL. Enlargement of lymph nodes and spleen. In: Longo DO, Fauci AS, Kasper DL, et al., eds. *Harrisons Hematology and Oncology*. 2nd ed. New York, NY: McGraw-Hill; 2013.

Hoffbrand, AV. Megaloblastic anemias. In: Longo DO, Fauci AS, Kasper DL, et al., eds. *Harrisons Hematology and Oncology*. 2nd ed. New York, NY: McGraw-Hill; 2013.

Hoots K, Shapiro A. Clinical manifestations and diagnosis of hemophilia. UpToDate. 2014. Available at: http://www.uptodate.com/contents/clinical-manifestations-and-diagnosis-of-hemophilia?source=search_result&search=hemophilia&selectedTitle=1%7E150. Accessed August 12, 2014.

Horwitz M. Hypercalcemia of malignancy. UpToDate. 2014. Available at: http://www.uptodate.com/contents/hypercalcemia-of-malignancy?source=search_result&search=hypercalcemia+of+malignancy&selectedTitle=1%7E150. Accessed August 15, 2014.

Kleinman S, Kor D. Transfusion related acute lung injury. 2014. UpToDate. Available at: http://www.uptodate.com/contents/transfusion-related-acute-lung-injury-trali?source=search_result&search=transfusion+related+acute+lung+injury&selectedTitle=1%7E43. Accessed August 23, 2014.

Konkle B. Disorders of platelets and vessel wall. In: Longo DO, Fauci AS, Kasper DL, et al., eds. *Harrisons Hematology and Oncology*. 2nd ed. New York, NY: McGraw-Hill; 2013.

Lee GM, Arepally GM. Diagnosis and management of heparin induced thrombocytopenia. *Hematol Oncol Clin North Am*. 2013;27:541–563.

Longo DL. Atlas of hematology and analysis of peripheral blood smears. In: Longo DO, Fauci AS, Kasper DL, et al., eds. *Harrisons Hematology and Oncology*. 2nd ed. New York, NY: McGraw-Hill; 2013a.

Longo DL. Malignancies of lymphoid cells. In: Longo DO, Fauci AS, Kasper DL, et al., eds. *Harrisons Hematology and Oncology*. 2nd ed. New York, NY: McGraw-Hill; 2013b.

Lyman GH, Khorana AA, Kuderer NM, et al. Venous thromboembolism prophylaxis and treatment in patients with cancer.

American Society of Clinical Oncology Clinical Practice Update. *J Clin Oncol*. 2013;31:2189–2204.

Morin PJ, Trent JM, Collins FS, Vogelstein B. Cancer genetics. In: Longo DO, Fauci AS, Kasper DL, et al., eds. *Harrisons Hematology and Oncology*. 2nd ed. New York, NY: McGraw-Hill; 2013.

Munshi NC, Longo DL, Anderson KC. Plasma cell disorders. In: Longo DO, Fauci AS, Kasper DL, et al., eds. *Harrisons Hematology and Oncology*. 2nd ed. New York, NY: McGraw-Hill; 2013.

Rajkumar SV, Melini G, San Miguel JF. Haematological cancer: redefining myeloma. *Nat Rev Clin Oncol*. 2012;9:494–496.

Rick M. *Clinical Presentation and Diagnosis of Von Willebrand Disease*. 2014. UpToDate. Available at: http://www.uptodate.com/contents/clinical-presentation-and-diagnosis-of-von-willebrand-disease?source=search_result&search=vwd&selectedTitle=1%7E150. Accessed August 22, 2014.

Rosenthal D. *Evaluation of the Peripheral Blood Smear*. 2014. UpToDate. Available at: http://www.uptodate.com/contents/evaluation-of-the-peripheral-blood-smear?source=search_result&search=red+cell+morphology&selectedTitle=1%7E14. Accessed August 13, 2014.

Sausville EA, Longo DL. Principles of cancer treatment. In: Longo DO, Fauci AS, Kasper DL, et al., eds. *Harrisons Hematology and Oncology*. 2nd ed. New York, NY: McGraw-Hill; 2013.

Schrier S. *Etiology and Clinical Manifestations of Vitamin B-12 and Folate Deficiency*. UpToDate. 2014. Available at: http://www.uptodate.com/contents/etiology-and-clinical-manifestations-of-vitamin-b12-and-folate-deficiency?source=search_result&search=HYPERSEGMENTED+NEUTROPHILS&selectedTitle=2%7E10#H2127027. Accessed August 25, 2014

Tefferi A. *Clinical Manifestations and Diagnosis of Polycythemia Vera*. UpToDate. 2014. http://www.uptodate.com/contents/clinical-manifestations-and-diagnosis-of-polycythemia-vera?source=search_result&search=PV&selectedTitle=1%7E106. Accessed August 28, 2014.

Van Etten R. *Clinical Manifestations and Diagnosis of Chronic Myeloid Leukemia*. 2014. UpToDate. Available at: http://www.uptodate.com/contents/clinical-manifestations-and-diagnosis-of-chronic-myeloid-leukemia?source=search_result&search=cml&selectedTitle=1%7E150. Accessed August 24, 2014.

Vinchinsky E. *Sickle Cell Trait*. 2014. UpToDate. Available at: http://www.uptodate.com/contents/sickle-cell-trait?source=search_result&search=sickle+cell+trait&selectedTitle=1%7E61. Accessed August 22, 2014.

Wetzler M, Marcucci G, Bloomfield CD. Acute and chronic myeloid leukemia. In: Longo DO, Fauci AS, Kasper DL, et al., eds. *Harrisons Hematology and Oncology*. 2nd ed. New York, NY: McGraw-Hill; 2013.

Xio RZ, Xiong MJ, Long ZJ, et al. Diagnosis of felty's syndrome, distinguished from hematological neoplasm: a case report. *Onco Lett*. 2014;3:713–716.

Young NS. Aplastic anemia, myelodysplasia, and related bone marrow failure syndromes. In: Longo DO, Fauci AS, Kasper DL, et al., eds. *Harrisons Hematology and Oncology*. 2nd ed. New York, NY: McGraw-Hill; 2013.

Zehnder J. *Clinical Use of Coagulation Tests*. 2014. UpToDate. Available at: http://www.uptodate.com/contents/clinical-use-of-coagulation-tests?source=search_result&search=ptt+mixing+study&selectedTitle=1%7E150#H1. Accessed August 10, 2014.

CHAPTER 7

Infectious Disease
Brenda L. Quincy, PhD, MPH, PA-C, DFAAPA

DIRECTIONS: Each of the numbered questions or incomplete statements is followed by possible answers or completions of the statement. Select the ONE-lettered answer or completion that is BEST in each case.

1. A 33-year-old woman presents with an itchy vaginal discharge for the past 2 days. She has been healthy other than a recent sinus infection for which she took a 10-day course of amoxicillin. Her husband is her only sexual partner and he has no symptoms. On examination, the vulva is noted to be slightly erythematous and swollen with some evidence of excoriation. Discharge is white and clumpy. Provided the most likely diagnosis is confirmed on microscopy, which of the following is first-line therapy?

   (A) Azithromycin (Zithromax) 250 mg four tablets by mouth once
   (B) Ceftriaxone (Rocephin) 250 mg intramuscularly once
   (C) Fluconazole (Diflucan) 150 mg one tablet by mouth once
   (D) Metronidazole (MetroGel) 500 mg four tablets by mouth once at night
   (E) Metronidazole (MetroGel) 500 mg one tablet by mouth twice daily × 7 days

2. A patient with known human immunodeficiency virus (HIV) infection presents with the gradual onset of a cough, shortness of breath on exertion, and a feeling of a "catch" on inspiration. The chest x-ray reveals a lobar infiltrate. His O_2 sat is 95% and purified protein derivative (PPD) is negative. CD4 cell count is 500. What is the most likely etiology?

   (A) Herpes simplex
   (B) Mycobacterium
   (C) *Pneumocystis jirovecii*
   (D) *Streptococcus pneumoniae*
   (E) *Toxoplasma gondii*

3. A 33-year-old HIV-positive woman presents with her second episode of oral thrush in the past 2 months. Her current CD4 count is 75. In addition to treatment for the thrush, which of the following should she receive as prophylactic therapy?

   (A) Amoxicillin 500 mg twice daily
   (B) Azithromycin 1,200 mg weekly
   (C) Clarithromycin 500 mg twice daily
   (D) Rifampin 600 mg daily
   (E) Trimethoprim/sulfamethoxazole double strength daily

4. A 55-year-old man presents with chest discomfort, shortness of breath, productive cough, and low-grade fever. He reports generalized malaise as well. He takes no medications and has no known allergies. Examination reveals a temperature of 102°F (oral), unremarkable head, ears, eyes, nose, throat, and few crackles anteriorly in the upper right lung field. Chest x-ray reveals a solitary nodule in the right upper lobe. Which of the following is the most likely etiology for his symptoms?

   (A) Candida species
   (B) Cryptococcosis
   (C) Influenza A
   (D) *Pneumocystis jirovecii*
   (E) *Streptococcus pneumoniae*

5. A 21-year-old male presents with cough and mild shortness of breath for three days. The cough is occasionally productive of yellowish mucus. He reports a low-grade fever with this episode but says that he has otherwise been healthy. He has spent the last month working in bat caves. He denies tobacco or alcohol use. Which of the following is the most likely diagnosis?

(A) Candidiasis

(B) Cryptococcosis

(C) Histoplasmosis

(D) Psittacosis

6. An 8-year-old girl is brought into the emergency department with abdominal cramps, nausea, and vomiting since early this morning. She has had two loose stools but denies melena or hematochezia. She has had a low-grade fever. In the past hour, her vision has become blurry and she feels increasingly weak. Her mother has had similar but milder symptoms. Twenty-four hour dietary recall includes only chicken broth today. Last night for dinner they had meatloaf (fully cooked), mashed potatoes, and green beans. Her mother cans all their vegetables. Her medical history is unremarkable. She takes no medications. No known drug allergies. Examination reveals a temperature of 99°F, clear lungs, and mildly tachycardic heart with no murmur audible. Abdomen-bowel sounds present, soft with mild diffuse tenderness, no guarding. Neurologic examination is significant for decreased visual acuity and decreased motor strength (2/5) in the upper and lower extremities. Which of the following is the most likely etiologic agent for the patient's illness?

(A) Cholera species

(B) Clostridium botulinum

(C) Enterotoxic Escherichia coli

(D) Pinworms

7. A 21-year-old bodybuilder presents with complaints of diarrhea, cramps, and low-grade fever for 24 hours. He has been training for a competition, eating large amounts of protein, including shakes made with raw eggs. He reports three loose stools with blood in the commode today. He denies nausea or vomiting and tolerates liquids and solids. Examination reveals a well-muscled man in no apparent distress; lungs and heart unremarkable; abdomen, with mildly hyperactive bowel sounds and no tenderness or organomegaly; no evidence of hemorrhoids or anal fissure, no masses, and no stool present for hemoccult. Based on the most likely diagnosis, which of the following is the most appropriate first-line management?

(A) Oral ciprofloxacin (Cipro)

(B) Intravenous metronidazole (Flagyl)

(C) Oral trimethoprim/sulfamethoxazole (Bactrim)

(D) Oral fluconazole (Diflucan)

(E) Supportive care

8. A 3-year-old male presents to the emergency department with 24 hours of fever and six episodes of diarrhea. He also had two episodes of vomiting and the most recent stool contained blood. His parents measured his temperature at 103.4°F (oral) last night. Other members of the family have had diarrhea in the last 24 hours but no one has been as sick as the 3-year old. When he arrived in the emergency room his temperature was nearly 105°F and he had a generalized seizure before the nursing staff was able to lower his temperature. Which of the following is the most likely etiologic agent of his diarrheal infection?

(A) Escherichia coli

(B) Salmonella species

(C) Shigella species

(D) Vibrio cholerae

9. A 32-year-old female presents with watery, non-bloody diarrhea and abdominal cramps for the past 2 days. She also reports a low-grade fever. She returned from a medical mission trip to South America yesterday. While on the trip she spent time in a remote area and is uncertain of the quality of the water she drank. She also ate shrimp one night for dinner. Which of the following is the most likely etiologic agent for her diarrhea?

(A) Giardia lamblia

(B) Hookworms

(C) Salmonella species

(D) Shigella species

(E) Vibrio cholerae

10. A 3-year-old African immigrant girl is brought into the emergency department with congestion and a sore throat. Her family has been in the United States for only 1 month. They were "rescued" from a refugee camp by a private relief organization. This is her first medical evaluation. On examination, she is noted to have a low-grade fever; tympanic membranes are pearly gray without injection or visible air–fluid levels. Throat is erythematous with enlarged tonsils covered by a grayish membrane. Tonsillar nodes are tender. Lungs are clear to auscultation. Rapid strep screen is negative. Which of the following is the most likely etiologic agent of her illness?

(A) *Bordetella pertussis*

(B) *Corynebacterium diphtheriae*

(C) *Haemophilus influenzae*

(D) *Streptococcus pyogenes*

11. A 23-year-old woman presents with pelvic discomfort and vaginal discharge for the past 3 days. She finished her period last week. She is taking oral contraceptives as directed. Her medical history is significant for a therapeutic abortion with no other hospitalizations or pregnancies. She has had three sexual partners in the past 6 weeks and does not use condoms. Her latest partner reported that he was treated recently for gonorrhea. On examination, she has a mucopurulent discharge with "strawberry" cervix on speculum examination with no cervical motion tenderness on bimanual examination. After collecting the appropriate specimens, which of the following is the best therapeutic option for this patient?

(A) Oral ofloxacin 400 mg once plus oral metronidazole 500 mg twice daily for 7 days

(B) Oral fluconazole 150 mg once

(C) Oral metronidazole 2 g once

(D) IM ceftriaxone 250 mg plus oral doxycycline 100 mg twice daily for 7 days

12. A 26-year-old homosexual male presents with multiple episodes of bloody diarrhea that began last night. He and his partner returned 2 days ago from a 2-month long humanitarian relief trip to a less developed country. During the final week of the trip, they travelled into a more remote region of the country. They spent more time than expected in this region with a limited water supply and poor sanitation. Which of the following organisms is the most likely cause of his diarrhea?

(A) *Entamoeba histolytica*

(B) *Giardia lamblia*

(C) Hookworm

(D) Salmonella species

(E) *Vibrio cholerae*

13. The organism shown in Figure 7-1 usually enters the body from infected soil through a break in the skin of the feet. It then is carried to the lungs, travels to the mouth, and is swallowed. Once in the gastrointestinal (GI) tract, it attaches to the wall and induces bleeding, leading to an iron deficiency anemia. Associated GI symptoms are uncommon. Additional symptoms include swelling and intense itching at the site in which the larva penetrates the skin. Which of the following organisms best fits this clinical picture and the organism shown in Figure 7-1?

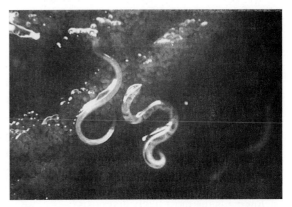

Figure 7-1. Centers for Disease Control and Prevention, National Center for Infectious Diseases, Division of Parasitic Diseases. (See also Color Insert).

(A) Hookworms

(B) Pinworms

(C) Strongyloides

(D) Whipworms

14. A 30-year-old male returning from a 2-week excursion into sub-Saharan Africa presents with fever, nausea, vomiting, and abdominal pain. He also reports significant muscle and joint pains making it difficult for him to get comfortable in any body position. He has no respiratory or urinary symptoms and reports one soft brown stool daily. His only medication has been acetaminophen 500 mg two pills every 4 to 6 hours as needed for fever and body aches. Last dose was 30 minutes ago. Vital signs: T: 101°F (oral), BP: 100/60, P: 92 bpm, regular. Examination: oropharynx with dry mucous membranes without erythema or exudate; lungs are clear to auscultation; heart–regular rate and rhythm; abdomen–positive bowel sounds with diffuse tenderness to palpation. Which of the following is the most common etiology of his presentation?

   (A) Dengue
   (B) Enteric fever
   (C) Leptospirosis
   (D) Malaria

15. A 16-year-old boy presents with complaints of a rash, low-grade fever, headache, and malaise. Symptoms began yesterday after he spent most of the past 4 days deer hunting in the woods around his house. He reports that he does check himself for ticks every night. He often finds them, but this season he has not noticed any that were latched on to his skin. On examination, his temperature is noted to be 99.9°F, his HEENT is unremarkable, and he has 1 to 2-mm red macules over wrists and ankles with remainder of skin clear. Heart, lungs, and abdomen are unremarkable. Which of the following is the most likely diagnosis?

   (A) Ehrlichiosis
   (B) Lyme disease
   (C) Q fever
   (D) Rocky Mountain spotted fever

16. A 3-year-old boy presents with 3 days of fever, runny nose, and injected conjunctiva. Initially his parents thought he had a cold so they managed it at home, but last night while bathing him they noted a maculopapular rash on his head. This morning it had progressed to his chest and back so they brought him in for evaluation. Physical examination confirms their report and reveals white spots in his mouth on the buccal mucosa. Which of the following childhood exanthems is the most likely explanation for this presentation?

   (A) Coxsackie virus
   (B) Herpes simplex infection
   (C) Measles
   (D) Rubella

17. An 8-year-old girl presents with painful skin lesions over the right side of her upper lip, extending onto her nose. The lesions appeared 3 days ago at the vermilion border of her lip. The first manifestation was a pink papule with associated tingling and burning, which evolved into a cluster of small, clear fluid-filled vesicles. Now the vesicles have extended onto her nose. The rash was accompanied by low-grade fever. Her parents report that she has had blisters on her lip twice before but they always resolved in a few days without spreading beyond her lip. Her family returned yesterday from a 1-week beach vacation during which she spent most of the day outdoors. Which of the following is the most likely diagnosis?

   (A) Herpes simplex virus
   (B) Herpesvirus 6
   (C) Parvovirus
   (D) Varicella zoster virus

18. A 6-year-old child with leukemia presents with a very painful vesicular rash as seen in Figure 7-2. This is the only dermatologic manifestation but is accompanied by fever and malaise. His medical history is significant for the leukemia, tonsillectomy, and adenoidectomy at age 3 and chicken pox 4 months later. He has had all his other childhood immunizations. The most likely diagnosis in this case is:

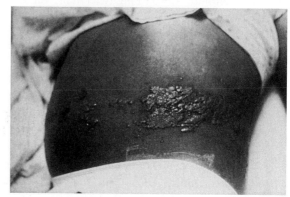

Figure 7-2. Centers for Disease Control and Prevention, National Immunization Program. (See also Color Insert).

(A) Herpes zoster

(B) Measles

(C) Molluscum contagiosum

(D) Recurrent varicella zoster

(E) Roseola

19. A 7-year-old girl is brought in by her mom for evaluation of a rash. She has had a fever for a few days and woke up this morning looking like she had been slapped on both cheeks. Other than supportive care, which instruction below represents the best patient education for this patient?

(A) She should remain out of school because she is contagious until the rash resolves.

(B) She may return to school but stay out of physical education class to avoid splenic injury.

(C) It spreads by the fecal–oral route, so she should wash her hands after using the bathroom.

(D) She may resume normal activities as her energy level improves.

20. A 22-year-old sexually active woman presents for her annual gynecologic evaluation. She reports one partner for the past 6 months and takes oral contraceptive pills as directed. Her periods have been regular. Her examination is unremarkable but her Pap smear returns with atypical squamous cells of undetermined significance and reflex testing is positive for human papillomavirus-16. Which of the following is the next most appropriate step for this patient?

(A) Colposcopy

(B) Repeat Pap smear in 12 months

(C) Repeat Pap smear in 24 months

(D) Schedule her for a loop electrosurgical excision procedure (LEEP)

21. A 55-year-old woman presents for a pre-employment physical for a nursing home where she will begin working as a certified nursing assistant. This is her first time working in a health care facility. She wonders about vaccines, specifically measles, mumps, and rubella (MMR). She does not think she has ever received any component of this vaccine but does remember having measles as a child. Which of the following is the first step in the management of this case?

(A) Tell the patient she does not need the vaccine at her age

(B) Draw titers of each component of the vaccine

(C) Give two MMR doses today and schedule for titer draw in one month

(D) Give one MMR dose today, return in 1 month for the second dose, delay employment by 1 month

22. A 25-year-old man presents for evaluation of diarrhea. He is generally healthy and reports he finished a 4-day hike about 2 weeks ago. He does mention that he ran out of water on day 3 and did not have a filter with him. Today he feels "ok" but has had 24 hours of abdominal bloating, increased flatulence, and loose stools. He denies melena or hematochezia. His physical examination is unremarkable but stool ova and parasite examination reveal ova and trophozoites. Based on the most likely diagnosis, which of the following is the most appropriate first-line therapy for this patient?

(A) No medicine needed; this is self-limiting and will resolve in 24 hours

(B) Ciprofloxacin (Cipro)

(C) Amphotericin b (Fungizone)

(D) Metronidazole (Flagyl)

23. A 2-year-old girl presents with a rash on her trunk and legs. Initially her parents state she developed a "cold" because she ran a fever for a few days. This morning her temperature was normal but she awoke with the rash. On examination, she has scattered discrete 2- to 3-mm macules on her torso with a few on her arms and legs. Her face is spared. Which of the following is the most likely cause?

(A) Measles

(B) Erythema subitum

(C) Erythema infectiosum

(D) Rubella

24. A 40-year-old male with Type 2 diabetes mellitus who was recently discharged from the hospital presents with a draining lesion on his back (see Fig. 7-3). Several days ago it began as a warm, erythematous, tender nodule. Yesterday it burst and drained copious amounts of purulent material. Which of the following is the preferred empiric therapy?

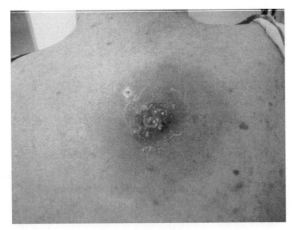

Figure 7-3. National Center for Emerging and Zoonotic Infectious Diseases, Centers for Disease Control and Prevention. Photographer: Gregory Moran, MD. (See also Color Insert).

(A) Clindamycin orally

(B) High-dose amoxicillin/clavulanate (Augmentin) orally

(C) Incision and drainage alone

(D) Incision and drainage plus high-dose amoxicillin

(E) Incision and drainage plus clindamycin

25. Which of the following purified protein derivative (PPD)-tested patients should receive antituberculosis prophylaxis?

(A) PPD of 13 mm in a person with no risk factors

(B) PPD of 8 mm in a foreign-born person from a country with a high prevalence of tuberculosis

(C) PPD of 3 mm in an HIV-positive person

(D) PPD of 6 mm in a Native American person

(E) PPD of 12 mm in an inmate at a correctional institution

26. A 32-year-old male states that he simply does not feel well. For the past several days he has experienced headache, fever, sore throat, and malaise. He reports that he is generally healthy with no chronic illnesses or history of hospitalizations or surgeries. He hesitantly reports that a couple of months ago, he developed a sore on his penis. He was embarrassed by the location, there was no urethral discharge and it did not hurt so he opted to watch and wait. It healed in about a week. He has had casual sexual encounters with two different women in the past 3 months but prior to that had the same female partner for 5 years. Which additional sign is the most commonly seen with the most likely diagnosis for this patient?

(A) Inguinal lymphadenopathy

(B) Kernig's sign

(C) Alopecia

(D) Generalized maculopapular rash

(E) Superficial painless gummas

27. A 30-year-old man presents for follow-up on an endoscopically diagnosed gastric ulcer. He was positive for *Helicobacter pylori* infection and has completed appropriate therapy. He has another refill available on the proton-pump inhibitor, but is currently asymptomatic. What is the most appropriate follow-up on the infection?

(A) No further testing is required

(B) Check urea breath test or fecal antigen today

(C) Repeat endoscopy with histologic testing for *H. pylori*

(D) Check *H. pylori* serology today

(E) Collect stool specimen for culture

28. An adult male, not previously vaccinated for rabies, presents to the emergency department after being bitten by an aggressive stray dog. The dog was captured and declared "probably rabid" by a local veterinarian. Which of the following treatment options should be administered for this patient?

(A) Human rabies immune globulin only

(B) Equine rabies antiserum only

(C) Human rabies immune globulin and equine rabies antiserum

(D) Human rabies immune globulin, equine rabies antiserum and human diploid cell rabies vaccine

(E) Human rabies immune globulin and human diploid cell rabies vaccine

29. An otherwise healthy, immunocompetent health care worker converts to a positive PPD. Which of the following drugs is the most optimal therapy for this person?

   (A) Ethambutol
   (B) Isoniazid
   (C) Pyrazinamide
   (D) Rifampin
   (E) Streptomycin

30. A 40-year-old male presents with persistent midepigastric discomfort that is most noticeable when he is hungry. Eating makes it feel better for awhile but highly spicy foods seem to aggravate it. He denies nausea or vomiting or changes in bowel habits. He does report darker than usual stools on two occasions but attributed it to something he had eaten. He is generally healthy. He does not smoke and takes no medications, prescription or over-the-counter. Upper endoscopy confirms a 1-cm ulcer in the gastric antrum with a positive campylobacter-like organism (CLO) test. Which of the following is the most effective treatment regimen for this patient?

   (A) Amoxicillin, bismuth subsalicylate and antacid
   (B) Bismuth subsalicylate, omeprazole and sucralfate
   (C) Clarithromycin, metronidazole and sucralfate
   (D) Metronidazole and omeprazole
   (E) Omeprazole, amoxicillin and clarithromycin

31. A 34-year-old woman with mitral valve prolapse is scheduled for a dental extraction. The patient has a history of penicillin allergy. Which of the following is an appropriate oral bacterial endocarditis prophylactic drug to give this patient?

   (A) Clarithromycin
   (B) Clindamycin
   (C) Doxycycline
   (D) Vancomycin

   (E) No prophylaxis for bacterial endocarditis is required for this patient

32. A 24-year-old male presents with abrupt onset of swelling, pain, redness, and increased warmth in his right knee. He denies any injury or previous joint issues. The symptoms began yesterday along with generally not feeling well and possible low-grade fever. His past medical history is unremarkable. He takes no medications and has no known drug allergies. He denies tobacco use, consumes alcohol socially with no recent episodes of heavy drinking, and follows a vegetarian diet. He is sexually active with a recent new partner. On physical examination, T: 100°F, right knee is edematous and erythematous with increased warmth and ROM decreased by pain. Left knee has no change in skin color or temperature with full pain-free ROM in flexion and extension. Examination of hip and ankle joints is unremarkable. Right knee synovial fluid analysis reveals increased leukocytes and absence of crystals. Which of the following is the most likely etiologic agent for this patient's knee pain?

   (A) *Neisseria gonorrhoeae*
   (B) *Staphylococcus aureus*
   (C) *Pseudomonas aeruginosa*
   (D) *Streptococcus pyogenes*
   (E) Bacterial etiology is not likely

33. A 30-year-old woman presents with 2 weeks of arthralgias, migrating from distal to proximal joints. It began with increased warmth and erythema in her right ankle and left knee. She has a low-grade fever and reports a history of sore throat and swollen glands about 1 month ago. Antistreptolysin O titer is positive. Which of the following is the most likely diagnosis for her joint pain?

   (A) New-onset rheumatoid arthritis
   (B) Rheumatic fever
   (C) Gonococcal arthritis
   (D) Gram-positive septic arthritis
   (E) Osteoarthritis

34. A sexually active 19-year-old woman presents with clusters of painful vesicles on an erythematous base on the vulva and cervix, accompanied by temperature of 100°F and mild malaise. She reports a history of a similar outbreak last month, which resolved in 10 days. Which of the following is most likely the finding on microscopic examination of cells from the basement of a blister treated with Giemsa stain?

(A) Gram-negative rods

(B) Gram-positive cocci in clusters

(C) Gram-positive cocci in chains

(D) Hyphae and buds

(E) Multinucleated giant cells

35. Which of the following characteristics is most helpful in distinguishing *Mycoplasma pneumoniae* as the etiologic agent in community-acquired pneumonia from other bacteria and viruses?

(A) Mycoplasma has a shorter incubation period than most viruses.

(B) Mycoplasma is more common in the elderly.

(C) Mycoplasma often follows exposure to cockroach infestation.

(D) Extrapulmonary manifestations often accompany the respiratory infection.

(E) Mycoplasma can only be diagnosed by polymerase chain reaction (PCR).

36. A 54-year-old male with a 30 pack-year smoking history presents with 2 days of fever, shortness of breath and cough productive of thick, purulent sputum. He also reports pleuritic chest pain that began today. He has hypertension that is well-controlled with HCTZ 25 mg once daily. He recalls no sick contacts though he spent the past 3 days at a conference in a hotel in another state. On physical examination, T: 101°F (oral), rest of vitals unremarkable. Lung examination reveals crackles at the left base with a few scattered wheezes throughout. Heart has regular rate and rhythm with no murmur, gallop, or rub. Initial laboratory tests demonstrate an elevated white blood cell count, decreased serum sodium and elevated liver transaminases. Sputum Gram stain does not show any organisms. Sputum culture is pending. Which of the following is the appropriate first-line empiric therapy for this patient?

(A) Ampicillin/sulbactam

(B) Azithromycin

(C) Ceftriaxone

(D) Clindamycin

(E) Vancomycin

37. A 16-year-old girl complains of a very sore throat, swollen lymph nodes, fever, and general malaise. Her examination reveals a temperature of 102.2°F (oral), enlarged exudative tonsils, tender cervical lymphadenopathy, and borderline enlarged spleen. Rapid strep screen is negative. Which of the following laboratory findings best supports the most likely diagnosis?

(A) Atypical lymphocytosis on white blood cell differential

(B) Decreased levels of antibody to Epstein–Barr viral capsid antigen

(C) Leukopenia

(D) Monocytosis on white cell differential

(E) Thrombocytosis

38. A 40-year-old farmer presents to the emergency department with shortness of breath and cough for the past 12 hours. He reports 4 to 5 days of fever, malaise, muscle aches, and headache. He denies chest pain but is experiencing marked shortness of breath with orthopnea. Until now he has been generally healthy. He reports recently cleaning out an old rat-infested hayloft to prepare for next season's hay crop. On examination, he is afebrile with crackles half way up from the bases bilaterally in posterior lung fields. Heart has a regular rate and rhythm. Abdomen is soft and nontender. Initial laboratory results include a white blood cell count of 50,000 with mildly elevated hematocrit. LDH, ALT, and AST are also elevated. Chest x-ray confirms pulmonary edema. Oxygen saturation by pulse oximetry is 86% on room air. Based on the patient's most likely diagnosis, what is the most likely etiology?

(A) Coronavirus

(B) Filovirus

(C) Flavivirus

(D) Hantavirus

(E) Human T-cell lymphotropic virus (HTLV)

39. Which of the following patients may receive a live, attenuated influenza immunization?

(A) 12-year old with hypersensitivity to eggs

(B) Otherwise healthy male on concomitant warfarin therapy

(C) 21-year old with Guillain–Barré syndrome

(D) Healthy 4-month old

(E) 6-year old with acute febrile illness

40. A 42-year-old male presents for an insurance physical examination. He reports having been hospitalized about 10 years ago after returning from a business trip to Hong Kong with a serious respiratory illness. His symptoms included fever, dry cough, and significant dyspnea. He ended up in the hospital on oxygen therapy. He was told that the doctors could not do much else for him but supportive care. Seemingly miraculously, he improved after several days and was discharged with no apparent sequelae. Which of the following was the most likely etiology for this respiratory illness?

(A) Coronavirus

(B) Flavivirus

(C) Hantavirus

(D) Respiratory syncytial virus

(E) West Nile virus

41. A 4-year-old boy presents with 5 days of fever, conjunctivitis, strawberry tongue, red lips, and injected throat. He has large, swollen, slightly tender lymph nodes in his neck and a peeling rash in the palms and soles. Which of the following is the most likely cause?

(A) Coxsackievirus

(B) Human parvovirus B19

(C) Kawasaki syndrome

(D) Measles

42. A 25-year-old woman presents not feeling well 1 week after returning from a trip to central Africa. She has had steadily increasing fever, abdominal distention, and diarrhea. She also has rashes on her abdomen, chest, and back, which are characterized by 3-mm pink papules that blanch with pressure. Heart rate is 60 beats/min. Blood culture is positive but final identification is pending. Which of the following is the most likely diagnosis?

(A) Hepatitis

(B) Malaria

(C) Shigellosis

(D) Typhoid fever

(E) Yellow fever

43. In a patient with high fever, malaise, and severe myalgias, which of the following additional pieces of history would raise the index of suspicion for plague?

(A) History of tick bite in the northeastern United States

(B) Exposure to wild rats in Southern California

(C) History of drinking stream water while hiking in the Appalachian mountains

(D) History of raising sheep in Wyoming

(E) Exposure to exotic birds in upper Midwest

44. A 14-year-old girl presents 1 week after the neighbor's cat bit her hand. In the first 3 days after the bite she developed a shallow ulcer at the bite site. Because her parents knew the cat was up to date on shots, they treated the ulcer with topical antibiotics and did not seek medical care. Now, the patient has low-grade fever and headache and feels tired. Axillary nodes on the affected side are swollen. The ulcer on the hand is nearly healed. Which of the following is the best treatment option at this time?

(A) Acyclovir

(B) Amoxicillin/clavulanate

(C) Azithromycin

(D) Doxycycline

(E) No therapy required

45. A 27-year-old woman presents with 3 days of fever, chills, headache, and a deep dry cough. She has been working at a pet store for the past month and thinks that one of the parakeets that came in 10 days ago may be sick. On examination, she has dullness to percussion of the right lung base and right-sided coarse crackles. Which of the following is the most likely diagnosis?

(A) Brucellosis

(B) Listeriosis

(C) Psittacosis

(D) Sarcoidosis

(E) Tularemia

46. A 35-year-old forest ranger presents with a rash on his back. It started 4 days ago as a red maculopapular lesion about 2 cm in diameter. The lesion is currently 14 cm in diameter with an area of central clearing. In addition to the rash, he has had a headache, fever, chills, and muscle aches. Based on the most likely diagnosis, which of the following is the gold standard test for diagnosis?

(A) Complete blood count

(B) ELISA followed by western blot

(C) Erythema migrans rash is pathognomonic; no laboratory test required

(D) Erythrocyte sedimentation rate

(E) Indirect immunofluorescence assay (IFA)

47. A 32-year-old, $G_3P_2Ab_0$ woman presents to the emergency department running a fever with a sore throat, headache, and significant malaise. She is 34 weeks' pregnant and has sole responsibility for her two small children and two cats. Since her divorce she has been uninsured and has had no prenatal care for this pregnancy. She has been working extra hours to make ends meet and states she feels like she did when she had mononucleosis in high school. The emergency room provider reassures her that her course of illness will likely resolve spontaneously. Which of the following has the greatest potential for harmful sequelae to the fetus?

(A) Brucellosis

(B) Echinococcosis

(C) Leishmaniasis

(D) Schistosomiasis

(E) Toxoplasmosis

48. A 42-year-old homeless man presents to the emergency department with fever, painful muscle spasms in his arms and legs, and difficulty eating because of painful spasms in his jaw muscles. Until a week ago, he was wandering around the city looking for food and work and taking shelter in a commercial construction site. He reports not having seen a medical professional in more than 15 years. Examination of his feet reveals shoes with holes in the soles and a small, puncture-type wound on the bottom of the right foot. It is surrounded by erythema and somewhat tender to touch. The patient is uncertain what he may have stepped on. X-ray is negative for any radiopaque foreign body. In addition to hospital admission, which of the following is the first-line therapy for this patient?

(A) Tetanus immune globulin, tetanus toxoid, and metronidazole

(B) Tetanus immune globulin and penicillin

(C) Tetanus toxoid and penicillin

(D) Tetanus immune globulin, tetanus toxoid, and penicillin

(E) Tetanus immune globulin and tetanus toxoid

49. A 73-year-old man is hospitalized for a prolonged period because his prostate surgery was complicated by pneumonia. After 10 days of broad-spectrum antibiotics, he developed fever, leukocytosis, and dysentery. Colonoscopy reveals pseudomembranes in his colon. Stool cultures are pending. Which of the following is the most likely etiology for his diarrhea?

(A) Enterobacteriaceae

(B) *Clostridium difficile*

(C) *Clostridium perfringens*

(D) *Norwalk virus*

(E) *Pseudomonas aeruginosa*

50. A 37-year-old male presents with fever, malaise, headache and cough and a skin lesion on his arm. He reports that the lesion began as a blister on his forearm that evolved into an ulcer. It oozed very little but he kept it covered with a bandage. He is a dairy farmer, milks cows daily and has been cleaning barns. He thought he scratched it on something and got a little infection because he gets so dirty by the end of his workday. Examination reveals a painless, black eschar around the area and swollen axillary lymph nodes. Gram stain of the fluid form the lesion reveals boxcar-shaped encapsulated rods in chains. Which of the following is the preferred first-line therapy for this patient?

(A) Amoxicillin

(B) Ciprofloxacin

(C) Dicloxacillin

(D) Erythromycin

(E) Metronidazole

Answers and Explanations

1. **(C)** The clinical presentation is consistent with vulvovaginal candidiasis. The recent oral antibiotic use increased her risk for developing the infection. The white clumpy discharge and relatively benign bimanual examination support the diagnosis, which is confirmed by 10% potassium hydroxide wet mount of the secretions. Treatment for an uncomplicated case may include topical or oral antifungals. Oral fluconazole in the one dose regimen is effective, convenient, and likely to increase compliance. The metronidazole regimens are appropriate for bacterial vaginosis and trichomoniasis, respectively. Ceftriaxone is an option for gonococcal infection and would likely worsen the candidiasis. Azithromycin is appropriate for suspected chlamydial infection. *(Morazzo & Holmes, 2012, Ch. 130)*

2. **(D)** Patients with HIV infections are at increased risk for ordinary bacterial pneumonias as their immune systems begin to decline in function. Community-acquired pneumonia (*S. pneumoniae* or *H. influenzae* among the most common etiologies) is the most common pulmonary disorder in HIV-infected patients. The clinical picture and lobar infiltrate on x-ray are consistent with typical community-acquired pneumonia, most often caused by *S. pneumoniae*. *P. jirovecii* pneumonia is unlikely until the CD4 count drops below 250 cells/mm^3. Mycobacterial pneumonia would likely be associated with a more chronic cough and the others are not likely to cause pulmonary disease. *(Katz & Zolopa, 2015, Ch. 31)*

3. **(E)** Prophylaxis against opportunistic infections is an important part of management in the HIV-infected patient. Prophylaxis for Pneumocystis pneumonia (PCP) with trimethoprim/sulfamethoxazole is initiated when the CD4 cell count drops below 200 cells/mm^3 or with recurrent episodes of thrush. Toxoplasma prophylaxis with trimethoprim/sulfamethoxazole is recommended when the CD4 count drops below 100 cells/mm^3. Mycobacterium avium prevention with azithromycin or clarithromycin and cytomegalovirus retinitis (CMV) prevention are considered when the CD4 count drops below 50 to 75 cells/mm^3, though in the case of CMV, the preferred approach is early initiation of effective antiretroviral therapy. Rifampin is recommended to prevent *Mycobacterium tuberculosis* infection in those resistant to isoniazid and with a tuberculin skin test reaction measuring greater than 5 mm. *(Katz & Zolopa, 2015, Ch. 31)*

4. **(B)** *Cryptococcus neoformans* is an opportunistic organism responsible for infections in immune-compromised hosts. *Cryptococcus gattii* is a second species that was formerly seen more often in immune-competent hosts in a tropical setting but is now being isolated in patients in the United States as well. The two most common areas for infection are the lungs and the central nervous system. Pulmonary involvement includes fever, productive cough, chest discomfort, and weight loss. Pleural effusions, lymphadenopathy, and solitary or multiple nodules can all be seen on chest x-ray. Central nervous system manifestations include meningitis and meningoencephalitis. Diagnosis is confirmed with India ink prep of cerebrospinal fluid showing yeast or histologic stains of tissue from the involved organs. Treatment is with oral or parenteral antifungal agents. Pneumocystis is an opportunistic organism causing an interstitial pneumonia in the immune compromised. The other options do not result in nodular lesions on chest x-ray. *(Lofland, Josephat & Kogut, 2014)*

5. **(C)** Histoplasmosis is found throughout the continental United States with greater concentration in the Ohio and Mississippi river valleys. It is found in soil, particularly in areas with large quantities of decaying wood or bird droppings. Bats also carry histoplasma. Histoplasma infection may be asymptomatic or present as a lung infection with cavitary lung lesions on chest x-ray. It may become disseminated in the immunocompromised host. Cryptococcus is most likely in people exposed to pigeons and is also found in soil enriched by bird droppings or in cockroach-infested environments. Parrots, parakeets, ducks, and turkeys are the usual hosts and most commonly infected species for psittacoccal infections as well. It is less common in humans. Candidal respiratory infections are more likely in immunocompromised hosts. *(Levinson, 2012, Ch. 49)*

6. **(B)** *C. botulinum* produces a neurotoxin that can lead to life-threatening illness including respiratory paralysis. Botulism infection is caused by the spore-forming bacteria that lives in soil and can be foodborne. In the latter case, home-canned foods are often the cause. After a 12-hour to 3-day incubation period, botulism begins with classic symptoms of abdominal pain, nausea, vomiting, and mild diarrhea and, if unchecked, evolves into a progressive neurologic disorder marked by double vision, motor weakness, and ptosis. Respiratory muscle involvement may occur ultimately and result in death. Because of the virulence of the neurotoxin it has been used as an agent of bioterrorism. Cholera and enterotoxigenic *E. coli* cause a foodborne diarrheal illness that can result in significant morbidity and mortality, but they do not have neurologic manifestations. Pinworm infection is usually found among younger children, is marked by severe anal itching, and fecal–oral transmission. *(Rosenthal, 2015, Ch. 35; Schwartz, 2015, Ch.33)*

7. **(E)** Salmonella enteritidis infection, caused by consuming raw eggs, is the most likely diagnosis in this case. It is one of several serotypes that cause nontyphoidal salmonellosis in the United States. Infection is characterized by fever, abdominal cramps, diarrhea (sometimes with blood) following a 6- to 48-hour incubation period. Most cases are self-limited, resolving within a week. For this reason, they are usually managed with supportive care only. In the rare case in which sepsis occurs, the patient should be hospitalized and treated with trimethoprim sulfamethoxazole or a fluoroquinolone. *(Pegues & Miller, 2012, Ch. 153)*

8. **(C)** Shigella and salmonella poisonings include fever, cramping, and bloody diarrhea but only shigella is known to progress to seizures in children. Salmonella is generally self-limited and resolves with supportive care. Cholera is a waterborne infection with large volume diarrhea and associated dehydration and also has the potential to result in sepsis. *Escherichia coli* presents with vomiting and crampy, watery diarrhea but not usually bloody stools nor does it cause seizures. *(Bernard et al., 2012, Ch. 25)*

9. **(E)** *V. cholerae* infection can be transmitted through wounds but the most often reported cause is eating undercooked shellfish or drinking contaminated water. The clinical picture most often includes a profuse, watery diarrhea that can lead to dehydration. In the immune compromised host, overwhelming sepsis is possible. First-line therapy includes azithromycin or doxycycline. Salmonella infection is associated with consumption of raw eggs and undercooked chicken or beef. Shigella is transmitted by the fecal–oral route, often because of poor hygiene. Giardia is waterborne and hookworms are found in the soil. *(Rosenthal, 2015, Ch. 35; Schwartz, 2015, Ch. 33)*

10. **(B)** The clues to the etiology of this presentation include the gray pseudomembranes on the tonsils and the lack of medical care resulting in missed childhood vaccines. *Corynebacterium diphtheriae* causes a respiratory and posterior pharyngeal infection with little likelihood of sepsis. However, the case fatality rate is high with mortality from neurologic impairment increasing the longer treatment is delayed. Because it releases a toxin into the local tissue in the throat, a tough gray colored pseudomembrane over the tonsils is the classic clinical finding. Although culture on special medium of a specimen collected from beneath the membrane confirms the diagnosis, therapy should be started based on clinical suspicion and includes parenteral penicillin or erythromycin. Vaccination with diphtheria toxin is preventive. *B. pertussis* infection is marked by the characteristic whooping cough. *S. pyogenes* usually manifests with tonsillar exudate

without membranes and palatal petechiae and in this case is ruled out by the negative rapid strep test. *H. influenzae* in a 3-year-old may result in an epiglottitis, ear infection, or pneumonia. *(Schwartz, 2015, Ch. 33)*

11. **(D)** The clinical presentation is consistent with cervicitis in a young woman with risk factors for sexually transmitted infection. She has likely been exposed specifically to *N. gonorrhoeae*. Coinfection with *Chlamydia trachomatis* is common. While test results are pending, the Centers for Disease Control and Prevention in its 2010 Guidelines for STI treatment recommend treating for both with ceftriaxone IM and either doxycycline or azithromycin first line. Quinolones no longer have a place in therapy because of resistance. Metronidazole is the appropriate therapy for trichomoniasis and fluconazole for vaginal candidiasis. *(Centers for Disease Control and Prevention (CDC), 2012, p. 590)*

12. **(A)** *E. histolytica* has two stages in its life cycle. In the active stage in the human intestine, it causes symptoms of dysentery, abdominal pain, stool mucus, and tenesmus. In the dormant stage, the cystic form is excreted in the stool and in developing nations frequently contaminates the supply of drinking water. When the amoeba is in the dormant stage, the cystic form can be excreted in the stool and, in the case of food handlers with poor personal hygiene, be transmitted to others. In addition, because of the cystic stage, individuals engaging in anal intercourse can transmit the infection unknowingly. The other choices are less likely to be transmitted sexually. Of the other options cholera is also transmitted through contaminated water but it causes larger volume watery diarrhea without blood. Salmonella also causes cramping and has a much shorter incubation period than *E. histolytica*. Hematochezia is also uncommon in Giardia infection. Diagnosis is made by microscopic evaluation of a stool wet prep and confirmed by serology. Treatment includes agents such as metronidazole or tinidazole. *(Rosenthal, 2015, Ch. 35; Schwartz, 2015, Ch. 33)*

13. **(A)** As described, hookworms generally enter through the skin and travel to the lungs. There they migrate to the mouth, are swallowed, and reproduce in the gut. Females lay thousands of eggs, which are subsequently excreted in the feces and mature in soil. The adult worms attach to the intestinal wall, causing bleeding and a subsequent anemia. They can also affect absorption, leading to nutritional deficiencies. Diagnosis is made through microscopic evaluation of a stool specimen and treatment is with albendazole. Whipworms (*Trichuris trichiura*) also lay eggs in the stool, which then reside in the soil. Many whipworm infections are asymptomatic. Strongyloides is different from other nematodes in that it can reproduce inside the intestine and persist for years. Pinworms (enterobiasis) are very small worms that exit the anus at night to lay eggs, causing intense itching and promoting the fecal–oral transmission. *(Weller & Nutman, 2012, Ch. 217)*

14. **(D)** Malaria is the most common cause of fever and hospitalization in travelers returning to the United States. Those with no history of exposure develop the most severe cases. There are four species of plasmodium causing human malarial infections in the United States, with *Plasmodium falciparum* and *Plasmodium vivax* being the most common and *P. falciparum* causing the most severe disease. Most U.S. travelers contract malaria in West Africa. *P. falciparum* has a shorter incubation period (up to 30 days). Symptoms are variable but may include fever, nausea, vomiting, abdominal pain, myalgias, and arthralgias. On physical examination, some patients will be tachycardic and hypotensive progressing to altered mental status. Complete blood cell count (CBC) may show erythrocytopenia and thrombocytopenia and atypical lymphocytosis on peripheral smear. Confirmation is obtained with Giemsa-stained peripheral smears. Treatment of uncomplicated cases includes atovaquone-proguanil when resistance is unknown or chloroquine phosphate for those who are sensitive. Dengue is the second most common cause of fever in returning travelers and has a much shorter incubation period. Clinical presentation usually includes fever, chills, headache, lymphadenopathy, and myalgias. Severe back pain may occur as well. Enteric fevers include typhoid and paratyphoid and are more common in those returning from the Indian subcontinent. Symptoms are constitutional and physical examination may include organomegaly. CBC shows pancytopenia and LFTs are often elevated. The organisms may be cultured from blood, urine, stool, or bone marrow. Treatment is with fluoroquinolones.

Leptospirosis is much less common. Transmission is through contact with infected animals' urine or body tissue. Cases have been reported in those who swam in infected water. Clinical pattern is often biphasic with two periods of fever and constitutional symptoms. Diagnosis is confirmed with serology or culture and treatment is with doxycycline or amoxicillin. *(CDC, 2013; Philip, 2015, Ch. 34; Schwartz, 2015, Ch. 33; Shandera & Kelly, 2015, Ch. 32)*

15. **(D)** Rocky Mountain spotted fever (RMSF) is a rickettsial infection caused by *Rickettsia rickettsiae.* The organism is transmitted to humans through the bite of the dog tick and is more common among those who spend time outdoors in a wooded area. The illness begins with generalized symptoms of fever, headache, nausea, vomiting, malaise, and myalgias. The rash of RMSF begins as a macular rash and progresses to nonblanching petechiae. The rash begins over the wrists and ankles and progresses to the arms, legs, and trunk. Untreated, it can progress to respiratory failure and/or central nervous system involvement. Serologic confirmation is not usually valid until 7 to 10 days after clinical symptoms begin so treatment is often started empirically. Drug of choice is doxycycline until the patient is afebrile and clinically better for 2 to 3 days. Lyme disease is distinguished from RMSF by the pattern of the rash. Lyme disease is characterized by the classic erythema chronicum migrans rash, usually on the trunk. Ehrlichiosis usually does not manifest with a rash. It begins with the same general symptoms but can progress to a toxic shock syndrome. Q fever can be transmitted by ticks, but it is often acquired through contact with sheep, cattle, and goats. It has similar generalized symptoms but can progress to a cough and pneumonia. It is usually without rash. *(Steere, 2012, Ch. 173; Walker, Dumler & Marrie, 2012, Ch. 174)*

16. **(C)** The description best fits that of measles. It has a 7 to 10 day incubation period followed by 3 days of coryza, fever, and conjunctival involvement. The prodrome dissipates as the characteristic rash develops first on the head and face and then the trunk. Koplik spots are the pathognomonic white spots that occur on the buccal mucosa in measles infection. Herpes simplex infection can present as painful vesicles on the mouth and lips (HSV-1) or genitalia (HSV-2). It is preceded by fever and a tingling or burning sensation at the site where the vesicle will develop. Coxsackievirus causes hand, foot, and mouth disease with lesion distribution in those three areas. Rubella has a longer incubation period (2–2.5 weeks) and is less contagious than measles. It is sometimes asymptomatic or produces a milder course than measles. *(Berger, 2015, Ch. 6; Shandera & Kelly, 2015, Ch. 32)*

17. **(A)** The description best fits that of herpes simplex. Serotype HSV-1 is usually acquired in childhood and may be asymptomatic or severe enough to produce a painful stomatitis. Subsequent outbreaks may be triggered by fever, other infection, stress, or excess sun exposure and are characterized by orolabial outbreak along the trigeminal nerve producing a painful vesicle which over 10 to 14 days crusts over and resolves. Treatment with topical or oral antivirals (such as acyclovir) shortens the course and lessens the severity if started early. Parvovirus and herpesvirus 6 do not have a period of latency. Varicella zoster does have a latency period but often in a spinal nerve or the ophthalmic branch of the trigeminal with rare orolabial involvement. *(Berger, 2015, Ch. 6; Shandera & Kelly, 2015, Ch. 32)*

18. **(A)** Herpes zoster outbreak (shingles) most often occurs in an elderly patient years after experiencing chicken pox (caused by varicella zoster virus) as a child or having received the immunization. The varicella zoster virus lies dormant in the spinal nerve root and later manifests as a very painful, skin-sensitive vesicular rash in a dermatomal distribution. Unlike chicken pox, a postherpetic neuralgia pain can persist for years and is, at times, debilitating. Although most common in the elderly, herpes zoster can occur in children in immunocompromised states such as those with malignancy or human immunodeficiency virus infection. Molluscum contagiosum presents with flesh colored, umbilicated papules and is typically not painful. Measles and roseola are maculopapular rashes. *(Berger, 2015, Ch. 6; Shandera & Kelly, 2015, Ch. 32)*

19. **(D)** The "slapped cheek" appearance to the rash is consistent with a Parvovirus B19 etiology for erythema infectiosum. It is a droplet infection that is no longer contagious once the rash breaks out. It generally has a benign course and patients recover

fully with supportive care. Splenic involvement is not typically a part of the course, so she may resume activities as she feels able. *(Shandera & Kelly, 2015, Ch. 32)*

20. **(B)** Human papillomavirus subtypes 6, 11, 16, and 18 increase risk for the development of cervical cancer. In a young woman over 21 years old with atypical squamous cells of undetermined significance (ASC-US) and positive HPV 16 subtype, the next step in evaluation is to repeat cytology in 12 months. If the results are negative, ASC-US or low-grade squamous intraepithelial lesion (LSIL) cytology is repeated once again in 12 months. At that point, a negative finding leads to a return to routine screening. If either cytology reports reveal a higher-grade lesion, the next step is colposcopy. *(American Society for Colposcopy and Cervical Pathology, 2013)*

21. **(B)** Adults born after 1957 need documentation of completion of the MMR series or serologic evidence of immunity to each component. In this case, the patient has a history of clinical measles, but no proof of mumps. The first step is to draw serologic titers of each component of the vaccine. If the titer does not demonstrate immunity to measles or mumps, two doses of MMR are recommended, 28 days apart. One dose of MMR is usually enough to confer rubella immunity if the rubella titer is the only one that does not demonstrate immunity. *(CDC, 2014)*

22. **(D)** The clinical picture is consistent with infection with *G. lamblia*, a parasite that can be picked up from contaminated water and infects the small intestine. It can be difficult to diagnose because it may be clinically asymptomatic. Nevertheless, an infected person passes the cysts in the stool and they can survive for weeks in cold water. Infection can also be transmitted by direct fecal–oral route, especially among small children and their caregivers. Clinical symptoms vary but often include bloating, loose stools or diarrhea, belching, and possibly weight loss. The course can be episodic. Diagnosis is made with stool specimen examined for ova and parasites or by stool antigen immunoassay. First-line therapy is metronidazole 250 mg orally every 8 hours for 5 days. Tinidazole is an effective alternative. *(Weller, 2012, Ch. 215)*

23. **(B)** Erythema subitum or roseola is caused by the human herpesvirus 6 and presents clinically as described. The fever resolves when the rash begins and the entire process is self-limiting with usual full recovery with supportive care. The key to this question is that the rash spares the face. Erythema infectiosum (fifth disease), rubella, and measles also begin with a febrile prodrome, but each of the associated rashes starts on the head or face before progressing to other parts of the body. *(Kaye & Kaye, 2012, Ch. 17)*

24. **(E)** In recent years, the prevalence of community-acquired methicillin-resistant *S. aureus* (CA-MRSA) infection has increased. CA-MRSA can manifest in a variety of ways but soft tissue abscess is among the more common. Controversy around treatment options exists but currently, for an uncomplicated abscess, incision and drainage alone is recommended. In prospective studies to date, adding antibiotics provided no additional benefit for uncomplicated infections. However, this patient may have contracted the infection during his recent hospitalization and his course is complicated by comorbid diabetes. For this reason, antibiotics are recommended in addition to incision and drainage. The Infectious Disease Society of America offers the following options for empiric therapy: clindamycin, trimethoprim-sulfamethoxazole, doxycycline, or linezolid. Regardless of empiric choice, sensitivity reports are key to definitive treatment. *(Schwartz, 2015, Ch. 33)*

25. **(E)** Recommendations by the Advisory Committee for the Elimination of Tuberculosis indicate that the following high-risk groups should receive preventive chemotherapy if their tuberculin skin test (PPD) is ≥10 mm: 1. Foreign-born persons from high-prevalence countries; 2. Medically underserved, low-income populations, including high-risk racial or ethnic minority populations; 3. Residents and employees of facilities for long-term care (e.g., correctional facilities, nursing homes); 4. Injection drug users who are HIV negative; 5. Children younger than 4 years or children and adolescents in contact with high-risk adults; and 6. Laboratory employees working in mycobacteriology. Patients who are HIV positive, those who have been in contact with others with active TB infection, those with fibrotic chest x-ray findings, and immunosuppressed patients

should be treated prophylactically when the area of induration following their PPD is ≥5 mm. For all others, a positive finding involves an indurated area ≥15 mm. *(Chesnutt & Prendergast, 2015, Ch. 9)*

26. **(D)** Secondary syphilis generally manifests a month or two after appearance of the primary chancre. Patients will complain of headache, fever, sore throat, and malaise and will exhibit generalized lymphadenopathy along with a maculopapular rash that begins at the sides of the trunk and later spreads over the rest of the body. The skin lesions may coalesce in warm moist areas, such as the perineum, and form large, flat-topped, pale papules termed *condyloma lata*. Skin and mucosal lesions are the most common signs of secondary syphilis. Kernig's sign (associated with aseptic meningitis) and alopecia may also occur in secondary syphilis. Formation of granulomatous nodules (*gummas*) is not a feature of secondary disease, but rather is the hallmark of tertiary syphilis. *(Philip, 2015, Ch. 34)*

27. **(D)** *H. pylori* is a spiral, gram-negative rod that resides in the gastric mucosa, where it causes PUD. It may be diagnosed by rapid urease test or by histology when endoscopy is performed. Noninvasive *H. pylori* testing options include the urease breath test, fecal antigen testing, and serology. Serological and fecal antigen tests are the most cost-effective methods. All three noninvasive tests have sensitivities and specificities greater than 90%. Proton-pump inhibitor therapy should be discontinued 1 to 2 weeks prior to the fecal antigen or breath tests because PPIs may increase the number of false negatives. In this case, serology is the least invasive, most cost-effective, and least likely to be invalidated by the proton-pump inhibitor therapy. *(McQuaid, 2014, Ch. 15)*

28. **(E)** Transmission of rabies to this patient must be seriously considered, and postexposure immunization should begin immediately by the administration of human rabies immune globulin (HRIG; 20 units/kg). About half the HRIG should be infiltrated around the bite wound, with the rest injected into a muscle in a location away from the injury. Human diploid cell rabies vaccine (HDCV) should also be given (1 mL IM in the deltoid), and again on days 3, 7, and 14. HDCV should be delivered in a different syringe and administered at a different site from HRIG. The role of equine antiserum is limited to situations in which HRIG is not available. Testing for sensitivity to horse serum should precede administration. *(Shandera & Kelly, 2015, Ch. 32)*

29. **(B)** The drug of choice for prophylaxis of tuberculosis is isoniazid (INH), given at a daily dose of 300 mg/day for 9 months (children: 10 to 14 mg/kg/day). The major risk of INH prophylaxis is drug-induced hepatitis, especially in the elderly. Therefore, periodic monitoring of liver function tests during the course of INH treatment is recommended for persons aged 35 and older. Minor transferase elevations (up to three times normal) are not indications to discontinue therapy. *(Chesnutt & Prendergast, 2015, Ch. 9)*

30. **(E)** Combination therapy is recommended for eradication of *H. pylori*-associated PUD. Administration of a proton-pump inhibitor (omeprazole or lansoprazole) and two antibiotics (clarithromycin and either amoxicillin or metronidazole) achieves eradication rates of over 80%. However, emerging resistance of *H. pylori* to metronidazole makes amoxicillin preferable for combination therapy. Regimens using bismuth compounds require two antibiotics plus a proton-pump inhibitor (quadruple therapy) to enhance efficacy. Also, bismuth regimens are associated with a higher incidence of side effects than are PPI regimens. Antacids and sucralfate are outdated as primary therapy for PUD. *(McQuaid, 2014, Ch. 15)*

31. **(E)** In 2007, the American Heart Association (AHA) updated its recommendations for bacterial endocarditis prophylaxis. Because of insufficient evidence for a decrease in morbidity or mortality with many cases in which prophylaxis was previously administered, the AHA now recommends antibiotic prophylaxis prior to dental procedures only for those with prosthetic heart valves, a personal history of infective endocarditis, unrepaired cyanotic heart disease, congenital heart disease repaired with prosthetic device, repaired congenital heart disease with residual problems or those with heart valve disease following heart transplant. Amoxicillin 2 g orally 1 hour before the procedure is the standard regimen. Patients who have a history of amoxicillin/penicillin allergy may be given clindamycin, cephalexin, azithromycin, or clarithromycin. For

adults, 600 mg of clindamycin is given orally 1 hour before the procedure. *(Schwartz, 2015, Ch. 33)*

32. **(A)** In otherwise healthy young adult patients, gonococcus is the most common cause of septic arthritis. When all patients are considered, *S. aureus* is the most common cause. Group B streptococcus is another important cause in adults. Patients with prevalent joint disease and intravenous drug users are especially susceptible to *Staphylococcus*. *Pseudomonas* is also a common cause of septic arthritis in intravenous drug users. *(Hellmann & Imboden, 2015, Ch. 20)*

33. **(B)** Rheumatic fever is an immune-mediated process occurring in response to prior infection with Group A *Streptococcus*. The arthritis often moves from one large joint to another in an asymmetrical pattern. In some cases there may be cardiac symptoms, skin rash (erythema marginatum), and subcutaneous nodules. Antistreptolysin O titer is often positive. It is important to quickly diagnose rheumatic fever because it requires long-term prophylaxis against *Streptococcus*. Osteoarthritis usually presents in an older patient, involving weight-bearing joints. Gonococcal and septic arthritis are likely to have a quicker onset and will not have the positive antistreptolysin O titer. For both rheumatoid and osteoarthritis, stiffness is an important symptom as well. *(Bashore et al., 2015, Ch. 10)*

34. **(E)** The clinical presentation is consistent with herpes simplex. The described microscopic study is a Tzanck smear, prepared by staining cells from the floor of an unroofed vesicle using Papanicolaou, Giemsa, or Wright methods. The Tzanck smear will show multinucleated giant cells. However, because the sensitivity is low and few clinicians are skilled in the procedure, the infection should be confirmed by identification of viral DNA or viral culture. Gram-positive cocci are consistent with staphylococcal or streptococcal infection and gram-negative rods are usually enteric pathogens. Hyphae and buds are seen on KOH prep with candidal infection. *(Corey, 2012, Ch. 179)*

35. **(E)** The incubation period for mycoplasma is actually longer than that of most viruses (weeks vs. days). Mycoplasma is much more common in adolescents and young adults than in the elderly. Exposure to

insects is associated with Q fever or tularemia, rather than mycoplasma. While extrapulmonary manifestations do occur, they usually happen in patients who do not have respiratory symptoms and they are rare relative to the incidence of *M. pneumoniae* pneumonia. The most commonly employed diagnostic test is polymerase chain reaction (PCR) of respiratory secretions. *(Hardy, 2012, Ch. 175)*

36. **(B)** The patient's presentation is consistent with Legionnaire's disease. Though often considered an atypical pneumonia because of the negative sputum Gram stain, it does present with high fever and pleuritic chest pain. Legionella infection is a relatively common cause of community-acquired pneumonia and is often transmitted through contaminated water or air-conditioning systems. It is more common in smokers, those with chronic lung disease and the immunocompromised. First-line therapy for legionella pneumonia (mild to moderate) in the immunocompetent host is oral azithromycin 500 mg once daily or oral clarithromycin 500 mg twice daily or oral levofloxacin 750 mg once daily for 10 to 14 days. Severe infection or treatment in the immunocompromised patient requires 21 days of therapy. *(Schwartz, 2015, Ch. 33)*

37. **(A)** With a negative rapid strep screen, the most likely explanation for this presentation is acute infectious mononucleosis. The fever, fatigue, tonsillar hypertrophy, and splenomegaly are all classic symptoms and signs. Laboratory evaluation often includes an elevated total white blood cell count with increased atypical lymphocytes on differential. Platelets may be decreased. Initially, IgM antibodies for the Epstein–Barr virus, and viral capsid antigen (VCA) levels will be elevated. Later, the IgG levels increase and IgM normalizes. *(Roig & Shandera, 2014, Ch. 32)*

38. **(D)** Hantavirus has a rodent vector and usually manifests in either hemorrhagic fever or Hantavirus pulmonary syndrome, which can rapidly progress to shock and adult respiratory distress syndrome; it may be fatal. In the United States, outbreaks are usually in the southwest. HTLV is a lymphotropic oncovirus associated with lymphoma. Dengue and yellow fever are both caused by Flaviviridae, which is carried by mosquitoes. Filoviruses cause Ebola fever and Marburg fever. The vector is unknown.

Coronavirus is the etiologic agent in severe acute respiratory syndrome. During the 2002 to 2003 epidemic that began in Southeast Asia, it was postulated that it was carried by the masked palm civet. *(Roig & Shandera, 2014, Ch. 32)*

39. **(B)** Influenza vaccine is an important adjunct to clinical and public health practice. The vaccine is produced from different components and is recommended yearly in the fall for anyone over 6 months of age. It is contraindicated in those with hypersensitivity to the vaccine or eggs and in patients with Guillain–Barré syndrome, or acute febrile illness. It may be administered following resolution of the fever. Patients on steroids or warfarin are able to take it if they have no other contraindication. The recombinant influenza vaccine (RIV) does not contain egg proteins. *(Roig & Shandera, 2014, Ch. 32)*

40. **(A)** SARS was first identified in 2003 in the Guangdong province in China and its etiologic organism is coronavirus. It appears to be transmitted when mucous membranes are contacted by respiratory droplets or fomites. SARS has been identified in people of all ages. It has an incubation period of less than 1 week and presents with symptoms consistent with atypical pneumonia, including fever, cough, dyspnea, headache, sore throat, myalgias and, in some, watery diarrhea. Rales and rhonchi may be heard on physical examination. None of the symptoms or physical examination findings is diagnostic. Several laboratory studies may return abnormal results including decreased WBCs and platelets. Liver functions and coagulation studies may also be abnormal. Arterial oxygen saturation is often low. Chest CT may show ground-glass opacifications. Supportive care, including oxygenation, is the treatment of choice. *(Roig & Shandera, 2014, Ch. 32)*

41. **(C)** Kawasaki syndrome occurs throughout the world, primarily in children. It is thought to be infectious but the etiologic agent has never been isolated. The syndrome is composed of fever and four of five of the following symptoms: bilateral conjunctivitis, some type of mucous membrane change, a peripheral extremity change, transverse grooves on the nails, a polymorphous rash, and cervical lymph nodes >1.5 cm. It can be complicated by arteritis. Treatment may include aspirin, immune

globulin, TNF blockers, or corticosteroids. Echocardiogram is indicated during the evaluation. If cardiac aneurysm is identified, anticoagulation with warfarin and/or heparin should be initiated as well. Measles commonly presents with pathognomonic Koplik spots (erythematous lesions with whitish center on buccal mucosa). Coxsackie virus manifests in a variety of clinical syndromes that may mimic coxsackievirus. However, the rash of coxsackie tends to be vesicular. There may also be a loss of fingernails and toenails and an oral stomatitis rather than the strawberry tongue and peeling rash of Kawasaki syndrome. Fifth disease (parvovirus B19) presents with a rash with a classic "slapped cheek" appearance. *(Shandera & Kelly, 2015, Ch. 32)*

42. **(D)** Typhoid fever is caused by *Salmonella typhus*. It is contracted by contaminated food or water. There are several endemic areas throughout Africa. Symptoms and signs may be nonspecific but often include blanchable, pink, papular rash over the trunk and a fever that increases in stepwise fashion. Blood culture is positive in 80% of cases in the first week. Abdominal symptoms may include distention and constipation, initially, followed by diarrhea and, possibly, splenomegaly. Prevention is not always accomplished but is recommended for close contacts with multidose oral or single-dose injectable vaccine. The predominant symptoms with shigellosis are diarrhea (often with blood and mucus) and constitutional symptoms without the skin involvement. Yellow fever begins with fever and constitutional symptoms and in its more advanced form, includes bradycardia, hypotension, and jaundice. Malaria presents with episodic bouts of high fever, chills and sweats, separated by relatively asymptomatic periods. As the infection progresses, other body systems may be involved including possible seizures. The course of illness for hepatitis varies from asymptomatic to severe illness but commonly involves fever and jaundice as the skin manifestation. *(Friedman, 2015, Ch. 16; Rosenthal, 2015, Ch. 35; Schwartz, 2015, Ch. 33; Shandera & Kelly, 2015, Ch 32)*

43. **(B)** The etiology of plague is the *Yersinia pestis* bacterium. Plague is transmitted by direct contact with wild rodents or fleabites by fleas that have bitten the rodents. Droplet transmission is also possible with exposure to an infected human host. Symptoms include high fever, increased heart rate, malaise, and headache. There may be signs of meningitis in addition to axillary, cervical, and inguinal adenopathy. Lymph nodes are very swollen and may drain purulent material. Central nervous system changes can progress to coma, and in "black plague," purpuras are visible on the skin. Blood and aspirate cultures confirm the diagnosis. Treatment is with streptomycin or gentamycin. *Y. pestis* must also be considered as a possible agent of bioterrorism. Southern California is one of the endemic areas for *Y. pestis*. A tick bite in the northeast puts the patient at risk for Lyme disease. Consuming unfiltered Appalachian stream water is a risk factor for Giardia infection. Q fever can be carried by sheep and psittacosis is carried by parrots and parakeets. *(Philip, 2015, Ch. 34; Rosenthal, 2015, Ch. 35; Schwartz, 2015, Ch. 33)*

44. **(E)** The history and course of illness are consistent with cat-scratch fever. It is caused by infection with *Bartonella henselae*. Cat scratch or bite transmits it to humans. Clinical course usually begins with papule or ulcer at the site within a few days of the bite. Fever, headache, and malaise develop 7 to 21 days later. Lymph drainage of the site may result in swollen, tender, and/or suppurative nodes. Diagnosis is typically made clinically, but special cultures or biopsies are possible. The symptoms usually resolve spontaneously with no specific therapy required. Complications may include encephalitis or disseminated disease in immunocompromised patients. *(Schwartz, 2015, Ch. 33)*

45. **(C)** The key piece of history in this question is the new exposure to parakeets. The symptoms and signs, including atypical pneumonia, are consistent with psittacosis but are not pathognomonic. Sarcoidosis is an illness of unknown cause. Listeriosis has been linked to exposures to contaminated food, particularly dairy products and hot dogs. Brucellosis can be caused by exposure to hogs, cattle, or goats. Tularemia is associated with contact with rabbits, other rodents, and biting arthropods. Psittacosis is usually treated with tetracycline. *(Schwartz, 2015, Ch. 33)*

46. **(B)** The description of the rash is consistent with the erythema chronicum migrans rash of Lyme disease. Lyme disease is caused by the spirochete, *Borrelia burgdorferi*, which is transmitted by tick bite. The course of Lyme disease usually involves progression through three stages. In stage 1, 80% to 90% of patients develop the rash, usually within a week of a tick bite. The rash begins with a maculopapular red lesion at the site. Over several days, the lesion can become much larger and develop central clearing. It is often described as looking like a bull's-eye. In addition to the rash, half of the patients will develop fever, chills, and myalgias. Diagnosis is based on exposure to tick habitat, clinical findings, and confirmed by laboratory testing. Leukocytosis, mild anemia, and an elevated erythrocyte sedimentation rate are common but not specific laboratory findings with Lyme disease. IFA is an option but it is not as sensitive and specific as ELISA followed by a confirmatory western blot. *(Philip, 2015, Ch. 34)*

47. **(E)** Cats are the definitive host for the parasite *Toxoplasma gondii*. It can exist in three forms but it is the oocyst that is found in cat feces. These oocysts can remain infective in soil for years. Human infections are frequently asymptomatic. In an otherwise healthy individual, symptoms resemble infectious mononucleosis. They may include swollen lymph nodes, malaise, arthralgias, headache, sore throat, and rash. Up to 1% of women are infected during pregnancy. Fetal effects are more severe if maternal infection occurs in the first trimester. Less than 15% of births among infected mothers result in severe brain or eye damage at birth but more than 85% manifest brain or eye effects later in their lives. Diagnosis can be made with serological tests. Treatment of pregnant women includes spiramycin 1 g by mouth every 8 hours until delivery. Spiramycin does not cross the placenta and so if the fetus is infected, sulfadiazine, pyrimethamine, and folinic acid should be used. *(Rosenthal, 2015, Ch. 35)*

48. **(D)** *Clostridium tetani* infection is a vaccine-preventable disease that results in approximately 50 cases per year in the United States. Even with modern medical resources, 20% to 25% of patients with generalized tetanus die. Almost all cases occur in individuals who are not properly immunized. Sixty percent of cases occur in older adults for whom immunity has waned. Tetanus presents in

different forms including generalized, localized, cephalad, and neonatal. Generalized is the most common and symptoms include mood changes, trismus, diaphoresis, dysphagia, and drooling. Later symptoms include painful flexion and adduction of the arms and pain with extension of the legs. Convulsions and spasms are possible, along with a variety of autonomic symptoms. Treatment includes airway protection, benzodiazepines for muscle spasm, tetanus immune globulin immediately, and three doses of tetanus toxoid given by the standard schedule. Penicillin is also administered to destroy the organism and prevent toxin production. *(Schwartz, 2015, Ch. 33)*

49. **(B)** Pseudomembranous colitis is caused by the toxin-producing *C. difficile*. It usually presents as fever, elevated WBC count, abdominal pain, and diarrhea (as many as 20 stools per day) following antibiotic therapy. Stools are occasionally bloody but usually watery and unformed. It is thought that *C. difficile*, which is generally harmless when colonized, overgrows when the normal balance of gut flora is altered by antibiotic use. In addition to making the diagnosis on colonoscopy, *C. difficile* can be cultured or the toxins detected by immunoassay. It can be treated by cessation of antibiotics and fluid replacement but most often an antibiotic targeted at the organism is employed. Metronidazole and vancomycin are the drugs of choice. In some areas, resistance to metronidazole is emerging. Oral therapy is preferred for

either agent. Though Pseudomonas is a common hospital-acquired pathogen, neither it nor any of the other incorrect choices results in the pseudomembranes that are characteristic of *C. difficile* infection. *(Gerding & Johnson, 2012, Ch. 129)*

50. **(B)** The patient's presentation is consistent with cutaneous anthrax. *Bacillus anthrax* infection manifests in three forms: cutaneous, gastrointestinal, and inhalational. The cutaneous form occurs in 95% of cases. The incubation period can last up to a week. The initial manifestation is papular and evolves over days to an ulcer. The ulcer is surrounded by swelling and redness and eventually becomes an eschar. The eschar falls off in 7 to 14 days. The cutaneous lesions are usually painless. Associated symptoms may include enlarged lymph nodes in the region of the lesion, fever, malaise, and nausea and vomiting. Because it may progress to meningitis or sepsis, it is usually treated with antibiotics. First-line therapy is ciprofloxacin or doxycycline. Gastrointestinal anthrax is caused by eating infected meat. It is very uncommon and can be highly lethal. Inhalational anthrax happens when spores are inhaled. The latency period may be up to 6 weeks. The symptoms may include fever, fatigue, body aches, chest discomfort, and, later, shortness of breath, shock, and death. Two months of therapy is the standard prevention after exposure to inhalational anthrax. *(Schwartz, 2015, Ch. 33)*

REFERENCES

American Society for Colposcopy and Cervical Pathology. Algorithms: Updated Consensus Guidelines for Managing Abnormal Cervical Cancer Screening Tests and Cancer Precursors, 2013. http://www.asccp.org/portals/9/docs/algorithms%207.30.13.pdf. Accessed August 7, 2014.

Bashore TM, Granger CB, Jackson K, Patel MR. Chapter 10: Heart disease. In: Papadakis MA, McPhee SJ, Rabow MW, eds. *CURRENT Medical Diagnosis and Treatment 2015*. 54th ed. New York, NY: McGraw Hill Education; 2015. http://accessmedicine.com. Accessed February 11, 2015.

Berger TG. Chapter 6: Dermatologic disorders. In: Papadakis MA, McPhee SJ, Rabow MW, eds. *CURRENT Medical Diagnosis and Treatment 2015*. 54th ed. New York, NY: McGraw Hill Education; 2015. http://accessmedicine.com. Accessed August 20, 2014.

Bernard TJ, Knupp K, Yang ML, Kedia S, Levisohn PM, Moe PG. Chapter 25: Neurologic & muscular disorders. In: Hay WW, Jr., Levin MJ, Deterding RR, Abzug MJ, Sondheimer JM, eds. *CURRENT Diagnosis & Treatment: Pediatrics*. 21th ed. New York, NY: McGraw-Hill; 2012. http://accessmedicine.com. Accessed August 20, 2014.

Centers for Disease Control and Prevention. Update to CDC's Sexually Transmitted Diseases Treatment Guidelines, 2010: Oral Cephalosporins No Longer a Recommended Treatment for Gonococcal Infections. Morbidity and Mortality Weekly Report. 2012;61(31):590–594. http://www.cdc.gov/mmwr/preview/mmwrhtml/mm6131a3.htm. Accessed February 25, 2015.

Centers for Disease Control and Prevention. Guidelines for treatment of malaria in the united states. Updated July 1, 2013. http://www.cdc.gov/malaria/resources/pdf/treatmenttable.pdf. Accessed August 7, 2014.

Centers for Disease Control and Prevention. Recommended vaccines for healthcare workers. 2014. http://www.cdc.gov/vaccines/adults/rec-vac/hcw.html. Accessed August 7, 2014.

Chesnutt MS, Prendergast TJ. Chapter 9: Pulmonary disorders. In: Papadakis MA, McPhee SJ, Rabow MW, eds. *CURRENT Medical Diagnosis & Treatment 2015*. New York, NY: McGraw-Hill; 2015. http://accessmedicine.com. Accessed February 11, 2015.

Corey L. Chapter 179: Herpes simplex virus infections. In: Longo DL, Fauci AS, Kasper DL, Hauser SL, Jameson J, Loscalzo J, eds. *Harrison's Principles of Internal Medicine*. 18th ed. New York, NY: McGraw-Hill; 2012. http://accessmedicine. com. Accessed August 20, 2014.

Friedman LS. Chapter 16: Liver, biliary tract, & pancreas disorders. In: Papadakis MA, McPhee SJ, Rabow MW, eds. *CURRENT Medical Diagnosis & Treatment 2015*. New York, NY: McGraw-Hill Education; 2015. http://accessmedicine.com. Accessed February 11, 2015.

Gerding DN, Johnson S. Chapter 129: Clostridium difficile infection, including pseudomembranous colitis. In: Longo DL, Fauci AS, Kasper DL, Hauser SL, Jameson J, Loscalzo J, eds. *Harrison's Principles of Internal Medicine*. 18th ed. New York, NY: McGraw-Hill; 2012. http://accessmedicine. com. Accessed August 20, 2014.

Hardy R. Chapter 175: Infections due to mycoplasmas. In: Longo DL, Fauci AS, Kasper DL, Hauser SL, Jameson J, Loscalzo J, eds. *Harrison's Principles of Internal Medicine*. 18th ed. New York, NY: McGraw-Hill; 2012. http://accessmedicine.com. Accessed August 20, 2014.

Hellmann DB, Imboden JB. Chapter 20: Rheumatologic & immunologic disorders. In: Papadakis MA, McPhee SJ, Rabow MW, eds. *CURRENT Medical Diagnosis and Treatment 2015*. 54th ed. New York, NY: McGraw Hill Education; 2015. http://accessmedicine.com. Accessed February 11, 2015.

Katz MH, Zolopa MA. Chapter 31: HIV Infection & AIDS. In: Papadakis MA, McPhee SJ, Rabow MW, eds. *CURRENT Medical Diagnosis and Treatment 2015*. 54th ed. New York, NY: McGraw Hill Education; 2015. http://accessmedicine. com. Accessed February 3, 2015.

Kaye ET, Kaye KM. Chapter 17: Fever and rash. In: Longo DL, Fauci AS, Kasper DL, Hauser SL, Jameson J, Loscalzo J, eds.

Harrison's Principles of Internal Medicine. 18th ed. New York, NY: McGraw-Hill; 2012. http://accessmedicine.com. Accessed August 20, 2014.

Levinson W. Chapter 49: Systemic mycoses. In: Levinson W, ed. *Review of Medical Microbiology & Immunology*. 12th ed. New York, NY: McGraw-Hill; 2012. http://accessmedicine.com. Accessed August 20, 2014.

Lofland D, Josephat F, Kogut A. Cryptococcus gattii expands its territory. *MLO Med Lab Obs.*, 2014;46(7)16,18.

McQuaid KR. Chapter 15: Gastrointestinal disorders. In: Papadakis MA, McPhee SJ, Rabow MW, eds. *CURRENT Medical Diagnosis & Treatment 2014*. New York, NY: McGraw-Hill; 2014. http://accessmedicine.com. Accessed August 20, 2014.

Morazzo JM, Holmes KK. Chapter 130: Sexually transmitted infections: overview and clinical approach. In: Longo DL, Fauci AS, Kasper DL, Hauser SL, Jameson J, Loscalzo J, eds. *Harrison's Principles of Internal Medicine*. 18th ed. New York, NY: McGraw-Hill; 2012. http://accessmedicine.com. Accessed February 3, 2015.

Pegues DA, Miller SI. Chapter 153: Salmonellosis. In: Longo DL, Fauci AS, Kasper DL, Hauser SL, Jameson J, Loscalzo J, eds. *Harrison's Principles of Internal Medicine*. 18th ed. New York, NY: McGraw-Hill; 2012. http://accessmedicine. com. Accessed August 20, 2014.

Philip SS. Chapter 34: Spirochetal infections. In: Papadakis MA, McPhee SJ, Rabow MW, eds. *CURRENT Medical Diagnosis & Treatment 2015*. New York, NY: McGraw-Hill; 2015. http://accessmedicine.com. Accessed February 3, 2015.

Roig IL, Shandera WX. Chapter 32: Viral & rickettsial infections. In: Papadakis MA, McPhee SJ, Rabow MW, eds. *CURRENT Medical Diagnosis & Treatment 2014*. New York, NY: McGraw-Hill; 2014. http://accessmedicine.com. Accessed August 20, 2014.

Rosenthal PJ. Chapter 35: Protozoal & helminthic infections. In: Papadakis MA, McPhee SJ, Rabow MW, eds. *CURRENT Medical Diagnosis & Treatment 2015*. New York, NY: McGraw-Hill Education; 2015. http://accessmedicine.com. Accessed February 3, 2015.

Schwartz BS. Chapter 33: Bacterial & chlamydial infections. In: Papadakis MA, McPhee SJ, Rabow MW, eds. *CURRENT Medical Diagnosis & Treatment 2015*. New York, NY: McGraw-Hill Education; 2015. http://accessmedicine.com. Accessed February 3, 2015.

Shandera WX, Kelly JD. Chapter 32: Viral & rickettsial infections. In: Papadakis MA, McPhee SJ, Rabow MW, eds. *CURRENT Medical Diagnosis & Treatment 2015*. New York, NY: McGraw-Hill Education; 2015. http://accessmedicine. com. Accessed February 3, 2015.

Steere AC. Chapter 173: Lyme borreliosis. In: Longo DL, Fauci AS, Kasper DL, Hauser SL, Jameson J, Loscalzo J, eds. *Harrison's Principles of Internal Medicine*. 18th ed. New York, NY: McGraw-Hill; 2012. http://accessmedicine.com. Accessed August 20, 2014.

Walker DH, Dumler J, Marrie T. Chapter 174: Rickettsial diseases. In: Longo DL, Fauci AS, Kasper DL, Hauser SL, Jameson J, Loscalzo J, eds. *Harrison's Principles of Internal Medicine*. 18th ed. New York, NY: McGraw-Hill; 2012. http://accessmedicine.com. Accessed August 20, 2014.

Weller PF. Chapter 215: Protozoal intestinal infections and trichomoniasis. In: Longo DL, Fauci AS, Kasper DL, Hauser SL, Jameson J, Loscalzo J, eds. *Harrison's Principles of Internal Medicine*. 18th ed. New York, NY: McGraw-Hill; 2012. http://accessmedicine.com. Accessed August 20, 2014.

Weller PF, Nutman TB. Chapter 217: Intestinal nematode infections. In: Longo DL, Fauci AS, Kasper DL, Hauser SL, Jameson J, Loscalzo J, eds. *Harrison's Principles of Internal Medicine*. 18th ed. New York, NY: McGraw-Hill; 2012. http://accessmedicine.com. Accessed August 20, 2014.

CHAPTER 8

Nephrology

Tricia A. Howard, MHS, PA-C, DFAAPA

Erica N. Davis, MHS, PA-C

Nancy Kim Zuber, MPAS, PA-C

DIRECTIONS: Each of the numbered questions or incomplete statements is followed by possible answers or completions of the statement. Select the ONE-lettered answer or completion that is BEST in each case.

1. The earliest sign of chronic kidney disease (CKD) is:

    (A) Microscopic hematuria

    (B) Hypertension (HTN)

    (C) Albuminuria

    (D) Abnormal creatinine

    (E) Hyperkalemia

2. A 49-year-old male complains of numbness and tingling around his mouth for the past 2 days following a parathyroidectomy performed 1 week ago. Physical examination reveals tetany of the masseter muscle with tapping of the facial nerve. Otherwise, the rest of the examination is unremarkable. Which of the following is the most likely diagnosis?

    (A) Hyperphosphatemia

    (B) Hypocalcemia

    (C) Hypophosphatemia

    (D) Hypercalcemia

    (E) Hypokalemia

3. A 52-year-old female is admitted to the hospital with complaints of chest pain for the past 24 hours. She denies any other symptoms. She has no known past medical history. A cardiac catheterization is performed which is normal. Forty-eight hours after the procedure, the patient becomes very lethargic and oliguric. Physical examination shows a lethargic patient who is arousable. Laboratory results include the following:

Sodium	Glucose	BUN
139 mEq/L	118 mg/dL	42 mg/dL
eGFR	Chloride	Potassium
12 mL/min/1.73 m^2	101 mEq/L	6.5 mEq/L
		Bicarbonate
		19 mEq/L

Urinalysis and microscopy reveal hematuria and myoglobin with the presence of renal tubular casts. Which of the following is the most likely diagnosis?

    (A) Acute interstitial nephritis

    (B) Acute tubular necrosis

    (C) Granulomatosis with polyangiitis

    (D) Goodpasture disease

    (E) Polycystic kidney disease

4. Which of the following urinary findings is suggestive of acute glomerulonephritis?

    (A) Red cells and red cell casts

    (B) White cells and white cell casts

    (C) Renal tubular epithelial cells

    (D) Oval fat bodies

    (E) Hyaline casts

5. In patients with known stage 5 chronic kidney disease, which of the following is an absolute indication to initiate dialysis?

    (A) Proteinuria >3 g/24 h

    (B) GFR of 10 mL/min

    (C) Hyperkalemia of 6.2 with a normal ECG

    (D) New-onset seizures

    (E) Anemia

6. A renal ultrasound would be most beneficial for diagnosing which of the following?

   (A) Nephrotic syndrome
   (B) Polycystic kidney disease
   (C) Glomerulonephritis
   (D) Acute tubular necrosis
   (E) Lupus nephritis

7. Which of the following is the most predictive of progression of kidney disease?

   (A) Systolic blood pressure
   (B) A1C levels
   (C) Urine albumin to creatinine ratio
   (D) Serum creatinine levels
   (E) Advancing age

8. Which of the following is diagnostic of nephrotic syndrome?

   (A) Hypoalbuminemia, hypolipidemia, proteinuria >10 g/24 h
   (B) Hyperalbuminemia, hyperlipidemia, proteinuria >1 g/24 h
   (C) Hypoalbuminemia, hyperlipidemia, proteinuria >2 g/24 h
   (D) Hypoalbuminemia, hyperlipidemia, proteinuria >3 g/24 h
   (E) Normal albumin, hyperlipidemia, proteinuria >10 g/24 h

9. Prolonged, heavy use of nonsteroidal anti-inflammatory drugs (NSAIDs) causes which type of kidney damage?

   (A) Glomerular
   (B) Tubulointerstitial
   (C) Autoimmune
   (D) Macrovascular
   (E) Chronic inflammatory

10. A 16-year-old girl is referred for a sports physical examination. Her blood pressure is 170/92 mm Hg. Urinalysis (UA) reveals 2+ protein. The girl's mother reports multiple episodes of urinary tract infections (UTIs) throughout childhood that were never investigated. The most likely diagnosis is:

   (A) Obstructive uropathy
   (B) Orthostatic proteinuria
   (C) Chronic reflux nephropathy
   (D) Nephrotic syndrome
   (E) Exercise-induced proteinuria

11. Which of the following best describes the mechanism of action of angiotensin-converting enzyme (ACE) inhibitors in controlling blood pressure and preventing or slowing kidney damage?

   (A) They result in systemic vasodilation.
   (B) They increase renal tubular excretion of sodium.
   (C) They result in dilation of the efferent arteriole, reducing glomerular pressure.
   (D) They block the angiotensin II receptor on the cell membrane.
   (E) They reduce production of angiotensinogen, the precursor to angiotensin I.

12. In which of the following settings could the use of an ACE inhibitor be contraindicated?

   (A) Diabetic nephropathy
   (B) Hypertensive nephrosclerosis
   (C) Lupus nephritis
   (D) Polycystic kidney disease
   (E) Significant renal artery stenosis

13. Which of the following is most useful in diagnosing renal artery stenosis?

   (A) Magnetic resonance angiography (MRA)
   (B) Computed tomography (CT) scanning
   (C) Captopril renal scan
   (D) Renal artery biopsy
   (E) Intravenous pyelogram (IVP)

14. Abnormal urinary albumin excretion is defined as:

   (A) >30 mg/24 h
   (B) >150 mg/24 h
   (C) >300 mg/24 h
   (D) >1 g/24 h
   (E) >3.5 g/24 h

15. Your patient known to have multiple myeloma would have what kind of protein found in their urine?

    (A) Bence Jones proteins
    (B) Tamm–Horsfall glycoproteins
    (C) Amyloid
    (D) Albumin
    (E) Microalbumin

16. Glucose will spill into the urine when the serum glucose reaches what level?

    (A) >126 mg/dL
    (B) >150 to 175 mg/dL
    (C) >180 to 200 mg/dL
    (D) >250 mg/dL
    (E) >400 mg/dL

17. Which of the following is MOST indicative of UTI?

    (A) Positive nitrite on dipstick
    (B) Positive leukocyte esterase on dipstick
    (C) Two to three white blood cells (WBCs) per high-power field (HPF) on urine dipstick
    (D) Urine culture revealing 10,000 to 20,000 colonies of *Lactobacillus*
    (E) Positive nitrite and leukocyte esterase on dipstick

18. A unilateral small kidney on ultrasound would suggest which of the following etiologies?

    (A) Polycystic kidney disease
    (B) Hypertensive nephrosclerosis
    (C) Diabetic nephropathy
    (D) Renal artery stenosis
    (E) Malignancy

19. An insulin-dependent 45-year-old male with chronic kidney disease (CKD 4: eGFR 20 mL/min/1.73 m^2) and a foot ulcer was treated with LEVAQUIN (levofloxacin) 750 mg/day. On day 3 of his antibiotic treatment, his wife comes home and finds him dead. What was the most likely cause of his demise?

    (A) Peaked T waves due to hyperkalemia
    (B) Sudden cardiac death in a diabetic
    (C) Increase in the QT interval
    (D) Pulmonary embolism in a high-risk patient
    (E) Wolff–Parkinson–White syndrome

20. Which of the following treatments for hyperkalemia works by redistributing potassium from the blood into the cell?

    (A) Oral sodium polystyrene sulfonate
    (B) Insulin and D50
    (C) Low potassium diet
    (D) Calcium gluconate IV
    (E) Hemodialysis

21. A 64-year-old female with CKD (eGFR 30 mL/min/1.73 m^2) and diabetes presents to the office with complaints of frequency and painful urination. Urine is sent for culture and sulfamethoxazole/trimethoprim DS is started while waiting for the culture results. The patient presents to the emergency room 72 hours later with lethargy and leg weakness. What is her metabolic abnormality?

    (A) Hyponatremia
    (B) Hyperkalemia
    (C) Metabolic alkalosis
    (D) Hypercalcemia
    (E) Rhabdomyolysis

22. A 56-year-old male with hypertension presents to the office after being referred for an elevated creatinine and hypertension. Patient states he has no complaints at this time. Physical examination reveals an S4; otherwise, the remainder of the examination is unremarkable. Laboratory work and ultrasound are ordered to assess for disease. Which of the following ultrasound findings demonstrate chronic kidney disease?

    (A) Kidney size <9 cm, with decreased echogenicity
    (B) Kidney size >9 cm, with increased echogenicity
    (C) Kidney size >9 cm, with normal echogenicity
    (D) Kidney size <9 cm, with increased echogenicity
    (E) Kidney size >9 cm, with decreased echogenicity

23. A 72-year-old man is transported via ambulance to the emergency department with severe chest pain and shortness of breath. Electrocardiogram (ECG) reveals STEMI. While in the emergency department, he loses consciousness and is found to be in ventricular fibrillation. Resuscitation is successful, and a pulse is restored within 3 minutes. He is taken to the cardiac catheterization laboratory, where he undergoes two-vessel stenting. Two days later, his creatinine has increased from a baseline of 1.1 to 2.2 mg/dL. The next day, the creatinine is 3.9 mg/dL. Fractional excretion of urinary sodium is ordered. You would expect this to be:

    (A) <1
    (B) >1
    (C) Unchanged from baseline
    (D) Undetectable
    (E) Equal to the serum creatinine level

24. When initially screening for chronic kidney disease (CKD), which of the following would be ordered?

    (A) Blood pressure measurement, serum creatinine level, 24-hour urine collection
    (B) Blood pressure measurement, serum creatinine level, spot urine albumin measurement
    (C) Blood pressure measurement, renal ultrasound, 24-hour urine collection
    (D) Blood pressure measurement, spot urine albumin measurement, abdominal CT scan
    (E) Blood pressure measurement, spot urine albumin measurement, renal angiogram

25. A 32-year-old construction worker presents to the emergency department after being involved in an accident at a job site. His left thigh was pinned under a 100-lb cement block. He is in moderate pain on presentation, and there is swelling and a large ecchymosis over the entire anterior thigh. Urine is rust-colored. Urine dip is positive for blood and protein, negative for glucose, ketones, nitrite, and leukocyte esterase. Urine sediment is negative for cells, organisms, and casts. What is the most likely cause of the positive urine dip for blood?

    (A) Hemoglobin due to hematoma formation
    (B) Contamination of the urine sample
    (C) Myoglobin due to rhabdomyolysis
    (D) Red cell casts due to glomerulonephritis
    (E) UTI

26. A hypertensive, diabetic 66-year-old female with chronic kidney disease (eGFR 32 mL/min/1.73 m^2) presents to the emergency room with shortness of breath. Her medications include hydrochlorothiazide, carvedilol, amlodipine, metformin, atorvastatin, and losartan. A STAT ECG shows peaked T waves with bradycardia. Which of the following is probably the offending medication?

    (A) Hydrochlorothiazide
    (B) Carvedilol
    (C) Losartan
    (D) Metformin
    (E) Atorvastatin

27. Which of the following best describes the pathophysiologic mechanism of distal renal tubular acidosis?

    (A) A defect in the ability of the distal renal tubule to excrete hydrogen ion
    (B) A defect in the ability of the distal renal tubule to reabsorb bicarbonate
    (C) A defect in the ability of the proximal renal tubule to excrete hydrogen ion
    (D) A defect in the ability of the proximal renal tubule to reabsorb bicarbonate
    (E) Inadequate aldosterone production

28. A reasonably healthy 35-year-old female is admitted in severe shock 1 week after being diagnosed with strep pharyngitis due to *Group B streptococcus*. She had little to no oral intake for the 4 days preceding her admission to the hospital. Upon arrival to the ED she was found to have a BUN of 117 mg/dL, Cr of 7.4 mg/dL, and blood pressure of 94/62 mm Hg. What would you expect to find on the patient's urine microscopy?

    (A) White blood cell casts
    (B) Hyaline casts
    (C) Gram positive cocci in chains
    (D) Muddy brown casts
    (E) Red blood cells

29. Most urinary tract infections (UTIs) are caused by:

(A) Gram-positive bacteria

(B) *Pseudomonas aeruginosa*

(C) *Staphylococcus aureus*

(D) *Escherichia coli*

(E) *Candida albicans*

30. Which of the following class of antihypertensive medications should be continuously monitored for potential hypokalemia?

(A) Angiotensin-converting enzyme inhibitors

(B) Angiotensin receptor blockers

(C) Loop diuretics

(D) Beta-blockers

(E) Calcium channel blockers

31. A 26-year-old male presents after an episode of gross hematuria that occurred approximately 2 weeks ago. His family history is significant for a father with polycystic kidney disease. Physical examination reveals a blood pressure of 150/92 mm Hg and is otherwise unremarkable. Which of the following is the most appropriate diagnostic test to order?

(A) Computed tomography

(B) Magnetic resonance imaging

(C) Ultrasound

(D) Intravenous pyelogram

(E) Abdominal plain film

32. Large numbers of epithelial cells on urine sediment indicate:

(A) UTI

(B) Acute tubular necrosis

(C) Sample contamination

(D) Vaginitis in women

(E) Prostatitis in men

33. Which of the following patients would require the LONGEST antibiotic treatment course for cystitis?

(A) A 28-year-old woman with a history of one urinary tract infection (UTI) 3 years ago

(B) A 74-year-old woman with a history of renal calculi but no previous history of UTI

(C) A 9-year-old girl with no previous history of UTI

(D) A 41-year-old man with no significant past medical history

(E) A 36-year-old woman who is sexually active

34. A 17-year-old male high school wrestler is brought into the emergency department after he collapsed at a wrestling match. He spent time fully clothed in a hot sauna prior to the match to try to "make weight." Labs are ordered, and results come back as follows:

Sodium	162 mEq/L	Glucose	108 mg/dL
Potassium	3.8 mEq/L	BUN	30 mg/dL
Chloride	121 mEq/L	Creatinine	2.0 mg/dL
Carbon dioxide	29 mEq/L	Urine sodium	>10 mEq/L
Weight	70 kg	Urine osmolality	428 mOsm/kg

Which IV fluid regimen would most effectively treat this patient's hypernatremia?

(A) Quarter normal (hypotonic) saline

(B) Half-normal saline

(C) Isotonic (normal) saline

(D) Dextrose 5% in water

(E) Lactated Ringer's

35. Which of the following diagnoses is the leading cause of end-stage renal disease in the United States?

(A) Polycystic kidney disease

(B) IGA nephropathy

(C) Diabetes mellitus

(D) Renal artery stenosis

(E) Glomerulonephritis

36. An 84-year-old man is admitted to the hospital after a fall and subsequent hip fracture. His creatinine at the time of presentation is at his baseline of 1.4 mg/dL. In the ED he receives three doses of IV pain medication, is started on normal saline and made NPO in preparation for surgery. He is assigned to you the following day and you note his creatinine has risen to 1.7 mg/dL. What is the most likely reason?

(A) His IV fluids were discontinued

(B) He was started on ketorolac for pain control

(C) He takes aspirin for his CAD

(D) He was started on enoxaparin for DVT prophylaxis

(E) He has minimal oral intake due to dementia

37. A 78-year-old male is brought to the emergency room by his son for mental status changes. His primary care practitioner started him on oxycodone and duloxetine (Cymbalta) for diabetic neuropathy. Past medical history (PMH) includes chronic kidney disease (CKD) with eGFR = 26 mL/min/1.73 m^2, peripheral vascular disease, gout, congestive heart failure, and coronary artery disease. He has been unable to eat due to nausea but has been able to take fluids. What metabolic abnormality will probably be seen on his labs?

(A) Hyponatremia

(B) Hyperkalemia

(C) Metabolic alkalosis

(D) Hypercalcemia

(E) Hyperchloremia

38. A 52-year-old male with kidney failure currently on hemodialysis presents to the dialysis clinic with complaints of low back pain that started 2 weeks ago and has gotten worse. He notes that pain shoots down his right leg as well. He further admits to numbness in the right leg. Physical examination demonstrates tenderness over the L3–L4 area, decreased sensation of the right leg, and a positive straight-leg raise. Imaging is recommended. Which of the following diagnostic studies has a risk of nephrogenic systemic fibrosis (NSF) and therefore should be avoided?

(A) Computed tomography with nonionic contrast

(B) Magnetic resonance imaging with gadolinium

(C) Lumbar plain x-ray

(D) Computed tomography with ionic contrast

(E) Bone density scan

39. A 72-year-old female with chronic kidney disease (CKD), with an eGFR = 28 mL/min/1.73 m^2, and heart failure by history presents to the office complaining of shortness of breath, vision changes (yellow lights), and increased lethargy. Her medication list includes simvastatin, digoxin, losartan, hydrochlorothiazide, and a multivitamin. Her pulse is 48 beats/min. What medication change is the first step?

(A) Stop the simvastatin

(B) Decrease the dose of the digoxin

(C) Increase the dose of the losartan

(D) Decrease the dose of hydrochlorothiazide

40. The most serious consequence of rapid correction of hyponatremia is which of the following?

(A) Brainstem herniation

(B) Central pontine myelinolysis

(C) Muscle cramps

(D) Hypernatremia

(E) Fluid overload

41. You are called by the emergency department to admit a patient with hyponatremia. You want to know if this patient's hyponatremia reflects hypo-osmolality of the plasma. What laboratory tests do you need to calculate estimated serum osmolality?

(A) Sodium, glucose, and BUN

(B) Sodium, glucose, and creatinine

(C) Sodium, chloride, and BUN

(D) Sodium, glucose, and chloride

(E) Sodium, glucose, and potassium

42. A 32-year-old male presents to the clinic with a pH of 7.48, PCO$_2$ 37 mm Hg, and HCO$_3$ 34 mEq/L. Which of the following best describes the primary acid–base disorder?

(A) Metabolic acidosis

(B) Metabolic alkalosis

(C) Respiratory acidosis

(D) Respiratory alkalosis

(E) No disorder

43. A 62-year-old man with a medical history of aortic stenosis is admitted to the hospital with increasing shortness of breath. Physical examination reveals a regular pulse of 120 beats/min, blood pressure: 90/60 mm Hg, and a respiratory rate of 28 breaths/ min. Physical examination reveals rales auscultated in the bases of the lung fields bilaterally, and a holosystolic murmur is heard at the apex. There is 2+ pretibial and pedal edema. Plain film x-ray of the chest reveals cardiomegaly and pulmonary edema. ECG is suggestive of left ventricular hypertrophy. Admission laboratory studies include the following:

Sodium	127 mEq/L	Potassium	3.8 mEq/L
Chloride	94 mEq/L	Bicarbonate	27 mEq/L
BUN	47 mg/dL	Creatinine	1.1 mg/dL
Urine sodium	12 mEq/L	Glucose	80 mg/dL
Serum osmolality	275 mOsm/kg		

What type of hyponatremia does this patient most likely have?

(A) Hypovolemic hypotonic

(B) Hypervolemic hypotonic

(C) Hypovolemic isotonic

(D) Hypervolemic hypertonic

(E) Hypovolemic hypertonic

44. A 52-year-old male with autosomal dominant polycystic kidney disease and hypertension sustains a Colles fracture and is scheduled for an open reduction and internal fixation. The preoperative labs show a total serum calcium of 10.9 mg/dL (nl 9–10.5 mg/dL). His medications include: Aspirin, hydrochlorothiazide, lisinopril, nifedipine, and atorvastatin. What is the mechanism of hypercalcemia caused by hydrochlorothiazide?

(A) Hydrochlorothiazide decreases urinary excretion in the distal tubule of the loop of Henle

(B) Hydrochlorothiazide increases calcium reabsorption at the proximal tubule of the loop of Henle

(C) Hydrochlorothiazide causes an increase in gastrointestinal absorption of calcium in the gut

(D) Hydrochlorothiazide causes a decrease in gastrointestinal excretion of calcium in the gut

(E) Hydrochlorothiazide promotes bone resorption

45. A 26-year-old woman presents to the emergency department after spending a week in Mexico for spring break. She noted onset of significant diarrhea about 4 days ago, accompanied by mild nausea but no vomiting. She hoped it would resolve on its own, but she is starting to feel worse with weakness and lightheadedness. Labs reveal the following results:

Sodium	139 mEq/L	pH	7.3
Potassium	2.8 mEq/L	PCO$_2$	15 mm Hg
Chloride	119 mEq/L	BUN	68 mg/dL
Bicarbonate	9 mEq/L	Creatinine	1.9 mg/dL

What is the nature of the acid–base disturbance?

(A) Respiratory acidosis

(B) Respiratory alkalosis

(C) Metabolic alkalosis

(D) High anion gap metabolic acidosis

(E) Nonanion gap metabolic acidosis

46. A 45-year-old female with chronic kidney disease comes to the office for routine follow-up. Three months ago, therapy with a statin (HMG-CoA reductase inhibitor) was initiated, and since that time, the patient says she has been having muscle pain. Physical examination shows tenderness to palpation over the quadriceps muscles. Results of laboratory studies include elevated serum creatine kinase level. Urinalysis shows the presence of myoglobin. Which of the following is the most likely diagnosis?

(A) Rhabdomyolysis

(B) Pyelonephritis

(C) Acute cystitis

(D) Diabetic ketoacidosis

(E) Compartment syndrome

47. Which of the following types of anemia are associated with chronic kidney disease (CKD)?

(A) Hypochromic, macrocytic

(B) Hyperchromic, microcytic

(C) Normochromic, macrocytic

(D) Hyperchromic, macrocytic

(E) Normochromic, microcytic

48. A 24-year-old male with no significant past medical history presents to urgent care with complaints of acute onset of hematuria. While taking his history he admits to having a viral upper respiratory infection to 2 days ago but did not seek treatment. What is the likely cause of his hematuria?

(A) Poststreptococcal glomerulonephritis

(B) Minimal change disease

(C) Acute interstitial nephritis

(D) Nephritic syndrome

(E) IgA nephropathy

49. What is the correct flow of blood through the glomerulus?

(A) Renal artery, afferent arterioles, glomerulus, efferent arterioles

(B) Renal artery, efferent arterioles, glomerulus, afferent arterioles

(C) Renal artery, afferent arteriole, arcuate artery, glomerulus

(D) Renal artery, efferent arteriole, afferent arteriole, renal vein

(E) Renal artery, efferent arteriole, arcuate artery, glomerulus

50. A 58-year-old female with chronic kidney disease (CKD) comes to the office for follow-up. Physical examination shows bilateral crackles in the lung bases and bilateral 2+ edema of the pretibial regions. Urinalysis shows fat oval bodies and 4+ protein. In this patient, serum chemistry laboratory studies are most likely to show which of the following abnormalities?

(A) Hypomagnesemia

(B) Hypercalcemia

(C) Hyperlipidemia

(D) Hypokalemia

(E) Hypoalbuminemia

51. Which of the following is a common sign or symptom of uremia?

(A) Anorexia

(B) Anxiety

(C) Diarrhea

(D) Thrombocytosis

(E) Fever

52. Autosomal dominant polycystic kidney disease (ADPKD) is a genetic disease follows what type of genetic inheritance?

(A) Single gene inheritance

(B) X-linked inheritance

(C) Y-linked inheritance

(D) Random mutation

(E) Mendelian trait inheritance

53. The most common type of acute kidney injury is which of the following?

(A) Postrenal azotemia

(B) Prerenal azotemia

(C) Intrinsic renal disease

(D) Drug induced

(E) Diabetic associated

54. In metabolic acidosis the lungs attempt to compensate by which of the following?

(A) Decreasing blood flow to the alveoli

(B) Increasing blood flow to the alveoli

(C) Increasing the respiratory rate

(D) Decrease the respiratory rate

(E) Increasing blood flow to the kidneys

55. A 35-year-old alcoholic presents to the emergency room with 5 days of cramps, lower abdominal pain, and nausea and vomiting. CT of the abdomen shows a 1.1 cm nonobstructing stone on the left. His serum creatinine is 2.2 mg/dL (baseline 0.6 mg/dL). What is the treatment of choice for this patient?

(A) IV saline 0.9%

(B) IV ketorolac

(C) IV morphine

(D) IV thiamine

(E) IV lactated Ringer's solution

56. A 27-year-old female presents with a pH of 7.29, PCO_2 56 mm Hg, and serum HCO_3 27 mEq/L. Which of the following best describes the primary acid–base disorder?

(A) Metabolic acidosis

(B) Metabolic alkalosis

(C) Respiratory acidosis

(D) Respiratory alkalosis

(E) No disorder

57. A 12-year-old boy presents to your office for a yearly physical examination. His mother reports that she has noticed he has gained about 17 lb over the first few months of summer break and his face is swollen upon awakening in the morning which resolves over the course of the day. The patient tells you his urine is bubbly. On examination he has 2+ bilateral lower extremity edema with a normal blood pressure for his age. Your preliminary testing shows:

| Creatinine | 0.7 mg/dL | Albumin | 1.7 g/dL |
| Urine protein | 5437 mg/day | Total cholesterol | 321 mg/dL |

What is the most likely diagnosis?

(A) Acute interstitial nephritis

(B) Minimal change disease

(C) Protein malnutrition

(D) Nephrotic syndrome

(E) Hereditary angioedema

58. A 35-year-old male baseball coach presents to the office after a hit in the back with a baseball. The kids on the team swear he was never hit by a baseball but the coach feels they are not telling the truth. He states he has been urinating blood and uses this to prove the kids are fibbing. He is agitated and his blood pressure is 160/96 bilaterally. If we believe his team, what is the more likely diagnosis?

(A) Polycystic kidney disease

(B) Rhabdomyolysis

(C) Bladder cancer

(D) Kidney stones

(E) Urinary tract infection

59. Acute kidney injury (AKI) can be classified by the RIFLE criteria. What does the acronym RIFLE stand for?

(A) Renal, infectious, function, loss, equation

(B) Risk, injury, failure, loss, end stage

(C) Risk, infectious, function, loss, end stage

(D) Renal, infiltrative, function, lower urinary, equation

(E) Renal, injury, failure, lower urinary, euvolemia

60. Which of the following is a typical complication of advanced chronic kidney disease?

(A) Hypophosphatemia

(B) Anemia

(C) Hypokalemia

(D) Hypoparathyroidism

(E) Metabolic alkalosis

Answers and Explanations

1. **(C)** "Albuminuria, tubular proteinuria, and renal tubular cell constituents are pathognomonic of kidney damage." The newest, international CKD guidelines (KDIGO) on the definition and classification of CKD state that albuminuria is the most predictive risk factor for the loss of kidney function. The term "proteinuria" is falling out of favor with the kidney community since protein can refer to multiple different diseases while albuminuria is the only "true" kidney protein. Studies of CKD progression have shown repeated relationships with albuminuria and progression of kidney disease. Serum creatinine can be effected by outside and/or laboratory factors (i.e., age, fluid/diet, medications) and is less predictive. "It (albuminuria) is the earliest marker of glomerular diseases, including diabetic glomerulosclerosis, where it generally appears before the reduction in GFR." *(KDIGO, 2013, pp. 21–22)*

2. **(B)** Hypocalcemia is one of the postoperative complications of parathyroidectomy. Hypocalcemia usually occurs within 24 hours of the procedure. Symptoms of hypocalcemia include irritability, carpopedal spasm, tingling of the circumoral area, hands, and feet. Chvostek sign, the contraction of the facial muscle elicited by the tapping of the facial nerve in front of the ear, is present with hypocalcemia. *(Cho, 2014, pp. 849–850)*

3. **(B)** Radiographic contrast media is the third leading cause of acute kidney injury in the hospitalized. It is theorized the injury results from direct renal tubular epithelial cell damage and ischemia of the medulla. Acute tubular necrosis will result in the presence of renal tubular epithelial cell casts and hemoglobin on microscopy and urinalysis respectively. *(Watnick & Dirkx, 2014, pp. 871–873)*

4. **(A)** Acute glomerulonephritis will demonstrate hematuria on urine dipstick. Microscopy will reveal red cell casts which are the hallmark of glomerulonephritis. Red cell casts are formed either in the distal tubule or the collecting duct. They are the result of concentrated amounts of red blood cells secondary to intraparenchymal bleeding. Stasis and an acidotic pH also contribute to the formation of casts. *(Watnick & Dirkx, 2014, p. 874)*

5. **(D)** Indicators for initiation are those that constitute uremic symptoms. Typical uremic symptoms include but are not limited to: dysgeusia, fatigue, anorexia and weight loss, nausea and emesis upon awakening. Patients nearing the need for dialysis may have abnormalities in their potassium and phosphorus levels as well as anemia and metabolic acidosis but they are often able to be effectively managed medically. Absolute indicators are those are imminently life threatening and include: neurologic dysfunction (i.e., encephalopathy, severely altered mental status, psychiatric disturbance, seizure, pleuritis, or pericarditis) without other explanation and bleeding diathesis manifested by prolonged bleeding time. *(Daugirdas, Blake, & Ing, 2007)*

6. **(B)** "Kidney imaging studies (i.e., ultrasound) remain the mainstay for diagnosing ADPKD." Lupus and nephrotic syndrome are diagnosed by the laboratory. Glomerulonephritis is often diagnosed by kidney biopsy. Acute tubular necrosis (ATN) is either a constellation of laboratory testing along with patient presentation or kidney biopsy. The ultrasound diagnosis of ADPKD is both dependent on the number of cysts, and the age of the patient. For those patients age 15 to 39 years, there must be three cysts found on ultrasound (can be in either one or two kidneys), whereas, for those patient older

than 40 years, only two cysts must be seen. If the patient is >60 years old, four cysts must be seen. The age-related definitions are due to the fact that cysts can develop in the young and old and so international diagnostic criteria were agreed upon for standardization worldwide. Confirmation is done with genetic testing to define PKD1 versus PDK2 genetic abnormality. *(Gilbert & Weiner, 2014)*

7. **(C)** Studies from 2002, when GFR nomenclature was first introduced to research, until 2013, when the newest KDIGO CKD guidelines were introduced, have shown that albuminuria is most predictive of progression of CKD. The albumin test of choice is the urine albumin to creatinine ratio (UACR) which is a "spot" urine looking for albumin. While the first morning urine is the best, a spot UACR can be done at any time. *(National Kidney Disease Education Program [NKDEP], 2010)*

8. **(D)** Nephrotic syndrome is characterized by massive proteinuria (>3 g/24 h/1.73 m^2), edema, hyperlipidemia, lipiduria, and hypoproteinemia, in particular hypoalbuminemia. Nephrotic syndrome that is severe enough also predisposes the patient to thrombosis due to loss of hemostasis control proteins (i.e., proteins C and S and antithrombin III) and infection due to the loss of immunoglobulins. It may also lead to accelerated atherosclerosis due to hyperlipidemia. *(Watnick & Dirkx, 2014, pp. 893–895)*

9. **(B)** The adverse effects of NSAIDs occur due to inhibition of prostaglandin synthesis leading to vasoconstriction and subsequent renal impairment in volume-depleted states. When this is unopposed it may lead to acute necrosis of the tubules and acute kidney injury. NSAIDs can also produce an interstitial nephritis secondary to minimal change disease, with or without nephrotic syndrome. Although this is typically an acute kidney injury it can progress into chronic kidney failure in some cases due to papillary necrosis. In patient on chronic NSAID therapy without kidney damage (acute or chronic), decreased creatitine clearance and/or a decreased ability to concentrate the urine have been shown to be present. While this subclinical dysfunction is reversible with cessation of the NSAIDs, some reports have suggested persistent dysfunction. *(Hellman & Imboden, 2014, pp. 788–789)*

10. **(C)** Reflux nephropathy may be silent for years and may only be discovered when chronic damage is already done to the kidney. The presenting symptom can be hypertension or repeated UTIs. Often a severe case is worked up in young childhood but the less severe cases can present at a much later age often with permanent tubular changes. Orthostatic proteinuria will give a false positive on a UA but due to the history of multiple UTIs, this is a less likely diagnosis. Nephrotic syndrome presents with hypertension but would also have florid edema which is not seen in this child. Exercise-induced proteinuria is also a possibility but the history of UTIs and the hypertension make this a less likely diagnosis. *(Lum, 2012, p. 722)*

11. **(C)** Angiotensin-converting enzyme inhibitors (ACEI) block the conversion of angiotensin I to angiotensin II. Angiotensin II is a potent vasoconstrictor. Blocking angiotensin II results in greater dilation of the efferent renal arteriole and subsequently reduces intraglomerular pressure by lowering the resistance of the outflow of blood from the glomerulus. Reducing intraglomerular pressure slows the decline of renal function in patients with chronic kidney disease. Though there is a risk for increase in serum potassium and creatinine with use of ACEIs, the incidence for hyperkalemia or acute kidney injury is low and renoprotection is provided. However, serum creatinine and potassium should be monitored for patients receiving an ACEI. *(Benowitz, 2009, pp. 181–183)*

12. **(E)** ACE inhibition is an excellent way to treat hypertension. ACE inhibitors cause systemic vasodilation, and thus lower systemic blood pressure, via the inhibition of the enzyme angiotensin II. ACE inhibitor-induced acute kidney injury occurs in settings where glomerular afferent arteriolar blood flow is reduced, and GFR is thus dependent on efferent arteriolar vasoconstriction, which is inhibited by the use of ACE inhibitors. In patients with bilateral renal artery stenosis it is usually impossible to use ACE inhibitor therapy without an unacceptable loss of renal function (greater than 30% from baseline). *(Benowitz, 2009, pp. 181–183)*

13. **(A)** Renal artery stenosis (RAS) is responsible for 1% to 5% cases of hypertension. Catheter angiography can be used to evaluate RAS, as can CT and

captopril renal scans but the test of choice is the MRA. CT angiography is more useful for anatomy and captopril renal scans have been found to have problems with sensitivity and specificity. While a biopsy is an excellent tool for intrinsic kidney disease, it is unable to elucidate any answers to renal blood flow. *(Watnick & Dirkx, 2014, pp. 883–884)*

14. **(A)** The first stage of diabetic nephropathy is the onset of albuminuria which is defined as >30 mg/24 h. Subsequently, the glomerular filtration rate will decline over time. It is recommended that patients with diabetes mellitus be screened for the presence of albuminuria. If albuminuria is present, an angiotensin converter enzyme inhibitor (ACEI) or angiotensin receptor blocker (ARB) should be started for its nephroprotective effects. If the albuminuria is negative, a repeat should be done annually. *(KDIGO 2012 Clinical Practice Guideline for the Evaluation and Management of Chronic Kidney Disease Guideline:1.4.4, p. 56)*

15. **(A)** Patients with multiple myeloma typically present with renal insufficiency due to cast nephropathy due to deposition of monoclonal light chains. These light chains are referred to as Bence Jones proteins. These patients typically have proteinuria on the order of >3 g/dL but will be negative when tested for albuminuria. Tamm–Horsfall is a type of urinary glycoprotein secreted by the tubules that forms the outer part of a cast. *(Watnick & Dirkx, 2014, pp. 902–903)*

16. **(C)** Glucose is not excreted in the urine until blood levels exceed approximately 180 to 200 mg/dL, termed the renal glucose threshold. *(Guyton & Hall, 2006, pp. 330–331)*

17. **(E)** Urinary tract infections are most common in women and urinalysis usually demonstrates pyuria and bacteriuria. Bacteria produce an enzyme known as reductase which reduces urinary nitrates to nitrites. The presence of pyuria results in a positive leukocyte esterase on the dipstick. *(Meng et al., 2014, pp. 906–907)*

18. **(D)** Polycystic kidney disease presents with cysts on either one or both kidneys. The name is both descriptive and diagnostic. Both hypertensive nephrosclerosis and diabetic changes will affect both kidneys equally. Malignancy may be unilateral or bilateral but often presents with a mass rather than a shrunken kidney. Approximately 30% of all primary renal cell cancers are found incidentally. Renal artery stenosis can be either unilateral or bilateral but the classical description is a unilaterally small kidney. *(Watnick & Dirkx, 2014, pp. 883–884)*

19. **(C)** "Hyperkalemia is usually associated with ACE inhibitors or ARBs. While a PE is possible, the patient is not at any higher risk of a PE as he was a week previously. Sudden cardiac death in a diabetic is always a possibility; it is more likely that the new prescription played a role in the death. Fluoroquinolones, including levofloxacin, gemifloxacin, and moxifloxacin, have been shown to be associated with prolongation of the QT interval on the electrocardiogram and infrequent cases of arrhythmia." Due to the need to renally dose fluoroquinolones, this is much more likely in CKD patients. *(Chambers & Deck, 2009, p. 821; Watnick & Dirkx, 2014, p. 880)*

20. **(B)** Administration of both bolus IV insulin and glucose in the form of D50 causes potassium to shift from the serum into the cells. Beta-2 agonists (albuterol) and sodium bicarbonate can also cause a shift; however, the treatment of choice is insulin and glucose. The effect of the potassium shifts is transient and treatments to remove potassium must also be used. Sodium polystyrene sulfonate (Kayexalate) ingestion (both orally and rectally) removes potassium by exchanging sodium ions for potassium ions in the intestine (especially the large intestine) before the resin is passed from the body. Thiazide or loop diuretics and dialysis remove potassium. Calcium gluconate is used to stabilize the cardiac membranes and should only be used for hyperkalemia with significant ECG findings (i.e., widened QRS, loss of P waves, but not peaked T waves alone) or severe arrhythmia thought to be caused by the hyperkalemia. The effect of calcium gluconate is transient and other modalities will also need to be employed. *(Cho, 2014, p. 847)*

21. **(B)** Sulfamethoxazole/trimethoprim, commonly known as bactrim or bactrim DS, has renal

medication dosing with decreased dosing below a creatinine clearance of 30 mL/min. Bactrim can also cause acute interstitial nephritis (AIN). Bactrim is a frequent cause of an increase in creatinine when the medication is first started due to catatonic transporting in the proximal convoluted tubule of the loop of Henle. The inhibition of the sodium channel in the loop of Henle can cause hyperkalemia. Thus, transient (reversible) hyperkalemia, decreases in serum creatinine and an increase in AIN, makes bactrim a poor choice in the CKD 4 patient. *(Cho, 2014, p. 847)*

22. **(D)** A kidney ultrasound is indicated in the initial workup of suspected kidney disease. A diagnosis of chronic kidney disease is most probable if one or both kidneys are observed to be less than 9 to 10 cm and echogenic by ultrasound. However, patients with normal to enlarged kidneys may still have chronic kidney disease with certain types of disease including polycystic kidney disease, diabetic nephropathy, obstructive disease, multiple myeloma, and amyloidosis. Other parameters to assess for the diagnosis of chronic kidney disease include estimated glomerular filtration rate and the presence of albuminuria. *(Watnick & Dirkx, 2014, p. 877)*

23. **(B)** Renal tubular necrosis secondary to a renal toxin results in tubular damage. Subsequently, in the setting of tubular damage, sodium is unable to be reabsorbed in the glomeruli resulting in an increase in urine fraction excretion of sodium of greater than 1%. It should be noted that in the presence of diuretics the urinary fractional excretion of sodium will be elevated regardless of disease. *(Cho, 2014, p. 837; Watnick & Dirkx, 2014, p. 870)*

24. **(B)** KDIGO updated the definitions of chronic kidney disease (CKD) in 2013. Albuminuria was added to the evaluation while little other changes were made. There is a time requirement of changes >3 months in order to distinguish from acute kidney injury (AKI), but screening remains the same. In order to determine a CKD stage, a serum creatinine would need to be reported, as would race and age. Some of the newer GFR calculators also use height and weight. However, CKD screening does not require any radiological evaluation.

KDIGO reiterated what KDOQI stated in 2002; a "spot" urine to creatinine ratio for albuminuria or proteinuria was more reliable than a 24-hour urine. Thus, the 2013 recommendations again state a "spot" urine is needed for staging of CKD. *(KDIGO, 2013, pp. 21–22)*

25. **(C)** This patient has a crush injury and resulting rhabdomyolysis. When the muscle is damaged myoglobin, a heme-containing protein, is released into the extracellular fluid and is subsequently excreted into the urine. It can cause the urine to take on a reddish brown color once the levels exceed approximately 100 to 300 mg/dL. The urine dip measures the presence of heme proteins (hemoglobin and myoglobin) and can be positive to varying degrees without the presence of red blood cells (normal <5 RBC/hpf) in the sediment on microscopy. Most urine dip sticks are sensitive to levels of red cells equivalent to less than 2 cells/hpf on microscopy. *(Hellman & Imboden, 2014, pp. 811–812)*

26. **(C)** Peaked T waves on an ECG are diagnostic of hyperkalemia. Both ACE inhibitors and ARBs can cause hyperkalemia. Thus, the most likely medication on this list is the losartan, an ARB. *(Cho, 2014, pp. 846–847)*

27. **(A)** Distal renal tubular acidosis, also known as type I RTA, is characterized by the inability of distal tubule to acidify the urine or secrete hydrogen ions and ammonium ions leading to abnormally high-urine pH of 5.5 or more. This can be acquired or congenital. In proximal (type 2) RTA, the proximal tubule is unable to reabsorb filtered bicarbonate due to a diminished threshold for bicarbonate reabsorption and thus bicarbonate wasting occurs. Hypoaldosteronism (type 4 RTA) is due to either aldosterone deficiency or tubular resistance to the action of aldosterone. These patients will typically have hyperkalemia as aldosterone is the main hormone that promotes potassium excretion. *(Cho, 2014, pp. 859–860)*

28. **(D)** This patient has developed acute tubular necrosis (ATN). ATN is an acute kidney injury that occurs due to epithelial tubular cellular injury in three settings; renal ischemia, sepsis, and nephrotoxin exposure. Most tubular epithelial cells will remain

viable after AKI but necrosis can occur in severe cases leading to cast formation. Muddy brown casts are coarse deeply pigmented granular (representing degenerated cellular material) casts and are also called heme-granular casts. Muddy brown casts are pathognomonic of ATN. Hyaline casts may be present due to hypovolemia, however one would expect the presence of significantly more muddy brown casts. Red blood cells would indicate glomerular injury not tubular injury. WBC casts would indicate interstitial injury and not tubular injury. *(Watnick & Dirkx, 2014, p. 872)*

29. **(D)** In the normal genitourinary (GU) tract, strains of *Escherichia coli* account for 75% to 95% of cases of UTI. The remaining gram-negative urinary pathogens are usually other *enterobacteria*, typically *Klebsiella* or *Proteus mirabilis*, and occasionally *Pseudomonas aeruginosa*. Among gram-positive bacteria, *Staphylococcus saprophyticus* is isolated in 5% to 10% of bacterial UTIs. Less common gram-positive bacterial isolates are *Enterococcus faecalis* (group D streptococci) and *Streptococcus agalactiae* (group B streptococci), which may be contaminants, particularly if they were isolated from patients with uncomplicated cystitis. *(Meng et al., 2014, pp. 906–907)*

30. **(C)** Hypokalemia is seen primarily with use of loop diuretics. Loop diuretics selectively inhibit Na^+ and Cl^- reabsorption in the ascending loop of Henle through the $Na^+/K^+/Cl^-$ transporter. Secondary to this action, K^+, Na^+, and Cl^- are excreted in the urine. Diuresis results from the process of water following Na^+ and Cl^-. Secondary to the loss of potassium via excretion, the serum potassium will be lowered. Angiotensin-converting enzyme inhibitors and angiotensin receptor blockers both increase serum potassium by increasing aldosterone via the renin angiotensin aldosterone system (RAAS). Beta-blockers and calcium channel blockers do not affect serum potassium. *(Ives, 2009, p. 259; Sutters, 2014, p. 429)*

31. **(C)** Autosomal dominant polycystic kidney disease (ADPKD) is the most common hereditary kidney disorder. It is equally represented in all ethnic groups. Approximately 5% of the total end-stage renal disease cases in the United States are a result of ADPKD. The disorder is characterized by cystic enlargement of kidneys. Hematuria, gross and microscopic, occurs in 35% to 50% of those affected by the disease secondary to cyst rupture. The diagnosis is confirmed by renal ultrasound. The criteria developed for the diagnosis of ADPKD include the following: individuals' ages 15 to 39 years old must have two to three renal cysts present either unilaterally or bilaterally, individuals' ages 40 to 59 years must have two renal cysts present bilaterally, and individuals 60 years and older must have four or more renal cysts present bilaterally. *(Watnick & Dirkx, 2014, pp. 901–902)*

32. **(C)** Urine samples containing large amounts of epithelial cells are contaminated. Urine that is to be cultured or examined microscopically must be obtained via clean catch. A clean-catch specimen is obtained midstream specimen; the first 5 mL of urine is not captured and the next 5 to 10 mL is collected in a sterile container. Prior to obtaining the sample the urethral opening should be washed with a mild disinfectant and air dried. Contact of the urinary stream with the mucosa should be minimized by spreading the labia in women and by pulling back the foreskin in uncircumcised men. *(Pagana & Pagana, 2006, p. 1013)*

33. **(D)** Men require a longer course of antibiotic treatment for cystitis. Duration of treatment is based on the etiology which may include prostatitis. Cystitis is rare in men and therefore the male patient should be evaluated for an underlying abnormality. Other populations are generally treated with an antimicrobial ranging from a single dose treatment to 9 days of therapy. Women who are sexually active are at increased risk for cystitis secondary to the shorter length of the female urethra and the ascending nature of the bacteria from the urethra. However, sexually active women do not require a longer duration of therapy. *Escherichia coli* is the most common pathogen. Drugs of choice for uncomplicated cystitis include cephalexin, nitrofurantoin, and fluoroquinolones. Trimethoprim–sulfamethoxazole may not be as efficacious in the treatment of cystitis secondary to emerging resistance of the organism. *(Meng et al., 2014, pp. 906–907)*

34. (C) This patient has acute hypernatremia due to volume loss from sweating and decreased oral fluid intake, also known as dehydration and hemoconcentration. In this case the most pressing issue is to correct his volume status which is best done by the administration of isotonic saline which contains 0.9% sodium. This will correct both the water deficit and serum osmolarity. The osmolarity of isotonic saline is 308 mOsm/kg and will likely be lower than that of someone who is significantly dehydrated. As the water deficit corrects the sodium will normalize. Quarter normal saline contains 0.24% sodium, half normal saline contains 0.45% sodium and the sodium content of lactated Ringer's is similar to that of half normal saline. Dextrose 5% in water contains no electrolytes and can be used to correct the hyponatremia after the water deficit is corrected. *(Cho, 2014, pp. 842–850)*

35. (C) The most common cause of chronic kidney disease (CKD) and end-stage renal disease (ESRD) is diabetic nephropathy. Hypertensive nephrosclerosis is the second cause. Approximately 50% of individuals with ESRD are secondary to diabetic nephropathy. In order to slow the progression to ESRD, the following management is recommended including: blood pressure control <130/80 in a diabetic or patient with CKD, proteinuria reduction, serum glucose control, hyperlipidemia treatment, and smoking cessation. *(Watnick & Dirkx, 2014, pp. 897–898)*

36. (B) Ketorolac is an NSAID commonly given to orthopedic patients. NSAID inhibition of cyclooxygenase enzymes with subsequent reduction in prostaglandin synthesis can lead to reversible renal ischemia, a decline in glomerular hydraulic pressure (the major driving force for glomerular filtration), and acute kidney injury. This occurs due to a decrease in renal vasodilation due to NSAIDs. In healthy patients, prostaglandins have little role in renal hemodynamics. However, synthesis of prostaglandins is increased in the setting of prolonged renal vasoconstriction, which serves to protect and increase the GFR. Prostaglandin synthesis is increased in several instances; in the elderly, those with chronic kidney disease (GFR <60 mL/min). Although aspirin is an NSAID, it typically does not cause renal injury at prophylactic doses. Enoxaparin does not cause kidney injury but must be dose adjusted for those with diminished GFRs. *(Hellman & Imboden, 2014, p. 789)*

37. (A) All SSRIs and SNRIs, as classes, can cause hyponatremia. The mechanism of action is felt to be syndrome of inappropriate antidiuretic hormone (SIADH). As this was a class issue after the medications were approved and used on a large, elderly population, the hyponatremia, which can be profound, is often missed in general practice. Reports from the FDA state that the incidence can be 9% of all SSRIs prescribed with a higher incidence of hyponatremia in the elderly and those with compromised kidney function. *(Mannesse, 2013, pp. 357–363)*

38. (B) Gadolinium-based contrast used in magnetic resonance imaging has been associated with a nephrogenic systemic fibrosis (NSF) in those patients with an estimated glomerular filtration rate below 30 mL/min/1.73 m^2. The mortality rate has been as high as 31%. Symptoms of the disease include sclerosing of the skin and organs. Patients may develop symptoms of the disease starting from day 1 of exposure to the gadolinium to months after exposure. *(Bernheisel, 2009, pp. 711–714; Watnick & Dirkx, 2014, pp. 903–904)*

39. (B) Simvastatin, as part of the family of statins, can cause rhabdomyolysis. Losartan, an angiotensin receptor blocker (ARB), is known for causing hyperkalemia. Hydrochlorothiazide can cause serum hypercalcemia. The only medication on this patient's medication list that can cause vision changes and bradycardia is digoxin. Digoxin, which is from the digitalis family, is renally cleared and must be dosed by creatinine clearance. Symptoms that show digoxin toxicity include bradycardia, confusion, loss of appetite with nausea and vomiting. Vision changes can also occur. These include blind spots, blurred vision, color changes, or seeing spots. *(Olson, 2009, p. 1023)*

40. (B) The neurologic manifestations associated with overly rapid correction have been called osmotic demyelination syndrome (formerly called central pontine myelinolysis). Almost all patients who develop ODS present with a serum sodium concentration of 120 mEq/L or less. In patients with true hyponatremia the decrease in serum osmolality causes movement of water into the brain which can lead to cerebral edema and neurologic symptoms. Therefore in response to hyponatremia, the brain makes adaptations that lower the cerebral volume toward normal to reduce the likelihood of neurologic complications. However, if these adaptations are chronic (present for more than 48 hours) the brain then becomes vulnerable to neurologic complications if the serum concentration is raised too quickly. Demyelination is most common and most severe when the serum sodium concentration in severe hyponatremia is raised more than 20 mEq/L in 24 hours and is rare at a rate below 9 mEq/L in 24 hours. The symptoms of ODS include dysarthria, dysphagia, paralysis, behavioral disturbances, changes in mental status including obtundation and coma; seizures may also be seen but are less common. Locked in syndrome can even occur in very severe cases. The symptoms are often irreversible or only partially reversible. *(Cho, 2014, p. 841; Singh et al., 2014, pp. 1443–1450).*

41. **(A)** Plasma osmolarity can be calculated from the serum sodium in mEq/L, glucose and BUN measured in mg/dL via the following formula *(Cho, 2014, pp. 837–38):*

$$P_{osm} = (2 \times \text{Serum } [Na^+]) + \text{Glucose}/18 + \text{BUN}/2.8$$

42. **(B)** The normal range for arterial blood pH is between 7.35 and 7.45. An acidosis is characterized as an arterial blood pH <7.35 and an alkalosis >7.45. The normal range for PCO_2 is 35 to 45 mm Hg. The normal range for serum bicarbonate is 24 to 31 mm Hg. This patient has a metabolic alkalosis based on the finding of a high pH (7.48) and a high HCO_3 (34 mm Hg). This patient's CO_2 is 37 mm Hg which is normal. The lungs will begin to compensate within minutes. CO_2 is a volatile acid produced in the tissues and must be removed by the lungs to maintain a normal pH. The respiratory rate will increase in the setting of an acidosis to reduce the amount of CO_2 via expiration and therefore increase the pH. Inversely, in the setting of alkalosis, the respiratory rate will decrease and retain CO_2 to lower the pH. The kidneys attempt to compensate within hours to days by retaining increased amounts of HCO_3 to increase the pH in a setting of acidosis. Inversely, the kidneys will decrease amounts of HCO_3 through excretion to decrease the pH in a

setting of alkalosis. There is no compensation noted at this point. *(Cho, 2014, pp. 856–864)*

43. **(B)** Hyponatremia is the most common electrolyte disorder in the hospitalized patient and is defined as serum sodium <135 mEq/L. Hyponatremia is a result of water versus sodium imbalance. Serum osmolality assists in identifying the potential etiology of hyponatremia. Recognizing whether serum osmolality is hypotonic (low osmolality), isotonic (normal osmolality), or hypertonic (high osmolality) is important in the treatment of this electrolyte disorder. Possible etiologies associated with isotonic hyponatremia include severe hyperlipidemia and hyperproteinemia. Hypertonic hyponatremia can occur with mannitol administration or hyperglycemia. Hypotonic hyponatremia is the most common and volume status (hypovolemic, euvolemic, hypervolemic) must be assessed in order to determine the cause. Hypovolemic hyponatremia is usually caused by extra renal salt loss defined as a urine sodium of <10 mEq/L or renal salt loss defined as urine sodium of >20 mEq/L. Extra renal salt losses occur with dehydration, diarrhea, or vomiting. Therapy includes restoring volume. Renal salt loss can be seen with use of diuretics, ACE inhibitors, nephropathies, and mineralocorticoid deficiency. Therapy is focused on reversing the underlying etiology.

   The patient in the scenario presents with signs and symptoms of heart failure. Serum osmolality is low, 275 mOsm/kg, therefore the patient is hypotonic. Evaluation of volume status is the next procedure. Based on physical examination, his volume overloaded indicated by the presence of rales and peripheral edema. Finally, the amount of sodium in the urine should be evaluated. Urinary sodium is 12 mEq/L which indicates there is neither a renal salt loss nor extra renal salt loss. Therefore, this patient has hypervolemic hypotonic hyponatremia secondary to heart failure. *(Cho, 2014, pp. 838–840)*

44. **(A)** Hydrochlorothiazide is not metabolized, but is rapidly excreted by, the kidney. Thiazides, as a class, decrease calcium excretion. This can cause an elevation of serum calcium by decreasing the urinary excretion of calcium. Since hypercalcemia can be a sign of parathyroid disease, all thiazides must be stopped before workup for parathyroid disease. *(Cho, 2014, p. 850; Ives, 2009, p. 260)*

45. (E) The normal range for arterial blood pH is between 7.35 and 7.45. An acidosis is characterized as a pH <7.35. This patient has a metabolic acidosis (low pH) secondary to loss of HCO_3 from diarrhea. The normal range for serum bicarbonate is 24 to 31 mm Hg. This patient's HCO_3 is 9 mEq/L and the pH is 7.32 and therefore indicates a metabolic acidosis. The PCO_2 is appropriately low as the body is attempting to compensate for the acidosis. The lungs begin to compensate within minutes to adjust the pH. The respiratory rate will increase in the setting of an acidosis to reduce the amount of CO_2 by expiration and therefore increase the pH. Anion gap calculation,

$$Na^+ - (Cl^- + HCO^{-3}),$$

should be obtained when a metabolic acidosis is present. A normal anion gap is 8 to 12 mEq/L. In the above scenario, the anion gap is 139–(119+9) = 11, which is in the normal range. Therefore the patient has a normal anion gap metabolic acidosis. The two major causes of normal anion gap metabolic acidosis are gastrointestinal HCO^3 bicarbonate loss (diarrhea, pancreatic drainage, and ureterosigmoidostomies) and renal tubular acidosis. (*Cho, 2014, pp. 856–864*)

46. (A) Myoglobin present in the urine is a result of rhabdomyolysis. Rhabdomyolysis is a clinical syndrome defined by muscle necrosis with subsequent release of intracellular contents into extracellular space. Myoglobin is filtered through the glomerulus and results in reabsorption by the renal tubules. Thus, distal convoluted tubule damage and obstruction can occur and result in acute kidney injury (AKI). Rhabdomyolysis symptoms include muscle pain and dark urine. Labs reveal an elevated serum creatinine kinase (CK 20,000–50,000 IU/L) and a false positive finding of hemoglobin on the urine dipstick. However, there will be very few or no red blood cells present on microscopy. Causes of rhabdomyolysis include crush injuries, overexertion, alcohol, and cocaine. Medications may also result in muscle necrosis and include statins, selective serotonin reuptake inhibitors, and psychotics. Treatment is focused on discontinuing the offending agent and fluid repletion. (*Hellman & Imboden, 2014, pp. 811–812*)

47. (C) According to the World Health Association, anemia is defined as a hemoglobin concentration of less than 12.0 g/dL. As the glomerular filtration rate declines, the incidence of anemia increases. A normochromic, normocytic anemia with chronic kidney disease is secondary to a lack of production of erythropoietin and loss of stimulatory effect on erythropoiesis. The cell has normal mean corpuscular hemoglobin (normochromic) and the cell is normal size (normal mean corpuscular volume). When the hemoglobin becomes less than 10 g/dL, patients may begin experiencing fatigue and have a decreased sense of well-being. Erythropoiesis-stimulating agents are the treatment of choice after all other types of anemia have been excluded. Recombinant human erythropoietin has been administered to patients since 1989. (*Watnick & Dirkx, 2014, p. 880*)

48. (E) IgA (immunoglobulin A) nephropathy is due to the deposition of IgA in the mesangium of the glomerulus in the absence of other diseases such as SLE. The most frequent presentation of IgA nephropathy in children and young adults in the western hemisphere is an episode of gross hematuria during or immediately (1–3 days) after an upper respiratory tract infection. Gross hematuria can also occur with poststreptococcal glomerulonephritis however it does not typically occur until 1 to 2 weeks after an untreated throat infection and is also typically accompanied by edema, proteinuria, and hypertension (nephritic syndrome). AIN can cause gross hematuria after an infection though it most often causes microscopic hematuria as well as sterile pyuria, eosinophiluria, and possibly red blood cell casts. (*Watnick & Dirkx, 2014, pp. 889–890*)

49. (A) Blood enters the kidney via the renal arteries and flows into the serial branches; the interlobar, arcuate, and interlobular arteries then into the afferent arterioles. From the afferent arterioles blood then flows into the glomerulus through Bowman capsule and out of the glomerulus through the efferent arterioles. (*Guyton & Hall, 2006, pp. 309–310*)

50. (E) Fat oval bodies present on urinalysis are specific for nephrotic syndrome. Nephrotic syndrome is defined as proteinuria greater than 3 g in 24 hours. The syndrome also includes hypoalbuminemia, peripheral edema, and hyperlipidemia. Fat oval bodies are formed secondary to tubular epithelial cells that have reabsorbed the excess lipids in the urine and have clumped off. Causes of nephrotic syndrome include minimal change disease which is more prevalent in children. In adults, membranous glomerulopathy is the most common cause in the Caucasian population while focal sclerosing glomerulonephritis (FSGS) is the primary cause of nephrotic syndrome in African Americans. *(Watnick & Dirkx, 2014, p. 894)*

51. **(A)** Anorexia and weight loss, fatigue, nausea, and vomiting are common symptoms of uremia. Sexual dysfunction is very common in men and disturbances in menstruation and infertility are common in women. Platelet dysfunction is common and leads to prolongation of the bleeding time. Fever is not a common sign of uremia, however patients with CKD are at much higher risk for infection, in particular those of the genitourinary tract and respiratory system. *(Watnick & Dirkx, 2014, pp. 868–869)*

52. **(E)** Autosomal dominant polycystic kidney disease (ADPKD) is a genetic disease that can be passed to either males or females in the family. Thus, there is no sex-linked inheritance pattern. While random mutation does play a role in ADPKD, the inheritance of the PKD1 or PKD2 gene follows the typical Mendelian pattern with the abnormal gene being the dominant player. Thus, if one was to inherit a PKD gene from one parent and a normal gene from the other parent, the PKD gene would be "dominant" and the offspring would show signs of ADPKD. ADPKD is the most common genetic disease and is manifested by hypertension and cyst growth in the kidney and often the liver. It is often undiagnosed in the general population. *(Watnick & Dirkx, 2014, pp. 901–902).*

53. **(B)** Intravascular volume depletion and the subsequent decreased renal perfusion, account for approximately 70% of acute kidney injury and are often reversible when treated appropriately and promptly. Obstructions of the urinary tract, or post renal failure, account for less than 5% of cases of AKI. Intrinsic renal failure occurs in the rest of the cases. Drug-induced AKI is often intrinsic in etiology and renal failure associated with diabetes is typically chronic in nature. *(Rahman et al., 2012, pp. 631–639; Watnick & Dirkx, 2014, p. 869)*

54. **(C)** Primary acid–base disturbances have a compensatory response; however, this response will not fully correct the pH. The lungs begin to compensate within minutes to adjust the pH. CO_2 is a volatile acid produced in the tissues and must be removed by the lungs to maintain a normal pH. The respiratory rate will increase in the setting of an acidosis to reduce the amount of CO_2 via expiration and therefore increase the pH. Inversely, in the setting of alkalosis, the respiratory rate will decrease and retain CO_2 to lower the pH. *(Cho, 2014, pp. 857–863)*

55. **(A)** Acute kidney injury (AKI) can be prerenal, intrarenal, or postrenal. As it was known that this patient has a previous normal serum creatinine but it is now elevated, a diagnosis of AKI is made. Once the diagnosis is made, a cause must be found. While the CT shows a stone, it is nonobstructing. Thus, it is unlikely that the stone is causing the AKI. There are no reports of medications and/or drugs, other than alcohol, in this patient. Thus, medication-induced acute tubular injury is unlikely. There is a history of 5 days of nausea and vomiting. Between the alcoholism and GI symptoms, the patient is most likely very dry. Reversal of the acute kidney injury will occur with IV fluids. Standard of care is replacement with isotonic saline (0.9%). *(Watnick & Dirkx, 2014, pp. 868–873)*

56. **(C)** The normal range for arterial blood pH is between 7.35 and 7.45. An acidosis is characterized as an arterial blood pH <7.35 and alkalosis >7.45. The normal range for PCO_2 is 35 to 45 mm Hg. The normal range for serum bicarbonate is 24 to 31 mm Hg. This patient has a respiratory acidosis based on the finding of a low pH (7.29) and a high PCO_2 (56 mm Hg). This patient's serum HCO_3 is 27 mEq/L, which is normal. The kidneys attempt to compensate within hours to days by retaining increased amounts of HCO_3 to increase the pH in a setting of acidosis. Inversely, the kidneys will decrease amounts of HCO_3 through excretion to decrease the pH in a setting of alkalosis. There is no compensation noted at this point. *(Cho, 2014, p. 863)*

57. **(B)** Minimal change disease is the single most common cause of nephrotic syndrome in children. Nephrotic syndrome is characterized by nephrotic range proteinuria (>3 g/D), significant edema that is often rapidly developing, hypoalbuminemia, and elevated cholesterol levels. Creatinine levels can be normal or abnormal. Although the patient in

this question has typical nephrotic syndrome, that is not a diagnosis in itself but a symptom of the disease. Hereditary angioedema is an immunologic disorder affecting the blood vessels and can cause rapid angioedema and other swelling; it has no other symptoms consistent with nephrotic syndrome. *(Lum, 2012, p. 725; Watnick & Dirkx, 2014, p. 895)*

58. **(A)** Hypertension can be primary or secondary. One of the most common secondary causes of hypertension is ADPKD (autosomal dominant polycystic kidney disease) with an incidence of 1 in 400 live births. Cysts will grow in the kidneys and can rupture with exertion, trauma, or without known precipitating factors. While both bladder cancer and a urinary infection can present with hematuria, the acute onset during exertion, along with the hypertension, lead one to ADPKD as the more likely cause. *(Watnick & Dirkx, 2014, pp. 901–902)*

59. **(B)** There are two complimentary, although sometimes competing, definitions for AKI: the *RIFLE* criteria and the *AKIN* criteria. The rifle criteria (risk, injury, failure, loss, and end stage) give a grading system dependent on serum creatinine, urinary output, and loss of GFR. The flaw with RIFLE is the requirement for a >25% loss in the GFR (serum creatinine increase ≥1.5 mL/min/1.73 m^2). Due to studies showing that small changes (defined as ≥3 mg/dL /1.73 m^2) can be associated with adverse outcomes, the acute kidney network introduced the AKIN criteria in 2007. In 2012, an international consensus body (KDIGO) combined RIFLE and AKIN into 1 definition to identify >95% of all AKI cases. *(KDIGO, 2013, pp. 14–15)*

60. **(B)** Advanced CKD (stage 3 or higher) can cause anemia, metabolic acidosis, and hyperkalemia as well as renal hyperparathyroidism and hyperphosphatemia. Volume overload, dyslipidemia, and hypertension are also common sequelae. *(Watnick & Dirkx, 2014, p. 878)*

REFERENCES

Benowitz NL. Antihypertensive agents. In: Katzung BG, Masters SB, Trevor AJ, eds. *Basic and Clinical Pharmacology.* 11th ed. New York, NY: McGraw-Hill Medical; 2009.

Chambers HF, Deck DH. Sulfonamides, trimethoprim & quinolones. In: Katzung BG, Masters SB, Trevor AJ, eds. *Basic and Clinical Pharmacology.* 11th ed. New York, NY: McGraw-Hill Medical; 2009.

Cho KC. Electrolyte & acid-base disorders. In: McPhee SJ, Papadakis MA, eds. *Current Medical Diagnosis and Treatment.* 53rd ed. New York, NY: McGraw-Hill; 2014.

Daugirdas J, Blake P, Ing T. *Handbook of Dialysis.* 4th ed. Lippincott Williams & Wilkins; 2007.

Gilbert S, Weiner D, eds. *National Kidney Foundation's Primer on Kidney Diseases.* 6th ed. Elsevier; 2014.

Guyton AC, Hall JE. *Textbook of Medical Physiology.* 11th ed. Philadelphia, PA: Elsevier Saunders; 2006.

Hellman DB, Imboden JB. Rheumatologic & immunologic disorders. In: McPhee SJ, Papadakis MA, eds. *Current Medical Diagnosis and Treatment.* 53rd ed. New York, NY: McGraw-Hill; 2014.

Ives HE. Diuretic agents. In: Katzung BG, Masters SB, Trevor AJ, eds. *Basic and Clinical Pharmacology.* 11th ed. New York, NY: McGraw-Hill Medical; 2009.

Jeffrey D, Bernheisel C. Gadolinium-associated systemic nephrogenic fibrosis. *Am Fam Physician.* 2009;80(7):711–714.

Kidney Disease: Improving Global Outcomes (KDIGO), CKD-MBD Work Group. KDIGO 2012 clinical practice guideline for the evaluation and management of chronic kidney disease. *Kidney Int Suppl.* 2013;3:1–150. http://www.kdigo.org/clinical_practice_guidelines/pdf/KDIGO%20AKI%20Guideline.pdf. Accessed on April 10, 2015.

Lum GM. Kidney and urinary tract. In: Hay WW, Levin MJ, Sondheimer JM, et al., eds. *Current Pediatric Diagnosis and Treatment.* 21st ed. New York, NY: McGraw-Hill; 2012.

Mannesse CK, Jansen PA, Van Marum RJ, et al. Characteristics, prevalence, risk factors, and underlying mechanism of hyponatremia in elderly patients treated with antidepressants: a cross-sectional study. *Maturitas.* 2013;76(4):357–363.

Meng MV, Walsh TJ, Stoller ML. Urologic disorders. In: McPhee SJ, Papadakis MA, eds. *Current Medical Diagnosis and Treatment.* 53rd ed. New York, NY: McGraw-Hill; 2014.

National Kidney Disease Education Program (NKDEP) of the National Institutes of Health. www.nkdep.nih.gov. NIH Publication No. 10–6286, 2010.

Olson KR. Management of the poisoned Patient. In: Katzung BG, Masters SB, Trevor AJ, eds. *Basic and Clinical Pharmacology*. 11th ed. New York, NY: McGraw-Hill Medical; 2009.

Pagana KD, Pagana TJ. *Mosby's Manual of Diagnostic and Laboratory Tests*. 3rd ed. Mosby's; 2006.

Rahman M, Shad F, Smith M. Acute kidney injury: a guide to diagnosis and management. *Am Fam Physician*. 2012;86(7):631–639.

Singh TD, Fugate JE, Rabinstein AA. Central pontine and extrapontine myelinolysis: a systematic review. *Eur J Neurol*. 2014;21(12):1443–1450.

Sutters M. Systemic hypertension. In: McPhee SJ, Papadakis MA, eds. *Current Medical Diagnosis and Treatment*. 53rd ed. New York, NY: McGraw-Hill; 2014.

Watnick S, Dirkx T. Kidney disease. In: McPhee SJ, Papadakis MA, eds. *Current Medical Diagnosis and Treatment*. 53rd ed. New York, NY: McGraw-Hill; 2014.

CHAPTER 9

Neurology

Les Swafford Jr., MPAS, PA-C
William Cody Black, MHS, PA-C

DIRECTIONS: Each of the numbered questions or incomplete statements is followed by possible answers or completions of the statement. Select the ONE-lettered answer or completion that is BEST in each case.

1. A 47-year-old male presents with a 3-month history of progressive bilateral leg weakness. Symptoms began in the left leg and eventually progressed to the right leg. The patient also reports associated muscle twitching and painful muscle cramps. He denies vision changes and any recent illnesses or immunizations. Physical examination reveals intact sensation bilaterally and a decrease in muscle strength of the lower extremities, more prominent on the left side than the right. Electromyography (EMG) testing reveals diffuse degenerative signs with normal nerve conduction. Which of the following is the most likely diagnosis?

    (A) Amyotrophic lateral sclerosis
    (B) Guillain–Barré syndrome
    (C) Multiple sclerosis
    (D) Myasthenia gravis
    (E) Nonparalytic poliomyelitis

2. A 25-year-old female presents with complaints of double vision and fatigue. These symptoms are generally better in the morning and progress throughout the day. She notes reading and watching television tend to bring on the double vision. She works long hours and states toward the end of her shift she is extremely fatigued and has difficulty completing her tasks. Which of the following is the most likely etiology?

    (A) Antibodies to acetylcholine receptors
    (B) Blockage of sodium-gated ion channels
    (C) Demyelination of peripheral nerves

    (D) Genetic defect of chromosomes
    (E) Inhibition of acetylcholine release

3. A 46-year-old HIV positive male is brought to the emergency department by his partner. Over the past few weeks, the patient has been having unexplainable headaches and episodes of confusion. This evening he became agitated and then suddenly dropped to the floor and began convulsing. This went on for 30 to 60 seconds. His partner reports that the patient has been unable to afford antiretroviral drugs since he quit his job over a year ago. Diagnostic testing reveals a CD4 count of $160/mm^3$, and a CT scan of the brain demonstrates ring-enhancing lesions. Which of the following is the most likely diagnosis?

    (A) Bacterial meningitis
    (B) Ischemic stroke
    (C) Infectious encephalitis
    (D) Status epilepticus
    (E) Subarachnoid hemorrhage

4. A 10-month-old girl is brought to your facility with a history of fever and a rash. The parents report she was in good health until this morning, when she developed poor feeding, fever, and irritability. In the afternoon her parents noticed bruises on her legs and trunk. On examination, she appears acutely ill with fever, tachycardia, cool hands and feet, and petechiae on her legs and trunk. Which of the following is the diagnostic test of choice?

    (A) Blood cultures
    (B) CBC with differential
    (C) Coagulation profile
    (D) CSF analysis
    (E) Serum electrolytes

5. A patient presents with progressive visual changes over the past 2 years. On physical examination, bitemporal hemianopsia is noted. A lesion in which of the following anatomic locations is most likely to cause these findings?

   (A) Optic tract
   (B) Optic nerve
   (C) Occipital cortex
   (D) Optic chiasm

6. A 69-year-old male is brought to your clinic by his wife. She states that his handwriting has become smaller and he has been progressively dropping things over the last year. He also has developed a mild shaking of the right hand over the last few months that is worse when he sits down to rest. Examination is significant for masked facies, hypophonia, and right-sided bradykinesia and rigidity. Which of the following class of drugs is most commonly used for treatment?

   (A) Cholinesterase inhibitor
   (B) Dopamine agonist
   (C) Monoamine oxidase inhibitors
   (D) Opioid agonist
   (E) Serotonin reuptake inhibitor

7. Recent vaccination is associated with the development of which of the following conditions?

   (A) Benign essential tremor
   (B) Guillain–Barré syndrome
   (C) Multiple sclerosis
   (D) Huntington disease
   (E) Parkinson disease

8. A 35-year-old male with a history of type I diabetes complains of a 4-week history of severe headaches that occur every evening. The headaches are sharp in nature and affect the left eye. He reports profuse watery discharge from the left nostril and the left eye with each headache. Eye examination is negative for myosis, ptosis, conjunctival injection, and papilledema. Which of the following is the most likely diagnosis?

   (A) Cluster headache
   (B) Horner syndrome
   (C) Intracranial tumor
   (D) Migraine with aura
   (E) Pseudotumor cerebri

9. A 46-year-old female reports feeling an uncomfortable deep crawling and aching sensation in her legs. The patient notes that she typically experiences this sensation at night when she gets into bed. Also associated is a strong urge to move her legs and she has to get up several times each night to relieve the feeling. She denies associated low back pain or recent blood donation. Neurologic and vascular examination is normal. Which of the following is the most likely diagnosis?

   (A) Lumbosacral radiculopathy
   (B) Nocturnal leg cramps
   (C) Periodic limb movements of sleep
   (D) Peripheral neuropathy
   (E) Restless leg syndrome

10. A 21-year-old female presents with blurred vision and pain with movement in one eye. In addition, she is concerned about an episode of numbness and tingling she had in both feet 6 weeks ago. Review of systems is positive for constipation, fatigue, and nocturnal leg cramps. She denies extremity weakness or urinary frequency. Which of the following is the test of choice in evaluation of this patient?

    (A) Serum antimyelin antibodies
    (B) Cerebrospinal fluid analysis
    (C) Computed tomography
    (D) Evoked potentials
    (E) Magnetic resonance imaging

11. A 75-year-old male is brought to your clinic by his daughter for evaluation of forgetfulness. The patient reports that he is doing well and, aside from occasional difficulty sleeping and hypertension, he does not have any other health problems. According to his daughter, over the last year his memory seems to be getting worse; he has difficulties finding words and remembering recent events. What is the next most appropriate step?

    (A) Electroencephalogram
    (B) Intelligence quotient testing
    (C) Mini–mental status examination
    (D) Noncontrast head CT
    (E) Rapid plasma reagin (RPR)

12. Which of the following seizure medications is associated with gingival hyperplasia?

(A) Carbamazepine (Tegretol)

(B) Clonazepam (Klonopin)

(C) Ethosuximide (Zarontin)

(D) Phenytoin (Dilantin)

(E) Valproic acid (Depakote)

13. Which of the following functions is controlled by the frontal lobe?

(A) Gait

(B) Writing

(C) Planning

(D) Smell

(E) Vision

14. A 65-year-old chronic alcoholic is found disoriented and stumbling. On examination, he is somnolent and confused. Neurologic examination reveals a horizontal gaze palsy and ataxia but normal extremity motor strength. Deficiency of which of the following vitamins is the most likely cause?

(A) Biotin

(B) Niacin

(C) Riboflavin

(D) Thiamine

(E) Vitamin C

15. Which of the following is the most common finding in a person presenting with a brain abscess?

(A) Fever

(B) Headache

(C) Nuchal rigidity

(D) Papilledema

(E) Vomiting

16. An otherwise healthy 40-year-old female presents to the emergency department with a severe headache, nausea, and vomiting. Physical examination is significant for bilateral papilledema. The remainder of the physical examination is completely normal. Which of the following interventions is indicated first?

(A) Carotid ultrasound

(B) Lumbar puncture

(C) Computed tomography of the head

(D) Temporal artery biopsy

(E) Visual field testing

17. A 10-year-old male is brought to the pediatrician by his parents. The parents are concerned about frequent symptoms of facial twitches and sudden uncontrollable outbursts of sounds. These symptoms have been going on since he was in kindergarten and he has become reluctant to go to school for fear of ridicule by his peers. Which of the following is the most likely diagnosis?

(A) Complex partial seizures

(B) Conduct disorder

(C) Huntington disease

(D) Myoclonic seizures

(E) Tourette disorder

18. For the past 4 days, a 77-year-old female has been crying easily, confused, and rambling incoherently. Her medical history is remarkable for mild dementia and well-controlled hypertension. She has never had anything like this in the past and she has not had any recent changes to her medications. When questioned, she has no difficulty articulating a sentence but difficulty remembering what she was asked. Laboratory testing is significant for leukocytosis. What is the most likely diagnosis?

(A) Alzheimer disease

(B) Depression

(C) Delirium

(D) Sundowning

(E) Wernicke aphasia

19. While doing an eye examination, it is noted that patient's left eye will not move lateral of the midline. Which cranial nerve is implicated?

(A) CN II

(B) CN III

(C) CN IV

(D) CN VI

(E) CN VII

20. A patient develops pain, numbness, and tingling in both the hands and feet 1 year after undergoing gastrectomy. She denies joint swelling and extremity weakness. Which of the following tests would be best for determining the etiology of her presenting symptoms?

(A) Antinuclear antibody
(B) Electromyography
(C) Lumbar puncture
(D) Nerve biopsy
(E) Serum B_{12} level

21. Which of the following seizures is associated with incontinence?

(A) Atonic
(B) Complex partial
(C) Psychogenic
(D) Simple partial
(E) Tonic–clonic

22. A 21-year-old male is observed by his girlfriend to have episodes during which he seems inattentive and unresponsive to stimulation. During these episodes he typically will pull on his shirt and make smacking noises with his mouth. The episodes last for 30 to 60 seconds. Afterward, he is confused and denies any recollection of the event. This scenario best describes which type of seizure disorder?

(A) Absence
(B) Atonic
(C) Complex partial
(D) Psychogenic
(E) Simple partial

23. A 35-year-old female with a history of chronic hepatitis develops progressive personality changes, clumsiness, and stuttering speech to the point of near incoherence over a 6-month period. On physical examination, you notice dysarthria, muscular rigidity in the lower extremities, and spasm of the arms. Slit-lamp examination reveals gold-brown rings that encircle the iris in both eyes. Which of the following is most likely to be decreased in the serum of this patient?

(A) Ammonia
(B) Calcium

(C) Ceruloplasmin
(D) Glucose
(E) Lactate

24. A 55-year-old female suffered a fracture of her right wrist after a fall. Two months after the cast was removed she presents with a burning pain over the radial aspect of her wrist and sharp shooting pains into her palm, which increase with movements of the wrist. One month later, she returns complaining of continued pain over the volar and lateral wrist, now with mild swelling and discoloration of her hand. Several months after her injury, symptoms worsen and she develops limitations in range of motion of the right shoulder and right wrist, and contractures of the digits. Repeat radiographs show demineralization. This scenario best describes which of the following?

(A) Complex regional pain syndrome
(B) de Quervain's tenosynovitis
(C) Thoracic outlet syndrome
(D) Ulnar nerve entrapment
(E) Median nerve entrapment

25. A 46-year-old female presents with a long history of headaches. She describes the pain as a generalized squeezing and tightness. The headaches occur almost daily. No over-the-counter medications that she has tried have helped. She denies nausea, vomiting, eye tearing, and nasal congestion. On examination, there is mild tenderness of her scalp and both trapezius muscles. Which of the following precipitants is most common with this type of headache?

(A) Foods
(B) Menstruation
(C) Odors
(D) Smoking
(E) Stress

26. A 6-year-old boy is struck by a car while riding his bicycle. He reportedly was wearing no helmet sustaining a soft tissue injury to the R temporal area of the head. He was reported to be unconscious for 2 minutes following the accident. He is conscious and alert upon arrival to the emergency department by EMS reporting anisocoria. Within 45 minutes of his ED arrival he begins to vomit and shortly thereafter he becomes completely unresponsive. Which of the following most likely explains this child's injury?

(A) Spinal cord transection

(B) Chronic subdural hematoma

(C) Acute epidural hematoma

(D) Acute subarachnoid hemorrhage

(E) Grade III concussion

27. A 75-year-old man is involved in a motor vehicle accident and strikes his forehead on the windshield. He complains of neck pain and severe burning in his shoulders and arms. His physical examination reveals weakness of his upper extremities. What type of spinal cord injury does this patient have?

(A) Anterior cord syndrome

(B) Central cord syndrome

(C) Brown-Séquard syndrome

(D) Complete cord transection

(E) Cauda equina syndrome

28. A 41-year-old woman presents to the emergency department complaining of a sudden "thunderclap" onset of the "worst headache of my life." She denies taking anticoagulants, oral contraceptives, or estrogen replacement therapy. There is no family history of brain aneurysm. A noncontrast, computed tomography (CT) scan of her brain was obtained and is read "normal." The next appropriate step in the diagnosis of this patient would be

(A) Outpatient magnetic resonance imaging (MRI) of the brain

(B) Complete blood cell count (CBC) with differential

(C) Injection of sumatriptan (Imitrex)

(D) Lumbar puncture

(E) Repeat CT scan in 48 hours

29. A 45-year-old woman with a known seizure disorder has been noncompliant with her anticonvulsant medication due to side effects she has been experiencing. While in your office, she starts to seize, and continues to convulse for longer than 5 continuous minutes. Which of the following is the most appropriate initial drug treatment?

(A) Lorazepam

(B) Phenytoin

(C) Phenobarbital

(D) Valproic acid

30. While performing a routine history and physical examination on a 70-year-old man, you note a right carotid bruit. He denies any symptoms suggestive of a transient ischemic attack (TIA) or cerebrovascular accident. A carotid Doppler ultrasound shows a 40% stenosis of the right common carotid artery. The next most appropriate step would be:

(A) STAT carotid arteriogram

(B) Initiate antiplatelet aggregating therapy with aspirin

(C) Anticoagulate with warfarin, or other direct Xa inhibitor

(D) Intra-arterial tissue plasminogen activator (tPA)

(E) Carotid endarterectomy

31. A cerebrospinal fluid analysis reveals the following results: opalescent color, increased protein, decreased glucose, and increased polymorphonuclear white blood cells (WBCs). The most likely diagnosis would be:

(A) Subarachnoid hemorrhage

(B) Bacterial meningitis

(C) Viral meningitis

(D) Multiple sclerosis

(E) Encephalitis

32. A 45-year-old man presents to the office with a 24-hour history of right facial droop, decreased tearing in the right eye, poor right eyelid closure, hyperacusis, dysgeusia, and drooling from the right side of his mouth. On examination, the patient is found to have a right facial droop, and he is unable to close his right eye and raise his right eyebrow. The remainder of the physical examination is completely normal. His vision is not affected. What would be the most appropriate therapy at this time?

(A) Prednisone for 1 week and re-evaluate in office

(B) Stat CT scan of the head and neurology consult

(C) Obtain Lyme disease titers

(D) Aspirin

33. A 30-year-old man presents complaining of back pain radiating down his right leg. On examination, you note that his knee jerk reflex is absent on the right. This finding suggests compression of which spinal nerve root?

(A) L1–L2

(B) L3–L4

(C) S1–S2

(D) T11–T12

(E) C5–C6

34. A 62-year-old obese woman presents with progressive numbness and tingling in her feet for the past 3 months. On physical examination, the patient is found to have decreased sensation to pinprick and vibration, absence of ankle reflexes, and difficulty with tandem walking. Which is the most common etiology of her symptoms?

(A) Diabetes mellitus

(B) Alcoholism

(C) Vitamin B_{12} deficiency

(D) Spinal cord tumor

(E) Rheumatoid arthritis

35. A 19-year-old woman presents to the emergency department complaining of headache. The headaches are generalized and increasing in intensity. They have not responded to over-the-counter (OTC) medications. She complains of approximately 1 week of blurred vision, intermittent diplopia, and vague dizziness. Her medical history includes obesity and acne. She takes accutane and oral contraceptives. She is found to have bilateral papilledema, visual acuity of 20/30 on physical examination, and a normal MRI of the brain. The next most appropriate step would be

(A) CT scan of the head

(B) Lumbar puncture

(C) Therapy with high-dose prednisone

(D) Stat cerebral arteriogram

(E) Reassurance and follow-up in the office in 6 months

36. A 12-year-old, left-hand dominant girl is being evaluated for "spells" that she has been experiencing. According to her parents, she was born following an uncomplicated pregnancy and was a healthy child until last year when she was struck by a drunk driver while walking home from a friend's house. The episodes begin by her complaining of an upset stomach and then she appears confused, turns her head to the left, and raises her left arm in the air. Each episode lasts for about 30 to 60 seconds, after which she is very tired for another hour. This scenario best describes which type of seizure disorder?

(A) Absence

(B) Tonic–clonic

(C) Simple partial

(D) Complex partial

(E) Pseudoseizures

37. A 65-year-old man presents to the emergency department with an acute ischemic stroke. His CT scan is normal. His blood pressure is 180/100 mm Hg. What is the most appropriate treatment for his hypertension?

(A) Labetalol (Normodyne) 20 mg IV

(B) Nifedipine (Procardia) 10 mg po

(C) Nitroprusside (Nipride) drip at 1 mg/kg/min

(D) Clonidine (Catapres) 0.1 mg po

(E) No antihypertensive at this time

38. A 78-year-old woman presents to the office complaining of a constant left-sided headache for 2 months. She has tried various over-the-counter (OTC) medications without relief. The patient admits to vision loss of her left eye last night for 10 minutes. The patient states that her vision then returned to normal. She denies pain in her eye. On review of systems, she relates several months of muscle aches and weight loss. On physical examination, she is found to have a tender, nonpulsatile superficial temporal artery. Her sedimentation rate is elevated at 90 mm/h. What is the next most appropriate step in the evaluation of this patient?

(A) Stat MRI/MRA of the brain and cranial vessels

(B) Aspirin therapy

(C) High-dose prednisone

(D) Lumbar puncture

(E) Sumatriptan (Imitrex) injection

39. An otherwise healthy 16-year-old girl presents to your office with a complaint of headache that began when getting ready for school today. Her mother, who has a history of migraine headaches herself, reports that her daughter had a similar headache a month ago lasting about 2 days. The pain continues to worsen on a pain scale of 9–10/10. It is generalized headache, throbs, and worsens when she moves. She is likely to vomit if she does not stop what she is doing and go lay down in a dark, quiet room. No over-the-counter medications that she tried have ever worked. The mother has migraines as well as the maternal grandmother. She is not on oral contraceptives, denies sudden "thunderclap" headache, and there is no family history of cerebral aneurysm. Her history is consistent with which of the following?

(A) Migraine with aura
(B) Cluster headache
(C) Tension-type headache
(D) Migraine without aura
(E) Medication withdrawal headache

40. After a carotid endarterectomy, a patient experienced a unilateral small pupil, mild ptosis with normal response to light and accommodation. This abnormality is called:

(A) Adie pupil
(B) Argyll Robertson pupil
(C) Horner syndrome
(D) Marcus Gunn pupil
(E) Light-near dissociation

41. A 73-year-old man is brought into your office by his adult children with a concern of memory loss. They report their father's memory has been declining since the death of their mother a few months ago but are now concerned because he is losing weight, sleeping during the daytime, and is not keeping up with current events like he usually does. This type of behavior is most associated with which of the following?

(A) Pick disease
(B) Creutzfeldt–Jakob disease
(C) Depression
(D) Alzheimer disease
(E) Vitamin B$_{12}$ deficiency

42. A postural tremor that occurs at rest and may be exacerbated by fear, anxiety, excessive physical activity, or sleep deprivation is consistent with which of the following?

(A) Wilson disease
(B) Intention tremor
(C) Asterixis
(D) Physiologic tremor
(E) Hemiballismus

43. Which of the following is the most appropriate initial disease-modifying treatment for a patient diagnosed with multiple sclerosis?

(A) Beta-interferon
(B) Methylprednisone
(C) Methotrexate
(D) Natalizumab

44. A 62-year-old man presents to the emergency department with aphasia and right lower extremity weakness that started about 4 hours ago. He now has progressive right upper extremity weakness, worsening right lower extremity weakness, and decreased sensation throughout his right side. This cerebral ischemia is best characterized as:

(A) Transient ischemic attack
(B) Stroke in evolution
(C) Completed stroke
(D) Subarachnoid hemorrhage
(E) Global cerebral ischemia

45. A 58-year-old man presents to your office with a complaint of tremor in his right hand at rest. Upon questioning, you discover that the tremor is getting worse and now seems to be in both arms especially when at his sides. He also complains that food doesn't smell as good now and he is having trouble eating with a fork and buttoning his shirt. On your physical examination, you notice a resting tremor, bradykinesia, rigidity, and a shuffling gait. What is your initial assessment?

(A) Essential tremor
(B) Wilson disease
(C) Huntington disease
(D) Parkinson disease
(E) Progressive supranuclear palsy

46. A 65-year-old man is brought to the clinic by his family noting increasing short-term memory loss, intermittent confusion, trouble handling money, and increased anxiety over the last 6 months. In the last couple weeks he seems to have an occasional problem recognizing people he should know, and a new unfamiliarity with performing tasks he normally would be accustomed to performing like simple use of the kitchen toaster. Recently, his decline has accelerated. This patient is most likely experiencing:

(A) Depression
(B) Delirium
(C) Hypothyroidism
(D) Normal pressure hydrocephalus
(E) Alzheimer dementia

47. A 52-year-old female bus driver presents to the clinic with a chief complaint of intense, shooting pains in her right cheek, each lasting for only a few seconds she avoids touching certain parts of her face and has started to chew food only on the right side of her mouth because she is afraid she will set off an attack of pain. In between attacks, the patient feels well. What is the most likely diagnosis?

(A) Cluster headache
(B) Tension-type headache
(C) Trigeminal neuralgia
(D) Giant cell arteritis
(E) Dental abscess

48. A 22-year-old woman, with no previous medical problems, suddenly cried out, fell to the ground, extended her legs, flexed her arms, and jerked her extremities for 30 seconds. There was associated tongue biting and urinary incontinence. She awoke slowly over a 10-minute period and recalled nothing about the episode. She remained lethargic for several hours but the rest of her neurologic examination was normal. What is the most likely etiology for this episode?

(A) Epilepsy
(B) Hyperventilation
(C) Cardiac arrhythmia
(D) Seizure
(E) Stroke

49. A 36-year-old auto mechanic presents to the emergency department after hurting his back on the job. While lifting an object, he experienced sudden pain in his lower back with radiation to the right buttock. He was initially treated for muscle strain with a nonsteroidal anti-inflammatory drug (NSAID) after x-rays of his lumbosacral spine demonstrated no pathology. He continued to complain of this low back pain now radiating posteriorly down his left leg to the midthigh. Physical examination is unremarkable. The most likely diagnosis is:

(A) Mechanical low back pain
(B) Left S1 radiculopathy
(C) Cauda equina syndrome
(D) L5–S1 disc herniation
(E) Lateral femoral cutaneous neuropathy

50. Midday, an 18-year-old woman is transferred to your emergency department from a local college infirmary. She presented to the infirmary complaining of headache beginning late the night before. At the infirmary her headache had worsened and she became confused. On examination, she was found to be febrile with a petechial rash. A lumbar puncture is done and the cerebrospinal fluid comes back with increased WBCs, increased protein, and decreased glucose. What is the most likely organism responsible for her meningitis?

(A) *Haemophilus influenzae*
(B) *Cytomegalovirus*
(C) *Neisseria meningitidis*
(D) *Mycobacterium tuberculosis*
(E) *Coxsackievirus B*

51. Which of the following is the most common etiology for a subarachnoid hemorrhage?

(A) Trauma
(B) Ruptured aneurysm
(C) Bleeding arteriovenous malformation
(D) Embolic stroke
(E) Primary intracerebral hemorrhage

52. A 63-year-old woman with a medical history of type II diabetes, hypertension, obesity, and *hyperlipidemia* presents to the clinic complaining of burning pain in her feet bilaterally *(dysautonomia)*.

Neurologic examination is normal except for hyperesthesia and loss of vibratory sensation bilaterally in her feet. Which of the following *may be the* preferred *initial* treatment for managing this patient's pain?

(A) Amitriptyline

(B) *Cetuximab (Erbitux)*

(C) Oxycodone (OxyContin)

(D) *Edrophonium (Tensilon)*

(E) *Vitamin D*

53. A 43-year-old woman presents complaining of a "pins and needles" sensation that started bilaterally in her feet 2 days ago. *Ten days prior she ate "on the road" and developed 4 days of nausea, vomiting, and diarrhea.* The sensation now extends up to her midthighs. On physical examination, she is noted to have mild sensory loss, *increasing difficulty with gait,* and absent reflexes bilaterally in her legs. Which of the following is the most likely diagnosis?

(A) Diabetic peripheral neuropathy

(B) Guillain–Barré syndrome

(C) Multiple sclerosis

(D) Myasthenia gravis

(E) Hypothyroidism

54. A 53-year-old man presents to the emergency department because of fever, headache, and confusion. On physical examination, you note an obtunded man who appears acutely ill with temperature of 104°F, blood pressure of 128/76 mm Hg, pulse of 98, and respiratory rate of 20. The patient has stomatitis, nuchal rigidity, and a positive Kernig sign. CSF examination shows increased opening pressure, 80 WBC/mL (normal <10/mL), mildly elevated protein, and normal glucose. Which of the following tests would confirm the most likely causative organism?

(A) CT of the head

(B) Polymerase chain reaction test for herpes simplex virus (PCR)

(C) Blood culture for herpes simplex virus

(D) Serum IgG for herpes simplex virus

(E) MRI of the head

55. A 62-year-old man is brought to the emergency department after being found unresponsive in his car. On physical examination, his pupils are noted to be 7 mm on the right and 3 mm on the left. Which of the following diagnostic tests is most likely to identify the cause of the patient's signs and symptoms?

(A) Straight catheter obtained urine drug screen

(B) STAT serum electrolytes

(C) MRI with contrast

(D) STAT liver function tests

(E) STAT skull x-rays

56. A 3-year-old girl is being followed by the neurologist to evaluate her motor spasticity that resulted from anoxia during labor and delivery. Which of the following is the most likely cause of this patient's spasticity?

(A) Cerebral palsy

(B) Congenital hypothyroidism

(C) Meningitis

(D) Multiple sclerosis

57. During physical examination, a 58-year-old man is instructed to hold his hands up as if he was attempting to stop traffic. After about 20 seconds of observation his wrists *demonstrate an* intermittent *sudden loss of postural tone that is translated into a flapping movement of flexion* and return to extension. This physical examination sign is known as:

(A) Asterixis

(B) Brudzinski sign

(C) Clonus

(D) Stereognosis

(E) *Hyperekplexia*

58. A 16-year-old girl presents to the clinic complaining of strong desires to sleep at inappropriate times. She is very concerned because she "felt paralyzed" while falling asleep on the couch last night. Which of the following is the best diagnostic test to confirm this patient's diagnosis?

(A) CT of the head

(B) Multiple sleep latency test

(C) Tensilon test

(D) Thyroid stimulating hormone

(E) Polysomnography

59. A 12-year-old boy presents to the clinic for follow-up regarding his recently diagnosed partial seizures. *Neither the parent nor the patient* reports *any interval* seizures or side effects since *he started taking* carbamazepine (Tegretol) 1 month ago. What study should be ordered to monitor this patient's treatment?

(A) Blood glucose

(B) Complete blood cell count, *liver function tests, sodium*

(C) Electroencephalogram

(D) Vitamin B_{12}

(E) Urinalysis

60. Which of the following findings is consistent with a lower motor neuron deficit?

(A) Aphasia

(B) Dysdiadochokinesia

(C) Sensory loss

(D) Weakness

(E) Hyperreflexia

61. A 78-year-old woman with a medical history of diabetes and hypertension presents to the emergency department complaining of left hand weakness and slurred speech. Which of the following tests is most likely to determine the source of an arterial thrombus?

(A) Carotid ultrasound

(B) CT of the brain

(C) Erythrocyte sedimentation rate

(D) Magnetic resonance angiography (MRA) of the vertebral arteries

62. It is not uncommon for premonitory symptoms of an impending cerebral aneurysm rupture to begin 10 to 20 days earlier to the event. The following lists are likely signs and symptoms that occur in order of prevalence, the first being the most common. Select the correct order of symptoms that can be found.

(A) Headache, sensory and motor disturbance, dizziness, diplopia, orbital pain

(B) Dizziness, headache, sensory and motor disturbance, diplopia, orbital pain

(C) Sensory and motor disturbance, diplopia, headache, dizziness, orbital pain

(D) Sensory and motor disturbance, dizziness, headache, orbital pain, diplopia

(E) Headache, dizziness, orbital pain, sensory and motor disturbance, diplopia

63. A 37-year-old woman presents to your office with the complaint of bouts of pain and tingling in dominant right hand most severe during hours of sleep. Sensation in the radial palm has been recurrent. On your examination, she demonstrates a positive Phalen sign, and positive Tinel sign with paresthesias consistently in the distribution of the median nerve. She states that the pain can sometimes wake her up at night and feels as if her thumb is falling asleep. What disease might be associated with this onset of symptoms?

(A) Myasthenia gravis

(B) Radial nerve compression

(C) Thoracic outlet syndrome

(D) Carpal tunnel syndrome

(E) Recent injury to the medial cord of the right brachial plexus

Answers and Explanations

1. **(A)** The diagnosis is amyotrophic lateral sclerosis. This is a degenerative motor neuron disease that is marked by weakness and wasting of affected muscles without accompanying sensory changes. Guillain–Barré syndrome most commonly follows infective illness, inoculations, or surgical procedures. It also typically involves lower extremity weakness but will have an ascending pattern and is associated with sensory changes. Multiple sclerosis will present with episodic weakness, numbness, tingling, or unsteadiness in a limb; optic neuritis and diplopia are also common. Myasthenia gravis presents with any combination of ptosis, diplopia, difficulty in chewing or swallowing, respiratory difficulties, and limb weakness. Nonparalytic poliomyelitis presents with fever, headache, and vomiting. Signs of meningeal irritation and muscle spasm occur in the absence of frank paralysis. *(Aminoff & Kerchner, 2013, pp. 1010, 1019, 1024, 1032, 1372)*

2. **(A)** Myasthenia gravis is due to antibodies directed at acetylcholine receptors. Demyelination of peripheral nerves is seen with multiple sclerosis. Inhibition of acetylcholine release is seen with botulism. A variety of disorders affecting muscle contraction and nerve function are due to chromosomal causes and/or gene mutations that affect sodium-gated ion channels. *(Aminoff & Kerchner, 2013, pp. 1010, 1032–1033)*

3. **(C)** The diagnosis is infectious encephalitis. Considering the advanced immunosuppression, an opportunistic infection is most likely. Toxoplasma is suggested by ring enhancement on CT. Bacterial meningitis typically presents with fever, headache, stiff neck, or altered mental status. Ischemic stroke would likely present with focal neurologic deficits and hemiplegia. Status epilepticus presents as prolonged seizure activity and is a medical emergency. Subarachnoid hemorrhage presents with sudden onset of the worst headache of life, which may lead rapidly to loss of consciousness. This would also be identified on a CT. *(Aminoff & Kerchner, 2013, pp. 970, 980, 1287; Koralnik, 2015)*

4. **(D)** A lumbar puncture will establish the diagnosis of meningitis and should be performed on any child in whom meningitis is suspected, unless specific contraindications to lumbar puncture are present. Isolation of a bacterial pathogen from the cerebrospinal fluid (CSF) confirms the diagnosis of bacterial meningitis. Blood tests are helpful in evaluation of bacterial meningitis but are nonspecific. Tests should include a complete blood count with differential and platelet count and two aerobic blood cultures. Serum electrolytes and glucose, blood urea nitrogen, and creatinine concentrations are helpful in determining the cerebrospinal fluid-to-blood glucose ratio, and in planning fluid administration. Evaluation of clotting function is indicated if petechiae or purpuric lesions are noted. *(Kaplan, 2015)*

5. **(D)** Bitemporal hemianopsia is caused by a chiasmatic lesion. An optic nerve lesion results in complete blindness in the eye affected. A homonymous hemianopia can result from lesions in multiple areas specifically the optic tract or occipital cortex. *(Ropper et al., 2014)*

6. **(B)** Pharmacologic options for Parkinson disease include dopamine agonists, anticholinergics, amantadine, monoamine oxidase type B inhibitors, levodopa/carbidopa, and catechol-O-methyltransferase inhibitors. The American Academy of Neurology determined that is reasonable to start treatment with levodopa, a dopamine precursor, or a dopamine

agonist. Cholinesterase inhibitors are used in treating Alzheimer disease and glaucoma. Opioid agonists are used in opioid dependence treatment. Monoamine oxidase inhibitors and selective serotonin reuptake inhibitors are used, in general, to treat depression and anxiety. *(Chisholm-Burns et al., 2013, pp. 596, 649, 681, 690–691, 722, 726)*

7. **(B)** Recent vaccination is one potential cause of Guillain–Barré syndrome (GBS). Patients can also develop GBS after another triggering event such as infection, surgery, trauma, or bone marrow transplantation. The cause of benign essential tremor is uncertain, but it is sometimes inherited in an autosomal dominant manner. Multiple sclerosis is likely autoimmune in nature and is more common in western Europeans who live in temperate zones. Huntington disease is caused by an inherited defect in a single gene on chromosome 4. Idiopathic Parkinson disease is due to dopamine depletion in the nigrostriatal system. Although, in contrast, parkinsonism has been linked to environmental triggers such as certain toxins and carbon monoxide. *(Aminoff & Kerchner, 2013, pp. 997–998, 1001, 1010; Vriesendorp, 2015)*

8. **(A)** The diagnosis is cluster headache as signified by episodes of severe unilateral periorbital pain accompanied by one or more of the following: ipsilateral nasal congestion, rhinorrhea, lacrimation, and redness of the eye. Horner syndrome presents with ptosis of the eyelid, meiosis or constriction of the pupil, and anhidrosis or reduced sweat secretion. Headaches associated with tumors may be worsened by exertion or postural change and may be associated with nausea and vomiting, but this is also true of migraine. Migrainous headaches generally are lateralized, may be dull or throbbing, and are sometimes associated with nausea, vomiting, photophobia, phonophobia, and blurring of vision. Migraine with aura denotes a migraine headache preceded by an abnormal sensory experience. Pseudotumor cerebri is suggested by headache, diplopia, and other visual disturbances due to papilledema and abducens nerve dysfunction. *(Aminoff & Kerchner, 2013, pp. 963, 965–966, 995)*

9. **(E)** The symptoms of voluntary leg movement prompted by an urge to move that is maximal at rest, worsens at night, and is relieved by movement

is classic for restless legs syndrome (RLS). Although symptoms of neuropathy and RLS can be partially overlapping, the discomfort of peripheral neuropathy is more commonly associated with sensory paresthesias and sensitivity to touching of the skin and typically not relieved by movement. Lumbosacral radiculopathy, unlike RLS, is often asymmetrical and associated with lower back pain and sensory paresthesias. Nocturnal leg cramps are typically a more localized pain characterized by sudden muscle tightness that is relieved by forceful muscle stretching rather than simple movement of the legs. *(Tarsey, 2015)*

10. **(E)** Multiple sclerosis (MS) can present in a myriad of ways but the most common presenting signs are optic neuritis and transverse myelitis. MRI is the test of choice to support the clinical diagnosis of MS. The McDonald diagnostic criteria include specific clinical and MRI findings needed for the demonstration of lesion dissemination in time and space. Current evidence suggests antimyelin antibodies are not associated with an increased risk of progression to MS or with MS disease activity. CSF analysis is not a requirement for the diagnosis of MS in patients with classic MS symptoms and brain MRI appearance, but it can be used to help rule out the diagnosis in equivocal cases. MRI detects many more MS lesions than CT, and it is able to detect plaques in regions that are rarely abnormal on CT such as the brainstem, cerebellum, and spinal cord. Evoked potentials may help with subclinical disease detection. Evoked potentials also may help define the anatomical site of the lesion in tracts not easily visualized by imaging, such as the optic nerve. *(Olek, 2015)*

11. **(C)** The mini-mental status examination is a useful screening test for dementia. Electroencephalogram is primarily utilized in the evaluation of seizure activity. Intelligence quotient (IQ) testing is not used in the diagnosis of dementia, although, estimating the premorbid mental ability may be useful to assess the extent of dementia present. Structural neuroimaging with a head CT or MRI scan is important for patients with acute onset of cognitive impairment and rapid neurologic deterioration. Screening for neurosyphilis with RPR is not recommended unless there is a high clinical suspicion. *(Aminoff & Kerchner, 2013, pp. 970–971; Shadlen & Larsen, 2015)*

12. (D) Phenytoin is associated with gingival hyperplasia, anemia, and hirsutism. Carbamazepine is associated with aplastic anemia, hyponatremia, and leukopenia. Clonazepam is associated with ataxia, sedation, and slowed thinking. Ethosuximide is associated with hepatotoxicity, neutropenia, and rash. Valproic acid is associated with hepatotoxicity, osteoporosis, and pancreatitis. *(Chisholm-Burns et al., 2013, pp. 567–572)*

13. (C) Functions of the frontal lobe include planning and initiating of activity, reasoning and abstraction, monitoring and shaping of behavior to ensure adaptive actions, prioritizing and sequencing actions, and problem solving. Function of the parietal lobe includes integrating sensory information from various senses, and in the manipulation of objects; portions of the parietal lobe are involved with visuospatial processing. Function of the occipital lobe includes sense of sight. Function of the temporal lobe includes sense of smell and sound, as well as processing of complex stimuli like faces and scenes. The cerebellum is involved in motor control. *(Silverthorn, 2007, pp. 308–311; Waxman, 2013)*

14. (D) Wernicke–Korsakoff syndrome is the best known neurologic complication of thiamine (vitamin B$_1$) deficiency. Nystagmus, ophthalmoplegia, and ataxia, along with confusion are common presenting signs and symptoms. This combination of symptoms is almost exclusively described in chronic alcoholics with thiamine deficiency. Symptoms of biotin deficiency are nonspecific and may include changes in mental status, myalgia, dysesthesias, anorexia, and nausea. Niacin deficiency, also known as pellagra, causes a symmetric hyperpigmented rash, similar in color to a sunburn. Other clinical findings are a red tongue and many nonspecific symptoms, such as diarrhea and vomiting. Neurologic symptoms include insomnia, anxiety, disorientation, delusions, dementia, and encephalopathy. Riboflavin deficiency is characterized by sore throat, hyperemia of pharyngeal mucous membranes, cheilitis, stomatitis, glossitis, normocytic-normochromic anemia, and seborrheic dermatitis. Scurvy (vitamin C deficiency) is characterized by ecchymoses, bleeding gums, petechiae, hyperkeratosis, arthralgias, and impaired wound healing. *(Pazirandeh et al., 2015)*

15. (B) Headache is the most common symptom of a brain abscess occurring in 69% of patients. The pain is usually localized to the side of the abscess, and its onset can be gradual or sudden. The pain tends to be severe and not relieved by over-the-counter pain medications. Neck stiffness occurs in 15% of patients. Fever is not a reliable indicator of brain abscess since only 45% to 53% of patients have this sign. Vomiting generally develops in association with increased intracranial pressure. Papilledema is found in 25% of patients with a brain abscess as a late manifestation of cerebral edema and usually takes days to develop. *(Southwick, 2015)*

16. (C) The first step in the evaluation of papilledema should be a neuroimaging study; although a brain MRI is preferred, a CT scan should be done if an MRI is not available, like in the emergency department. Lumbar puncture with measurement of opening pressure and analysis of cerebrospinal fluid should follow a normal neuroimaging study. Measurements of visual acuity and visual field testing are important while following the course of papilledema and response to treatment. Carotid ultrasound is recommended in patients with neurologic symptoms, hemiparesis, paresthesia, and acute speech and visual field defects. Temporal artery biopsy is used in the evaluation of headache associated with giant cell arteritis. *(Aminoff & Kerchner, 2013, pp. 846, 978; Bienfang, 2015)*

17. (E) Tourette disorder is most likely. Motor tics are the initial manifestation in 80% of cases and most commonly involve the face, whereas in the remaining 20%, the initial symptoms are phonic tics; ultimately a combination of different motor and phonic tics develop in all patients. These are noted first in childhood, generally between the ages of 2 and 15. Complex partial seizures involve impaired consciousness. Myoclonic seizures consist of single or multiple muscle jerks and are not associated with vocal outbursts. Huntington disease is characterized by onset of chorea and dementia between 30 and 50 years of age. The disease is progressive and usually leads to a fatal outcome within 15 to 20 years. *(Aminoff & Kerchner, 2013, pp. 969, 1001, 1004–1005)*

18. (C) Delirium is the most likely diagnosis. Delirious individuals have cognitive and perceptual problems, including memory loss, disorientation, and difficulty with language and speech. Delirium may be the only finding suggesting acute illness in older demented patients. Infections are common precipitators of delirium and the underlying leukocytosis in this patient is key. In contrast to delirium, cognitive change in Alzheimer disease is typically insidious, progressive, without much fluctuation, and occurs over a much longer time. Delirium is commonly misdiagnosed as depression. Both are associated with poor sleep and difficulty with attention or concentration but depression will not cause a leukocytosis. Sundowning presents as behavioral deterioration seen in the evening hours, typically in demented, institutionalized patients. Patients with Wernicke aphasia may appear delirious in that they do not comprehend or obey and seem confused. However, the problem is restricted to language, while other aspects of mental function are intact. *(Francis & Young, 2015)*

19. **(D)** Three cranial nerves provide efferent control of the extraocular muscles. The abducens nerve (CN VI) controls the lateral rectus. The trochlear nerve (CN IV) controls the superior oblique. The oculomotor nerve controls the superior rectus, inferior rectus, and medial rectus. This can be summarized as SO4, LR6, and the remainder 3 which means that superior oblique muscle is innervated by the trochlear nerve, the lateral rectus muscle is innervated by the abducens nerve, and the remainder of the eye muscles is innervated by the oculomotor nerve. *(Chung & Chung, 2008, pp. 381–382)*

20. **(E)** Gastrectomy can produce vitamin B_{12} deficiency which subsequently can cause a distal neuropathy. Laboratory tests with the highest yield for detecting abnormalities in patients with polyneuropathy are blood glucose and serum B_{12} level. Antinuclear antibodies are used to diagnose autoimmune disease which is unlikely with this presentation. Electromyography and/or nerve conduction is useful when there is no clear etiology or when symptoms are severe or rapidly progressive. Nerve biopsy is occasionally useful for diagnosing the underlying etiology of polyneuropathy. Nerve biopsy generally is reserved for patients in whom it is difficult to define whether the process is predominantly axonal or demyelinating. Lumbar

puncture is helpful in identifying patients with inflammatory demyelinating polyneuropathies. *(Pagana & Pagana, 2007, p. 90; Rutkove, 2015; Schrier, 2015)*

21. **(E)** Tonic–clonic seizures are associated with cessation of breathing and incontinence. Atonic seizures are typically associated with loss of muscle tone and collapse to the ground. In complex partial seizures (focal seizure with loss of consciousness) there are focal motor or autonomic symptoms, or subjective sensory or psychic symptoms that may precede, accompany, or follow the period of altered responsiveness. Psychogenic nonepileptic seizures (PNES) resemble tonic–clonic seizures, but there may be obvious preparation before a PNES occurs. Moreover, there is usually no tonic phase. Simple partial seizures (focal seizure with no loss of consciousness) present with focal motor, sensory, psychic and/or autonomic symptoms but the patient does not lose consciousness. *(Aminoff & Kerchner, 2013, pp. 969–972)*

22. **(C)** The scenario describes a complex partial seizure (focal seizure with loss of consciousness). Observable focal motor or autonomic symptoms, or subjective sensory or psychic symptoms may precede, accompany, or follow the period of altered responsiveness. Atonic seizures are typically associated with loss of muscle tone and collapse to the ground. Clinically, psychogenic nonepileptic seizures (PNES), resemble tonic–clonic seizures, but there may be obvious preparation before a PNES occurs. Moreover, there is usually no tonic phase; instead, there may be an asynchronous thrashing of the limbs, which increases if restraints are imposed and rarely leads to injury. Postictally, there are no changes in behavior or neurologic findings. Simple partial (focal seizure with no loss of consciousness) present with focal motor or autonomic symptoms, or subjective sensory or psychic symptoms but the patient does not lose consciousness. *(Aminoff & Kerchner, 2013, pp. 969–972)*

23. **(C)** Approximately 80% to 90% of patients with Wilson disease have low serum ceruloplasmin levels and a serum ceruloplasmin concentration less than the laboratory lower limit for normal. Decreased levels of ammonia are seen with essential or malignant hypertension and hyperornithinemia.

Hypocalcemia is seen in multiple diseases but commonly with hypoparathyroidism and renal failure. Hypoglycemia is seen with diseases such as insulinoma. A decreased lactate dehydrogenase is not clinically significant but can be caused by drugs such as ascorbic acid. *(Pagana & Pagana, 2007, pp. 53, 225, 491, 583; Schilsky, 2015)*

24. **(A)** Complex regional pain syndrome (formerly called reflex sympathetic dystrophy) is a rare disorder of the extremities characterized by autonomic and vasomotor instability. The cardinal symptoms and signs are pain localized to an arm or leg, swelling of the involved extremity, disturbances of color and temperature in the affected limb, dystrophic changes in the overlying skin and nails, and limited range of motion. Most cases are preceded by direct physical trauma, often of relatively minor nature, to the soft tissues, bone, or nerve. Radiographs eventually reveal severe generalized osteopenia. Compression of the ulnar nerve is the second most common entrapment neuropathy after carpal tunnel syndrome. The most frequent site of compression is at the elbow. Symptoms usually begin with tingling in the fourth and fifth digits of the hand. Patients suffering from thoracic outlet syndrome have pain that radiates from the point of compression to the base of the neck, axilla, arm, forearm, and hand. Paresthesias are common and distributed to the volar aspect of the fourth and fifth digits. Sensory symptoms may be aggravated at night or by prolonged use of the extremities. Weakness and muscle atrophy are the principal motor abnormalities. Vascular symptoms consist of arterial ischemia characterized by pallor of the fingers on elevation of the extremity. There is no associated osteopenia in thoracic outlet syndrome. With de Quervain's tenosynovitis, patients experience pain on grasping with their thumb. Swelling and tenderness are often present over the radial styloid process. The usual cause is repetitive twisting of the wrist. *(Aminoff & Kerchner, 2013, pp. 818–819, 823–825; Josephson & Samuels, 2012; Langford & Gilliland, 2012)*

25. **(E)** Stress and mental tension are reported to be the most common precipitants for tension headache. Foods, hunger, menstruation, and odor are significantly more common triggers in patients with migraine headache. *(Taylor, 2015)*

26. **(C)** This is the classic history of an epidural hematoma. The typical presentation is that of a child who sustains a blow to the head and experiences a brief loss of consciousness, followed by a lucid interval, when the child is awake and alert. As the hematoma expands, the patient experiences a headache followed by vomiting, lethargy, ipsilateral anisocoria, and contralateral hemiparesis. This condition may progress to coma and/or death if left untreated. This injury usually results from a temporal bone fracture with a laceration of the middle meningeal artery or vein and less often a tear in a dural venous sinus. Intracranial epidural hematoma may be acute (58%), subacute (31%), or chronic (11%). Epidural hematomas are treated with surgical evacuation of the clot and ligation of the bleeding vessel. Spinal cord transection should not present initially as a loss of consciousness and will affect distal motor and sensory function. Chronic subdural hematomas present more than 20 days after the trauma. Subarachnoid hemorrhage typically presents as a generalized headache without associated trauma. A grade III concussion usually involves continued improvement after consciousness is gained. The lucid period followed by worsening symptoms in this question is worrisome of more severe intracranial pathology. *(Aminoff et al., 2005, p. 329; McBride, 2013)*

27. **(B)** The central cord syndrome involves loss of motor function that is more severe in the upper extremities than in the lower extremities, and is more severe in the hands. There is typically hyperesthesia over the shoulders and arms. Anterior cord syndrome presents with paraplegia or quadriplegia, loss of lateral spinothalamic function with preservation of posterior column function. Brown-Séquard syndrome consists of weakness and loss of posterior column function on one side of the body distal to the lesion with contralateral loss of lateral spinothalamic function one to two levels below the lesion. Complete cord transection would affect motor and sensory function distal to the lesion. Cauda equina syndrome typically presents as low back pain with radiculopathy. *(Hauser & Ropper, 2008, p. 2580)*

28. **(D)** The hallmark of a subarachnoid hemorrhage is the very sudden onset of a severe headache. The headache is often described as the "worst headache

of my life." A CT scan will detect a subarachnoid hemorrhage in about 93% to 100% of cases within 24 hours if a fifth-generation CT scanner is used. Studies show that small bleeds may not be found on CT scan. Furthermore, the accuracy of CT scanning finding a bleed may reduce to approximately 58% by 5 days from initial bleed. When the history suggests SAH and the CT scan fails to detect a bleed, a lumbar puncture is mandatory. The lumbar puncture may yield bloody cerebrospinal fluid indicating a subarachnoid hemorrhage, or possibly, a bloody tap. Cell counts in tubes #1 and #4 often help to clarify this point. Following neurologic consultation, admission most often occurs to allow for additional workup and management. CBC with differential, chemistries, and PT/PTT/INR may be ordered. Treatment with Imitrex is contraindicated in the presence of a potential cerebrovascular syndrome. *(Singer, Ogilvy & Rordorf, 2013)*

29. **(A)** Status epilepticus is defined as a continuous seizure or repeated seizures for longer than 5 minutes without the patient regaining consciousness. This is a medical emergency that calls for prompt intervention to stop the seizure activity. An intravenous infusion of a longer acting benzodiazepine, such as lorazepam, has been shown to be effective in terminating a seizure. If the seizures persist, then other potential agents to use after the initial lorazepam infusion include fosphenytoin (phenytoin), phenobarbital, or valproic acid (depakote). *(Lowenstien, 2015)*

30. **(B)** The patient exhibits an asymptomatic carotid bruit. The most appropriate step would be to initiate antiplatelet aggregating therapy with daily aspirin. Arteriography would not be indicated for an asymptomatic carotid bruit. Anticoagulation with warfarin (coumadin), or any Xa inhibitor drug should be limited to symptomatic bruits manifested as multiple TIAs. Carotid endarterectomy is reserved for carotid artery stenosis that is greater than 50% to 70% in patients who have had recurrent TIAs on medical therapy. *(Aminoff et al., 2005, pp. 308–310; McCarron, Goldstein & Matchar, 2015)*

31. **(B)** The cerebrospinal fluid (CSF) analysis in bacterial meningitis includes a cloudy appearance with a markedly elevated protein and white cell content. The white cells are predominantly polymorphonuclear (PMN) leukocytes. Bacterial utilization of CSF glucose causes it to be low. Gram stain may or may not be positive for bacteria. The diagnosis of bacterial meningitis requires a culture of the CSF. CSF pressures at the time of the lumbar puncture are elevated in 90% of cases. In viral meningitis, the CSF white count is usually 1,000/mL. The cell types are lymphocytes or monocytes but early in the disease PMN leukocytes may predominate. CSF glucose is normal in viral meningitis and protein is elevated. Gram stain will be negative and the culture will show no growth. The CSF in multiple sclerosis may have a mild lymphocytosis with an increased protein concentration. CSF protein electrophoresis in multiple sclerosis shows discrete bands of IgG called *oligoclonal bands*. These oligoclonal bands are present in 90% of patients with multiple sclerosis. The CSF in subarachnoid hemorrhage may be grossly bloody. Because bleeding can be caused by a traumatic puncture, the red blood cell (RBC) count should be done on the first and last tubes and the counts compared. In subarachnoid hemorrhage, the RBC count will be the same, whereas in a traumatic lumbar puncture, the RBCs will not be present, or, may be markedly diminished in the last tube that is collected. The CSF in subarachnoid hemorrhage may reveal xanthochromia. This is a yellow appearance in the centrifuged CSF supernatant caused by the degradation of RBCs in the CSF. The CSF becomes xanthochromic after it has been exposed to blood for several hours. *(Aminoff et al., 2005, p. 12)*

32. **(A)** This is a typical presentation of Bell's palsy. Bell's palsy is an idiopathic facial nerve palsy that results in unilateral weakness or paralysis of the facial muscles. This results in facial drooping, decreased tearing, aching in the ear or mastoid of the affected side, taste alteration, tingling or numbness involving the cheek/mouth of the affected side, and, an inability to close the eye and to raise the affected eyebrow. Facial weakness caused by a stroke does not affect the ability to close the affected eye or to move the forehead. This weakness is characteristic of peripheral seventh nerve palsy. In a stroke, there are often other abnormalities beyond the facial nerve. Bell's palsy is often

preceded or accompanied by pain around the ear. It is more common in pregnancy and in diabetics. It is believed that starting prednisone within 5 days of the onset of symptoms increases the number of patients who recover completely. The weakness or paralysis is usually maximal between 2 and 5 days. Eighty percent of patients recover in several weeks. In some cases, it may take up to 2 months to resolve. Improvement in facial motor function within the first 5 to 7 days is the most favorable prognostic sign. A CT scan of the head and neurologic consult are not indicated in this patient. Lyme disease would be a rare cause of facial nerve paralysis and is not part of the routine evaluation. Aspirin is not indicated, since this is not caused by cerebrovascular disease. *(Aminoff et al., 2005, p. 182; Ronthal, 2015)*

33. **(B)** The absence of the knee jerk reflex suggests compression of the L3–L4 spinal nerve root. The four most commonly tested deep tendon reflexes are the Achilles (ankle jerk) reflex, quadriceps (knee jerk) reflex, triceps reflex, and biceps reflex. The nerve roots that each tests in ascending order are S 1 and 2, L 3 and 4, C 5 and 6 (biceps), and C 7 and 8 (triceps). One only needs to remember that the ankle jerk is a sacral nerve root, the knee jerk is a lumbar nerve root, and the biceps and triceps are cervical nerve roots. *(Aminoff et al., 2005, p. 367)*

34. **(A)** Peripheral neuropathy is a syndrome that is manifested by muscle weakness, paresthesias, decreased deep tendon reflexes, and autonomic disturbances most commonly in the hands and feet, such as coldness and sweating. There are many causes of peripheral neuropathy ranging from metabolic conditions to malignant neoplasm, rheumatoid arthritis, and drug and alcohol use. The increase in non–insulin-dependent diabetes mellitus due to obesity in the American population has increased the incidence of associated disease states. *(Aminoff et al., 2005, pp. 213–214)*

35. **(B)** The presence of headache associated with papilledema raises the concern for a brain tumor. The MRI excluded a mass lesion, raising a strong suspicion of pseudotumor cerebri. This is also known as *benign intracranial hypertension.* It is not a benign condition, however, since it causes severe

headache and may result in visual loss. It is particularly frequent in obese adolescent girls and young women. The etiology is unknown but may be associated with the use of oral contraceptives, vitamin A, and tetracycline. The presentation consists of headaches caused by an increase in intracranial pressure and blurring of vision. There may be diplopia, but the remainder of the neurologic examination is unremarkable. Papilledema is virtually always part of the presentation. The mental status examination is normal. The differential diagnosis includes venous sinus thrombosis, sarcoidosis, and tuberculosis or carcinomatous meningitis. The last two are excluded by lumbar puncture. An abnormal cerebrospinal fluid is not consistent with pseudotumor cerebri. The diagnosis is made by excluding mass lesions with CT scan or MRI and demonstrating markedly increased intracranial pressure by lumbar puncture. The treatment involves weight loss, diuretics, and steroids. Repeat lumbar punctures to remove cerebrospinal fluid and decrease intracranial pressure are usually effective. In cases that are unresponsive to these measures, lumbar-peritoneal shunting is effective, as is unilateral optic nerve sheath fenestration. Effective treatment can improve headaches and prevent vision loss. *(Horton, 2008, p. 188)*

36. **(D)** Complex partial seizures are often preceded by some type of sensory aura. This is followed by an impairment of consciousness (but not total loss of consciousness) along with an involuntary motor activity. The seizure will resolve in about 30 minutes and is followed by postictal confusion. Simple partial seizures have no alteration of consciousness. Absence and tonic–clonic seizures are generalized seizure disorders in which consciousness is lost. Absence seizures are characterized by staring spells without motor involvement, whereas tonic–clonic seizures involve strong muscle extension and contraction in many major muscle groups. Pseudoseizures are a diagnosis of exclusion. All tests results including an electroencephalogram (EEG) are normal, and the seizures may be a manifestation of an underlying psychiatric disturbance. *(Aminoff et al., 2005, pp. 267–278)*

37. **(E)** Blood pressure is typically elevated at the time of presentation in acute ischemic stroke. It will decline without medication in the first few hours to

days. Aggressively lowering blood pressure in an acute ischemic stroke may decrease the blood flow to the ischemic but salvageable brain tissue. This potentially salvageable brain tissue is referred to as the *penumbra*. Decreasing blood flow to the ischemic penumbra by acutely lowering blood pressure may result in eventual infarction of this brain tissue. Treatment of previously undiagnosed hypertension should be deferred for several days. Blood pressure should be treated if there are other indications, such as angina or heart failure. Control of blood pressure is appropriate in patients who are receiving tissue plasminogen activator (tPA) for their stroke. Blood pressure should be lowered cautiously to a systolic of less than 185 mm Hg and a diastolic of less than 110 mm Hg. This is thought to decrease the incidence of intracerebral hemorrhage in these patients. *(Wells et al., 2009, p. 158)*

38. **(C)** The diagnosis is temporal arteritis. This is an arteritis of the temporal branch of the external carotid artery characterized by unilateral or bilateral headaches that may be localized to a tender temporal artery. The temporal artery may be thickened and tender and may be thrombosed and nonpulsatile late in the disease. Many patients present with malaise and have anemia and a low-grade fever. Fifty percent of patients report generalized muscle aches consistent with polymyalgia rheumatica. The most severe complication of temporal arteritis is blindness resulting from thrombosis of the ophthalmic artery. In some cases, this may be preceded by previous episodes of amaurosis fugax before the blindness becomes irreversible. Once blindness occurs in one eye, it may be prevented in the other by initiating treatment. The diagnosis is based on recognizing the clinical picture and obtaining a temporal artery biopsy. Treatment should not be delayed pending the biopsy. Early treatment with prednisone may prevent irreversible blindness. The efficacy of treatment can be measured with serial sedimentation rates. MRI and MRA have no value in establishing the diagnosis of temporal arteritis. Antiplatelet aggregating therapy would not be inappropriate but is inadequate for this diagnosis. The potentially unilateral headache should not be confused with a migraine for which Imitrex therapy would be appropriate. Lumbar puncture has no role in establishing this diagnosis. *(Langford & Fauci, 2008, p. 2127)*

39. **(D)** The history is consistent with migraine without aura. Migraine is a headache that is defined by a pain that is usually unilateral, is pounding or will take on a pounding quality with activity, can be made worse with physical activity, and may be associated, nausea, vomiting, photophobia, and phonophobia. If the headache is preceded by an abnormal sensory experience such as a visual disturbance that lasts no longer than 60 minutes and totally remits, it is classified as a migraine with aura. Cluster headaches are usually unilateral as well but tend to be periorbital and are of shorter duration but greater intensity, often described as a stabbing pain. In addition, patients may experience ipsilateral autonomic symptoms such as epiphora, rhinorrhea, and ptosis. Tension-type headaches are mostly due to contraction of cranial and cervical muscles and are described as bilateral, tight, or squeezing in nature, and are sometimes relieved by physical activity. Medication withdrawal headaches typically present as daily, constant headaches. *(Aminoff et al., 2005, pp. 85–92)*

40. **(C)** Horner syndrome is defined by a unilateral, small pupil with mild ptosis in which pupillary response to light and accommodation is preserved. It may also be associated with ipsilateral anhydrosis. It is usually caused by some interruption in the oculosympathetic pathway. An Adie pupil is characterized by a unilateral-dilated pupil that is sluggish to direct light stimuli. An Argyll Robertson pupil usually affects both eyes, is irregular in shape, and is poorly reactive to light. A Marcus Gunn pupil constricts slower to direct light stimulation than to the consensual stimulation. Light-near dissociation is usually bilateral and consists of preserved constriction to accommodation but impaired response to light. *(Aminoff et al., 2005, pp. 138–139)*

41. **(C)** This patient's symptoms are most consistent with situational depression over the loss of his spouse. Transient memory problems can be a component of depression as a result of decreased attention and interest. Dementia is a progressive impairment of higher cognitive function, and initially, the patient's social graces are preserved. It has many causes, of which Pick disease, Creutzfeldt–Jakob disease, and Alzheimer disease are irreversible. Vitamin B_{12} deficiency can cause

reversible form of cognitive impairment, in which the elderly are susceptible, so serum analysis of vitamin B_{12} should be performed in diagnostic evaluations of dementia in this population. *(Aminoff et al., 2005, pp. 44–51)*

42. **(D)** Physiologic tremor is a postural tremor that may be exacerbated by the factors outlined in this question. Both asterixis and intention tremor are also postural tremors; however, asterixis is seen in the context of metabolic encephalopathy and intention tremor during activity. Wilson disease occurs with other abnormal cerebellar findings. Hemiballismus is a choreiform movement disorder and not an oscillatory movement. *(Aminoff et al., 2005, pp. 234–236)*

43. **(A)** The goal of the treatment of multiple sclerosis is to reduce the frequency and severity of recurrent attacks. Most data agree that the use of beta-interferons as early as possible in the diagnosis of multiple sclerosis is the treatment of choice for attaining this goal. Corticosteroids may be used to lessen the severity of an acute attack but have not been shown to be effective in suppressing further attacks. Methotrexate and natalizumab are not first-line agents. The use of amantadine and physical therapy can help with energy and mobility issues. *(Hauser & Goodin, 2008, pp. 2618–2619)*

44. **(B)** During a stroke in evolution, symptoms will worsen or new symptoms will appear. A completed stroke is one in which neurologic symptoms have stabilized, whereas a transient ischemic attack produces deficits that resolve over time. This patient's symptoms do not match those of an acute subarachnoid hemorrhage. Global cerebral ischemia as seen in sudden cardiac arrest would involve loss of consciousness. *(Aminoff et al., 2005, pp. 286–297)*

45. **(D)** The symptoms of a resting tremor, bradykinesia or hypokinesia, postural instability, and rigidity are *the cardinal symptoms* for Parkinson disease. Difficulty with activities of daily living will usually prompt a patient to seek medical attention. Essential tremor and Wilson disease are postural tremors with different characteristics than the tremor seen in Parkinson disease. Huntington

disease produces choreiform movements and has a much earlier age of onset. Progressive supranuclear palsy is characterized by an ophthalmoplegia in addition to tremor. *(Aminoff et al., 2005, pp. 241–250; Chou, 2015)*

46. **(E)** This presentation is classic for Alzheimer dementia. Increasing short-term memory loss, anomia, apraxia are all significant components to the constellation of progressive symptoms. There is no history of urinary incontinence, which would suggest normal pressure hydrocephalus. Depression is a possibility along with his any dementia, however, dementia would be the primary suspect to account for these symptoms. There are no other historical or examination findings suggestive of hypothyroidism. *(Aminoff et al., 2005, pp. 47–49; Wolk & Dickerson, 2015)*

47. **(C)** Trigeminal neuralgia is characterized by sharp, brief pain often described as "shooting, jabbing, electric shock, or stabbing." It occurs more frequently in women than men, with advancing age, and more likely on the right than left. The history given for cluster headache (typically ipsilateral ocular headaches with tearing, and lasting for 2 hours) and tension-type headache is unlike this patient's complaints. The history for temporal arteritis is generally includes ocular symptoms, but a sedimentation rate may be justified. This pain pattern is different than that of a focal dental problem. *(Beal & Hauser, 2008, p. 2583; Brazis et al., 2001, pp. 280–281)*

48. **(D)** This event represents a well-demarcated episode affecting some combination of consciousness, motor, and/or sensory function consequent to abnormal electrical discharges in the brain. This is consistent with the definition of a seizure. Epilepsy refers to multiple, recurrent seizures. This history is not consistent with hyperventilation, stroke, or cardiac arrhythmia, which would typically include chest pain, shortness of breath, dyspnea on exertion, or focal neurologic deficits. *(Aminoff et al., 2005, p. 265)*

49. **(A)** Low back pain is one of the more common presenting neurologic complaints to a primary care provider. Most acute pain syndromes are benign, self-limiting conditions, with pain arising from myofascial sources. Patients with back pain and normal neurologic examinations are unlikely to have any serious underlying pathology and further diagnostic testing is usually unrevealing. *(Engstrom, 2008, p. 110)*

50. **(C)** *Neisseria meningitidis* and *Streptococcus pneumoniae* are the most common etiologic agents for bacterial meningitis in this patient's age group. So much so that many colleges and universities require a vaccine for students who live in dormitories. Her fever and the cerebrospinal fluid values are consistent with a bacterial and not a viral infectious source for the meningeal irritation. *(Aminoff et al., 2005, pp. 20–30)*

51. **(B)** Up to 80% of subarachnoid hemorrhages can be attributed to the rupture of saccular or berry aneurysms in nontraumatic subarachnoid hemorrhages. Most of these aneurysms arise from the anterior circulation. Most are in the anterior communicating artery. Twenty-five percent of patients will have more than one aneurysm. Because of cerebrovascular anatomy, the blood is usually confined to the subarachnoid space. Blood from a ruptured arteriovenous malformation can be intraparenchymal and cause focal neurologic symptoms. Trauma is more likely to cause epidural or subdural hematoma. *(Aminoff et al., 2005, pp. 74–76; Toy et al., 2012, p. 103)*

52. **(A)** The patient most likely is suffering from diabetic peripheral neuropathy (pending further testing to rule out other causes). Amitriptyline is *one of several medications that may be* effective in some cases of diabetic neuropathy. *Cetuximab is a chemotherapeutic drug for metastatic colorectal carcinoma.* Oxycodone would not be used as initial treatment of this *likely* chronic *condition especially because of increasing drug dependence and increasing fall risk. Edrophonium is a drug used for the evaluation of myasthenia gravis. And,* vitamin D is not closely associated with peripheral neuropathy. *(Aminoff et al., 2005, pp. 211–212; Toy et al., 2012, p. 137)*

53. **(B)** The pattern of sensory, motor, and reflex findings occurring over an acute time period is consistent with Guillain–Barré Syndrome. *Campylobacter jejuni bacterial infection often*

precedes the development of this syndrome. Diffuse diabetic peripheral neuropathy develops more insidiously than this case scenario. Multiple sclerosis presents with central nervous system (CNS) lesions that are unlikely to occur in this pattern. Myasthenia gravis causes intermittent motor symptoms without sensory involvement. Hypothyroidism may cause weakness and delayed reflexes, but is not the single best answer for this question. *(Aminoff et al., 2005, p. 212; Toy et al., 2012, pp. 331–333)*

54. **(B)** The patient's presentation is consistent with viral meningitis with potential encephalitis. The presence of active stomatitis indicates herpes simplex virus as the most likely causative organism. A CT of the head could be considered prior to performing a lumbar puncture and may show temporal lobe abnormalities that support a diagnosis of herpes virus encephalitis, but like an MRI will not identify the causative organism and has limited sensitivity. Of the three herpes tests described, the PCR technique is the most likely to identify the herpes simplex virus as the causative organism in the CSF due to its high sensitivity and specificity. Serum IgG indicates prior infection from herpes simplex virus but does not confirm the causative organism of the patient's encephalitis. Viral blood cultures for herpes simplex would likely show no growth even in the presence of herpes simplex virus encephalitis. *(Aminoff et al., 2005, p. 30)*

55. **(C)** The patient's unilateral symptoms are best explained by a local anatomical cause (e.g., tumor) that would be detected with an imaging study (MRI). An MRI is preferred over skull x-rays to assess directly for intracranial pathology. CNS abnormalities arising from systemic causes are more likely to be symmetric. *(Aminoff et al., 2005, p. 138)*

56. **(A)** Cerebral palsy is caused by perinatal injury to the nervous system and results in motor spasticity. The history of perinatal anoxia is consistent with cerebral palsy. Congenital hypothyroidism is typically asymptomatic at birth and diagnosed through routine screening tests. Neonatal meningitis may result in anoxia, but this patient's anoxia is attributed to the birthing process. Multiple sclerosis is caused by inflammation, demyelination, and scarring. *(Sudarsky, 2008, p. 151)*

57. **(A)** The test described is known as asterixis, and is a finding associated with metabolic encephalopathy *specifically affecting the thalamus*. Brudzinski sign is performed by passively flexing the neck of a supine patient *and is more specific for ruling in/out meningeal irritation*. Clonus is assessed by rapid passive plantar-dorsiflexion of the ankle followed by sustained dorsiflexion. *A positive test indicates an upper motor neuron lesion.* Stereognosis is assessed by having the patients recognize a familiar object placed in their hand. Hyperekplexia is the sudden loss of postural tone following a startling stimuli as may be exacerbated in thalamic lesions. *(Bickley, 2009, p. 704; Brazis et al., 2001, p. 573; Fuller et al., 2004, pp. 154, 204)*

58. **(B)** Narcolepsy is characterized by hypersomnolence, loss of muscle tone prior to sleep, hallucinations upon initiating or arising from sleep, and episodes of sleep paralysis. The diagnostic test that is used in conjunction with clinical history to establish the diagnosis is the multiple sleep latency test. The tensilon test is utilized to assess for the presence of myasthenia gravis. Polysomnography can be useful in excluding other sleep disorders, but it does not assess sleep latency time necessary to support the diagnosis of narcolepsy. *(Czeisler et al., 2008, pp. 177–178)*

59. **(B)** Carbamazepine is an antiepileptic drug that potentially causes *aplastic anemia, agranulocytosis, or hyponatremia. Therefore, baseline and periodic CBC, LFT, and Na testing are required.* Disorders of carbohydrate metabolism, vitamin B_{12} deficiency, or renal toxicity are not commonly reported. EEG is used to help establish a diagnosis of a seizure disorder. *(Aminoff et al., 2005, pp. 275–277; Schachter, 2015)*

60. **(D)** Weakness is one potential finding of a lower motor neuron process. When these axons are damaged, the innervated muscles will show some combination of the *following signs: weakness or paralysis of the involved muscles, flaccidity, hypotonia, diminished or absent muscle stretch reflexes (hypo or areflexia), and eventually atrophy.* Aphasia results from injury to the speech pathways within the brain. Sensory loss arises from many causes, but it is not a motor issue. Dysdiadochokinesia

(impaired performance of rapidly alternating movements) is consistent with cerebellar pathology. Hyperreflexia is typically a signal of upper motor neuron disease. *(Bickley, 2009; Brazis et al., 2001, pp. 12, 376)*

61. **(A)** The patient's symptoms are consistent with pathology arising from the anterior cerebral circulation including the carotid arteries. A CT should be ordered to rule out acute hemorrhage and an erythrocyte sedimentation rate may be useful if giant cell arteritis was suspected. An MRA of the vertebral arteries would likely show deficits but is not likely to demonstrate the etiologic location of this stroke. *(Aminoff et al., 2005, pp. 287–291)*

62. **(E)** In order of prevalence, headache (48%) is most common, followed by dizziness (10%), orbital pain (7%), sensory and motor disturbance (6%), and diplopia (4%). The collections of prodromal signs and symptoms are sentinel leaks, mass effect, and possible emboli. Sentinel leaks are usually small amounts of blood loss from the aneurysm occurring in 30% to 50% of subarachnoid headaches (SAHs). A sentinel leak produces a sudden focal or generalized head pain and is usually severe. This may occur a few hours to a few months with an average of 2 weeks before discovery of the SAH. The mass effect occurs from the expanding aneurysm size and its location within the brain vascular. Emboli are the result of the formation of intra-aneurysmal thrombus leading to transient ischemic attacks (TIA). *(Singer, Oglilvy & Rordorf, 2013)*

63. **(D)** Carpal syndrome is composed of four major components including bouts of pain in the affected wrist/hand especially prevalent during sleep hours, paresis and atrophy of the abductor pollicis brevis muscles, etc., sensory loss in the affected radial palm, and often positive Tinel/Phalen (flexion and extension of the wrist testing). Myasthenia gravis is characterized by weakness then recovery with rest. Radial nerve compression usually occurs as a result of entrapment following a crush or twisting injury to the wrist and forearm as occurs with certain jobs. And, a medial cord injury to the right brachial plexus is consistent with an ulnar nerve anomaly. Thoracic outlet syndrome may be purely vascular, purely neuropathic, or, rarely, mixed. *(Brazis et al., 2001, pp. 38, 50, 83–84)*

REFERENCES

Aminoff MJ, Greenberg DA, Simon RP. *Clinical Neurology.* 6th ed. New York, NY: McGraw-Hill; 2005.

Aminoff M, Kerchner G. Chapter 24: Nervous system disorders. In: McPhee SJ, Papadakis MA, eds. *Current Medical Diagnosis and Treatment.* 52th ed. New York, NY: McGraw-Hill; 2013.

Beal MF, Hauser SL. Trigeminal neuralgia, Bell's palsy and other cranial nerve disorders. In: Fauci AS, Braunwald E, Kasper DL, et al., eds. *Harrison's Textbook of Medicine.* 17th ed. New York, NY: McGraw-Hill; 2008.

Bickley LS. *Bates' Guide to Physical Examination and History Taking.* 10th ed. Philadelphia, PA: Lippincott Williams & Wilkins; 2009.

Bienfang DC. Overview and differential diagnosis of papilledema. In: Brazis P, ed. *UpToDate,* Waltham, MA: UpToDate; 2015. www.uptodate.com. Accessed May 6, 2015.

Brazis PW, Masdeu JC, Biller J. *Localization in Clinical Neurology.* 4th ed. Philadelphia, PA: Lippincott Williams & Wilkins; 2001.

Chisholm-Burns MA, Wells BG, Schwinghammer TL, et al. *Pharmacotherapy Principles and Practice.* New York, NY: McGraw-Hill; 2013.

Chou L. Clinical manifestations of Parkinson disease. In: *UpToDate,* 2015.

Chung KW, Chung HM. Chapter 8: Head and neck. In: Chung KW, Chung HM, eds. *Gross Anatomy.* 6th ed. Baltimore, MD: Lippincott Williams and Wilkins; 2008.

Czeisler CA, Winkelman JW, Richardson GS. Sleep disorders. In: Fauci AS, Braunwald E, Kasper DL, et al., eds. *Harrison's Textbook of Medicine.* 17th ed. New York, NY: McGraw-Hill; 2008.

Engstrom JW. Back and neck pain. In: Fauci AS, Braunwald E, Kasper DL, et al., eds. *Harrison's Textbook of Medicine.* 17th ed. New York, NY: McGraw-Hill; 2008.

Francis J, Young GB. Diagnosis of delirium and confusional states. In: Aminoff M, Schmader K, eds. *UpToDate,* Waltham, MA: UpToDate; 2015. www.uptodate.com. Accessed May 2, 2015.

Fuller G. *Neurological Examination.* 3rd ed. New York, NY: Churchill-Livingstone; 2004.

Hauser SL, Goodin DS. Multiple sclerosis and other demyelinating diseases. In: Fauci AS, Braunwald E, Kasper DL, et al., eds. *Harrison's Textbook of Medicine.* 17th ed. New York, NY: McGraw-Hill; 2008.

Hauser SL, Ropper AH. Diseases of the spinal cord. In: Fauci AS, Braunwald E, Kasper DL, et al., eds. *Harrison's Textbook of Medicine.* 17th ed. New York, NY: McGraw-Hill; 2008.

Horton CH. Disorders of the eye. In: Fauci AS, Braunwald E, Kasper DL, et al., eds. *Harrison's Textbook of Medicine.* 17th ed. New York, NY: McGraw-Hill; 2008.

Josephson S, Samuels MA. Chapter 47: Special issues in inpatient neurologic consultation. In: Longo DL, Fauci AS, Kasper DL, Hauser SL, Jameson J, Loscalzo J, eds. *Harrison's Principles of Internal Medicine.* 18th ed. New York, NY: McGraw-Hill; 2012. http://accessmedicine.mhmedical.com/content.aspx?bookid=331&Sectionid=40727206. Accessed May 6, 2015.

Kaplan SL. Bacterial meningitis in children older than one month: Clinical features and diagnosis. In: Edwards MS, Nordli DR, eds. *UpToDate,* Waltham, MA: UpToDate; 2015. www.uptodate.com. Accessed May 6, 2015.

Koralnik I. Approach to HIV-infected patients with central nervous system lesions. In: Bartlett J, Mittey J, eds. *UpToDate,* Waltham, MA: UpToDate; 2015. www.uptodate.com. Accessed May 2, 2015.

Langford CA, Fauci AS. The vasculitis syndromes. In: Fauci AS, Braunwald E, Kasper DL, et al., eds. *Harrison's Textbook of Medicine.* 19th ed. New York, NY: McGraw-Hill; 2015.

Langford CA, Gilliland BC. Chapter 337: Periarticular disorders of the extremities. In: Longo DL, Fauci AS, Kasper DL, Hauser SL, Jameson J, Loscalzo J, eds. *Harrison's Principles of Internal Medicine.* 18th ed. New York, NY: McGraw-Hill; 2012. http://accessmedicine.mhmedical.com/content.aspx?bookid=331&Sectionid=40727140. Accessed May 6, 2015.

Lowenstein DH. Seizures and epilepsy. In: Fauci AS, Braunwald E, Kasper DL, et al., eds. *Harrison's Textbook of Medicine.* 19th ed. New York, NY: McGraw-Hill; 2015.

McBride W. Intracranial epidural hematoma in adults. In: *UpToDate,* 2014.

McCarron M, Goldstein L, Matchar D. Screening for asymptomatic carotid artery stenosis. In: *UpToDate,* 2015.

Olek M. Diagnosis of multiple sclerosis in adults. In: Gonzelez-Scarano F, ed. *UpToDate,* Waltham, MA: UpToDate; 2015. www.uptodate.com. Accessed May 2, 2015.

Pagana KD, Pagana TJ. *Mosby's Diagnostic and Laboratory Test Reference.* 8th ed. Edinburgh: Mosby; 2007.

Pazirandeh S, Lo C, Burns D. Overview of water-soluble vitamins. In: Lipman T, ed. *UpToDate,* Waltham, MA: UpToDate; 2015. www.uptodate.com. Accessed May 2, 2015.

Ronthal M. Bell's palsy: Pathogenesis, clinical features, and diagnosis in adults. In: *UpToDate,* 2015.

Ropper AH, Samuels MA, Klein JP. Chapter 13: Disturbances of vision. In: Ropper AH, Samuels MA, Klein JP, eds. *Adams & Victor's Principles of Neurology.* 10th ed. New York, NY: McGraw-Hill; 2014. http://accessmedicine.mhmedical.com/content.aspx?bookid=690&Sectionid=49251500. Accessed May 4, 2015.

Rutkove SB. Overview of polyneuropathy. In: Shefner JM, ed. *UpToDate,* Waltham, MA: UpToDate; 2015. www.uptodate.com. Accessed May 6, 2015.

Schachter S. Overview of the management of epilepsy in adults. In: *UpToDate*, 2015.

Schilsky ML. Wilson disease: Diagnostic tests. In: Rand EB, Runyon BA, Aminoff MJ, eds. *UpToDate*, Waltham, MA: UpToDate; 2015. www.uptodate.com. Accessed May 6, 2015.

Schrier SL. Etiology and clinical manifestations of vitamin B12 and folate deficiency. In: Mentzer WC, ed. *UpToDate*, Waltham, MA: UpToDate; 2015. www.uptodate.com. Accessed May 6, 2015.

Shadlen M, Larson EB. Evaluation of cognitive impairment and dementia. In: Steven T, DeKosky ST, Schmader KE, eds. *UpToDate*, Waltham, MA: UpToDate; 2015. www.uptodate.com. Accessed May 6, 2015.

Silverthorn DU. Chapter 9: The central nervous sytem. In: Silverthorn DU, ed. *Human Physiology: An Integrated Approach*. 4th ed. San Francisco, CA: Pearson/Benjamin Cummings; 2007.

Singer R, Ogilvy C, Rordorf G. Clinical manifestations and diagnosis of aneurysmal subarachnoid hemorrhage. In: *UpToDate,* 2013.

Southwick FS. Pathogenesis, clinical manifestations, and diagnosis of brain abscess. In: Calderwood SB, ed. *UpToDate*, Waltham, MA: UpToDate; 2015. www.uptodate.com. Accessed May 6, 2015.

Sudarsky L. Gait and balance disorders. In: Fauci AS, Braunwald E, Kasper DL, et al., eds. *Harrison's Textbook of Medicine*. 17th ed. New York, NY: McGraw-Hill; 2008.

Tarsey D. Clinical manifestations and diagnosis of restless legs syndrome in adults. In: Hurtig H, Benca R, eds. *UpToDate*, Waltham, MA: UpToDate; 2015. www.uptodate.com. Accessed May 2, 2015.

Taylor FR. Tension-type headache in adults: pathophysiology, clinical features, and diagnosis. In: Swanson JW, ed. *UpToDate*, Waltham, MA: UpToDate; 2015. www.uptodate. com. Accessed May 6, 2015.

Toy EC, Simpson E, Tintner R. *Case Files Neurology*. 2nd ed. New York, NY: McGraw-Hill; 2012.

Vriesendorp F. Pathogenesis of Guillain-Barré syndrome. In: Shefner J, Targoff I, eds. *UpToDate*, Waltham, MA: UpToDate; 2015. www.uptodate.com. Accessed May 2, 2015.

Waxman SG. Chapter 21: Higher cortical functions. In: Waxman SG, ed. *Clinical Neuroanatomy*. 27th ed. New York, NY: McGraw-Hill; 2013. http://accessmedicine.mhmedical.com/content.aspx?bookid=673&Sectionid=45395986. Accessed May 5, 2015.

Wells BG, DiPiro JT, Schwinghammer TL, et al. *Pharmacotherapy Handbook*. 7th ed. New York, NY: McGraw-Hill; 2009.

Wolk D, Dickerson B. Clinical features and diagnosis of Alzheimer disease. In: *UpToDate,* 2015.

CHAPTER 10

Pulmonology

Randy D. Danielsen, PhD, PA-C, DFAAPA

DIRECTIONS: Each of the numbered questions or incomplete statements is followed by possible answers or completions of the statement. Select the ONE-lettered answer or completion that is BEST in each case.

1. A 19-year-old male college student presents with a 4-day history of fever, headache, sore throat, myalgia, malaise, and a nonproductive cough. On examination, you note an erythematous pharynx without exudate. The lung examination is unimpressive. A chest x-ray reveals a right-sided lower lobe patchy infiltrate. Which of the following is the most likely cause?

   (A) *Klebsiella pneumoniae*
   (B) *Mycoplasma pneumoniae*
   (C) *Staphylococcus aureus*
   (D) *Streptococcus pneumoniae*
   (E) Viral pneumonia

2. A 40-year-old woman presents with the sudden onset of cough productive of blood-speckled sputum, chest pain with cough, shaking chills, high fever, and myalgias for the last 12 hours. On examination, she appears acutely ill, is tachypneic, and is coughing. Auscultation of the chest reveals rales and chest x-ray reveals unilateral lobar consolidation consistent with pneumonia. Which of the following is the most likely cause?

   (A) Aspiration pneumonia
   (B) *Chlamydia pneumoniae*
   (C) *M. pneumoniae*
   (D) *S. aureus*
   (E) *S. pneumoniae*

3. A 3-year-old patient presents with sudden onset of coughing and wheezing, which began at the dinner table this evening. Vital signs are pulse 120, respirations 26, and temperature 98.6°F. The most likely diagnosis is a partial obstruction secondary to tracheal foreign body. What is the next step in the management of this patient?

   (A) Bronchoscopy
   (B) Chest physiotherapy
   (C) Fluid challenge
   (D) Intubation
   (E) Tracheostomy

4. An otherwise healthy 30-year-old patient presents with a 3-week history of cough and malaise. The history reveals that prior to this episode he had an upper respiratory tract infection that was treated with acetaminophen, bed rest, and fluids. The physical examination reveals a normal lung examination and no fever. The patient is coughing while in the office. The chest x-ray is normal. What is the most effective treatment for this patient?

   (A) Albuterol HFA
   (B) Clarithromycin
   (C) Flumadine
   (D) Fluticasone
   (E) Prednisone

5. A 32-year-old patient with a 3-week history of fever, malaise, weight loss, joint pain, and dry cough presents to your office. The chest x-ray reveals bilateral hilar adenopathy with no parenchymal abnormalities. You suspect and would like to rule out sarcoidosis. How can the definitive diagnosis be made?

(A) Administer an intradermal purified protein derivative
(B) Biopsy of the mediastinal nodes
(C) Measure serum angiotensin-converting enzyme
(D) Perform a bronchoalveolar lavage
(E) Serologic tests for coccidioidomycosis

6. What is the most common mode of transmission of the *Mycobacterium tuberculosis* bacteria?

(A) Aerosolized droplets
(B) Blood borne
(C) Enteric
(D) Transdermal
(E) Transplacental

7. A 65-year-old alcoholic male patient presents with the acute onset of fever, cough productive of purulent sputum, hemoptysis, chest pain, and shortness of breath. On examination, he is noted to be confused and hypotensive. Chest x-ray shows bilateral infiltrates and cavitations. Sputum smear reveals gram-negative rods. Which of the following is the most likely cause of this pneumonia?

(A) *C. pneumoniae*
(B) Coccidioidomycosis
(C) *K. pneumoniae*
(D) *M. pneumoniae*
(E) *Pneumocystis jirovecii*

8. What is the drug treatment of choice for *M. pneumoniae*?

(A) Aminoglycosides
(B) Cephalosporins
(C) Macrolides
(D) Penicillin
(E) Sulfamethoxazole/trimethoprim

9. What is the empirical drug treatment of choice for a known case of community-acquired pneumonia?

(A) Clarithromycin
(B) Gentamycin
(C) Penicillin
(D) Sulfamethoxazole/trimethoprim
(E) Vancomycin

10. A 50-year-old man presents with a history of persistent cough, hemoptysis, and weight loss over the past 6 months. He has smoked 2 packs per day for 30 years and also complains of shoulder and chest pain. On examination, he is noted to be pale, febrile, and dyspneic upon exertion. The chest x-ray shows hilar adenopathy. What is the most likely diagnosis?

(A) Asthma
(B) Bronchiectasis
(C) Bronchogenic carcinoma
(D) Chronic obstructive pulmonary disease (COPD)
(E) Vocal cord dysfunction

11. A 43-year-old woman with a history of COPD presents to the office with worsening dyspnea, especially at rest. She also complains of dull, retrosternal chest pain. On examination, she has narrow splitting of S1. Radiographic findings demonstrate peripheral "pruning" of the large pulmonary arteries. What is the most likely diagnosis?

(A) Congestive heart failure
(B) Pericarditis
(C) Pulmonary artery aneurysm
(D) Pulmonary embolus
(E) Pulmonary hypertension

12. What radiologic finding(s) is/are most suggestive of chronic silicosis?

(A) Atelectasis
(B) Eggshell calcification of enlarged hilar lymph nodes
(C) Pneumothorax and atelectasis
(D) Large nodules that appear primarily in the lower lobes
(E) Pleural thickening and plaques

13. A 50-year-old patient presents with a fever of 102°F, productive cough, mild chest pain on deep breathing and coughing, and general malaise for the last 2 days. Prior to the onset of these symptoms, the patient had a "bad cold" for 5 days. What physical finding would be most consistent with this history?

(A) Decreased transmitted voice sounds

(B) Diffuse hyperresonance

(C) Inspiratory crackles

(D) Inspiratory wheezes

(E) Vesicular breath sound

14. Which histological type of lung cancer has the lowest 5-year survival rate?

(A) Adenocarcinoma

(B) Bronchioalveolar

(C) Large cell

(D) Small cell

(E) Squamous cell

15. A 43-year-old female patient who is HIV negative is recently diagnosed with pulmonary tuberculosis via a positive purified protein derivative (PPD) and culture. She receives annual PPD testing and prior to this test has been negative. What is the current recommended treatment?

(A) 6 months of isoniazid (INH), rifampin (RIF), and an additional 2 months of pyrazinamide (PZA) and ethambutol (EMB).

(B) 2 months of INH, RIF, PZA, and streptomycin (SM) followed by one month of INH and RIF.

(C) 2 months of INH, RIF, PZA, and EMB followed by four months of INH and RIF.

(D) 6 months single treatment with INH

(E) 6 months of INH and RIF

16. A 35-year-old man who is HIV positive presents to the emergency department (ED) complaining of high fever, pleuritic chest pain, and grossly purulent sputum. History also reveals that he was recently at a local conference and spent most of the time indoors. The ED has seen three other patients this week with the same complaints. On examination, he is toxic appearing with a temperature of 103°F.

The chest film demonstrates focal patchy infiltrates. Of the following, what is the treatment of choice?

(A) Doxycycline

(B) Erythromycin

(C) Levofloxacin

(D) Penicillin

(E) Sulfamethoxazole/trimethoprim

17. A 19-year-old woman, post motor vehicle accident, is hospitalized with a femur fracture. She develops sudden onset of dyspnea, cough, and anxiety with retrosternal chest pain. On examination, her pulse is 120, respirations 32, and blood pressure 120/80 mm Hg. Chest x-ray shows mild bilateral atelectasis. Electrocardiogram (ECG) is normal. What is the most likely diagnosis?

(A) Aortic dissection

(B) Nosocomial pneumonia

(C) Pneumothorax

(D) Pulmonary thromboembolus

(E) Pneumonia

18. What imaging study is the "gold standard" used to confirm the diagnosis of deep vein thrombosis?

(A) Arteriography

(B) Contrast venography

(C) D-Dimer

(D) Doppler ultrasound

(E) Ventilation–perfusion scan

19. A 70-year-old patient with a long history of COPD presents to the office for a regular office visit. The patient's history is unchanged and the physical examination is consistent with a long-term history of COPD. One of the findings is distal phalanges that are rounded and bulbous. Upon palpation, the proximal nail folds feel spongy. This finding is consistent with what condition?

(A) Acute dyspnea

(B) Chronic hypoxia

(C) Chronic hyponatremia

(D) Psoriasis

(E) Transient hypercapnia

20. What is the mainstay bronchodilator treatment for mild intermittent asthma?

    (A) Beta-aminophylline
    (B) Beta-adrenergic agonists
    (C) Adrenergic agents
    (D) Ipratropium
    (E) Theophylline

21. A 29-year-old patient with a history of HIV presents to the emergency department with signs and symptoms consistent with *P. jirovecii* pneumonia. What chest x-ray findings are considered the "classic" pattern associated with this diagnosis?

    (A) Diffuse interstitial infiltrates
    (B) Focal consolidation
    (C) Kerley B lines
    (D) Multiple pulmonary nodules
    (E) Upper lobe cavitation

22. What is considered the primary therapy for patients with pulmonary thromboembolism (PTE) who are hemodynamically unstable?

    (A) Anticoagulation with heparin
    (B) Antiembolization stockings
    (C) Insertion of an inferior vena cava filter
    (D) Thrombolysis with tissue plasminogen activator (t-Pa)
    (E) Aspirin 325 mg

23. A 79-year-old woman who is 7 days post a total hip replacement complains of sudden onset of dyspnea, cough, and retrosternal chest pain. On examination, she appears anxious with vital signs as follows: pulse 120, respirations 32, and blood pressure 138/92 mm Hg. A chest x-ray demonstrates mild bilateral atelectasis and other than tachycardia a normal ECG. What imaging modality will best confirm the diagnosis?

    (A) Arteriography
    (B) Contrast venography
    (C) Doppler ultrasound
    (D) Helical CT scan
    (E) Ventilation–perfusion scan

24. A 17-year-old girl presents complaining of a nonproductive cough, postnasal drip, and nasal congestion. Examination reveals inflamed nasal turbinates, cobblestoning of the posterior pharynx, and diffuse bilateral end expiratory wheezes. Which laboratory test will provide the best information to assist in making the diagnosis?

    (A) Arterial blood gas
    (B) Chest x-ray
    (C) Peak flow measurements
    (D) Pulse oximetry
    (E) Spirometry

25. A 7-year-old boy with a history of asthma presents with nocturnal cough occurring every night along with daily exacerbations of wheezing and shortness of breath. How would his asthma be classified?

    (A) Exercise-induced
    (B) Mild intermittent
    (C) Mild persistent
    (D) Moderate persistent
    (E) Severe persistent

26. A 13-year-old girl presents complaining of intermittent episodes of wheezing, which occur only when she is exercising. Which of the following medications is most appropriate to prevent her symptoms?

    (A) Ipratropium
    (B) Fluticasone
    (C) Prednisone
    (D) Salmeterol
    (E) Terbutaline

27. A 35-year-old woman with a history of severe persistent asthma has been treated with inhaled corticosteroids, a long-acting bronchodilator, and prednisone tablets for several years. In order to decrease the severity of side effects of this treatment regimen, which of the following should be prescribed?

    (A) Benzodiazepines
    (B) Beta-blockers
    (C) Folic acid
    (D) Vitamin B
    (E) Vitamin D and calcium

28. A 17-year-old girl with a history of cystic fibrosis presents with a chronic cough productive of copious, foul smelling, purulent sputum. The patient is afebrile and the lung examination reveals crackles at the lung bases bilaterally. What is the most likely diagnosis?

(A) Asthma

(B) Bronchiectasis

(C) Bronchiolitis

(D) Pneumonia

(E) Pneumonitis

29. Which of the following disorders of the large bronchioles is characterized by the destruction of bronchial walls?

(A) Asthma

(B) Bronchiectasis

(C) Cystic fibrosis

(D) COPD

(E) Pneumonia

30. A 35-year-old man is suspected of having a small right-sided pleural effusion. What imaging modality is most sensitive to detect a small amount of pleural fluid?

(A) Chest CT

(B) Lateral chest film

(C) Left lateral decubitus chest film

(D) Standard upright chest film

(E) VQ scan

31. A 58-year-old man with a history of hypertension and left ventricular hypertrophy presents with shortness of breath. Examination reveals dullness to percussion bilaterally with decreased breath sounds. Pleural fluid is aspirated and analyzed. Which of the following results is consistent with his most likely diagnosis?

(A) Glucose 40 mg/dL

(B) LDH 300 IU/L

(C) Protein 2.5 mg/dL

(D) WBC 2,000/mm³

32. A 75-year-old male smoker presents with hemoptysis, weight loss, and chronic cough. Chest film reveals a hilar mass greater than 5 cm and fluid in the costophrenic sulcus. An analysis of the pleural fluid is completed. Which of the following results is consistent with his most likely diagnosis?

(A) Glucose 40 mg/dL

(B) LDH 100 IU/L

(C) Protein 2.9 g/dL

(D) Serum sodium 134

(E) WBC 787/mm³

33. A 14-year-old healthy boy presents to the emergency department complaining of an acute onset of unilateral chest pain and dyspnea that occurred without a precipitating event. Examination reveals unilateral chest expansion and decreased breath sounds. What is the most likely diagnosis?

(A) Atypical pneumonia

(B) Pericarditis

(C) Pulmonary embolus

(D) Spontaneous pneumothorax

(E) Vocal cord dysfunction

34. A 25-year-old patient with a history of tobacco use presents complaining of the acute onset of right-sided chest pain and dyspnea. He has no other symptoms. Examination reveals a tall, thin man, who is mildly anxious and short of breath. An expiratory film shows a visceral pleural line. What chest examination findings are consistent with this patient's diagnosis?

(A) Decreased tactile fremitus; hyperresonant to percussion

(B) Egophony

(C) Increased tactile fremitus; dullness to percussion

(D) Decreased tactile fremitus; dullness to percussion

(E) Increased tactile fremitus; hyperresonant to percussion

35. Which of the following chest films will best demonstrate a small pneumothorax?

(A) Expiratory

(B) Inspiratory

(C) Lateral decubitus

(D) Lordotic

(E) Oblique

36. A 65-year-old man presents with a chronic productive cough, dyspnea, and wheezing. Examination reveals cyanosis, distended neck veins, and a prominent epigastric pulsation. What is the most likely diagnosis?

(A) Asthma

(B) Cor pulmonale

(C) Chronic bronchitis

(D) Emphysema

(E) Pneumonia

37. A 4-year-old child is brought to the emergency department with a low-grade fever, barking cough, and respiratory stridor with activity but not at rest. On examination, you note the cough and the absence of drooling. What is the most appropriate treatment for this child?

(A) Dexamethasone IM

(B) Endotracheal intubation and IV antibiotics

(C) Inhaled budesonide

(D) Nebulized racemic epinephrine

(E) Supportive therapy with oral hydration

38. An otherwise healthy 2-year-old is brought to your office in late winter with a low-grade fever, wheezing, and cough. On physical examination, you note diffuse wheezing and retractions. The patient is not having any trouble feeding or swallowing. This is the fifth child you have seen this week with the same symptoms. What is the most likely diagnosis?

(A) Bronchiolitis due to respiratory syncytial virus

(B) Epiglottitis due to *Haemophilus influenzae* type B

(C) Pharyngitis due to Group A *Streptococcus*

(D) Pneumonia due to *M. pneumoniae*

(E) Tracheitis due to *S. aureus*

39. What is a common initial presentation of cystic fibrosis?

(A) Biliary cirrhosis

(B) Bronchiolitis

(C) Congestive heart failure

(D) Failure to thrive

(E) Ulcerative colitis

40. Which viral illness is transmitted via the respiratory route by droplet nuclei?

(A) Arbovirus

(B) Influenza

(C) Respiratory syncytial virus (RSV)

(D) Rhinovirus

(E) Severe acute respiratory syndrome (SARS)

41. A 4-year-old child presents with a 2-week history of cough, rhinitis, and sneezing without fever. In the last 2 days, the cough has become more severe and is now paroxysmal (10–20 forceful coughs at a time). The paroxysms are accompanied by a loud high-pitched inspiratory sound. The child's medical history reveals that immunizations were not completed in infancy. What is the most likely diagnosis?

(A) Diphtheria

(B) *H. influenzae* type B

(C) Legionella

(D) Pertussis

(E) RSV

42. A 37-year-old man who recently immigrated to the United States and is otherwise well presents to the office complaining of severe paroxysms of cough that have persisted for the past 4 weeks. He describes the cough as severe, causing him to have difficulty catching his breath and making him feel as if he will vomit. He states that before the onset of cough, he was fatigued and complained of symptoms of a head cold. What is the treatment of choice for the most likely diagnosis?

(A) Ceftriaxone

(B) Erythromycin

(C) Isoniazid

(D) Penicillin

(E) Sulfamethoxazole/trimethoprim

43. Which laboratory/diagnostic finding is consistent with coal workers' pneumoconiosis (CWP)?

(A) CT scan showing predominance of ground-glass abnormality

(B) Chest x-ray with eggshell calcifications in hilar lymph nodes

(C) Decreased FEV1

(D) Positive antinuclear antibodies

(E) Positive rheumatoid factor

44. What is the most commonly prescribed initial treatment of idiopathic pulmonary fibrosis (IPF)?

(A) Colchicine in combination with a broad-spectrum antibiotic

(B) Corticosteroids in combination with immunosuppressive agents

(C) Hospitalization, intubation, and broad-spectrum antibiotics

(D) Lung transplantation

(E) Methotrexate in combination with low-dose corticosteroids

45. A patient diagnosed with lung cancer presents with a 4-cm tumor in the mainstem bronchus. The tumor is not within 2 cm of carina. There is no invasion of the visceral pleura or associated atelectasis. There are no distant metastases or nodal involvement. The TNM descriptor is T2N0M0. Given these findings, what is the correct stage of the patient's disease?

(A) 0

(B) IA

(C) IB

(D) IIA

(E) IIB

46. A preterm infant (33 weeks) presents at 10 days of age. The mother complains that the infant is experiencing an increasing number of apneic episodes of 20 to 30 seconds associated with cyanosis. After a careful history, physical examination, and workup, the decision is made to treat the infant. What is the appropriate treatment for this infant?

(A) Corticosteroids alone

(B) Corticosteroids in combination with broad-spectrum antibiotics

(C) Dexamethasone

(D) IV glucose and careful electrolyte management

(E) Methylxanthines

47. Which of the following combination of findings would provide a definitive diagnosis of cystic fibrosis (CF)?

(A) Family abnormal PFT; pancreatic insufficiency

(B) Abnormal chest x-ray; family history of CF

(C) Abnormal sweat test; pancreatic insufficiency

(D) Abnormal spirometry; abnormal chest x-ray

(E) History of CF; abnormal PFT

48. A premature infant is born at 32 weeks and after several hours develops rapid shallow respirations at 60/min, grunting retractions, and duskiness of the skin. The chest x-ray reveals diffuse bilateral atelectasis, ground glass appearance, and air bronchograms. What is the most likely diagnosis?

(A) Cystic fibrosis

(B) Hyaline membrane disease

(C) Meconium aspiration

(D) Tetralogy of Fallot

(E) Ventral septal defect

49. A child presents to the office with respiratory symptoms consistent with influenza. What would be most helpful in supporting the diagnosis?

(A) Chest x-ray with air bronchograms

(B) Elevated WBC count

(C) Epidemiologic and overall clinical data

(D) History of no influenza immunization

(E) Presence of pneumonia

50. A 5-month-old patient is diagnosed with bronchiolitis, which occurred during an annual outbreak in the early spring. You are now concerned about the sequelae of this infection. What etiologic agent is most likely to cause persistent airway reactivity later in life?

(A) Coxsackievirus

(B) Influenza A

(C) Parvovirus

(D) Respiratory syncytial virus

(E) Rotavirus

51. Which of the following recommendations for annual influenza immunization is correct?

(A) Healthy children aged 0 to 6 months should be immunized.

(B) Live attenuated vaccine (nasal spray) is contraindicated in children younger than 12 years.

(C) Pregnant women in the second or third trimester should be immunized.

(D) One dose of vaccine is recommended for adults over 60 years of age if they have had a Pneumovax.

(E) Two doses of vaccine are recommended for children older than 9 years who are receiving vaccine for the first time.

52. What antiviral agent is indicated for the treatment of influenza A?

(A) Acyclovir

(B) Famciclovir

(C) Lamivudine

(D) Oseltamivir

(E) Vidarabine

53. A 50-year-old man presents to the office complaining of progressive dyspnea over the past few years. History reveals that he has worked in construction for the past 20 years demolishing and refurbishing old buildings. He rarely uses any protective breathing equipment. Physical examination demonstrates an afebrile man in mild respiratory distress with inspiratory crackles. The chest x-ray reveals a reticular linear pattern with basilar predominance, opacities, and honeycombing. What is the most likely diagnosis?

(A) Acute hypersensitivity pneumonitis

(B) Asbestosis

(C) Coal workers' pneumoconiosis (CWP)

(D) Silicosis

(E) Small cell carcinoma

54. Classically, pertussis is an illness that lasts for weeks and is divided into stages. A patient who presents with 5 days of congestion, rhinorrhea, low-grade fever, and sneezing is in which stage?

(A) Catarrhal

(B) Convalescent

(C) Paroxysmal

(D) Postdromal

(E) Prodromal

55. A 30-year-old patient presents to the office complaining of an acute onset of fever of 101°F, chills, productive cough, and chest pain. The pain is described as severe, knife-like, and worsened by coughing and/or deep inspiration. What is the name given to this type of chest pain?

(A) Ischemic

(B) Neuralgic

(C) Pleuritic

(D) Somatic

(E) Visceral

56. A 47-year-old man is admitted to the ICU in shock following a near-drowning 3 hours ago. While in the ICU, he suddenly develops dyspnea. Examination reveals labored breathing, tachypnea, and rales. The chest film demonstrates air bronchograms and patchy bilateral infiltrates that spare the costophrenic angles. There is no cardiomegaly or pleural effusions. What is the most likely diagnosis?

(A) Asthma

(B) ARDS

(C) Congestive heart failure

(D) Pneumothorax

(E) Embolism pulmonary

57. A 7-year-old previously healthy patient presents with acute onset of respiratory distress following ingestion of a piece of candy. Which of the following signs or symptoms is most ominous?

(A) Aphonia

(B) Cough

(C) Drooling

(D) Stridor

(E) Wheezing

58. A 55-year-old smoker with lung cancer presents with ptosis and miosis. What is the third clinical finding that comprises this syndrome found in patients with lung cancer?

(A) Anhidrosis

(B) Pericarditis

(C) Pneumonitis

(D) Systemic acidosis

(E) Systemic alkalosis

59. A 32-year-old African-American woman with a history of erythema nodosum presents with nonspecific complaints such as fatigue and malaise. Based on the fact that she is a smoker with these symptoms, a chest x-ray is ordered that demonstrates bilateral hilar adenopathy. A transbronchial lung biopsy reveals noncaseating granulomas. What is the most likely diagnosis?

(A) Asbestosis

(B) Bronchogenic carcinoma

(C) Mesothelioma

(D) Sarcoidosis

(E) Tuberculosis

60. A 25-year-old man presents for preadmission testing (PAT) to correct a ventral hernia. The PAT includes a chest x-ray, which reveals a single, smooth, well-defined node with dense central calcification of approximately 2 cm in diameter. What is the most appropriate next step in the management of this patient?

(A) Obtain a CT scan

(B) Obtain old films for comparison

(C) Proceed directly to biopsy

(D) Repeat CXR

(E) Watchful waiting

61. A 47-year-old patient with a history of HIV presents with fever, tachypnea, shortness of breath, and a nonproductive cough. Bronchoalveolar lavage reveals *P. jirovecii*. What is the treatment of choice?

(A) Amoxicillin/clavulanate

(B) Azithromycin

(C) Ciprofloxacin

(D) Doxycycline

(E) Trimethoprim–sulfamethoxazole

62. A 61-year-old woman who was recently diagnosed with COPD presents with an acute exacerbation of chronic bronchitis. She is allergic (anaphylaxis) to penicillin and develops a rash when she takes Bactrim. What is the most appropriate antibiotic to prescribe?

(A) Augmentin

(B) Azithromycin

(C) Ceftriaxone

(D) Cefuroxime

(E) Trimethoprim–sulfamethoxazole

63. A 3-year-old child presents to the emergency department with a sudden onset of fever, difficulty swallowing, drooling, and dyspnea. Examination reveals a febrile child who is sitting, leaning forward with his neck extended. Chest examination reveals soft stridor with inspiratory retractions. What is the next step in the management of this patient?

(A) Inspection and intubation under controlled conditions

(B) IV cephalosporin therapy

(C) IV corticosteroids

(D) Treatment with nebulized albuterol

(E) Treatment with nebulized epinephrine

64. In which gender and age group is a spontaneous pneumothorax most likely to occur?

(A) Male between 2 and 10 years of age

(B) Female between 2 and 10 years of age

(C) Male between 20 and 40 years of age

(D) Female between 20 and 40 years of age

(E) No gender difference

65. A 32-year-old patient with a history of Wilson disease is 14 months status post liver transplant. The result of a routine pre-employment PPD is induration of 7 mm. What is the recommended management?

(A) Isoniazid

(B) Isoniazid and rifampin

(C) Isoniazid, rifampin, pyrazinamide, and ethambutol

(D) No treatment

(E) Rifampin only

66. A 59-year-old patient presents complaining of a daily productive cough for the last 3 years, which is worse in the winter months. He has also noted some shortness of breath with moderate to heavy exertion. He has no other symptoms. The patient admits to smoking a pack of cigarettes per day for 38 years but quitting 9 months ago. Physical examination is normal. What is the most likely diagnosis?

    (A) Asthma
    (B) Bronchiectasis
    (C) Chronic bronchitis
    (D) Tuberculosis
    (E) Vocal cord dysfunction

67. A 60-year-old patient presents with the insidious onset of dyspnea with exertion and a nonproductive cough and fatigue. The physical examination reveals bi-basilar inspiratory crackles and clubbing of the fingers. The chest x-ray shows a reticular pattern of densities in the lower lung fields. What is the most definitive method of establishing a diagnosis in this patient?

    (A) CT scan
    (B) MRI
    (C) Pulmonary function tests
    (D) Surgical lung biopsy
    (E) Ventilation–perfusion scan

68. Which disease entity is defined as a condition of the lung characterized by abnormal permanent enlargement of the air spaces distal to the terminal bronchioles accompanied by destruction of their walls and without obvious fibrosis?

    (A) Asthma
    (B) Emphysema
    (C) Hyaline membrane disease
    (D) Sarcoidosis
    (E) Silicosis

69. An 82-year-old male has a long history of chronic obstructive pulmonary disease (COPD). His resting oxygen saturation is 84% on room air. Treatment includes oral bronchodilators, inhaled corticosteroids, inhaled beta-agonists, inhaled cholinergics, oral corticosteroids, and home oxygen. Which one of the treatments has been shown to prolong survival in cases such as this?

    (A) Inhaled cholinergics
    (B) Inhaled corticosteroids
    (C) Home oxygen
    (D) Oral bronchodilators
    (E) Oral corticosteroids

70. A 25-year-old male smoker presents to your office with the complaint of cough for 3 weeks. Physical examination and chest x-ray are normal. What is the most logical next step to determine a cause for the cough?

    (A) Ask the patient to stop smoking and return for reevaluation in four weeks
    (B) Ask the patient to enter a smoking cessation class and return in 3 months
    (C) Prescribe antibiotic active against streptococcal pneumonia
    (D) Prescribe a short acting bronchodilator
    (E) Prescribe 4 weeks of proton-pump inhibitor therapy

Answers and Explanations

1. **(B)** *M. pneumoniae* often presents after days of constitutional symptoms and a nonproductive cough. Generally, the examination reveals little more than a reddened throat and rarely, bullous myringitis. Diagnosis is made on clinical grounds. Cold agglutinins are a common confirmatory test. *(Chesnutt et al., 2014)*

2. **(E)** *S. pneumoniae* is the most common cause of pneumonia. Classically it presents with the abrupt onset of fever, cough (productive of rusty sputum), and pleuritic chest pain. Chest x-ray usually reveals a lobar consolidation. *(Chesnutt et al., 2014)*

3. **(A)** Upper airway obstruction usually causes pronounced stridor (obstruction of inspiratory airflow equal to or greater than expiratory airflow), which may be accentuated by forced ventilatory efforts. The stridor may be accompanied by intercostal, suprasternal, or supraclavicular retractions or other signs of increased respiratory effort. The diagnosis can be made with lateral softtissue x-rays of the neck. In some cases, fiberoptic laryngoscopy is helpful. In most cases, the definitive diagnosis is made by endoscopy, and treatment can be accomplished at the same time by removal of the object. *(Stone, 2011)*

4. **(A)** In patients with acute bronchitis, bronchodilators may give symptomatic relief. Studies show that bronchodilator therapy may lead to quicker resolution of cough and return to normal functioning. Antibiotics have not been shown to be effective in patients with acute bronchitis. Corticosteroid therapy (both oral and inhaled) and antiviral therapy are not appropriate for acute bronchitis. *(Hueston & Casey, 2011)*

5. **(B)** Diagnosis is confirmed by finding well-formed noncaseating granulomas in affected tissues. Because the lung is involved so commonly, the routine chest x-ray is almost always abnormal but cannot be used as the sole criteria. *(Baughman & Lower, 2012)*

6. **(A)** *M. tuberculosis* is most commonly transmitted from a patient with infectious pulmonary tuberculosis to other persons by droplet nuclei, which are aerosolized by coughing, sneezing, or speaking. Crowding in poorly ventilated rooms is one of the most important factors in the transmission of tubercle bacilli, since it increases the intensity of a contact with a case. *(Ryan et al. 2010)*

7. **(C)** *K. pneumoniae* is the most likely cause. It is common, along with other gram-negative bacilli, in alcoholic and in debilitated patients. It typically causes the acute onset of cough, chest pain, and shortness of breath. Cavitations are likely to be seen in pneumonias caused by *Klebsiella*. *(Chesnutt et al., 2014)*

8. **(C)** Macrolides such as erythromycin or tetracyclines are the drugs of choice in treating *M. pneumoniae*. Gastrointestinal intolerance is common with erythromycin. Doxycycline, azithromycin, or clarithromycin may be used as alternatives. *(Chesnutt et al., 2014)*

9. **(A)** The pneumococcus is the most common cause of community-acquired pyogenic bacterial pneumonia. The prevalence of penicillin-resistant pneumococci is increasing in the United States; therefore, macrolides are the class of choice (Level I evidence) and may be used in penicillin-allergic patients. *(Chesnutt et al., 2014)*

10. **(C)** The clinical manifestations of bronchogenic carcinoma can vary and are largely based on the location of the tumor and extent of disease. Anorexia, weight loss, asthenia, and cough are some of the more common clinical manifestations. Chest x-ray may demonstrate hilar adenopathy, infiltrates, or single or multiple nodules. Asthma and chronic obstructive pulmonary disease usually reveal hyperinflation of the lungs and flattened diaphragms. The medical history is not consistent with bronchiectasis where the chest film may demonstrate dilated, thickened bronchi, scattered opacities, and atelectasis. *(Chesnutt et al., 2014)*

11. **(E)** Peripheral "pruning" of the large pulmonary arteries is characteristic of pulmonary hypertension in severe emphysema. *(Chesnutt et al., 2014)*

12. **(B)** Eggshell calcification of hilar or mediastinal lymph nodes is characteristic of silicosis. The disease may also be recognized by the presence of small nodules, which appear predominately in the upper lobes. Pneumothorax, atelectasis, and pleural thickening and plaques are not radiologic features of silicosis. *(Balmes & Speizer, 2012)*

13. **(C)** In a patient with pneumonia, inspiratory crackles along with bronchial breath sounds, increased tactile fremitus and transmitted voice sounds (the presence of egophony, bronchophony, and/or whispered pectoriloquy), and dullness to percussion over the involved area would be consistent findings on physical examination. *(Kritek & Choi, 2012)*

14. **(D)** The prognosis for each type of lung cancer varies according to the pathologic stage. However, in general, small-cell lung carcinoma has the worst prognosis, with the median survival period of 12 to 16 months with only 5% to 25% surviving 2 years, whereas patients with extensive disease have a median survival period of only 7 to 11 months, with only 1% to 3% surviving 2 years. *(Theodore & Jablons, 2010)*

15. **(A)** The Centers for Disease Control and Prevention currently recommends a minimum of 6 months of INH and RIF with initial 2 months of PZA and SM or EMB for immunocompetent persons. *(Iseman, 2003)*

16. **(C)** The treatment of choice for immunocompromised patients with legionella infection is either azithromycin or clarithromycin, or a fluoroquinolone such as levofloxacin. Erythromycin and doxycycline are acceptable treatments for immunocompetent patients with legionella. Penicillin is ineffective against legionella. *(Schwartz & Chambers, 2009, p. 1278)*

17. **(D)** Pulmonary thromboembolism is most often caused by the embolization of thrombus from the deep veins of the lower extremities. People at risk for pulmonary embolus are those with hypercoagulable states, which may arise from the use of birth control pills, local stasis, immobilization that may be the result of an accident or illness, fractures, obesity, and congestive heart failure. Signs and symptoms often begin abruptly and include dyspnea, cough, and chest pain (frequently pleuritic in nature). Hemoptysis may occur; tachypnea and tachycardia are common in this illness. A low-grade fever, wheezing, rales, or pleural rub are also signs of pulmonary embolism. *(Goldhaber, 2012)*

18. **(B)** Contrast venography, although expensive, is the imaging study of choice to diagnose a deep vein thrombosis. Currently however it is rarely used due to improvements in ultrasound screening and other imaging modalities. Arteriography and V/Q scans would not be appropriate studies to diagnose deep vein thrombosis. *(Stern, 2010)*

19. **(B)** This description is consistent with digital clubbing. It accompanies chronic hypoxia associated with conditions such as COPD, lung cancer, heart disease, and cirrhosis. *(Usatine et al., 2013)*

20. **(C)** Beta-adrenergic agonists are the mainstay bronchodilator treatment for mild asthma. Theophylline and aminophylline are bronchodilators of moderate potency and are usually reserved for patients with moderate to severe asthma. Antileukotrienes are controller medications, not bronchodilators. *(Boushey, 2012)*

21. **(A)** Chest radiographs most often show diffuse "interstitial" infiltration, which may be heterogeneous, miliary, or patchy early in infection. There may also be diffuse or focal consolidation, cystic

changes, nodules, or cavitation within nodules. *(Shelburne & Hamill, 2014)*

22. **(D)** Primary therapy consists of clot dissolution with thrombolysis or removal of PTE by embolectomy and is reserved for patients at high risk of death from right heart failure and for those patients at risk of recurrent PTE despite adequate anticoagulation. Anticoagulation with heparin is useful to prevent further clot development, but it does not directly dissolve thrombi or emboli. The use of filters is considered a preventative measure, as is the recommended use of antiembolism stockings. *(Chesnutt et al., 2014)*

23. **(A)** Pulmonary arteriography is the "gold standard" for the diagnosis of PTE. An intraluminal defect in more than one projection establishes a definitive diagnosis. Contrast venography is the reference standard for the diagnosis for deep vein thrombosis. Helical CT is replacing V/Q scans as the initial diagnostic study for suspected PTE but is less sensitive than pulmonary arteriography. V/Q scans are helpful for screening especially if they are either normal or indicate high probability of PTE. *(Chesnutt et al., 2014)*

24. **(E)** Evaluation for asthma should include spirometry before and after the administration of a short-acting bronchodilator to determine whether airflow obstruction is immediately reversible. Peak expiratory flow meters are designed for home use to assess severity and provide objective data to guide treatment. Arterial blood gas measurement may be normal in mild exacerbations, but respiratory alkalosis is also common in severe cases. Chest films may show only hyperinflation and are indicated only if pneumonia or pneumothorax is expected. *(Chesnutt et al., 2014)*

25. **(E)** In this case, the nighttime symptoms and daily exacerbations would classify his asthma as severe persistent. The National Asthma Education and Prevention Program has outlined the classification of severity of chronic asthma, which is useful in directing asthma therapy. The classification is based on the frequency of symptoms, nighttime severity, and peak flow measurements. *(Chesnutt et al., 2014)*

26. **(D)** Long-acting bronchodilators, such as salmeterol, are indicated for long-term prevention of asthma symptoms and nocturnal symptoms, and for the prevention of exercise-induced bronchospasm. It is critical to educate the patient that this should not be used as a treatment for acute bronchoconstriction. Fluticasone is an inhaled corticosteroid that can be used as part of the treatment strategy for mild persistent, moderate persistent, and severe persistent asthma. Ipratropium is an anticholinergic agent used to reverse vagally mediated bronchospasm but not allergen or exercise-induced bronchospasm. Theophylline is a phosphodiesterase inhibitor that is not recommended for therapy of asthma exacerbation. *(Chesnutt et al., 2014)*

27. **(E)** Concurrent treatment with calcium supplements, vitamin D, and bisphosphonates can be prescribed to prevent steroid-induced bone mineral loss that occurs with long-term use of steroids. Benzodiazepines, folic acid, and bile acid sequestrants are not indicated for patients on long-term steroids. *(Chesnutt et al., 2014)*

28. **(B)** Symptoms of bronchiectasis include chronic cough, purulent sputum, hemoptysis, and recurrent pneumonia. In addition, weight loss, anemia, and other systemic manifestations are common. Cystic fibrosis causes about half of all cases. Asthma can cause cough but is generally characterized as nonproductive and presents with expiratory wheezes. Bronchiolitis is common in infants and children and is most commonly caused by respiratory syncytial virus or adenovirus. Pneumonitis is a general term for inflammation of the lung (alveolitis) and may be the result of an infectious or environmental insult. *(Chesnutt et al., 2014)*

29. **(B)** Bronchiectasis is characterized by permanent, abnormal dilation and destruction of bronchial walls. Asthma is a chronic inflammatory disorder of the airways. Cystic fibrosis causes altered chloride transport and water flux across the apical surface of epithelial cells. Pneumonia is caused by the infiltration of the lower respiratory tract by microorganisms. *(Chesnutt et al., 2014)*

30. **(A)** A chest CT can identify as little as 10 mL of fluid. On the lateral view, at least 75 to 100 mL of pleural fluid must accumulate in the posterior sulcus to be visible. To make fluid in the right side become visible, the patient must be in the right lateral

decubitus position. The frontal view requires that at least 175 to 200 mL must be present. *(Chesnutt et al., 2014)*

31. **(C)** The patient is most likely in congestive heart failure, which would result in a transudative effusion. Pleural findings consistent with a transudate include glucose greater than 60 mg/dL; protein less than 3.0 g/dL; WBCs less than 1,000 µL; LDH less than 200 IU/L. *(Usatine et al., 2013)*

32. **(A)** The patient most likely has carcinoma, which would result in an exudative effusion. Pleural findings consistent with an exudate include glucose less than 60 mg/dL; protein greater than 3.0 g/dL; WBCs less than 1,000 µL; LDH greater than 200 IU/L. *(Usatine et al., 2013)*

33. **(D)** These findings are most consistent with a spontaneous pneumothorax, which is primarily found in tall, thin men between the ages of 10 and 30. Pericarditis is an acute inflammatory process of the pericardium due to either an infectious process or systemic disease, neoplasm, radiation, drug toxicity, or other processes. The clinical presentation includes chest pain, which is relieved by leaning forward. Pulmonary embolus presents as acute onset of chest pain with tachycardia. Breath sounds are usually normal and fremitus is symmetrical. *(Chesnutt et al., 2014)*

34. **(A)** This patient has a pneumothorax. Because of the accumulation of air in the pleural space, fremitus on the affected side will be decreased and percussion will be hyperresonant. *(Chesnutt et al., 2014)*

35. **(A)** Small pneumothoraces may only be seen on an expiratory film. Other findings include a visceral pleural line on a chest film and a "deep sulcus sign" on a supine film. *(Chesnutt et al., 2014)*

36. **(B)** Cor pulmonale is right ventricular hypertrophy and failure resulting from pulmonary disease. It is most commonly caused by chronic obstructive pulmonary disease, which is this patient's underlying disorder precipitating the failure. While the other three diagnoses may have similar symptoms, none of them would present with distended neck veins and prominent epigastric pulsations. *(Chesnutt et al., 2014)*

37. **(E)** Viral croup is the most likely diagnosis in the patient. It is most often caused by the parainfluenza virus. This patient displays mild symptoms: low-grade fever, cough, and stridor only with activity. In this case, the most appropriate treatment is supportive. If this patient was more seriously ill and had stridor at rest, other treatment including inhaled, oral, or intramuscular (IM) steroids and/or epinephrine would be appropriate. Intubation is reserved for the most severe patients with impending respiratory failure. The use of intravenous (IV) antibiotics is inappropriate in a viral illness. *(Candice, Bjornson & Johnson, 2013)*

38. **(A)** Bronchiolitis due to respiratory syncytial virus is the best answer. Respiratory syncytial virus peaks in late winter and is common in young children. It is often a diagnosis made on the basis of symptoms, particularly during an outbreak. Epiglottitis presents more acutely with sudden onset of fever, dysphagia, drooling, and cyanosis. Tracheitis is also more severe; patients develop high fever, toxicity, and upper airway obstruction. Pneumonia due to mycoplasma is not usually seen in this age group; generally, patients with mycoplasma are older than 5 years. Pharyngitis generally presents with sore throat and fever; cough and wheezing are not part of the clinical presentation. *(Ryan & Ray, 2010)*

39. **(D)** More than 40% of patients with cystic fibrosis present in infancy with failure to thrive, and respiratory compromise. The age of presentation may be variable from infancy into adulthood. Biliary cirrhosis becomes symptomatic in only 2% to 3% of patients. Congestive heart failure is not usually part of the initial presentation. Gastrointestinal disease is equally common and most commonly caused by distal intestinal obstruction syndrome, not by ulcerative colitis. *(Boucher, 2012)*

40. **(B)** Influenza is transmitted via droplet nuclei. RSV, rhinovirus, and SARS are transmitted via fomites or large particle aerosols. Arbovirus is transmitted by arthropods or ticks and produces a variety of encephalitides including West Nile fever, St. Louis encephalitis, and California encephalitis. *(Boucher, 2012)*

41. **(D)** The most likely diagnosis is pertussis, which is typically preceded by 2 to 3 weeks of cough and coryza without fever: the characteristic "whooping"

cough is a high-pitched inspiratory sound. Diphtheria typically presents with sore throat, fever, and malaise and produces a pseudomembrane, most often in the pharynx. *H. influenzae* type B causes a severe febrile illness that presents with meningitis, epiglottitis, septic arthritis, and cellulitis. Legionella causes abrupt onset with fever, chills, and headache, which progress rapidly to pneumonia. *(Halperin, 2012)*

42. **(B)** This is a classic presentation of pertussis. Although the classic posttussive "whoop" is described in the literature, it is a more common symptom in children and found less frequently in adults. Because of the waning of immunity to pertussis in adults who are not receiving booster vaccinations, the incidence of pertussis is increasing. Treatment of pertussis is erythromycin, clarithromycin, or azithromycin. Household contacts should also be treated. The other drugs listed would not be appropriate for the treatment of pertussis. *(Halperin, 2012)*

43. **(C)** A decreased FEV1 is typically found in patients with CWP. Chest x-ray with eggshell calcifications is found in a small percentage of patients with silicosis. A CT scan showing a ground-glass abnormality may be found in nonspecific interstitial pneumonia. A positive antinuclear antibody may be found in silicosis but is nonspecific. A positive rheumatoid factor may be found in rheumatoid arthritis with pulmonary involvement. *(Balmes & Speizer, 2012)*

44. **(B)** No treatment to date has demonstrated improvement in survival; however, oral corticosteroids with an immunosuppressive agent is the most commonly prescribed treatment. Lung transplantation is considered only if medical therapy fails. Colchicine, methotrexate, and broad-spectrum antibiotics are not used in the treatment of IPF. Initial treatment does not generally require hospitalization or intubation. *(Prendergast et al., 2010)*

45. **(C)** The TNM International Staging System provides useful prognostic information and is used to stage all patients with NSCLC. The various T (tumor size), N (regional node involvement), and M (presence or absence of distant metastasis) are combined to form different stage groups. This is stage IB. Stage IA is T1N0M0; stage IIA is T1N1M0; and stage IIB is T2N1M0 or T3N0M0. *(Horn et al., 2012)*

46. **(E)** Signs and symptoms of sepsis in the newborn can be very subtle and nonspecific, such as temperature instability, hypoglycemia or hyperglycemia, apnea, poor feeding, or tachypnea. Methylxanthines in the form of caffeine citrate (20 mg/kg as loading dose and 5 to 10 mg/kg/day) is the drug of choice. The other treatments offered play no role in treating apnea in the preterm infant. *(Raab & Kelly, 2013)*

47. **(C)** An elevated quantitative pilocarpine iontophoresis sweat test is one of the most consistent findings in CF. Only 2% of CF patients have a normal result. Genetic testing may also be performed. *(Murray & Gross, 2012)*

48. **(B)** Hyaline membrane disease is the most common cause of respiratory distress in the preterm infant. It is caused by a deficiency in surfactant that results in poor lung compliance and atelectasis. Meconium aspiration causes a chest x-ray characterized by patchy infiltrates and coarse streaking, with flattening of the diaphragms. In an infant with ventral septal defect (VSD), the chest x-ray would be normal or show cardiomegaly depending on the size of the VSD. Tetralogy of Fallot does not usually cause symptoms at birth. *(Thilo & Rosenberg, 2012)*

49. **(C)** Epidemiologic and clinical data are most helpful. Influenza is otherwise indistinguishable from any number of acute respiratory illnesses. Leukocytosis may be present but does not assist in making the diagnosis. Chest x-ray findings are nonspecific and may reveal atelectasis and/or an infiltrate in about 10% of children. Lack of vaccination may contribute to the diagnosis but would not by itself be diagnostic. Pneumonia is a common complication of influenza but is not diagnostic. *(Dolin, 2012)*

50. **(D)** Respiratory syncytial virus is a common cause of bronchiolitis and is most often associated with reactive airway disease later in life. Coxsackievirus usually occurs in the summer months. Influenza A is usually transmitted in the fall or winter and would not cause concern for airway reactivity later in life. Parvovirus rather than bronchiolitis is the cause of erythema infectiosum in children. *(Chesnutt et al., 2014)*

51. **(C)** Pregnant women in the second and third trimester are among the groups targeted for influenza vaccine. The vaccine should not be given to children

younger than 6 months. The live virus vaccine should not be given to children younger than 5 years. Two doses of vaccine are recommended for children younger than 9 years who are vaccinated for the first time. *(Dolin, 2012)*

52. **(D)** Influenza A may be treated with inhaled zanamivir or oral oseltamivir. Acyclovir, famciclovir, lamivudine, and vidarabine are all antiviral agents used to treat other viral illnesses but are not recommended to treat influenza. *(Dolin, 2012)*

53. **(B)** The clinical presentation described best fits asbestosis. CWP and silicosis cause a nodular pattern with upper lobe predominance. Acute hypersensitivity pneumonitis would not be a likely diagnosis in this patient who presents with a chronic condition and not an acute process. *(Chesnutt et al., 2014)*

54. **(A)** Catarrhal: the first stage of illness. The second stage—paroxysmal—is marked by the onset of coughing. The third and final stage is the convalescent stage where the number, severity, and duration of coughing episodes diminish. There is no formal prodromal phase in pertussis. *(Levinson, 2012)*

55. **(C)** The description best fits pleuritic chest pain. Visceral pain is poorly localized and usually described as aching or heaviness. Ischemic pain and neurologic pain can be very variable in presentation. Neither would fit the description above. *(Bickley & Szilagyi, 2007, pp. 268–269)*

56. **(B)** This is a classic presentation of acute respiratory distress syndrome (ARDS). Common risk factors for ARDS include sepsis, shock, and trauma. Air bronchogram on chest x-ray is found in 80% of patients with noncardiogenic acute respiratory distress syndrome. There may also be peripheral distribution of infiltrates that typically spare the costophrenic angles. Kerley B lines and flattened diaphragms are not part of the picture. The heart is usually of normal size. *(Chesnutt et al., 2014)*

57. **(A)** Aphonia, the inability to vocalize, is a sign of a complete obstruction of the airway as is an inability to cough. Signs and symptoms of a partial obstruction include cough, stridor, and drooling. *(Isaacson, 2003)*

58. **(A)** Horner syndrome (ipsilateral ptosis, miosis, and anhidrosis) is due to involvement of the inferior cervical ganglion and the paravertebral sympathetic chain. Pericarditis, pneumonitis, and systemic acidosis are not components of Horner syndrome. *(Riordan, 2011)*

59. **(D)** Sarcoidosis is a systemic disease of unknown etiology, which is generally characterized by granulomatous inflammation of the lung. In the United States, the incidence is highest in blacks. Symptoms may include malaise, fatigue, and dyspnea but can also include others. Erythema nodosum is not an uncommon finding. Bronchogenic carcinoma may also present with bilateral hilar adenopathy and a biopsy would also confirm such a diagnosis. Mesothelioma and tuberculosis do not present with these signs or symptoms. *(Baughman & Lower, 2012)*

60. **(B)** The findings mentioned are highly suggestive of a benign lesion and evaluation of old radiographs would be warranted to determine stability. A CT should be ordered if it is determined that there is an increase in size. Rapid progression (doubling times less than 30 days) suggests infection; long-term stability (doubling time over 465 days) suggests benignity. *(Chesnutt et al., 2014)*

61. **(E).** The treatment of choice for *P. jirovecii* is trimethoprim–sulfamethoxazole. It is a pneumonia-causing fungus found in mammals and humans worldwide. Patients with HIV and other immunosuppressive disorders are at high risk for developing this infection. Amoxicillin/clavulanate, azithromycin, and doxycycline are not appropriate for the treatment of *P. jirovecii*. *(Parks et al., 2012)*

62. **(B)** First-line agents for the treatment of acute exacerbations of chronic bronchitis include macrolides, fluoroquinolones, and Augmentin. Considering that this patient is allergic to penicillin, the best choice would be azithromycin. Because both cefuroxime and ceftriaxone are cephalosporins, these would be contraindicated given the patient's severe allergy (anaphylaxis) to penicillin. *(Chesnutt et al., 2014)*

63. **(A)** In a patient with suspected epiglottitis, the definitive diagnosis is made by direct inspection of the epiglottis by an experienced specialist under

controlled conditions (such as an OR). The most common finding is a red and swollen epiglottis. After intubation, IV antibiotics can be started. Treatment with albuterol and epinephrine is not appropriate. *(Gunn, 2011)*

64. **(C)** Spontaneous pneumothorax is secondary to intrinsic abnormalities of the lung, and the most common cause is rupture of an apical subpleural bleb. The cause of these blebs is unknown, but they occur more frequently in smokers and males (between 20 and 40 years of age), and they tend to be seen predominately in young postadolescent males with a tall, thin body habitus. *(Nason et al., 2010)*

65. **(C)** The combination of isoniazid, rifampin, pyrazinamide, and ethambutol is the appropriate treatment for a recently converted and previously untreated patient. Although the PPD induration is only 7 mm, in this patient with recent organ transplantation, induration of greater than or equal to 5 mm is considered positive. *(Chesnutt et al., 2014)*

66. **(C)** This clinical picture best fits a diagnosis of chronic bronchitis, which characteristically presents in the 50s and 60s with chronic cough. Asthma is more likely to present with episodic wheezing and chest tightness along with episodic cough. Bronchiectasis would be more likely to present with recurrent pneumonia, hemoptysis, and digital clubbing on physical examination. Tuberculosis is more likely to present with weight loss, fever, night sweats, and cough. *(Chesnutt et al., 2014)*

67. **(D)** The most likely diagnosis in this patient is interstitial pulmonary fibrosis (IPF). The definitive diagnostic test for IPF is a surgical lung biopsy. CT scan may show marked peripheral and subpleural distribution of the interstitial densities but this does not make a definitive diagnosis. Pulmonary function tests may show decreased lung volume and flow rates but these findings are nonspecific. Ventilation–perfusion lung scans are not recommended as a routine part of the evaluation of IPF. *(Chesnutt et al., 2014)*

68. **(B)** This definition best fits the description of emphysema. Permanent enlargement of distal air spaces is not seen in hyaline membrane disease, sarcoidosis, or silicosis. *(Huang, 2012)*

69. **(C)** If patients remain hypoxemic at the time of discharge, they will require home oxygen therapy. To meet the Centers for Medicare and Medicaid Services (CMS) criteria for 24 hours per day long-term home oxygen therapy, patients must have resting, room air PaO_2 of 55 mm Hg or less or PaO_2 of 59 mm Hg or less with coexisting congestive heart failure, peripheral edema, hematocrit >56%, or cor pulmonale. Long-term oxygen therapy improves mortality for COPD patients that have resting hypoxemia. *(Staton & Satterwhite, 2012)*

70. **(A)** Ask the patient to stop smoking and return for reevaluation in four weeks. The most common causes of chronic cough are (1) smoking, often with chronic bronchitis; (2) upper airway cough syndrome (formerly postnasal discharge); (3) asthma; (4) gastroesophageal (GE) reflux; and (5) angiotensin-converting enzyme (ACE) inhibitor or angiotensin II receptor blocker (ARB) therapy. *(Sarko & Stapczynski, 2011)*

REFERENCES

Balmes JR, Speizer FE. Chapter 256: Occupational and environmental lung disease. In: Longo DL, Fauci AS, Kasper DL, Hauser SL, Jameson J, Loscalzo J, eds. *Harrison's Principles of Internal Medicine*. 18th ed. New York, NY: McGraw-Hill; 2012.

Baughman RP, Lower EE. Chapter 329: Sarcoidosis. In: Longo DL, Fauci AS, Kasper DL, Hauser SL, Jameson J, Loscalzo J, eds. *Harrison's Principles of Internal Medicine*. 18th ed. New York, NY: McGraw-Hill; 2012.

Bickley LS, Szilagyi PG. Chapter 17: The nervous system. In Bates' Guide to Physical Examination and History Taking (11th ed., pp. 708–719, 758–759). Philadelphia: Lippincott Williams & Wilkins; 2013.

Boucher RC. Chapter 259: Cystic fibrosis. In Longo DL, Fauci AS, Kasper DL, Hauser SL, Jameson J, Loscalzo J, eds. *Harrison's Principles of Internal Medicine*. 18th ed. New York, NY: McGraw-Hill; 2012.

Boushey HA. (2012). Chapter 20: Drugs used in asthma. In Katzung BG, Masters SB, Trevor AJ, eds. *Basic & Clinical Pharmacology*, 12th ed.

Candice L. Bjornson, David W. Johnson. Croup in Children. *Canadian Medical Association Journal*. 2013;185(15):1317–1323.

Chesnutt MS, Prendergast TJ, Tavan ET. Chapter 9: Pulmonary disorders. In Papadakis MA, McPhee SJ, Rabow MW, eds. *Current Medical Diagnosis & Treatment 2014*. New York, NY: Lange, McGraw-Hill; 2014.

Dolin R. Chapter 187: Influenza. In: Longo DL, Fauci AS, Kasper DL, Hauser SL, Jameson J, Loscalzo J, eds. *Harrison's Principles of Internal Medicine*, 18th ed. New York, NY: McGraw-Hill; 2012.

Goldhaber SZ. Chapter 262: Deep venous thrombosis and pulmonary thromboembolism. In: Longo DL, Fauci AS, Kasper DL, Hauser SL, Jameson J, Loscalzo J, eds. *Harrison's Principles of Internal Medicine*. 18th ed. New York, NY: McGraw-Hill; 2012.

Gunn JD, III. Chapter 119: Stridor and drooling. In: Tintinalli JE, Stapczynski J, Ma O, Cline DM, Cydulka RK, Meckler GD, eds. *Tintinalli's Emergency Medicine: A Comprehensive Study Guide*. 7th ed. New York, NY: McGraw-Hill; 2011.

Halperin SA. Chapter 148: Pertussis and other bordetella infections. In: Longo DL, Fauci AS, Kasper DL, Hauser SL, Jameson J, Loscalzo J, eds. *Harrison's Principles of Internal Medicine*. 18th ed. New York, NY: McGraw-Hill; 2012.

Horn L, Pao W, Johnson DH. Chapter 89: Neoplasms of the lung. In: Longo DL, Fauci AS, Kasper DL, Hauser SL, Jameson J, Loscalzo J, eds. *Harrison's Principles of Internal Medicine*. 18th ed. New York, NY: McGraw-Hill; 2012.

Huang HJ. Chapter 17: The respiratory system. In: Janson LW, Tischler ME, eds. *The Big Picture: Medical Biochemistry*. New York, NY: McGraw-Hill; 2012.

Hueston WJ, Casey BR. Chapter 27: Respiratory problems. In: South-Paul JE, Matheny SC, Lewis EL. eds. *Current Diagnosis & Treatment in Family Medicine*. 3th ed. New York, NY: Lange, McGraw-Hill; 2011.

Isaacson, G; Developmental Anatomy and physiology of the Larynx, Trachea, and Esophagus. Chapter 74: The Larynx, Trachea, Bronchi, Lungs, and Esophagus. Bluestone, et al. *IN Pediatric Otolaryngology*, Vol. 2 (2003) [online]

Iseman MD, Iseman MD. Chapter 39: Mycobacterial diseases of the lungs. In: Hanley ME, Welsh CH. eds. *Current Diagnosis & Treatment in Pulmonary Medicine*. New York, NY: Lange, McGraw-Hill; 2003.

Jacobs R, et al. Common problems in infectious disease. In: McPhee S, Papadakis M, eds. *Current Medical Diagnosis and Treatment*. New York, NY: McGraw-Hill; 2009.

Kritek P, Choi A. Chapter 251: Approach to the patient with disease of the respiratory system. In: Longo DL, Fauci AS, Kasper DL, Hauser SL, Jameson J, Loscalzo J, eds. *Harrison's Principles of Internal Medicine*, 18th ed. New York, NY: McGraw-Hill; 2012.

Levinson W. Part IX: Brief summaries of medically important organisms. In: Levinson W, eds. *Review of Medical Microbiology & Immunology*. 12th ed. New York, NY: Lange, McGraw-Hill; 2012.

Murphy TF. Chapter 145: Haemophilus and moraxella infections. In: Longo DL, Fauci AS, Kasper DL, Hauser SL, Jameson J, Loscalzo J, eds. *Harrison's Principles of Internal Medicine*. 18th ed. New York, NY: McGraw-Hill; 2012.

Nason KS, Maddaus MA, Luketich JD. Chapter 19: Chest wall, lung, mediastinum, and pleura. In: Brunicardi F, Andersen DK, Billiar TR, et al, eds. *Schwartz's Principles of Surgery*. 9th ed. New York, NY: McGraw-Hill; 2010.

Parks C, Berkowitz DM, Bechara R. Chapter 243: Pleural diseases. In: McKean SC, Ross JJ, Dressler DD, Brotman DJ, Ginsberg JS, eds. *Principles and Practice of Hospital Medicine*. New York, NY: McGraw-Hill; 2012.

Prendergast TJ, Ruoss SJ, Seeley EJ. Chapter 9: Pulmonary disease. In: McPhee SJ, Hammer GD, eds. *Pathophysiology of Disease*. 6th ed. New York, NY: Lange, McGraw-Hill; 2010.

Raab EL, Kelly LK. Chapter 22: Neonatal resuscitation. In: DeCherney AH, Nathan L, Laufer N, Roman AS, eds. *Current Diagnosis & Treatment: Obstetrics & Gynecology*. 11th ed. New York, NY: Lange, McGraw-Hill; 2013.

Riordan-Eva P, Hoyt WF. Chapter 14: Neuro-ophthalmology. In: Riordan-Eva P, Cunningham ET Jr, eds. *Vaughan & Asbury's General Ophthalmology*. 18th ed. New York, NY: Lange, McGraw-Hill; 2011.

Ryan KJ, Ray C. Chapter 9: Influenza, parainfluenza, respiratory syncytial virus, adenovirus, and other respiratory viruses. In: Ryan KJ, Ray C, eds. *Sherris Medical Microbiology*. 5th ed. New York, NY: McGraw-Hill; 2010.

Sarko J, Stapczynski J. Chapter 65: Respiratory distress. In: Tintinalli JE, Stapczynski J, Ma O, Cline DM, Cydulka RK, Meckler GD, eds. *Tintinalli's Emergency Medicine: A Comprehensive Study Guide*. 7th ed. New York, NY: McGraw-Hill; 2011.

Schwartz B, Chambers H. Bacterial and chlamydial infections. In: McPhee S, Papadakis M, eds. *Current Medical Diagnosis and Treatment*. New York, NY: Lange, McGraw-Hill; 2009.

Shelburne SA, Hamill RJ. Chapter 36: Mycotic infections. In: Papadakis MA, McPhee SJ, Rabow MW. eds. *Current Medical Diagnosis & Treatment 2014*. New York, NY: Lange, McGraw-Hill; 2014.

Staton GW, Satterwhite L. Chapter 239: Chronic obstructive pulmonary disease. In: McKean SC, Ross JJ, Dressler DD, Brotman DJ, Ginsberg JS, eds. *Principles and Practice of Hospital Medicine*. New York, NY: McGraw-Hill; 2012.

Stern SC, Cifu AS, Altkorn D. Chapter 14: I have a patient with dyspnea. How do I determine the cause?. In: Stern SC, Cifu AS, Altkorn D, eds. *Symptom to Diagnosis: An Evidence-Based Guide*. 2nd ed. New York, NY: Lange, McGraw-Hill; 2010.

Stone C. Chapter 13: Respiratory distress. In: Stone C, Humphries RL, eds. *Current Diagnosis & Treatment Emergency Medicine*. 7th ed. New York, NY: Lange, McGraw-Hill; 2011.

Theodore PR, Jablons D. Chapter 18: Thoracic wall, pleura, mediastinum, & lung. In: Doherty GM, eds. *Current Diagnosis & Treatment: Surgery*. 13th ed. New York, NY: Lange, McGraw-Hill; 2010.

Thilo EH, Rosenberg AA. Chapter 2: The newborn infant. In: Hay WW, Jr, Levin MJ, Deterding RR, Abzug MJ, Sondheimer JM, eds. *Current Diagnosis & Treatment: Pediatrics*. 21th ed. New York, NY: Lange, McGraw-Hill; 2012.

Usatine RP, Smith MA, Chumley HS, Mayeaux EJ, Jr. Chapter 51: Clubbing. In: Usatine RP, Smith MA, Chumley HS, Mayeaux EJ, Jr, eds. *The Color Atlas of Family Medicine*. 2nd ed. New York, NY: McGraw-Hill; 2013.

CHAPTER 11

Obstetrics and Gynecology

Aleece Fosnight, MSPAS, PA-C, CSC, CSE

DIRECTIONS: Each of the numbered questions or incomplete statements is followed by possible answers or completions of the statement. Select the ONE-lettered answer or completion that is BEST in each case.

1. A 25-year-old nullipara female presents for consultation because she suddenly stopped menstruating. On questioning her further it is found that she recently lost 19 lb after starting long-distance running. The MOST appropriate step in her evaluation is measurement of

    (A) human chorionic gonadotropin (hCG) concentration.
    (B) serum estradiol-17b concentration.
    (C) serum prolactin concentration.
    (D) serum testosterone concentration.
    (E) serum thyroid stimulating hormone (TSH) concentration.

2. A man and woman in their 20s have been trying unsuccessfully to conceive for the last year. The woman has regular menses and a 28-day cycle. In the initial evaluation, which of the following tests or evaluations should be considered first line?

    (A) Endometrial biopsy
    (B) Hysterosalpingogram
    (C) Postcoital testing
    (D) Semen analysis
    (E) Transvaginal ultrasound

3. A 39-year-old woman, G3P3, complains of severe, progressive secondary dysmenorrhea and menorrhagia. Pelvic examination demonstrates a tender, diffusely enlarged uterus with no adnexal tenderness. Endometrial biopsy findings are normal. Which diagnostic examination is needed next?

    (A) Computed tomography (CT) scan of the pelvis
    (B) Hysterosalpingography
    (C) Laparoscopy
    (D) Magnetic resonance imaging (MRI)
    (E) Transvaginal and abdominal ultrasound

4. Which of the following elements of a patient's history is the greatest risk factor for endometrial cancer?

    (A) Age greater than 70 years
    (B) Combination progestin and estrogen hormone therapy
    (C) Obesity
    (D) Postmenopausal bleeding
    (E) Tobacco use

5. A 36-year-old G2P2 complains of heavy menstrual bleeding for the past year. The patient is bleeding through a super tampon and a heavy pad every hour of the first 3 days of her cycle. Her cycle lasts 5 days and the cycle length has decreased to having a period every 20 days. She complains of fatigue. Her physical examination and laboratory work-up are normal (negative β-hCG, luteinizing hormone [LH], follicle stimulating hormone [FSH], prolactin, clotting times, liver function, and renal function tests), except for the complete blood cell count (CBC) and further labs indicating she has iron deficiency anemia. The patient's weight is 298 lb. In addition to iron supplementation, which of the following is the BEST INITIAL therapy for this patient?

    (A) Daily dosing of aspirin
    (B) Dilation & curettage of the endometrium
    (C) Hysterectomy
    (D) Long-term conjugated estrogen therapy
    (E) Oral contraceptives

6. A 26-year-old patient is complaining of depression and anxiety just prior to her menses. The symptoms have been going on for more than 1 year, but are now starting to interfere with her relationships and her productivity at work. One week prior to menses each month she experiences a depressed mood, a feeling of being on edge, increased irritability, difficulty sleeping, a feeling of being overwhelmed, and is easily fatigued. She charted her symptoms daily in a log and returned to the office two cycles later. The log is consistent with the history. Her physical examination and general laboratory profile showed no abnormalities. Which of the following is the MOST effective treatment choice for this patient?

(A) Alprazolam (Xanax)
(B) Fluoxetine (Prozac)
(C) Ibuprofen
(D) Progestin-only oral contraceptive
(E) Spironolactone (Aldactone)

7. A 25-year-old nulliparous woman complains of dysmenorrhea that has become progressively worse over the past 2 years. Her pain is described as a constant, aching pain. It begins 2 to 7 days prior to onset of bleeding and does not subside until the menstrual flow decreases. In addition, she complains of pain with intercourse. She has never been pregnant and uses condoms and foam for contraception. Which of the following is the BEST way to confirm the most likely diagnosis definitively?

(A) Laparoscopy
(B) MRI
(C) Pelvic examination
(D) Pelvic ultrasound
(E) Trial of prostaglandin synthetase inhibitors

8. A 47-year-old G3P3 woman comes into the office complaining of heavy, painful, and irregular menstrual bleeding that has been going on for the past 6 months to a year. She has not been sexually active for the past year. On physical examination, her uterus is estimated to be the size of a uterus at 12 weeks' gestation. Pelvic ultrasound confirms the presence of a leiomyoma. Her hematocrit is 29%, mean corpuscular volume (MCV) is 68 fL, and serum ferritin is 10 g/L. What should be the first-line therapy?

(A) Ablation therapy
(B) Depot methodroxyprogesterone acetate (Depo-Provera)
(C) Hysterectomy
(D) Myomectomy of leiomyoma
(E) Oral contraceptive therapy in standard doses

9. A 26-year-old woman has undergone a suction curettage for a hydatidiform mole and was diagnosed with benign gestational trophoblastic neoplasia (GTN). Following this INITIAL treatment, which choice of monitoring should be done for patients in order to prevent the development of choriocarcinoma?

(A) Administer prophylactic chemotherapy
(B) Follow-up every 2 weeks with a urine pregnancy test
(C) Monitor serum β-hCG once per week until three to four normal values are obtained, and then monthly for a year
(D) Monitor serum hCG levels after 6 months and again at 1 year
(E) Monitor serum hCG levels monthly accompanied by chest x-ray to rule out metastases

10. A 20-year-old nulligravida presents with pelvic pain and irregular menstrual bleeding. She denies sexual activity, and her β-hCG urine test is negative. She has never been on oral contraceptives. On pelvic examination, unilateral tenderness on the left side and a palpable cystic mass approximately 4 to 5 cm in size are present. The MOST likely diagnosis is

(A) choriocarcinoma.
(B) ectopic pregnancy.
(C) functional ovarian cyst.
(D) molar pregnancy.
(E) sarcoma.

11. A 40-year-old G2P2 complains of postcoital bleeding. Her last Pap smear was 15 years ago. On examination, she had a friable lesion on her cervix and her cytology demonstrates squamous cell carcinoma. At this point, the MOST appropriate step in this patient's management is which of the following?

(A) Biopsy visualized lesion and refer patient for gynecologic consult

(B) Colposcopy with endocervical curettage and directed biopsy

(C) Loop electrosurgical excision procedure (LEEP) or cervical conization

(D) Radical hysterectomy and radiation therapy

(E) Repeat Pap smear in 4 to 6 months

12. A 25-year-old G1P1 presents to the clinic for her annual examination. She has no history of abnormal Pap smears, but the results from today's test show low-grade squamous intraepithelial lesions (LSIL). Which of the following is the BEST option for what should be done next?

(A) Colposcopy

(B) HPV testing

(C) Recheck Pap in 1 year

(D) Repeat Pap smear in 4 to 6 months, using traditional slide method

(E) Repeat Pap smear in 4 to 6 months, using liquid-based cytology

13. A 58-year-old woman who is 8 years postmenopausal complains of urinary urgency, frequency, and occasional incontinence. On pelvic examination, her vaginal mucosa appears shiny, pale pink with white patches, and bleeds slightly to touch. Her urinalysis and urine cultures are negative. Which of the following is the BEST treatment for this patient?

(A) Oral antibiotics

(B) Surgical procedure

(C) Topical testosterone cream to affected areas

(D) Topical vaginal estrogens

(E) Vaginal suppositories containing sulfa antibiotics

14. A 26-year-old mother who is nursing presents to clinic complaining of right breast tenderness and fever. Upon physical examination, she has a 2-cm fluctuant mass at the site of erythema and tenderness. The patient had been seen 4 days ago and was placed on oxacillin, which she has been taking. At this point, the BEST treatment is

(A) changing antibiotic to vancomycin and discontinuing nursing.

(B) discontinuation of nursing and hot soaks.

(C) hot packs and manual emptying of breasts.

(D) incision and drainage, hot soaks, antibiotics, and breast emptying.

(E) surgical drainage and continuation of nursing.

15. At 8 weeks' gestation, a 24-year-old primipara was seen a week prior complaining of vaginal bleeding and lower abdominal cramping. Her β-hCG level was 1,000 mIU/mL at that time. Today, she has no abdominal pain or evidence of tissue passed per vagina. Transvaginal ultrasound (TVUS) shows no adnexal masses as well as no intrauterine pregnancy. Her repeat β-hCG level is 1,100 mIU/mL. What can be concluded from this information?

(A) The patient has a pregnancy that is nonviable but its location is unknown.

(B) She has had a spontaneous abortion and must have a dilation & curettage.

(C) The hCG level needs to be repeated in 48 hours for more information on viability.

(D) This is definitely an ectopic pregnancy.

(E) This is a molar pregnancy.

16. A 24-year-old Hispanic woman, G3P2, presents for routine prenatal care at 20 weeks' gestation. Her urine is positive for glycosuria (2+). This finding would likely indicate

(A) gestational diabetes.

(B) need to follow-up with a 3-hour glucose tolerance test.

(C) need for a 50-g, 1-hour glucose challenge test.

(D) need for instituting dietary control.

(E) normal increase in renal threshold for glucose.

17. Which of the following risk factors places a woman at the highest risk of developing an ectopic pregnancy?

(A) Advanced maternal age

(B) Amenorrhea

(C) History of spontaneous abortion

(D) History of oral contraceptive use

(E) History of pelvic inflammatory disease

18. A 35-year-old primipara at 39 weeks' gestation is in the labor and delivery suite for a nonstress test. She has had an uneventful pregnancy but has not felt the fetus moving much in the past 24 hours. A subsequent external fetal monitor tracing demonstrates a repetitive late heart rate deceleration. The first step in managing this patient is

(A) administration of a tocolytic agent.

(B) checking maternal oxygen saturation.

(C) evaluation of maternal hypotension.

(D) evaluation of fetal acid–base status.

(E) repositioning the patient.

19. A 30-year-old woman who is nursing presents to the clinic complaining of breast tenderness. Physical examination reveals a warm, erythematous, tender area with induration of the right breast. The next step in management would be to

(A) culture breast drainage to determine causative organism.

(B) discontinue nursing, empty breasts, and apply hot soaks to affected breast.

(C) observe for fever and rest while continuing breastfeeding without medication.

(D) prescribe dicloxacillin (Dynapen).

(E) prescribe topical mupirocin and continue breastfeeding.

20. A 30-year-old woman presents with bilateral breast pain and nodularity. The tenderness and size of the nodules increase premenstrually. She has no family history of breast cancer. On physical examination, multiple tender "rope-like" nodules are palpated. There is no dominant mass and the lymph nodes are not palpable. After reassuring the patient regarding cancer probability, which of the following is recommended for INITIAL management?

(A) 200-mg danazol daily during luteal phase of menses

(B) Decreasing use of caffeine and tobacco

(C) Fine-needle aspiration to determine atypia

(D) Galactography to determine if lesions are focal

(E) Ultrasound for definitive diagnosis

21. A 32-year-old woman, G2P1, with gestational diabetes is delivering at 39 weeks' gestation. The fetus appears to be about 4,100 g. The woman has experienced 5 hours of stage 1 labor and currently is in her second hour of stage 2 labor. The head is delivering but the shoulders are not. Which of the following descriptions includes the BEST option for delivering this infant?

(A) Flexing of the mother's thighs, pitocin augmentation, and suprapubic pressure

(B) Flexing of the mother's thighs, suprapubic pressure, and cutting an episiotomy

(C) Elevation of the mother's legs, suprapubic pressure, and oxygen for the mother

(D) No elevation of the mother's legs, pitocin, and fundal pressure

(E) No elevation of the mother's legs, suprapubic pressure, and cutting an episiotomy

22. A 32-year-old woman, G2P1, at 35 weeks' gestation presents with a complaint of intermittent bleeding over the past week; however, she has had no evident pain or cramping. Upon physical examination, fetal heart rate is noted to be normal. These clinical characteristics are MOST consistent with which of the following?

(A) Placental abruption

(B) Placenta previa

(C) Premature labor with bloody mucous discharge

(D) Premature rupture of membranes

(E) Vasa previa

23. At 33 weeks' gestation, a 28-year-old patient, G1P0, calls the office with a complaint of a fluid gush from her vagina. She is not having contractions or evidence of bleeding. She is advised to go to labor and delivery to be examined. Which of the following procedures should be performed first?

(A) Administration of antibiotics to prevent infection

(B) Digital cervical examination to determine whether patient is in labor

(C) Induction of labor

(D) Sterile speculum examination or nitrazine testing

(E) Ultrasound to estimate amniotic fluid volume

24. At 16 weeks' gestation, a 19-year-old G1P0 Asian patient presents with a complaint of vaginal bleeding. She also has been experiencing severe nausea and vomiting. Her quantitative β-hCG is much higher than expected and her fundal height is approximately at 18- to 20-week size. Although she denies a past history of hypertension, her blood pressure is 140/90 mm Hg. No fetal heart sounds can be heard on Doppler and there is no sign of a fetus on ultrasound. What is the MOST likely diagnosis?

    (A) Fetal demise at 16 weeks
    (B) Hydatidiform mole
    (C) Incomplete abortion
    (D) Threatened abortion
    (E) Twin gestation

25. A 20-year-old sexually active woman complains of a profuse, whitish gray vaginal discharge with a fishy odor that becomes stronger after intercourse and during menses. She denies any irritation and states that her sexual partner has no symptoms. Microscopic evaluation of the discharge reveals granular-appearing epithelial cells. Which of the following is the BEST therapy?

    (A) Ciprofloxacin (Cipro)
    (B) Doxycycline
    (C) Fluconazole (Diflucan)
    (D) Metronidazole (Flagyl)
    (E) Miconazole cream (Monistat)

26. A 17-year-old complains of severe dysmenorrhea since her first menses at age 13. The dysmenorrhea is often accompanied by nausea and vomiting the first 2 days of her menstrual period; analgesics or heating pads do not relieve the pain. She is sexually active and does not want to get pregnant. Her pelvic examination is normal. Which of the following medications is MOST appropriate for this patient?

    (A) Luteal progesterone
    (B) Narcotic analgesics
    (C) Oral contraceptives
    (D) Oxytocin
    (E) Prostaglandin synthetase inhibitors

27. A 26-year-old female at 34 weeks' gestation presents concerned about lack of fetal movement. An ultrasound and stress test is ordered. Which of the following nonstress tests results is most reassuring?

    (A) No change in the fetal heart rate with fetal movements over a 30-minute period
    (B) Two decelerations with fetal movements over a 40-minute period
    (C) One acceleration with fetal movements over a 1-hour period
    (D) Five decelerations with fetal movements over a 20-minute period
    (E) Two accelerations with fetal movements over a 20-minute period

28. A 28-year-old primigravida woman at 42 weeks' gestation delivers a 4,000-g (8 lb 13 oz) newborn. Labor stages are as follows: first stage, 17 hours; second stage, 4 hours; third stage, 35 minutes. After an episiotomy was performed, the baby was delivered with low forceps. The placenta appeared to be intact. Ten minutes after delivery, she experiences vaginal bleeding estimated to be 500 mL over a 5-minute period. Upon examination, her uterus feels soft and boggy. Which of the following is the MOST likely cause of the hemorrhage?

    (A) Disseminated intravascular coagulation
    (B) Genital tract laceration
    (C) Retained placental tissue
    (D) Uterine atony
    (E) Uterine inversion

29. A previously desensitized Rh-negative woman in her second pregnancy is seen in her 26th week. She complains of edema in her legs and some tingling in her left hand. What is the next step in managing this patient?

    (A) Amniocentesis
    (B) Analysis of the husband's blood type
    (C) Intramuscular Rho (anti-D) immune globulin
    (D) Rh antibody titer
    (E) Ultrasonic evaluation of amniotic fluid volume

30. A 26-year-old G1P0 at 28 weeks' gestation presents to labor and delivery complaining of low abdominal pain. Her contractions are regular and occur every 15 minutes. The fetal heart rate is 139 bpm and the nonstress test is reassuring. Cervical dilation is 1 cm with no effacement. Patient denies any fluid loss via the vagina. Which of the following medications should be administered next?

   (A) Betamethasone
   (B) Magnesium sulfate
   (C) Nifedipine
   (D) Ritodrine
   (E) Terbutaline

31. A 36-year-old woman at 22 weeks' gestation presents for her regular check-up. Her hemoglobin level is 10.8 g/dL. Which of the following statements regarding this patient's hemoglobin level is TRUE?

   (A) This patient has iron deficiency anemia
   (B) This patient has physiologic anemia of pregnancy, no further work-up necessary
   (C) This patient should receive ferrous sulfate 300 mg 1–2 × a day
   (D) Repeat hemoglobin in 2 months when more accurate reading can be obtained
   (E) A complete evaluation of the anemia, including serum ferritin, needs to be done

32. When counseling a 53-year-old postmenopausal female regarding the risks and benefits of a short course (<5 years) of hormone replacement therapy (HRT), which of the following is a documented risk of HRT that should be discussed?

   (A) Increased risk of endometrial cancer
   (B) Increased risk of breast cancer
   (C) Decreased bone mineral density
   (D) Increased risk of thromboembolism
   (E) Increased risk of colon cancer

33. A 30-year-old G2P1 woman whose last menses was 8 weeks ago presents with heavy vaginal bleeding and left lower quadrant (LLQ) pain. She noted passage of something that "looked like liver" the previous day. Pelvic examination reveals a 2-cm cervical dilation. Which of the following is the MOST likely diagnosis?

   (A) Complete abortion
   (B) Incompetent cervix
   (C) Incomplete abortion
   (D) Missed abortion
   (E) Threatened abortion

34. A 44-year-old G2P2 woman who had two normal pregnancies (13 and 11 years ago) presents with the complaint of amenorrhea for 8 months. She has remarried and would like to become pregnant again. A pregnancy test is negative. Her physical examination is normal. Which of the following tests is next indicated in the evaluation of this patient's amenorrhea?

   (A) Endometrial biopsy
   (B) Hysterosalpingogram
   (C) Luteinizing hormone, follicle-stimulating hormone, and estradiol levels
   (D) Ovarian antibody assay
   (E) Testosterone and dehydroepiandrosterone levels

35. A 27-year-old G1P0 woman has received regular prenatal care throughout her pregnancy. She presents to the ED at 34 weeks with facial edema, severe headache, and epigastric pain. On physical examination, she has a blood pressure of 160/110 mm Hg, elevated liver function tests, and a platelet count of 60,000/uL. The baby is noted to be alive. Urinalysis indicates 4+ proteinuria. Which therapeutic measure should be taken next in managing this patient?

   (A) Colloid solution for plasma volume expansion
   (B) Intravenous immunoglobulin therapy
   (C) Magnesium sulfate therapy and induction of labor
   (D) Oral antihypertensive therapy
   (E) Platelet transfusion

36. A 28-year-old primigravida presents for routine prenatal care at 32 weeks' gestation. Her pregnancy has been uneventful and she has been receiving regular prenatal care. At her visit today, the fundal height measurement is 36 cm. Of the possibilities below, which of the following is the LEAST likely cause for the increased fundal height?

(A) Fetal macrosomia

(B) Fetal position

(C) Fibroid uterus

(D) Multiple gestation

(E) Oligohydramnios

37. A 25-year-old female at 10 weeks' gestation presents to an outpatient clinic concerned about vaginal bleeding and passing pieces of tissue. Which of the following is the most likely etiology of her spontaneous abortion?

(A) An incompetent cervix

(B) Chromosomal anomalies

(C) Inadequate progesterone

(D) Maternal drug abuse

(E) The presence of maternal lupus anticoagulant

38. A 45-year-old female, G4P4, presents concerned about increased pelvic pressure and a large bulge protruding from her vaginal introitus. Examination reveals a large uterine prolapse. Surgical repair of her prolapse will most likely involve repairing which of the following structures?

(A) Detrusor muscles

(B) Levator ani muscle

(C) Obturator internus muscle

(D) Sacral nerve

(E) Transverse and uterosacral ligaments

39. A healthy 20-year-old woman is using a low-dose triphasic contraceptive pill for birth control. She experiences breakthrough bleeding during the third week of each cycle for the past few months. Her pregnancy test is negative. The physical examination is normal. There is no infection or thyroid problem. The patient desires to stay on oral contraceptives. What is the BEST way to manage her therapy?

(A) Continue current oral contraceptive pill (OCP), but add extra estrogen during the third week

(B) Change to a pill with a higher progestin component

(C) Prescribe a progestin-only pill

(D) Reassure her and have her return in 1 month

(E) Switch to a pill with a higher estrogenic component

40. A 28-year-old female has had several recurrent spontaneous abortions secondary to an incompetent cervix. At her most recent office visit, her pregnancy test was positive and a viable pregnancy was seen on ultrasound at 8 weeks and 3 days. Which of the following is the BEST way to avoid a miscarriage or a premature birth for this patient?

(A) Bed rest

(B) Cerclage

(C) Magnesium sulfate

(D) Pessary

(E) Terbutaline

41. A 23-year-old female presents to the outpatient clinic with irregular menses and abnormal menstrual bleeding. Based on the most likely diagnosis of dysfunctional uterine bleeding in this patient's age group, which of the following symptoms would likely be elicited during the history?

(A) Deep thrust dyspareunia, pelvic pain, and headache

(B) Dysmenorrhea, headache, insomnia, and pelvic pain

(C) Dysuria, introital dyspareunia, insomnia, pelvic pain

(D) Dysmenorrhea, deep thrust dyspareunia, and pelvic pain

(E) Dysmenorrhea, introital dyspareunia, constipation, and dysuria

42. A 32-year-old nulliparous woman is seeking contraceptive advice. She is in a monogamous relationship and is a nonsmoker and has a history of one ectopic pregnancy 5 years ago. She wishes to consider childbearing in the future. Her history includes mild, well-controlled hypertension, and frequent urinary tract infections. Which one of the following contraceptive options would be contraindicated?

(A) Condoms and spermicide

(B) Diaphragm

(C) Intrauterine device

(D) Low-dose combined oral contraceptive

(E) Progesterone-only oral contraceptive

43. A 15-year-old female presents to the local health department concerned about several pruritic fleshy raised lesions on her labia. The patient is diagnosed with genital warts upon examination. She is counseled on the low-risk human papillomavirus (HPV) types and the rare association with cancer. Which of the following subtypes of HPV was she most likely exposed to?

(A) 6 and 11

(B) 11, 12, and 73

(C) 31 and 58

(D) 22 and 78

(E) 39 and 82

44. Given a healthy woman, with no history of abnormal Paps and no history of abnormal mammograms, what is the minimum age a female can stop getting Pap smears and mammograms?

(A) 65

(B) 68

(C) 70

(D) 72

(E) 75

45. A 27-year-old G3P3 presents to an outpatient clinic for her wellness examination. Last year her Pap smear was normal. This year, however, her Pap results indicate atypical squamous cells of undetermined significance (ASCUS) and the reflex HPV testing results show high-risk (HR) HPV. What is the most appropriate next step in her evaluation?

(A) Colposcopy

(B) Endometrial biopsy

(C) Loop electrosurgical excision procedure (LEEP)

(D) Repeat cytology at 6 and 12 months

(E) Repeat reflex HPV testing

46. A 20-year-old female college student presents complaining of recent onset vaginal pruritis, discharge, and odor. On physical examination, a thin yellow discharge is observed along with "strawberry spots" on the cervix. The wet prep reveals a pH of 6.0, positive whiff test, and mobile protozoan. What is the best treatment for this patient?

(A) Acyclovir 400 mg by mouth, 3 times daily, for 7 days

(B) Fluconazole 150 mg by mouth, one dose

(C) Metronidazole 500 mg by mouth, twice daily, for 7 days

(D) Metronidazole 2 g by mouth, one dose

(E) Miconazole 2% cream, 5 g intravaginally, for 7 days

47. A 27-year-old female complains of multiple painful labial ulcerations that appeared about 48 hours ago. A genital swab was obtained and was found to be herpes simplex viral polymerase chain reaction (HSV PCR) positive. Which of the following would be the BEST treatment option for this patient?

(A) Acyclovir 400 mg orally, three times a day for 7 days

(B) Ceftriaxone 1 g intramuscular, one dose

(C) Ciprofloxacin 250 mg orally, twice daily for 5 days

(D) Ibuprofen 800 mg orally, three times a day for 3 days

(E) Penciclovir 1% topical every two hours for 3 days

48. A 22-year-old nulliparous woman presents with a chief complaint of heavy, irregular menstrual bleeding over the past year. Patient has a body mass index (BMI) of 35 with hirsutism, acne and borderline hypertension. Patient denies any vaginal dryness, mood changes, hot flashes, hot or cold intolerance, diarrhea, or heart palpitations. She is currently not sexually active. Which of the following would be the BEST diagnostic tool for the most likely diagnosis?

(A) CT scan of abdomen and pelvis

(B) History and physical examination

(C) Labs—estradiol, luteinizing hormone, and follicle stimulating hormone

(D) Transvaginal ultrasound

(E) Wet mount

49. A 37-year-old G2P2 woman presents to your office complaining of low libido for the past year. She is currently in a monogamous relationship with her husband and denies any vaginal dryness, dyspareunia, or anorgasmia. Current medications include meto-prolol (Lopressor), sertraline (Zoloft), omeprazole (Prilosec), cetirizine (Zyrtec OTC) and multivitamin. Which of her medications is most likely contributing to the patient's symptoms?

(A) Cetirizine

(B) Metoprolol

(C) Multivitamin

(D) Omeprazole

(E) Sertraline

50. A 34-year-old African-American female presents to the office concerned about worsening lower abdominal bloating, pelvic pressure, mild deep dyspareunia, and heavy menstrual bleeding. On pelvic examination, a 20-week size uterus is palpated and transvaginal ultrasound confirms a large leiomyoma. The patient and her husband have been trying to conceive over the past year and have been unsuccessful. What treatment option would be the BEST course for this patient?

(A) Endometrial ablation

(B) Laparoscopic-assisted myomectomy

(C) Leuprolide acetate (Lupron Depot)

(D) Oral contraceptives

(E) Total abdominal hysterectomy

51. A 21-year-old female presents to the family planning clinic at her local health department for an annual examination. Patient is currently sexually active and has had three new partners over the past year. She uses oral contraceptives, however rarely uses condoms during her sexual encounters. Other than increased vaginal discharge, patient is asymptomatic. Speculum examination shows a mildly friable, erythematous cervix with no active discharge. Pregnancy test is negative and no cervical motion tenderness or adnexal masses. Two weeks later, her vaginal nucleic acid amplification test (NAAT) comes back positive. What is the MOST likely pathogen causing the positive test?

(A) *Candida albicans*

(B) *Chlamydia trachomatis*

(C) *Escherichia coli*

(D) Herpes simplex virus

(E) *Neisseria gonorrhoeae*

52. At her annual examination, a 36-year-old woman is concerned about worsening abdominal bloating, urinary urgency and anorexia over the past 6 months. Upon pelvic examination, a very firm, right ovarian mass is palpated. Which of the following interventions should be considered first with this patient?

(A) Chemotherapy

(B) Exploratory laparoscopy

(C) Oral contraceptives

(D) Radiation therapy

(E) Surgical oncologist consult

53. A 44-year-old female presents for cancer testing after her mother was recently diagnosed with breast cancer 6 months ago. Her laboratory work confirms a positive result for *BRCA1* gene mutation. Which of the following types of cancer is she at MOST increased risk for developing?

(A) Cervical cancer

(B) Endometrial cancer

(C) Ovarian cancer

(D) Vaginal cancer

(E) Vulvar cancer

54. During a routine well woman examination on a 34-year-old female patient, cervical cysts are noted while performing a Papanicolaou test. The MOST likely treatment is

(A) loop electrosurgical excision procedure (LEEP).

(B) metronidazole (Flagyl) 500 mg orally, twice daily for 14 days.

(C) miconazole vaginal suppository twice daily for 3 days.

(D) no treatment is needed.

(E) trichloroacetic acid topical weekly until gone.

55. A 47-year-old female presents to the clinic concerned about a growing mass on her left labia that is now causing discomfort while sitting. Patient denies any fever, chills, or vaginal discharge. On physical examination, a 3-cm fluctuant mass is palpated at the 7 o'clock position. Her BEST course of treatment would be which of the following?

(A) Amoxicillin/clavulanate (Augmentin) 875 mg orally, twice daily for 7 days
(B) Catheter drainage
(C) Cephalexin (Keflex) 500 mg orally, three times daily for 7 days
(D) Conservative management with warm compress
(E) Surgical removal

56. A 14-year-old female presents to the emergency department complaining of fullness in her lower abdomen, lower back pain, urinary urgency, and constipation. Patient is not sexually active and denies menarche. Urinalysis and complete blood count (CBC) are within normal limits. On physical examination, she has suprapubic discomfort to palpation and pelvic examination shows a thin, bulging, dark bluish membrane covering her vaginal introitus. What would be the BEST initial intervention for this patient?

(A) Biopsy
(B) Incision and drainage (I&D)
(C) General surgical consult
(D) Gynecology consult
(E) Papanicolaou test

57. An 18-year-old female college student presents to the emergency department stating that she was sexually assaulted 2 hours earlier. Appropriate INITIAL medical professional intervention for the patient should be

(A) provide acute medical care.
(B) prophylaxis therapy for sexually transmitted infections and pregnancy.
(C) psychology consult.
(D) referral to counseling services.
(E) reporting to local authorities.

58. A 28-year-old patient presents for annual well woman physical. She is concerned about a 1-cm right breast mass she found on a self-breast examination last month. During the clinical breast examination, the mass is easily mobile, firm, painless upon palpation, and rubbery in consistency. What diagnostic study should be considered first in this patient?

(A) Fine-needle aspiration biopsy
(B) Magnetic resonance imaging
(C) Mammogram
(D) Open breast biopsy
(E) Ultrasound

59. A 52-year-old woman comes in for her annual physical examination. A thorough medical history shows no family history of breast cancer or cervical cancer. Her physical examination reveals no breast skin changes however a firm 1-cm mass can be palpated on the left breast lateral to her areola. Her screening and diagnostic mammogram confirms the mass as suspicious for breast cancer. What is the next best step in the management of this patient?

(A) Core needle biopsy
(B) Fine-needle aspiration biopsy
(C) Open surgical biopsy
(D) Lumpectomy
(E) Ultrasound

60. A 62-year-old female presents to clinic complaining about a bulge from her vagina. She states that the area has grown in size over the past 6 months and has had worsening pelvic pressure after a vaginal hysterectomy over 1 year ago. Patient does complain of vaginal dryness and the feeling that she does not empty her bladder to completion with each void. On physical examination, there is a bulge from the upper one-third of the vagina and 1-cm protrusion from the vaginal introitus with valsalva as well as weak pelvic floor muscles and vaginal atrophy. What is her BEST course of treatment?

(A) Oral anticholinergics
(B) Oral estrogen therapy
(C) Pessary insertion
(D) Surgical intervention
(E) Vaginal estrogen therapy

61. A 32-year-old, G2P0 presents to an outpatient clinic at 34 weeks' gestation. Her prenatal care has been routine for twin gestations without any complications. Today, she is complaining of low pelvic

"cramping." While at the office she has had four cramping episodes in the last 20 minutes and upon pelvic examination is at least 2 cm dilated. What is of greatest concern for this patient at this time?

(A) Incompetent cervix

(B) Intrauterine fetal demise

(C) Gestational diabetes

(D) Preeclampsia

(E) Preterm labor

62. A 36-year-old female presents to an outpatient clinic complaining of burning pain on her left labia radiating to her inner thigh. Patient states that the pain is worsened with tight fitting clothes and prolonged sitting. She states that her primary care provider could not find anything abnormal on physical examination and her urinalysis was negative. Labs performed today are negative for candida, sexually transmitted infections, and vaginal atrophy. She does tell you that 6 months ago she had a motorcycle accident and bruised her pelvis. What is the next best step to confirm the most likely diagnosis?

(A) CT scan

(B) CT scan of pelvis

(C) MRI of pelvis

(D) Q-tip test

(E) Wet mount

63. Which of the following is the most significant risk factor for the development of abruption placentae?

(A) Abdominal trauma

(B) Advanced maternal age

(C) Gestational diabetes

(D) Maternal hypertension

(E) Previous miscarriage

64. At an outpatient clinic, a 24-year-old female 16 weeks' gestation presents complaining of copious amounts of white vaginal discharge for the past 3 days. She is also complaining of vulvar irritation, dysuria, and pruritis. Wet mount reveals hyphae and budding yeast. Her BEST course of treatment would be

(A) ciprofloxacin 250 mg orally, twice daily for 7 days.

(B) clindamycin 300 mg orally, twice daily for 7 days.

(C) clotrimazole 100 mg vaginal suppository, once daily for 7 days.

(D) fluconazole 150 mg orally, one dose only.

(E) metronidazole 500 mg orally, twice daily for 7 days.

65. A 37-year-old female in her third week postpartum presents complaining of recent onset of breast pain with firmness to her right upper outer quadrant. She is lactating however has noticed decreased milk production despite continuing breastfeeding. Upon examination, her breast is firm, warm, edematous, and erythematous. Which of the following is the most common pathogen causing this patient's diagnosis?

(A) *Enterococcus faecalis*

(B) *Escherichia coli*

(C) Group B Streptococcus

(D) *Staphylococcus aureus*

(E) *Streptococcus pyogenes*

66. A 27-year-old G1P0 presents to labor and delivery with progressively severe and frequent contractions over the past 10 hours. Her contractions are lasting about 50 seconds with 4 minutes in between each contraction. Cervical examination shows dilation to 6 cm with 75% effacement. The stage of labor for this patient would be assessed as

(A) first stage, latent phase.

(B) first stage, active phase.

(C) first stage, transition phase.

(D) second stage.

(E) third stage.

67. A 23-year-old female, G1P0, at 12 weeks' gestation presents for routine prenatal care with a normal medical history. Which of the following should be done at today's visit?

(A) 3 hour glucose tolerance test after 100 g oral glucose load

(B) Complete blood count, HIV testing, and urinalysis

(C) Chorionic villus sampling

(D) Trichomonas vaginalis screening

(E) X-ray pelvimetry

68. A 35-year-old female presents to an outpatient clinic for evaluation of amenorrhea. All of her laboratory work came back normal except for a positive pregnancy test. Her last menstrual cycle was August 4, 2015. Her estimated date of delivery will be

(A) April 26, 2016.

(B) May 3, 2016.

(C) May 10, 2016.

(D) May 17, 2016.

(E) June 3, 2016.

69. A 17-year-old female patient presents to an outpatient clinic and is requesting emergency contraception after having unprotected intercourse 4 days ago. Should this patient receive emergency contraception based on her time frame for the greatest effectiveness in preventing a pregnancy?

(A) No, time frame should be 0 to 24 hours

(B) No, time frame should be 24 to 48 hours

(C) No, time frame should be 48 to 72 hours

(D) No, time frame should be 72 to 96 hours

(E) Yes, time frame should be less than 120 hours

70. A 50-year-old postmenopausal woman presents to the clinic complaining of vulvar pruritis for the past year. Upon examination, the patient has whitening patches of her vulvar skin in the shape of a figure eight down to her anus. Which of the following is the best course of treatment for this patient?

(A) Clobetasol topical to area twice daily for 14 days

(B) Miconazole topical to area twice daily for 14 days

(C) Oral conjugated estrogens daily

(D) Prednisone 5 mg orally, twice daily for 14 days

(E) Vaginal estrogen therapy daily

71. A 46-year-old perimenopausal woman presents to an outpatient clinic complaining of hot flashes affecting her quality of life. Her menstrual cycles have been irregular for the past year and is currently on no medications. Patient retains all of her female reproductive organs. She has tried lifestyle modification however nothing has improved her symptoms and is interested in hormonal replacement therapy. What would be her BEST treatment option?

(A) Alpha agonists

(B) Oral estrogen only

(C) Oral progesterone only

(D) Oral combination estrogen/progesterone

(E) Serotonin selective reuptake inhibitors (SSRI's)

72. A 58-year-old female presents to clinic complaining of a pruritic bump she found on her labia. She has not had a pelvic examination in 10 years since her vaginal hysterectomy. On exam, there is a 1-cm irregularly shaped raised brown lesion on her left labia. What is the BEST initial intervention for this patient?

(A) Biopsy of lesion

(B) Oral prednisone

(C) Pelvic MRI

(D) Topical corticosteroids

(E) Vaginal estrogen therapy

73. A 36-year-old female presents to family planning clinic at her local health department inquiring about birth control options. She is a ½ pack-day smoker and the only medication she is taking is lisinopril for her hypertension. Which of the following contraceptives is MOST appropriate for this patient?

(A) Combined oral contraceptive pills

(B) Depot medroxyprogesterone acetate

(C) Intrauterine device

(D) Transdermal contraceptive patch

(E) Vaginal ring (NuvaRing)

74. A 44-year-old female presents to an outpatient clinic with her 14-year-old daughter and is interested in the HPV vaccine. Which of the following should be discussed with the patient and her daughter?

(A) The vaccine only protects against external genital warts

(B) The vaccine only protects against cervical cancer

(C) The vaccine must be given in three separate doses: 0, 2, and 6 months

(D) The vaccine cannot be given until age 18

(E) Once the vaccine is given, Papanicolaou testing is not necessary

75. A 27-year-old female, 38 weeks' gestation presents to the clinic complaining of abdominal cramping for the past 2 hours and spontaneous rupture of membranes. Upon pelvic examination, cervix is dilated to 7 cm. After 4 hours of active labor, the external fetal monitor shows several decelerations and fetal distress is a major concern. What is the BEST course of action for this patient?

(A) Immediate cesarean delivery

(B) Reposition patient to left lateral decubitus

(C) Start intravenous oxytocin

(D) Start an epidural

(E) Wait until she has dilated to 10 cm for vaginal delivery

Answers and Explanations

1. **(A)** Although exercise-induced secondary amenorrhea may seem apparent in this case, it is imperative that pregnancy is ruled out as a cause of the amenorrhea. All amenorrheic women of reproductive age should be assumed to be pregnant until proven otherwise. Therefore, an hCG test is indicated as a first step in the evaluation of this patient. Sudden weight loss and increased physical activity can cause secondary amenorrhea, as can hypothyroidism and hyperprolactinemia. If ordering serum estradiol concentrations, an FSH level should also be ordered. Serum estradiol levels alone are less useful than FSH in deciphering cause of amenorrhea. Decreased estradiol occurs with either hypothalamic–pituitary axis failure or ovarian failure. Decreased FSH indicates hypothalamic–pituitary axis failure whereas elevated FSH indicates ovarian failure. Ordering serum testosterone levels should only be considered if the patient has symptoms of PCOS or androgen excess. *(Halvorson, 2012a, pp. 440–459)*

2. **(D)** Generally, infertility is defined as the inability for a couple to conceive after reasonably frequent unprotected intercourse for 1 year. In approaching the diagnostic work-up for infertility, with a thorough physical examination and history of both partners, the clinician should establish the following points: (1) does the woman ovulate? (if not, why not); (2) does the semen have normal characteristics? (3) is there a female reproductive tract abnormality? Noninvasive tests should be done first line. For the male partner, semen analysis is noninvasive and helpful, though not diagnostic. In the initial evaluation of the female partner, noninvasive procedures, such as the measurement of LH and midluteal phase progesterone (to determine ovulatory function) and transvaginal ultrasound (to rule out the possibility of fibroids or polycystic ovaries), are first-line investigations. Pelvic ultrasound should also be part of the routine gynecologic evaluation because it allows a more precise evaluation of the position of the uterus within the pelvis and provides more information about its size and irregularities. Hysterosalpingography is an invasive procedure and therefore not first line in the evaluation. Endometrial biopsy and postcoital testing are no longer recommended for the routine infertility evaluation because they have poor predictive value. *(Halvorson, 2012b, pp. 400–439)*

3. **(E)** It is important to evaluate why this patient has an enlarged and tender uterus; therefore, the next step in evaluation would be ultrasound. Common causes of secondary dysmenorrhea in this age group are endometriosis, adenomyosis, and the presence of an intrauterine device. For this patient, it would be important also to rule out leiomyomas, endometrial polyps, and tumors. Given the most common causes, endometriosis and adenomyosis, noninvasive studies with transvaginal and abdominal ultrasound would be a reasonable (and economical) first choice. The imaging diagnosis of adenomyosis is usually made by using TVUS or, more expensively, by MRI. Abdominal ultrasound alone can be highly sensitive for detecting masses, but often lacks specificity for the diagnosis of adenomyosis or endometriosis. Hysterosalpingography is more invasive and is used to exclude endometrial polyps, leiomyomas, and congenital abnormalities of the uterus. The inability to resolve subtle differences in soft tissue attenuation limits the usefulness of computed tomography (CT). Laparoscopy is often needed as a last resort to make the diagnosis of endometriosis where surgical correction can occur simultaneously. *(Hoffman, 2012, pp. 219–245)*

4. (D) More than 90% of patients with endometrial cancer present with postmenopausal bleeding, thus making it the hallmark history component. In the United States, endometrial cancer is the most common gynecologic cancer. There are approximately 39,000 cases of endometrial cancer diagnosed each year and about 7,400 patients die from the disease. Of all endometrial cancer cases, 75% are type I and 25% are type II. There are several risk factors for developing type I endometrial cancer, but in general excessive estrogen is the cause. Therefore, women who are taking postmenopausal unopposed estrogen replacement or tamoxifen and women who are 50 lb above their ideal body weight are at risk for endometrial hyperplasia and endometrial cancer. Type II endometrial cancers tend to occur in older, thinner women without exogenous estrogen exposure. *(Miller, 2012, pp. 817–838)*

5. (E) Oral contraceptives are the best treatment for this patient. Treatment for premenopausal abnormal uterine bleeding is varied. Once infection, fibroid tumors, pregnancy, neoplasm, and iatrogenic causes (e.g., medication related) are ruled out, a woman may be treated hormonally to control bleeding. In this patient, the most likely cause of the bleeding is anovulatory cycles caused by estrogen excess due to her obesity; in addition, the iron deficiency anemia also can cause menometrorrhagia. In patients with irregular cycles, secondary to chronic anovulation, or oligoovulation, combined oral contraceptive (COC) pills help to prevent the risks associated with prolonged unopposed estrogen stimulation of the endometrium. Treatment with cyclic progestins for days 16 through 25 following the first day of the most recent menstrual flow is preferred when OCP use is contraindicated, such as in smokers older than age 35 and women at risk for thromboembolism. *(Hoffman, 2012, pp. 219–245)*

6. (B) Although approximately 40% of menstruating women experience one or more of the cluster of physical, emotional, or behavioral symptoms associated with the luteal phase of the menstrual cycle (premenstrual syndrome or premenstrual tension), a small percentage have symptoms so severe that they meet the DMS-V diagnosis of premenstrual dysphoric disorder (PMDD). For the treatment of mild to moderate symptoms, lifestyle and dietary changes may be effective. Therefore, a trial of regular aerobic exercise, decrease in caffeine and alcohol intake, 1,200 mg of dietary calcium with 800 IU of vitamin D per day, and eating complex carbohydrates as opposed to simple sugars could be initiated. For patients whose symptoms affect jobs and relationships, it is warranted to prescribe serotonin reuptake inhibitors such as fluoxetine. Fluoxetine 20 mg can be taken daily or only premenstrually. *(MacKay & Woo, 2014, pp. 726–758)*

7. (A) Diagnostic laparoscopy is the only definitive way to diagnose endometriosis. Ultrasound and MRI may be helpful in the diagnostic work-up, but laparoscopy is the most certain method of diagnosing endometriosis. *(Beshay & Carr, 2012, pp. 281–303)*

8. (B) This patient has a leiomyoma of the uterus (or fibroid tumors), which is the most common benign neoplasm, but she is also significantly anemic. The labs suggest iron deficiency anemia. It is important to control her bleeding and treat her anemia prior to surgery. The heavy bleeding that typically accompanies fibroid tumors can be minimized by using intermittent progestin supplementation (depot methodroxyprogesterone acetate 150 mg IM every 28 days) and/or prostaglandin synthetase inhibitors. In general, the size of the mass can be decreased and the bleeding can be lessened, but the only curative treatment is a myomectomy or hysterectomy. *(MacKay & Woo, 2014, pp. 726–775)*

9. (C) Gestational trophoblastic neoplasia (GTN) consists of benign GTN, most often a hydatidiform mole and malignant GTN, which includes nonmetastatic and metastatic GTN. Approximately, 15% to 20% of women who have a complete hydatidiform mole and 2% to 4% of partial moles, will go on to develop some form of malignant GTN. Complete and partial molar pregnancies differ clinically, genetically, and histologically. Because of the risk for progression to malignancy, these patients must be monitored. After molar evacuation, serum radioimmunoassay β-hCG levels should be monitored weekly until they have become undetectable. Historically, monitoring has continued monthly after the undetectable levels for at least 6 additional months. However, studies have shown that it is safe to cease monitoring after a single blood sample demonstrates undetectable levels of β-hCG. Urine pregnancy tests are inadequate, and a sensitive radioimmunoassay is mandatory. Prophylactic chemotherapy is controversial because of significant drug toxicity and possible lack of efficacy; it is usually reserved for the highest risk cases or for patients who are unable to return for regular follow-up. Routine chest x-ray at every visit is not warranted unless hCG values rise. *(Schorge, 2012, pp. 898–917)*

10. **(C)** A functional ovarian cyst is a much more likely diagnosis than any of the others listed. A follicular cyst develops when an ovarian follicle fails to rupture. The granulosa cells lining the cyst continue to enlarge and fluid continues to accumulate. Symptoms associated with a functional ovarian cyst include mild to moderate unilateral pain and alteration in the menstrual cycle. On occasion, rupture of the follicular cyst causes acute pelvic pain and may need laparoscopic surgery for complete evaluation. In most cases, pain control for 4 to 5 days is what is indicated as well as the consideration of contraception to suppress future ovarian cyst formation. *(Heinzman & Hoffman, 2012, pp. 246–280)*

11. **(A)** There is no generalized clinical picture of cervical carcinoma, but there are two symptoms often associated with it. They are postcoital bleeding and abnormal uterine bleeding. The average age at diagnosis is 50. Lesions on the cervix that should be considered for immediate biopsy include new exophytic, friable, or bleeding lesions. In this patient, the lesion should have been biopsied at initial examination and this would have helped to make the diagnosis. When lesions are visualized and the biopsy confirms carcinoma, no colposcopic assessment is needed. This patient should definitely not wait 4 to 6 months for a repeat Pap smear. The gynecologic oncologist should stage the cancer and decide on appropriate therapy. *(Richardson, 2012, pp. 769–792)*

12. **(A)** On the basis of the 2012 Consensus Guidelines for the Management of Women with cervical cytological abnormalities, it is recommended that colposcopy be done following LSIL on Pap smears. Viewing the cervix and its transformation zone with 10–20× magnification of colposcopy allows for visual assessment. Two solutions are used to further enhance visualization and determination of normal from abnormal tissue. When a dilute solution of

acetic acid is applied to the cervix, abnormal areas will look white. After painting the cervix with Lugol solution (a strong iodine solution), the normal squamous epithelial will take on the stain whereas the abnormal tissue will not. All abnormal-appearing tissue is biopsied. *(Griffith & Werner, 2012, pp. 730–768)*

13. **(D)** The patient's symptoms describe postmenopausal atrophic changes affecting the vagina, bladder, and urethra. In women with more severe changes, vaginal irritation, dyspareunia, and fragility may become problems. Atrophy is diagnosed by the presence of a thin, clear, or bloody discharge; a vaginal pH of 5 to 7; loss of vaginal rugae; and the finding of parabasal epithelial cells on microscopic examination of a wet-mount preparation. These symptoms are all due to estrogen depletion. Treatment with topical estrogen preparations (cream, tablet, or ring) appears equally effective. Complete relief of symptoms usually occurs within weeks; in the interim, patients may obtain relief through use of vaginal lubricants and moisturizers (e.g., Astroglide, Replens). Rarely, endometrial hyperplasia can be a side effect of vaginal estrogen treatment. *(Nathan, 2013, pp. 953–956)*

14. **(D)** A true abscess will require surgical drainage and therapy with antibiotics, rest, warm soaks, and complete emptying of the breasts every 2 hours. The abscess drainage should be cultured and sensitivities determined. There have been no formal studies of treatment of lactation mastitis associated abscesses. However, incision and draining is recommended along with parenteral antibiotics administered with added coverage for anaerobic bacteria. As soon as the pain of the wound permits, breastfeeding or pumping should be resumed in order to drain the affected breast. *(Euhus, 2012, pp. 333–355)*

15. **(A)** This is a nonviable pregnancy, but whether or not the pregnancy was located intrauterine or ectopic is not something that can be concluded with the data presented. Because there is a plateau in the hCG level after 1 week (48 hours is usually sufficient), the pregnancy is nonviable. The hCG level need not be repeated at this point. TVUS appears to demonstrate no visualized products of conception. It should be noted, however, that this could represent

an incomplete abortion. An ectopic pregnancy cannot be ruled in or out yet. If β-hCG levels are 1,500 mIU/mL and the uterus is empty, a live uterine pregnancy is very unlikely. When β-hCG is less than 1,500 IU/L and an ectopic pregnancy is not seen, progesterone level needs to be determined. If the progesterone level is greater than 25 ng/mL then an ectopic pregnancy is unlikely. At this point, a D&C should be considered. The low hCG levels and lack of findings on ultrasound (e.g., "snowstorm" appearance) would help rule out a molar pregnancy. *(Cunningham et al., 2014, pp. 167–193)*

16. **(C)** Although glycosuria is more common during pregnancy because of the lowering of the renal threshold for glucose excretion, this patient may be at an increased risk for gestational diabetes (GDM) because of her ethnicity. Normal screening for GDM occurs at 24 weeks' gestation. Because glycosuria has been detected, screening with a 50-g, 1-hour glucose challenge test would be indicated at this time. Patients do not have to fast for this test. To be considered normal, serum or plasma glucose values should be less than 130 mg/dL (7.2 mmol/L) or less than 140 mg/dL (7.8 mmol/L). Using a value of 130 mg/dL or higher will increase the sensitivity of the test from 80% to 90% and decrease its specificity, compared with using the 140 mg/dL cutoff. An abnormal 1-hour screening test should be followed by a 100-g, 3-hour venous serum or plasma glucose tolerance test. Normal blood sugars at 0, 1, 2, and 3 hours, respectively, are:

- fasting blood sugar 95 mg/dL or less
- 1-hour blood sugar 180 mg/dL or less
- 2-hour blood sugar 155 mg/dL or less
- 3-hour blood sugar 140 or less

A diagnosis of GDM is made if two or more samples are increased or if any is greater than 200 mg/dL and the patient should be advised regarding dietary control, regardless. *(Cunningham et al., 2014, pp. 1125–1146)*

17. **(E)** Women with a prior history of PID are at 7 to 10 times increased risk in having an ectopic pregnancy. In decreasing order, the next most common risk factors include tubal surgery, intrauterine contraceptive devices, previous ectopic pregnancy, in vitro fertilization, smoking, previous abdominal surgery, and induced abortions. *(Gala, 2012, pp. 198–218)*

18. **(E)** Fetal heart rates by fetal monitoring are described by rate and pattern of variability. Baseline is defined as 120 to 160 bpm. Late decelerations are a symmetrical fall in fetal heart rate (FHR) beginning at or after the peak of the uterine contraction and returning to baseline only after the contraction has ended. They indicate possible uteroplacental insufficiency and imply some degree of fetal hypoxia. Remedial techniques are empirically designed to overcome uteroplacental insufficiency or to decrease cord compromise and improve placental and fetal oxygenation. Changing maternal position to right/left side lying recumbent or knee–chest position is a reasonable and quick first step. Late FHR decelerations, however, are an ominous sign and should be evaluated quickly and seriously. Persistent nonreassuring tracings indicate the need for emergent delivery. Other remedial techniques include the following: IV infusion, mask oxygen, stopping oxytocics, subcutaneous terbutaline, and amnioinfusion. *(Cunningham et al., 2014, pp. 433–454)*

19. **(D)** Mastitis is an inflammation of the breast that is common in breastfeeding women. In order to make a diagnosis of mastitis, there must be an area of hardness, pain, redness, and swelling in the breast. It can be caused by engorgement, a blocked milk duct, or a cracked nipple that allows bacteria to enter. The most common pathogen in infective mastitis is penicillin-resistant *S. aureus*. Less common pathogens are *Streptococcus* or *E. coli*. The preferred antibiotics are usually penicillinase-resistant penicillins such as dicloxacillin, with patients usually responding within 24 to 26 hours. In addition to antibiotic treatment, regular emptying of the breast by breastfeeding and/or pumping is necessary to prevent more bacteria from collecting in the breast. There is no evidence of risk to the healthy, term infant from continuing breastfeeding. Symptomatic treatment such as application of heat (e.g., a shower or a hot pack) to the breast prior to feeding may help with the milk flow. *(Cunningham et al., 2014, pp. 668–681)*

20. **(B)** Cyclic mastalgia in usually managed symptomatically and requires no evaluation. Fibrocystic breast changes are the most common type of benign breast mass. Clinically they are often described as "rope-like," meaning they have the characteristic on palpation of feeling like a coiled rope. There is

often diffuse nodularity, although solitary cysts may range in size. Also, the size of an individual cyst may fluctuate throughout the menstrual cycle. Pain is the most common presenting symptom of fibro-cystic breast change. Often, women will respond to dietary changes, such as decreased caffeine and/or tobacco. Danazol as well as bromocriptine, tamoxifen, and GnRH agonists are usually reserved for women with the most severe symptoms. *(Euhus, 2012, pp. 333–355)*

21. **(B)** Shoulder dystocia is a complication associated with macrosomia. Although there is no evidence that any one maneuver is superior to another in releasing an impacted shoulder or reducing the chance of injury, American College of Obstetricians and Gynecologists guidelines recommend performance of the McRoberts maneuver, as described by choice B, as a reasonable initial approach. Fundal pressure should never be attempted. *(Cunningham et al., 2014, pp. 433–454)*

22. **(B)** Placenta previa can be distinguished from abruptio placentae by many factors. Placenta previa is most commonly characterized by painless hemorrhage, which usually does not present until the end of the second trimester or later. No abdominal discomfort, a normal FHR, and no significant maternal history are usually associated with the problem. Abruptio placentae, on the other hand, is associated with severe pain, abnormal FHR, usually continuous bleeding, and associated with a history in the mother such as cocaine use, abdominal trauma, maternal hypertension, multiple gestations, and polyhydramnios. In this case, one will need to rule out early labor (accompanying contractions, bloody mucus discharge), coagulopathy, hemorrhoids, vasa previa, cervical or vaginal lesion, or trauma. Vasa previa also occurs late in pregnancy, with vaginal bleeding occurring concomitantly with rupture of membranes. Vasa previa occurs when umbilical cord blood vessels transverse the membranes and cross the cervical os below the fetus. Fetal distress will also accompany vasa previa because the blood loss will be fetal; it requires immediate delivery and is accompanied by a high rate of fetal death. *(Cunningham et al., 2014, pp. 780–828)*

23. **(D)** The accurate diagnosis of spontaneous rupture of membranes is important in order to ascertain whether the patient has begun labor or if the patient has premature rupture of membranes (this patient is 33 weeks). To evaluate for spontaneous rupture of membranes, a sterile speculum examination is performed with the patient in the dorsal lithotomy position. Evidence of rupture of membranes would be clear when blood-tinged fluid in the posterior fornix of the vagina, or pooling, and escape of clear fluid from the cervical os occurs when the patient coughs. Nitrazine testing can distinguish amniotic fluid from urine or vaginal secretion samples from speculum examination. If the pH is 7.1 to 7.3, it will show positive on nitrazine paper (dark blue). False positives can occur, however, with cervical mucus, blood, or semen in the sample. Until rupture of membranes has been ascertained, this patient should not be induced because of risk of prematurity in the fetus. Ultrasound determination of amniotic fluid volume is an important means of evaluating premature and preterm rupture of membranes, but it is not a means of diagnosing rupture of membranes. Digital cervical examination should not be performed because this would increase the risk of ascending infection. *(Cunningham et al., 2014, pp. 433–454)*

24. **(B)** Hydatidiform mole is one component of gestational trophoblastic neoplasm (GTN). Moles occur in a gestation in which there is a proliferation of trophoblastic tissue. It can be a complete mole, in which there is no sign of a fetus, or a partial mole, in which the fetus may be viable, or there are findings consistent with a nonviable fetus. Young pregnant women (20) and older (>40) reproductive ages have increased incidence as do patients with Asian, Latino, or Filipino ethnicity. The most common symptom of hydatidiform mole is several episodes of vaginal bleeding. A size-to-dates discrepancy also is common. Severe nausea and vomiting may occur as well. When signs and symptoms of preeclampsia present earlier than 24 weeks' gestation, molar pregnancy should be high on the differential. The trophoblast is responsible for production of human chorionic gonadotropin (hCG); therefore, the levels of β-hCG in the serum are greater than expected for the weeks of gestation. Ultrasound demonstrates a characteristic "snowstorm" appearance and is the best means of diagnosing a mole. An incomplete abortion usually occurs prior to 12 to 14 weeks and is often characterized by a decreasing β-hCG level. A fetal demise at 16 weeks would also

have decreasing β-hCG levels and would not be associated with hypertension. In twin gestation, there would be a higher level of β-hCG and a larger fundal height, but at 16 weeks, fetal heart tones should be heard. *(Schorge, 2012, pp. 898–917)*

25. **(D)** The most likely diagnosis of this vaginitis is bacterial vaginosis (BV) and the treatment is metronidazole 500 mg twice daily for 7 days. Other treatments include vaginal preparations of metronidazole and also vaginal preparations of clindamycin. The other treatments would be inappropriate for the treatment of BV. Ciprofloxacin is a treatment for a urinary tract infection. Miconazole cream and fluconazole are treatments for yeast vaginitis. Doxycycline is the treatment for *chlamydia trachomatis. (MacKay, 2014, pp. 701–731)*

26. **(C)** Conservative measures for treating dysmenorrhea include heating pads, mild analgesics, and outdoor exercise. Evidence suggests that primary dysmenorrhea is due to prostaglandin F2 alpha (PGF2 alpha), a potent myometrial stimulant and vasoconstrictor, in the secretory endometrium. Prostaglandin synthetase inhibitors such as naproxen, ibuprofen, indomethacin, and mefenamic acid can be very effective. However, for patients with dysmenorrhea who are sexually active, oral contraceptives will provide needed protection from unwanted pregnancy and generally alleviate the dysmenorrhea. The OCPs minimize endometrial prostaglandin production during the concurrent administration of estrogen and progestin. *(Hoffman, 2012, pp. 219–245)*

27. **(E)** A reactive stress test (normal) is defined as two or more fetal heart rate increases in 20 minutes. The accelerations increase by 15 beats for 15 seconds and are related to fetal movement. A nonreactive stress test (abnormal) requires monitoring for two 20-minute periods where neither period yields adequate accelerations. *(Cunningham et al., 2014, pp. 433–454)*

28. **(D)** Uterine atony is responsible for ~50% of postpartum hemorrhage (PPH). Several factors may predispose to uterine atony including conditions that enlarge the uterus (e.g., multiple gestations, multiparity, microsomy, hydramnios), abnormal labor (e.g., precipitous or prolonged delivery,

general anesthesia, prolonged labor, use of forceps), and conditions that interfere with uterine contraction (e.g., uterine leiomyomas, magnesium sulfate use). Vaginal and cervical lacerations are less common than uterine atony, but are serious and require prompt surgical attention. Retained placenta, secondary to lack of complete separation from the uterus and abnormally adherent placenta, such as placenta accreta, are less common causes of PPH. Although coagulation studies should be part of the work-up, in the immediate postpartum period, disorders of the coagulation system and platelets do not usually result in excessive bleeding. Fibrin deposition over the placental site and clots within supplying vessels play a significant role in the hours and days following delivery, and abnormalities in these areas can lead to late PPH or exacerbate bleeding from other causes, most notably, trauma. Uterine inversion is a rare condition. *(Poggi, 2013, pp. 349–368)*

29. **(D)** An Rh-negative woman must be tested for the presence of antibodies at the beginning of the third trimester (usually at 28 weeks) so that the rare Rh sensitization of that pregnancy can be detected. If she is negative she is given Rho (anti-D) immune globulin. If she is positive for Rh sensitization, she may require intrauterine blood transfusion to prevent erythroblastosis fetalis. In mothers who receive Rh immunoglobulin, the risk of isoimmunization is reduced from 16% to 0.2%. *(Roman, 2013, pp. 250–266)*

30. **(A)** Corticosteroids accelerate lung maturation and are given to expectant mothers who are less than 34 weeks' gestation and are in preterm labor. Some clinicians believe it is appropriate to use tocolytics to stop preterm contractions, but this is controversial. Tocolytics may temporarily stop contractions, but they do not consistently prevent preterm labor and they carry a significant risk. Examples of tocolytics are terbutaline, magnesium sulfate, ritodrine, and nifedipine. In general, if tocolytics are given they should be given with corticosteroids and generally not after 34 weeks. *(Cunningham et al., 2014, pp. 829–861)*

31. **(B)** In healthy pregnant women who are not deficient in iron or folate, a modest fall in hemoglobin levels at this point of gestation is usually due to the relative greater expansion of plasma volume

compared with the increase in hemoglobin mass and red blood cell volume that accompanies normal pregnancy. In healthy nonpregnant women, anemia is defined as a hemoglobin of less than 12 g/dL. During pregnancy, a patient is not considered anemic until the hemoglobin falls below 10 g/dL. In the first trimester and at term, the hemoglobin level for most healthy women is 11 g/dL or greater. During the second trimester, women experience a nadir in their hemoglobin between 22 and 24 weeks and anemia is not considered until the hemoglobin is 10.5 g/dL or less. *(Cunningham et al., 2014, pp. 167–193)*

32. **(D)** Currently, hormone replacement therapy (HRT) is indicated only for the treatment of vasomotor symptoms of menopause, vaginal atrophy, and for the treatment and prevention of osteoporosis. HRT increases an older woman's risk of CHD, and in all women it increases their risk of breast cancer, stroke, and thromboembolism. Increased risks of breast cancer are seen in women who use HRT for longer than 5 years. Estrogen-only therapy given to women with an intact uterus increases the risk of endometrial hyperplasia (thickening of the lining of the uterus) and eventually endometrial cancer. Daily estrogen combined with progesterone given for 10 to 14 days per month (sequential HRT) reduces this risk but does not eliminate it. *(Euhus, 2012, pp. 333–355)*

33. **(C)** In the classification of spontaneous abortions, an incomplete abortion is characterized by the passage of tissue and an open cervical os. A complete abortion would have a similar history of passing tissue; however, pain or cramping would have subsided and the cervix would be closed. In a threatened abortion, there will be bleeding but no passage of tissue, and the cervical os would be closed. A missed abortion is defined by no symptoms and a closed os. With an incompetent cervix, women present with painless cervical dilation. The treatment of an incomplete abortion is dilation and curettage. Serum-hCG levels are useful to follow after spontaneous abortion; hCG levels should halve every 48 to 72 hours, and a plateau could indicate residual retained tissue. *(Cunningham et al., 2014, pp. 350–376)*

34. **(C)** This patient has secondary amenorrhea. The most common reason for amenorrhea in a woman of reproductive age is pregnancy, which has been ruled out. In the differential diagnosis for her secondary amenorrhea, possibilities include (among others) endometriosis, hypothyroidism, and premature ovarian failure (if patient is aged less than 40), and ovarian failure or menopause if patient is older than 40. For a patient of this age, ovarian failure is more likely. Studies for establishing the diagnosis of ovarian failure are as follows: (1) serum FSH level, (2) serum LH, and (3) serum estradiol. Persistently elevated gonadotropin levels (especially when accompanied by low serum estradiol levels) are diagnostic of ovarian failure. Ovarian antibody assay is a test with low sensitivity and specificity for determining the diagnosis of autoimmune ovarian failure. Serum testosterone and DHEAS levels should be ordered only if the patient shows symptoms of androgen excess (acne, hirsutism, male pattern balding, clitoromegaly) or hypertension. The hysterosalpingogram is part of an infertility work-up that may demonstrate Asherman syndrome, but is more invasive and not indicated until ovarian failure has been excluded. *(Halvorson, 2012a, pp. 440–459)*

35. **(C)** This patient has preeclampsia (BP $\geq 140/90$ mm Hg, proteinuria, platelets $< 100,000$, increased liver enzymes, headache, and epigastric pain). Because gestational hypertension also referred to commonly as pregnancy-induced hypertension has been associated with raised rates of maternal morbidity and mortality and with many increased risks to the fetus, patients with moderate to severe preeclampsia should be delivered if the disease develops after 34 weeks' gestation. Magnesium sulfate is the treatment of choice for preeclampsia as it reduces the risk of eclampsia and probably maternal death. Hypertensive disease is classified into five types: gestational (also called pregnancy-induced), preeclampsia, eclampsia, preeclampsia superimposed on chronic hypertension, and chronic hypertension. Oral hypertensive drug therapy, though decreasing the risk of severe hypertension, has not been associated with decreased risk in the infant or mother. There is insufficient evidence for any effects of plasma volume expansion. Intravascular volume expansion carries a serious risk of volume overload, which could lead to pulmonary or cerebral edema. Patients with a platelet count greater than $40,000/mm^3$ are unlikely to bleed and do not require transfusion unless the platelet count drops to less than $20,000/mm^3$. *(Cunningham et al., 2014, pp. 455–472)*

36. **(E)** Oligohydramnios, diminished amniotic fluid volume, may be associated with intrauterine growth retardation, and would result in a fundal height lower than expected. The fundal height directly correlates with gestational age in weeks from 20 to 32 weeks' gestation—for example, at 32 weeks it should measure 32 cm. This measurement, however, is subject to measurement problems. A full bladder can cause an increase of 3 cm and obesity can also distort the correlation. *(Cunningham et al., 2014, pp. 167–193)*

37. **(B)** The most common cause of spontaneous abortion in the first 12 weeks of pregnancy is chromosomal anomalies (accounting for about half of abortions). Maternal lupus anticoagulant, incompetent cervix, maternal tobacco abuse, and inadequate progesterone during the luteal phase can also be associated with early abortion. Maternal disease is more likely to be responsible in second trimester miscarriage. *(Cunningham et al., 2014, pp. 350–376)*

38. **(E)** Childbirth can injure the pelvic floor muscles resulting in a prolapsed uterus. The transverse and uterosacral ligaments are particularly affected. The degree of protrusion of the uterus in relationship to the introitus determines the classification. Grade 0 is normal position of the uterus. Grade 1 or slight prolapse is when the uterus descends toward the introitus, but is still in the vagina. Grade 2 or moderate prolapse is when the uterus and cervix descend to the introitus, and grade 3 or marked prolapse is when the cervix and uterus descend past the hymen halfway. Grade 4 is when the uterus is at the maximum descent. When the prolapse interferes with daily life or quality of life, a surgical repair is indicated. *(Schaffer, 2012, pp. 633–658)*

39. **(B)** During the initial 3 months of oral contraceptive use, breakthrough bleeding is a common side effect and can be best managed by encouraging the patient to continue on the contraceptives. After initiating therapy, when breakthrough bleeding occurs during the third week of the cycle, it is due to a lack of progestin and is best managed by changing to a pill with a higher progestin component. *(Beckman et al., 2014, pp. 237–252)*

40. **(B)** Although all the methods listed (bed rest, devices, and pharmacologic agents and surgery)

work to some degree to treat an incompetent cervix, the generally accepted treatment is surgical. A cervical cerclage is a suture or bands that are placed surgically on the cervix to keep it closed prior to delivery. The sutures are removed after fetal maturity has been achieved (about 37 weeks). Labor and delivery occurs rapidly after the removal of the cerclage. The terbutaline and magnesium sulfate are pharmacologic agents used for the medical management of preterm labor with a competent cervix. *(Cunningham et al., 2014, pp. 167–193)*

41. **(D)** There is great variability in the symptoms with which endometriosis will present. Some women may even be asymptomatic, but endometrial lesions may be found during laparoscopy for other gynecologic reasons. The classic symptoms of endometriosis are dysmenorrhea, deep thrust dyspareunia, infertility, abnormal bleeding, and pelvic pain. Thorough history taking greatly helps in the diagnosis, but the definitive diagnosis is made when the lesions are visualized during laparoscopic surgery or by tissue biopsy. *(Beckman et al., 2014, pp. 295–300)*

42. **(C)** A prior tubal pregnancy contraindicates IUD use. Condoms and spermicides are free of hormonal side effects and, if used in combination, are reasonably effective. This patient's hypertension is mild and controlled and unlikely to be negatively affected by either low-dose or progesterone-only oral contraceptives. Although there can be an association between urinary tract infections and diaphragm use in susceptible women, this would not be an absolute contraindication to diaphragm use. *(Cunningham & Stuart, 2012, pp. 132–169)*

43. **(A)** Low-risk human papillomavirus types 6 and 11 cause almost all genital warts. Although they are very prevalent, they are not associated with malignancy or neoplasia. The HR HPV types 16, 18, 31, 33, 35, 45, and 58 are associated with 95% of all cervical cancers worldwide. Gardasil, a recombinant quadrivalent HPV vaccine is for prophylactic protection from HPV types 6, 11, 16, and 18. *(Griffith & Werner, 2012, pp. 730–768)*

44. **(A)** The minimal accepted age for women to stop getting yearly Pap smears and mammograms is 65 years old. A woman must have documented three consecutive normal Pap smears and no history of

preinvasive lesions and also no risk factors that would put her at increased risk for cervical cancer. In women of any age who have undergone a hysterectomy and who have no history of invasive or preinvasive cervical disease, Pap smears may be discontinued. Similarly, women may elect to stop having mammography at age 70 years as well. *(Saslow et al., 2012)*

45. **(A)** The most appropriate evaluation of this patient is for her to be referred for a colposcopy. A Pap smear is a medical consultation that interprets a laboratory test. The interpretation is not a diagnosis. The final diagnosis is made in conjunction with clinical and often histological data. In this patient, it would be inappropriate to repeat the HPV test or repeat the Pap smear. The 2012 ASCCP guidelines for the management of abnormal Pap smears recommend that following the results of atypical cells of undetermined significance (ASCUS), there are three evaluation possibilities: HPV DNA testing, repeat cytology at 6 and 12 months, and colposcopy. If either the HPV testing or the repeat cytology is abnormal, then immediate referral for colposcopy is recommended. ASCUS has about a 5% chance of progressing to cervical intraepithelial neoplasia (CIN) 2 or 3. *(Griffith & Werner, 2012, pp. 730–768)*

46. **(D)** This patient would be diagnosed with trichomoniasis based on her symptoms and positive wet mount with protozoans. Women with trichomoniasis may notice pruritis, burning, genital erythema, dysuria, yellow-greenish frothy vaginal discharge. Upon speculum examination a strawberry cervix with vaginal discharge can also be appreciated. The CDC recommends treatment with metronidazole 2 g orally as a single dose. Alcohol consumption should be avoided during treatment and for 24 thereafter. Sexual partners should also be treated and offered screening for other sexually transmitted infections. The metronidazole 500 mg dose listed is for the treatment of bacterial vaginosis. The fluconazole and miconazole are for the treatment of vaginal candidiasis. The acyclovir is for the treatment of an initial herpes outbreak. *(Hemsell, 2012, pp. 64–109)*

47. **(A)** A positive HSV PCR indicates genital herpes diagnosis and according to the CDC, the recommended treatment is oral therapy 400 mg three times a day for at least 7 days. Topical antiviral therapy has been shown to not be as affected as oral therapy for symptomatic ulcers. Ibuprofen can be used for pain control however will not treat the ulcers. *(Workowski & Berman, 2010)*

48. **(B)** Polycystic ovarian syndrome (PCOS) is suggested by her being moderately overweight and having hirsutism and acne. Eighty percent to 90% of the diagnosis can be made from the medical history. Clinically, the most common signs of PCOS are hirsutism (90%), menstrual irregularity (90%), and infertility (75%). *(Wilson, 2012, pp. 460–480)*

49. **(E)** The medication most responsible for the patient's low libido is sertraline secondary to its increased serotonin levels, which create negative effects on the limbic system in the brain, therefore lowering a patient's sexual desire. Metoprolol also has negative effects on sexual functioning however beta blockers decrease the compliancy of blood vessels affecting blood flow causing decreased arousal, not decreased libido. *(Clayton et al., 2014)*

50. **(B)** For women desiring to preserve their fertility, myomectomy is an option if the number and size of the fibroids is limited. Surgical approach depends on the location and a magnetic resonance imaging (MRI) can localize and estimate the volume of the myoma. *(Nelson & Gambone, 2010, p. 244)*

51. **(B)** Chlamydial genital infections are the most frequently diagnosed sexually transmitted infection in the United States. More than 50% of the time, the patient is asymptomatic. In women, the infection tends to occur in the endocervical canal with symptoms that may include intramenstrual or postcoital bleeding, an odorless mucoid vaginal discharge, pelvic pain, or dysuria. Untreated or inadequately treated infections can lead to a more serious problem such as pelvic inflammatory disease, ectopic pregnancy, and infertility. *(Centers for Disease Control & Prevention, 2014)*

52. **(E)** The size and firmness of the ovarian mass suggests endometrioid carcinoma, a tumor in which the potential for malignancy is 100%. Referral to a gynecologic oncologist should be considered first whenever an ovarian malignancy is suspected.

Standard of care is complete surgical staging, excision of all visible masses, and abdominal hysterectomy and bilateral salpingo-oophorectomy followed by chemotherapy. Radiation oncology could also be considered. *(MacKay & Woo, 2014, pp. 726–758)*

53. **(C)** About 1.4% of women will develop ovarian cancer sometime during their lives. However, 39% of women who inherit a harmful *BRCA1* mutation will develop ovarian cancer. This patient is also at increased risk of ovarian cancer because her mother was diagnosed with breast cancer and testing for *BRCA2* mutation should be recommended if not already completed. Increased risk of cervical cancer would include a positive HPV cytology. Women who have had breast cancer or ovarian cancer may have an increased risk of developing endometrial cancer, however this patient is only *BRCA1* mutation positive and does not yet have the active disease. *(Euhus, 2012, pp. 333–355)*

54. **(D)** The cervical cysts seen during the Pap test are Nabothian cysts which are a very common benign finding. They result from the process of squamous metaplasia where a layer of superficial squamous epithelium entraps an invagination of columnar cells beneath the surface. The underlying columnar cells continue to secrete mucus and a mucous retention cyst is created. Nabothian cysts are opaque with a yellowish or bluish hue, varying in size from 0.3 to 3 cm. *(Nelson & Gambone, 2010, p. 246)*

55. **(B)** The mass on the patient's left labia would be diagnosed as a Bartholin cyst and is the most common vulvovaginal tumor. They are mostly clinically diagnosed by history and physical. Since she is symptomatic and the size of the cyst is greater than 3 cm treatment with a catheter insertion and drainage would be the most appropriate course of action at this time and can be performed in the office. If abscess is a concern, adjunct therapy with broad-spectrum antibiotics should also be implemented. Surgical intervention should only be an option for recurrent Bartholin cysts. *(Bornstein, 2013, pp. 620–645)*

56. **(D)** Based on patient's history and physical examination, an imperforate hymen should be her diagnosis. If not detected until after menarche, an imperforate hymen may be seen as a thin, dark bluish or thicker clear membrane blocking menstrual flow at the introitus. There are no imaging studies that would help to validate the diagnosis and a gynecology consult should be implemented for immediate surgery with an elliptical excision of the membrane followed by evacuation of the obstructed material. A general surgery consult would not be the most appropriate referral since this type of procedure is generally not performed by a general surgeon. *(Domany et al., 2013)*

57. **(A)** Unfortunately, one in six women in America will be a victim of sexual assault in their lifetime and will often present to the emergency room for help. As a medical provider, the initial point of contact is to ensure the patient is stable and provide acute medical care. Often victims have been beaten or injured. Although providing prophylaxis therapy for sexually transmitted infections and prevention of pregnancy be offered, this would not be the first step in treating this patient. A consult with the local sexual assault agency should be made and it is up to the victim to report the crime unless child abuse or human trafficking is suspected. *(Ettinger & Gambone, 2010, p. 324)*

58. **(E)** A fibroadenoma is the most common benign tumor found in the female breast. Clinically, these tumors are sharply circumscribed, freely mobile, may occur at any age, but are more common in women younger than 30 years of age. An ultrasound should be performed first to determine consistency of the tumor and may be followed with a mammogram if the ultrasound is inconclusive. A biopsy may be done to get a definite diagnosis, especially for women over the age of 30. Women with fibroadenomas have a slightly higher risk of breast cancer and follow up with watchful waiting and monthly self-breast examinations is recommended. If there are changes to the tumor, a biopsy or surgical removal may be warranted. *(Katz & Dotters, 2012, pp. 301–334)*

59. **(A)** Although a fine-needle aspiration biopsy may be a good choice, a core needle biopsy would be a better diagnostic test for this patient secondary to the size of the mass and mammography changes that make this mass suspicious for breast cancer. A large, hollow needle is used to withdraw small cylinders or cores of tissue from the abnormal area in the breast. The needle obtains anywhere from three

to six samples and is more likely to give a clear result versus a fine-needle aspiration because more tissue is taken to be evaluated by the pathologist. Usually this procedure is performed with ultrasound or fluoroscopy to guide the needle in the correct place, however if the area is easily palpated, those extras are not necessary if the provider feels confident in guiding the needle to the correct location. *(Katz & Dotters, 2012, pp. 301–334)*

60. **(C)** This patient would be diagnosed with a cystocele or anterior vaginal wall prolapse. A cystocele may result from muscle straining during vaginal delivery or with heavy lifting and is often seen after pelvic surgeries, such as a vaginal hysterectomy. Cystoceles are graded—grade 1 when the bladder droops only a short way into the vagina, grade 2 when the bladder sinks far enough to reach the opening of the vagina and the most advanced, grade 3 when the bladder bulges out through the opening of the vagina. This patient would be diagnosed with a grade 2 cystocele because during rest, the cystocele does not protrude past the vaginal introitus. Large cystoceles may require surgery especially if there is urinary retention, however for this patient a pessary would be the best initial therapy. Adjunct therapy should also include vaginal estrogen therapy to avoid ulceration of the vaginal wall from the pessary. *(Lentz, 2012, pp. 453–474)*

61. **(E)** Multiple gestations are at a higher risk for preterm labor and this patient is already eliciting signs and symptoms of preterm labor. The American College of Obstetricians and Gynecologists defines preterm labor as regular contractions associated with cervical change before 37 weeks' gestation. The following are criteria to diagnose preterm labor: (1) four contractions in 20 minutes or 8 contractions in 60 minutes; (2) cervical dilation greater than 1 cm; (3) cervical effacement of greater than 80%. Multiple gestations include various complications for the mother and fetus. For the mother, twin pregnancies are associated with higher risk of pregnancy-induced hypertension, anemia, hyperemesis, abruption, placenta previa, postpartum hemorrhage, and increased risk of operative delivery. For the fetus, twin pregnancy increases risk of intrauterine death, spontaneous abortion, congenital anomalies, cerebral palsy, and intrauterine growth retardation. Twin pregnancies have a similar risk of gestational

diabetes compared to singleton pregnancies, and so this is not a risk for this patient at all. *(Cunningham et al., 2014, pp. 473–503)*

62. **(D)** Vulvodynia is chronic vulvar pain without an identifiable cause. The location, constancy and severity of the pain vary among sufferers. The most common symptom reported is burning. Vulvodynia is broken down into two main subtypes: localized and generalized. After taking a thorough medical history a careful examination of the vulvar should be performed along with a Q-tip test with a cotton-swab, according the National Vulvodynia Association. A vulvar biopsy is not necessary on a routine basis, but is helpful to diagnose suspected skin disorders. It is also important to rule out other possible causes such as infections, skin disease, trauma, systemic disease, skin precancer and cancer, and irritants. The Q-tip test is a simple diagnostic test—imagine the vestibule as the face of a clock with 12 just above the urethra and the 6 at the bottom. Touching around the vestibule "clock" with a cotton swab produces pain in one or more places with the 6 o'clock position eliciting the most pain. *(Haefner, 2013)*

63. **(D)** Abruptio placentae or premature separation of the normally implanted placenta, complicates 0.5% to 1.5% of all pregnancies. The most common risk factor associated with abruptio placentae is maternal hypertension, either chronic or as a result of preeclampsia. Other risk factors include prior placental abruption, trauma, polyhydramnios with rapid decompression, premature rupture of membranes, short umbilical cord, tobacco use, and folate deficiency. The diagnosis of an abruptio placentae is based on painful vaginal bleeding in association with uterine tenderness, hyperactivity, and increased tone. *(Kim et al., 2010, pp. 130–131)*

64. **(C)** Based on patient's history, physical, and wet mount, vaginal candidiasis is diagnosed and is very common during pregnancy due to hormonal changes, especially during the second trimester. Vaginal creams or suppositories are the recommended course of treatment since oral antifungals have not been proven safe during pregnancy or lactation. *(Workowski & Berman, 2010)*

65. **(D)** The patient is suffering from mastitis. In most cases, lactation mastitis occurs within the first

4 weeks. First symptoms are usually slight fever and chills followed by redness of a segment of the breast which becomes indurated and painful. The etiologic agent is usually *S. aureus*, which originates from the infant's oral pharynx. Milk should be obtained from breast for culture and sensitivity. The mother should be immediately placed on penicillinase-resistant antibiotic, such as dicloxacillin. Breastfeeding may be discontinued but is not contraindicated. *(Hobel & Zakowski, 2010, p. 110)*

66. **(B)** The first stage of labor is divided into two stages: latent and active. The latent stage refers to cervical effacement and early dilation. The active phase occurs when dilation has reached 3 to 4 cm or greater. The second stage of labor begins when cervical dilation is complete and ends with delivery of the infant. The third stage of labor begins after the infant is delivered and ends with placental expulsion. *(Cunningham et al., 2014, pp. 433–454)*

67. **(B)** During the first trimester, several diagnostic tests are routine. For this patient with a normal medical history and no risk factors, a CBC, HIV testing and urinalysis is performed at the first obstetrics appointment. A CBC is performed to evaluate for any anemias or platelet disorders that would mean a blood clotting disorder. HIV testing is important to diagnosis and treat to improve the health of the mother and dramatically reduce the transmission of HIV from mother to fetus. A urinalysis should be performed to evaluate for glycosuria, proteinuria and hematuria which would all be signs of possible complications during pregnancy. If the patient has increased risk factors such as multiple sexual partners, other sexually transmitted infections should be screened. A 3-hour glucose tolerance test should only be performed if the patient fails the 1 hour glucose tolerance test between 26 and 28 weeks, so for this patient, it is too early for any glucose tolerance testing. Chorionic villus sampling is performed to detect chromosomal abnormalities and genetic disorders, and is usually done between 10 and 12 weeks' gestation, but is not routine in a normal pregnancy. *(ACOG Committee on Obstetric Practice, 2012, pp. 105–168)*

68. **(C)** The estimated date of confinement (EDC) or due date is calculated after obtaining a thorough menstrual history. The date of the last onset of normal menses is key in determining EDC. If the patient is unaware of last menstrual cycle, an ultrasound should be performed for dating purposes. A "normal" pregnancy lasts 40 ± 2 weeks. Calculated from the first day of the last normal menses, add 7 days to the first day of the last normal menstrual flow and subtract 3 months. *(Cunningham et al., 2014, pp. 167–193)*

69. **(E)** Emergency contraception (EC) can stop a pregnancy before it starts. There are four types of EC and they all work up to 5 days or 120 hours after unprotected intercourse, however, effectiveness can decrease each day and should be used sooner rather than later. Types of EC include Paragard IUD, ulipristal (Ella), levonorgestrel-based pills (Plan B One-Step, Next Choice One Dose, Next Choice, My Way), and Yuzpe Regimen (using certain birth control pills as EC). *(Hatcher et al., 2011, pp. 277–290)*

70. **(A)** This patient has lichen sclerosis and can be identified on examination with the classic figure eight white patch around the vulvar skin and down to the anus. A biopsy can also be performed for diagnosis. Treatment should include topical clobetasol propionate 0.05% ointment twice daily for 14 weeks then daily thereafter for at least 12 weeks. Other treatments should include avoiding skin irritants and well-ventilated clothing. In all patients with lichen sclerosis, regular follow-up is needed because of the increased risk of developing squamous cell carcinoma. *(Bornstein, 2013, pp. 620–645)*

71. **(D)** The patient is experiencing vasomotor symptoms associated with menopause. Hot flashes are the second most frequently reported perimenopausal symptom, after irregular menses, and are considered the hallmarks of perimenopause. Nearly 25% of women experience severe discomfort from vasomotor symptoms and seek help from a healthcare provider. Lifestyle modifications should be initiated first, however, this patient has failed lifestyle changes and would benefit from hormonal replacement therapy. A combination estrogen and progesterone regimen would be appropriate treatment option for this patient. Since the patient retains her uterus, progesterone needs to be added with the estrogen as this reduces the risk of endometrial adenocarcinoma compared to unopposed estrogen. Use of this therapy should be limited to the shortest duration consistent with treatment goals, benefits,

and risks for the individual woman. Initiating combination therapy during the perimenopausal period is associated with lower risk than starting therapy several years after menopause. *(Bradshaw, 2012, pp. 554–580)*

72. **(A)** The irregular lesion on the patient's vulva is questionable for vulvar intraepithelial neoplasia or vulvar cancer. Patients may be without symptoms or complain of pruritis or burning. Raised brown, red, pink, white, or gray lesions of various colors may be present. Tests to diagnose include colposcopy and biopsy of lesion. Treatment depends on the degree of the disease, sometimes requiring surgical or laser removal. Patients should have regular follow-ups with a healthcare provider and self-vulvar examinations should be recommended monthly. The human papillomavirus (HPV) has been shown to increase risk of VIN and vulvar cancer. *(Edge et al., 2010, pp. 379–381)*

73. **(C)** In patients over the age of 35, contraception options can be tricky. It is an absolute contraindication to oral contraceptive use in women over the age of 35 and a smoker. The risk of stroke, pulmonary embolism, and hypertension outweighs the benefits. Even the vagina ring (NuvaRing) or the transdermal contraceptive patch causes an increased risk for vascular events. Depot medroxyprogesterone acetate should be used with caution secondary to the patient's history of hypertension and tobacco use. The most appropriate contraceptive option for this patient would be an intrauterine device (IUD). Either IUD, levonorgestrel IUD or the copper IUD, would be a suitable option for this patient and poses no increased risks. *(Frieden et al., 2010, pp. 1–86)*

74. **(C)** There are currently three vaccines approved by the Food and Drug Administration (FDA): quadrivalent (Gardasil), 9-valent (Gardasil 9), and Bivalent (Cervarix). The vaccines target various subtypes of HPV which help to prevent against cervical cancer and precancer, vulvar and vaginal cancer, penile, anal, and oropharyngeal cancers as well as external genital warts. The vaccine is indicated in females and males aged 9 to 26. Although the vaccine helps to prevent against these types of cancers and warts, it is still vital to have routine Pap testing. The vaccine must be given in three separate intramuscular injection doses, 0, 2, and 6 months which is the correct response to this question. *(Food and Drug Administration, 2014)*

75. **(A)** The patient is considered full term and signs of labor have started with spontaneous rupture of membranes. The patient has not completed stage one of labor since she is only dilated to 7 cm and there is a concern for her failure to progress. The most common cause of fetal distress is lack of oxygen to the baby, which can cause fetal brain injury. When fetal monitoring detects decelerations or decrease in fetal heart rate below normal levels, an emergency cesarean should be considered the most appropriate next step. Waiting until she has dilated to 10 cm and starting IV Pitocin may cause increased fetal distress. Starting an epidural can slow down labor and delivery of baby is of utmost importance with decelerations on fetal monitoring. Changing the mother's position may help, however ACOG recommends quick decisions within 30 minutes to prevent trauma to mother and baby. *(Cunningham et al., 2014, pp. 473–503)*

REFERENCES

ACOG Committee on Obstetric Practice. Preconception and antepartum care. In: Riley LE, Kilpatrick SJ, Papile L, eds. *Guidelines for Perinatal Care.* 7th ed. Washington, DC: The American College of Obstetrics and Gynecology; 2012.

Beckman CR, Ling FW, Herbert WN, et al. *Obstetrics and Gynecology.* 7th ed. Philadelphia, PA: Lippincott, Williams & Wilkins; 2014.

Beshay VE, Carr BR. Endometriosis. In: Hoffman BL, Schorge JO, Schaffer JI, et al., eds. *Williams Gynecology.* New York, NY: McGraw Hill; 2012.

Bornstein J. Benign disorders of the vulva and vagina. In: Decherney AH, Nathan L, Goodwin TM, et al., eds. *Lange Current Diagnosis and Treatment Obstetrics and Gynecology.* 11th ed. New York, NY: McGraw Hill; 2013.

Bradshaw KD. Menopausal transition. In: Hoffman BL, Schorge JO, Schaffer JI, et al., eds. *Williams Gynecology*. New York, NY: McGraw Hill; 2012.

Centers for Disease Control and Prevention. Sexually transmitted disease surveillance 2013. Centers for Disease Control and Prevention. Web site: http://www.cdc.gov/std/stats13/chlamydia.htm. Published December 2014. Accessed December 27, 2014.

Clayton AH, Haddad ES, Iluonakhamhe JP, et al. Sexual dysfunction associated with major depressive disorder and antidepressant treatment. *Expert Opinion Drug Safety*. 2014; 10:1361–1374.

Cunningham FG, Leveno KJ, Bloom SL, et al. *Williams Obstetrics*. 24th ed. New York, NY: McGraw-Hill; 2014.

Cunningham FG, Stuart GS. Contraception and sterilization. In: Hoffman BL, Schorge JO, Schaffer JI, et al., eds. *Williams Gynecology*. New York, NY: McGraw-Hill; 2012.

Domany E, Gilad O, Shwarz M, Vulfsons S, Garty BZ. Imperforate hymen presenting as chronic low back pain. *Pediatrics*. 2013;132:768–770.

Edge SB, et al. Vulva. In: Edge SB, Fritz AG, Byrd DR, Greene FL, Trotti A, Compton CC, eds. *AJCC Cancer Staging Manual*. 7th ed. New York, NY: Springer; 2010.

Ettinger BB, Gambone JC. Family and intimate partner violence, and sexual assault. In: Hacker NF, Gambone JC, Hobel CJ, eds. *Hacker and Moore's Essentials of Obstetrics and Gynecology*. 5th ed. Philadelphia, PA: Elsevier; 2010.

Euhus DM. Breast disease. In: Hoffman BL, Schorge JO, Schaffer JI, et al., eds. *Williams Gynecology*. New York, NY: McGraw Hill; 2012.

Food and Drug Administration. Gardasil vaccine safety: information from CDC and RDA on the safety of Gardasil vaccine. Website: http://www.fda.gov/BiologicsBloodVaccines/Vaccines/ApprovedProducts/ucm172678.htm. Published December 11, 2014. Accessed December 28, 2014.

Frieden TR, Briss PA, Stephens JW, Thacker SB. U.S. Medical Eligibility Criteria for Contraceptive Use. In: Shaw FE, Casey CG, Rutledge TF, et al., eds. *Centers for Disease Control MMWR*. Vol 59; 2010.

Gala RB. Ectopic pregnancy. In: Hoffman BL, Schorge JO, Schaffer JI, et al., eds. *Williams Gynecology*. New York, NY: McGraw Hill; 2012.

Griffith WF, Werner CL. Preinvasive lesions of lower genital tract. In: Hoffman BL, Schorge JO, Schaffer JI, et al., eds. *Williams Gynecology*. New York, NY: McGraw Hill; 2012.

Hacker NF, Gambone JC, Hobel CJ, eds. *Hacker and Moore's Essentials of Obstetrics and Gynecology*. 5th ed. Philadelphia, PA: Elsevier; 2010.

Haefner HK. Vulvodynia. Website: http://obgyn.med.umich.edu/patient-care/womens-health-library/vulvardiseases/information. Published March 14, 2013. Accessed December 27, 2014.

Halvorson LM. Amenorrhea. In: Hoffman BL, Schorge JO, Schaffer JI, et al., eds. *Williams Gynecology*. New York, NY: McGraw Hill; 2012a.

Halvorson LM. Evaluation of the infertile couple. In: Hoffman BL, Schorge JO, Schaffer JI, et al., eds. *Williams Gynecology*. New York, NY: McGraw Hill; 2012b.

Hatcher R, Trussell J, Nelson A, Cates W. Emergency contraception. In: Kowal D, Hatcher R, eds. *Contraceptive Technology*. 20th ed. New York, NY; Ardent Media; 2011.

Heinzman AB, Hoffman BL. Pelvic mass. In: Hoffman BL, Schorge JO, Schaffer JI, et al., eds. *Williams Gynecology*. New York, NY: McGraw Hill; 2012.

Hemsell DL. Gynecologic infections. In: Hoffman BL, Schorge JO, Schaffer JI, et al., eds. *Williams Gynecology*. New York, NY: McGraw Hill; 2012.

Hobel CJ, Zakowski M. Normal labor, delivery and postpartum care: anatomic considerations, obstetric analgesia and anesthesia, and resuscitations of the newborn. In: *Hacker and Moore's Essentials of Obstetrics and Gynecology*. 5th ed. Philadelphia, PA: Elsevier; 2010.

Hoffman BL. Abnormal uterine bleeding. In: Hoffman BL, Schorge JO, Schaffer JI, et al., eds. *Williams Gynecology*. New York, NY: McGraw Hill; 2012.

Katz VL, Dotters D. Breast diseases: diagnosis and treatment of benign and malignant disease. In: Katz VL, Lentz GM, Lobo RA, Gershenson DM, eds. *Comprehensive Gynecology*. 6th ed. Philadelphia, PA: Elsevier Mosby; 2012.

Kim M, Hayashi RH, Gambone JC. Obstetric hemorrhage and puerperal sepsis. In: Hacker NF, Gambone JC, Hobel CJ, eds. *Hacker and Moore's Essentials of Obstetrics and Gynecology*. 5th ed. Philadelphia, PA: Elsevier; 2010.

Lentz GM. Anatomic defects of the abdominal wall and pelvic floor. In: Katz VL, Lentz GM, Lobo RA, Gershenson DM, eds. *Comprehensive Gynecology*. 6th ed. Philadelphia, PA: Elsevier Mosby; 2012.

MacKay G. Sexually transmitted diseases and pelvic infections. In: McPhee SJ, Papadakis MA, eds. *Lange 2014 Current Diagnosis and Treatment*. 53rd ed. New York, NY: McGraw Hill; 2014.

MacKay HT, Woo J. Gynecologic disorders. In: McPhee SJ, Papadakis MA, eds. *Lange 2014 Current Diagnosis and Treatment*. 53rd ed. New York, NY: McGraw Hill; 2014.

Miller DS. Endometrial cancer. In: Hoffman BL, Schorge JO, Schaffer JI, et al., eds. *Williams Gynecology*. New York, NY: McGraw Hill; 2012.

Nathan L. Menopause and postmenopause. In: Decherney AH, Nathan L, Goodwin TM, et al., eds. *Lange Current Diagnosis and Treatment Obstetrics and Gynecology*. 11th ed. New York, NY: McGraw Hill; 2013.

Nelson AL, Gambone JC. Congenital anomalies and benign conditions of the uterine corpus and cervix. In: Hacker NF, Gambone JC, Hobel CJ, eds. *Hacker and Moore's Essentials of Obstetrics and Gynecology*. 5th ed. Philadelphia, PA: Elsevier; 2010.

Poggi SB. Postpartum hemorrhage and the abnormal puerperium. In: Decherney AH, Nathan L, Goodwin TM, et al., eds. *Lange Current Diagnosis and Treatment Obstetrics and Gynecology*. 11th ed. New York, NY: McGraw Hill; 2013.

Richardson DL. Cervical cancer. In: Hoffman BL, Schorge JO, Schaffer JI, et al., eds. *Williams Gynecology*. New York, NY: McGraw Hill; 2012.

Roman AS. Late pregnancy complications. In: Decherney AH, Nathan L, Goodwin TM, et al., eds. *Lange Current Diagnosis and Treatment Obstetrics and Gynecology*. 11th ed. New York, NY: McGraw Hill; 2013.

Saslow D, Solomon D, Lawson HW, et al. American cancer society, American society for colposcopy and cervical pathology, and American society for clinical screening guidelines for prevention and early detection of cervical cancer. *Journal of Lower Genital Tract Disease*. 2012;16(3): 175–204.

Schaffer JI. Pelvic organ prolapse. In: Hoffman BL, Schorge JO, Schaffer JI, et al., eds. *Williams Gynecology*. New York, NY: McGraw Hill; 2012.

Schorge JO. Gestational trophoblastic disease. In: Hoffman BL, Schorge JO, Schaffer JI, et al., eds. *Williams Gynecology*. New York, NY: McGraw Hill; 2012.

Wilson EE. Polycystic ovarian syndrome and hyperandrogenism. In: Hoffman BL, Schorge JO, Schaffer JI, et al., eds. *Williams Gynecology*. New York, NY: McGraw Hill; 2012.

Workowski KA, Berman S; Centers for Disease Control and Prevention (CDC). Sexually transmitted diseases treatment guidelines, 2010. *MMWR Recommendations and Reports*. 2010;59:1–110.

CHAPTER 12

Pediatrics

Camilla E. Hollen, MMS, PA-C
Anne E. Schempp, MPAS, PA-C

DIRECTIONS: Each of the numbered questions or incomplete statements is followed by possible answers or completions of the statement. Select the ONE-lettered answer or completion that is BEST in each case.

1. Which of the following symptoms is a manifestation of late lead exposure?

   (A) Ataxia
   (B) Convulsions
   (C) Irritability
   (D) Personality changes
   (E) Vomiting

2. Upon newborn screening, a neonate is found to have microcytic anemia. The subsequent hemoglobin electrophoresis is positive for Bart's hemoglobin. Which of the following is the most likely diagnosis?

   (A) α-Thalassemia
   (B) β-Thalassemia minor
   (C) β-Thalassemia major
   (D) Hemophilia A
   (E) Sickle cell trait

3. In the United States, tonsillitis is most commonly caused by which of the following pathogens?

   (A) Adenovirus
   (B) *Corynebacterium diphtheriae*
   (C) Epstein–Barr virus
   (D) Group A beta-hemolytic *Streptococcus pyogenes*
   (E) *Mycoplasma pneumoniae*

4. A child born with the genetic abnormality trisomy 21 has the greatest risk for which of the following congenital heart disorders?

   (A) Bicuspid atresia
   (B) Patent ductus arteriosus
   (C) Tetralogy of Fallot
   (D) Transposition of the great vessels
   (E) Ventricular septal defect

5. In the pediatric population, which of the following malignant disorders is most common?

   (A) Acute lymphoblastic leukemia
   (B) Astrocytoma
   (C) Hodgkin lymphoma
   (D) Nephroblastoma
   (E) Osteosarcoma

6. Which of the following is the most common etiologic agent of bacterial meningitis in the pediatric population of the United States?

   (A) *Haemophilus influenzae* type B
   (B) *Listeria monocytogenes*
   (C) *Neisseria meningitidis*
   (D) *Staphylococcus aureus*
   (E) *Streptococcus pneumoniae*

7. A 9-year-old patient presents with a new-onset early decrescendo diastolic murmur with joint swelling and pain in the knee and wrists for the past 2 weeks. He has no known drug allergies. An antistreptolysin titer is positive. Which of the following is the drug of choice for this patient?

   (A) Ampicillin
   (B) Azithromycin (Zithromax)
   (C) Benzathine penicillin (Bicillin L-A)
   (D) Clarithromycin (Biaxin)
   (E) Clindamycin (Cleocin)

8. A 12-year-old boy presents for a coagulation evaluation after multiple episodes of hemarthroses and easy bruising. His activated partial thromboplastin time (aPTT) is increased and prothrombin time (PT) is normal. Which of the following disorders is consistent with his clinical picture?

   (A) Antiphospholipid antibody syndrome
   (B) Disseminated intravascular coagulation
   (C) Factor V deficiency
   (D) Hemophilia A
   (E) Vitamin K deficiency

9. Upon physical examination of a 12-year-old girl, dark, coarse, curly pubic hair spread sparsely over the pubic symphysis is present. She has elevation of the breast and areola without separation of their contours. At what tanner stage of sexual maturation is this patient classified?

   (A) Stage I
   (B) Stage II
   (C) Stage III
   (D) Stage IV
   (E) Stage V

10. During the first year of life, what is the expected average growth for an infant who weighs 8 pounds (lb) at birth?

   (A) 7 lb at 2 weeks, 14 lb at 6 months, 21 lb at 12 months
   (B) 7 lb at 2 weeks, 21 lb at 4 months, 28 lb at 12 months
   (C) 8 lb at 2 weeks, 16 lb at 4 months, 24 lb at 12 months
   (D) 8 lb at 2 weeks, 20 lb at 4 months, 30 lb at 12 months
   (E) 8 lb at 2 weeks, 24 lb at 6 months, 32 lb at 12 months

11. Which of the following orthopedic disorders, when seen in a child, is suspicious for child abuse?

   (A) Dislocation of the patella
   (B) Nontraumatic knee effusion
   (C) Slipped capital femoral epiphysis
   (D) Subluxation of the radial head
   (E) Talipes equinovarus

12. A 10-month-old infant is diagnosed with rotavirus. Which of the following treatment regimens is appropriate for this patient?

   (A) Clear liquids × 5 days
   (B) Lactose rich diet
   (C) Loperamide
   (D) Oral immunoglobulin
   (E) Oral rehydration solution

13. Which of the following bone tumors occurs most commonly in the pediatric population and is benign?

   (A) Chondroblastoma
   (B) Ewing sarcoma
   (C) Osteochondroma
   (D) Osteosarcoma
   (E) Osteoid osteoma

14. Which of the following is the first sign of normal male sexual maturation?

   (A) Appearance of axillary hair
   (B) Appearance of facial hair
   (C) Appearance of pubic hair
   (D) Deepening of the voice
   (E) Enlargement of the testes

15. Huntington disease follows which of the following patterns of genetic inheritance?

   (A) Autosomal dominant
   (B) Autosomal recessive
   (C) X-linked dominant
   (D) X-linked recessive
   (E) Y-linked

16. A 10-year-old female presents with complaints of recurrent, episodic migraine headaches. They occur about two to three times a month and have started to interfere with schoolwork when they occur. Which of the treatments is FDA approved for abortive therapy for this patient?

   (A) Almotriptan (Axert)
   (B) Coenzyme Q10
   (C) Dihydroergotamine (Migranal)
   (D) Rizatriptan (Maxalt)
   (E) Topiramate (Topamax)

17. A 5-year-old child presents for a school physical examination. His medical history is unremarkable, including normal growth and development. His physical examination is normal except for a grade II/VI high-pitched, vibratory, systolic ejection murmur heard best at the left lower sternal border with radiation to the apex. When the child is in a supine position, the murmur is louder. Which of the following etiologies is the MOST likely cause of this clinical picture?

   (A) Patent ductus arteriosus
   (B) Physiologic peripheral pulmonic stenosis
   (C) Pulmonary ejection murmur
   (D) Still's murmur
   (E) Venous hum

18. Which of the following sleeping positions reduces the risk for sudden infant death syndrome?

   (A) Left lateral decubitus
   (B) Prone position
   (C) Seated position
   (D) Side position
   (E) Supine position

19. Which of the following items, if swallowed by a child, is safe to pass on its own as long as the child remains symptom free?

   (A) Button battery
   (B) Multiple magnets
   (C) Open safety pin
   (D) Straight pin
   (E) Wooden toothpick

20. In the initial evaluation of a child with newly diagnosed hypertension, which of the following evaluations will help rule in the most common etiology?

   (A) Chest radiography
   (B) Electrocardiogram
   (C) Renal ultrasonography
   (D) Serum uric acid
   (E) Urinalysis

21. Which of the following congenital infections causes neonatal microcephaly, jaundice, and hepatosplenomegaly?

   (A) Cytomegalovirus
   (B) Parvovirus B19
   (C) Rubella
   (D) Toxoplasmosis
   (E) Varicella

22. When evaluating a 4-month-old infant, which of the following findings is most concerning for child abuse?

   (A) Bruising on abdomen
   (B) Dry, scaly rash on cheeks
   (C) Tearful affect
   (D) Unilateral absence of red reflex
   (E) Weight in 25th percentile

23. A 2-year-old is brought to the emergency department by her parent for evaluation of jerking motions that lasted for about 2 minutes. Her temperature is 39°C rectal; pulse 120/min; respirations 32/min; blood pressure 110/64 mm Hg. On physical examination, she is sleepy but arousable with negative Kernig and Brudzinski signs. Which of the following seizures did this patient most likely experience?

   (A) Absence
   (B) Complex partial
   (C) Febrile
   (D) Psychogenic nonepileptic
   (E) Simple partial

24. A 6-month-old male infant presents with a 2-day history of a fever, vomiting, and poor feeding. He is uncircumcised. Temperature is 39.6°C (rectal) and urinalysis of a catheterized specimen reveals 50 to 100 white blood cells per high-power field and moderate bacteria. Two days later, the urine culture results are available. Which of the following pathogens is most likely responsible for this infant's urinary tract infection?

   (A) *Enterococcus faecalis*
   (B) *Escherichia coli*
   (C) *Klebsiella pneumoniae*
   (D) *Proteus* species
   (E) *Staphylococcus saprophyticus*

25. What is the leading cause of death in the adolescent population?

(A) Cancer

(B) Heart disease

(C) Homicide

(D) Suicide

(E) Unintentional injury

26. A previously well, 15-month-old baby boy is brought to the emergency department with increased irritability and severe paroxysmal colicky abdominal pain followed by vomiting. On physical examination, a tubular mass is palpated in the abdomen. The rectal examination reveals bloody mucus. Which of the following is the MOST likely diagnosis?

(A) Appendicitis

(B) Celiac disease

(C) Infectious enteritis

(D) Intussusception

(E) Pyloric stenosis

27. At what age (in years) can children begin to brush teeth without assistance from an adult?

(A) 2

(B) 4

(C) 6

(D) 8

(E) 10

28. Which of the following is the recommended treatment for a 4-year-old child with presumed bacterial meningitis?

(A) Ampicillin plus chloramphenicol

(B) Cefotaxime (Claforan) or ceftriaxone (Rocephin) plus ampicillin

(C) Cefotaxime (Claforan) or ceftriaxone (Rocephin) plus vancomycin (Vancocin)

(D) Gentamicin plus ampicillin

(E) Rifampin (Rifadin) plus dexamethasone (Decadron)

29. At a 2-month-old well-child checkup, a female infant is noted to have the following physical findings: widely open anterior and posterior fontanels, large protruding tongue, coarse facial features, low-set hair line, and an umbilical hernia. In her newborn period, she had a history of prolonged physiologic icterus. Which of the following diagnoses is consistent with this clinical picture?

(A) Congenital adrenal hyperplasia

(B) Congenital hypothyroidism

(C) Crigler–Najjar syndrome

(D) Galactosemia

(E) Gilbert syndrome

30. Within hours of birth, a healthy newborn develops the following finding:

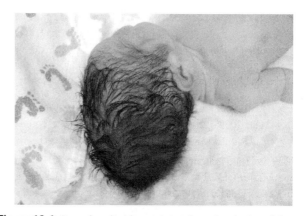

Figure 12-1. Reproduced, with permission, from Cunningham FG, Leveno KJ, Bloom SL, et al. *Williams Obstetrics.* 24th ed. New York, NY: McGraw-Hill Education, 2014. Figure 22–19.

Which of the following identifies this condition?

(A) Caput succedaneum

(B) Cephalohematoma

(C) Craniotabes

(D) Skull fracture

(E) Subgaleal hemorrhage

31. A 2-year-old male child is brought to the emergency department by his mother with a sudden onset of choking, gagging, coughing, and wheezing. Vital signs are: temperature 37°C; pulse 120 bpm, reg; respirations 28/min, shallow. The physical examination reveals decreased breath sounds over the right lower lobe with inspiratory rhonchi and localized expiratory wheezing. The chest radiography reveals normal inspiratory views but expiratory views show localized hyperinflation with mediastinal shift to the left. Which of the following is the MOST likely diagnosis?

(A) Asthma

(B) Epiglottitis

(C) Foreign-body aspiration

(D) Pulmonary embolism

(E) Tracheomalacia

32. A 16-year-old girl is brought to the emergency department by ambulance after reportedly ingesting a bottle of aspirin about 12 hours before. Vital signs are temperature 37.8°C oral; pulse 94 bpm, reg; respirations 30/min, shallow; blood pressure 100/68 mm Hg. Based on this history, what is the expected result of her arterial blood gas analysis?

(A) Anion gap metabolic acidosis with respiratory acidosis

(B) Nonanion gap metabolic acidosis with respiratory alkalosis

(C) Anion gap metabolic acidosis with respiratory alkalosis

(D) Nonanion gap metabolic acidosis with respiratory acidosis

(E) Arterial blood gas within normal limits

33. A 16-year-old boy presents 4 hours after sustaining an abrasion to his knee after a fall while skateboarding on the playground. His school immunization record reveals that his last diphtheria, tetanus, and acellular pertussis (DTaP) booster was administered at age 4. In this situation, which of the following is MOST appropriate to be administered to this patient?

(A) Adult tetanus and diphtheria toxoid (Td)

(B) Diphtheria, tetanus, and acellular pertussis (DTaP) vaccine

(C) Diphtheria, tetanus toxoid, and acellular pertussis (Tdap) vaccine

(D) Tetanus immune globulin

(E) Tetanus toxoid

34. Which of the following newborn reflexes should still be present at the 9-month checkup?

(A) Galant reflex

(B) Moro reflex

(C) Parachute reflex

(D) Placing reflex

(E) Rooting reflex

35. A 3-day-old neonate has bilateral copious, yellow-green eye discharge and conjunctival inflammation. A Gram stain of this discharge reveals gram-negative intracellular diplococci. Which of the following antibiotics is the drug of choice for this infection?

(A) Acyclovir (Zovirax)

(B) Ceftriaxone (Rocephin)

(C) Cephalexin (Keflex)

(D) Erythromycin (Ilotycin)

(E) Gentamicin (Garamycin)

36. A 10-year-old boy presents complaining of a painful, swollen area along his right jaw and neck. His parents elected not to vaccinate him as a child. On physical examination, he is febrile and has diffuse tenderness over the right parotid gland. Serum amylase is elevated. Based on the most likely diagnosis, this patient is at risk for which of the following complications?

(A) Blindness

(B) Deafness

(C) Hepatitis

(D) Pneumonitis

(E) Testicular torsion

37. Which of the following physical examination findings in a neonate should cause the clinician to suspect a genetic disorder?

(A) Café au lait spots

(B) Hemangioma

(C) Miliaria

(D) Subconjunctival hemorrhages

(E) Vernix caseosa

38. Calculate the Apgar score for the following patient at 1 minute: Heart rate of 120 bpm, reg, strong cry, some flexion in the upper extremities, sneezing with nasal catheter suction, bluish hands and feet with the remainder of the body pink.

(A) 6

(B) 7

(C) 8

(D) 9

(E) 10

39. Which of the following is the most common congenital heart malformation?

(A) Atrial septal defect

(B) Atrioventricular septal defect

(C) Tetralogy of Fallot

(D) Transposition of the great vessels

(E) Ventricular septal defect

40. A 5-year-old male child presents for a kindergarten physical examination. Assuming that his prior immunizations have followed the recommended schedule, which of the following immunizations should the patient receive today?

(A) Hepatitis A, diphtheria, tetanus, acellular pertussis (DTaP), measles, mumps, rubella (MMR), varicella

(B) Hepatitis B, inactivated poliovirus (IPV), DTaP, MMR, varicella

(C) IPV, DTaP, MMR, pneumococcal (PCV)

(D) IPV, DTaP, MMR, *Haemophilus influenzae* type B (Hib)

(E) IPV, DTaP, MMR, varicella

41. Which of the following is an absolute contraindication to breastfeeding?

(A) Human immunodeficiency virus of the mother

(B) Infant with cystic fibrosis

(C) Maternal smoking

(D) Methadone treatment (20 mg/d)

(E) Tuberculosis of the mother

42. A 4-month-old infant is brought for her well-child visit after missing her 2-month visit. The parents state that they have no concerns and think she is doing well. She breastfeeds every 4 to 6 hours, has four wet diapers a day, and stools twice a day. Her birth weight was 7 pounds (lb) 7 ounces (oz) (50th percentile). Today, she weighs 11 lb 5 oz (5th percentile). This scenario is concerning for which of the following disorders?

(A) Beckwith–Wiedemann syndrome

(B) Dwarfism

(C) Growth deficiency

(D) Lactose intolerance

(E) Laron syndrome

43. During influenza season, a 15-year-old boy presents to the emergency department, unresponsive. The parents state that when they tried to wake him up in the morning he would not get up and was barely breathing. They deny any drug or alcohol use and state that he had cold symptoms the past few days. A spinal tap shows decreased glucose, increased pressure, and normal cell counts. The rest of the blood work shows elevated liver enzymes, but normal serum bilirubin and alkaline phosphatase. A liver biopsy demonstrates microvesicular steatosis with absent glycogen and large mitochondria. Which of the following is the best treatment for this patient?

(A) Antiviral therapy

(B) Broad-spectrum antibiotics until the cultures come back

(C) High-dose steroids

(D) Liver transplant

(E) Maintenance fluids and hyperventilation

44. The common finding of physiologic jaundice of the newborn occurs due to which of the following mechanisms?

(A) Congenital hepatic hypofunction

(B) Hemolysis due to G6PD deficiency

(C) Normal digestion of breast milk

(D) Rh-isoenzyme incompatibility

(E) Slow GI motility and absence of normal gut flora

45. A 24-month-old infant presents for his routine well-child visit. The parents state that he has been in line with all of the developmental milestones for his age. On examination, a grade II/VI murmur is auscultated along the left sternal border that radiates into the left axilla and the left side of the back. Femoral pulses are decreased bilaterally. Based on this clinical presentation, which of the following is expected on chest radiography?

(A) Absence of the main pulmonary artery

(B) Boot-shaped heart

(C) Dextrocardia

(D) Narrowed mediastinum

(E) Notching of the ribs

46. An 8-year-old female presents to the emergency department with her parents. She has been coughing all night the past few nights, to the point she sounds like she is choking. Pulse oximetry is 92% on room air and the child is afebrile. On examination, she has mild chest retractions at rest but during auscultation of the lung fields, retractions worsen and she develops diffuse stridor. Which of the following is the recommended treatment for this patient?

    (A) Intramuscular (IM) dexamethasone (Decadron)
    (B) Intravenous (IV) antibiotics, with gram-negative coverage
    (C) Nebulized budesonide (Pulmicort)
    (D) Nebulized racemic epinephrine (Asthmanefrin) and oral dexamethasone (Decadron)
    (E) Supportive care only—mist therapy

47. A neonate presents with meconium ileus that is successfully unobstructed. As an infant, she presents to her 4-month well-child evaluation with signs of failure to thrive. Which of the following is the most likely diagnosis for this patient?

    (A) Cystic fibrosis
    (B) Distal intestinal obstruction syndrome
    (C) Intussusception
    (D) Volvulus
    (E) Wilson disease

48. Which of the following is an acyanotic heart lesion?

    (A) Atrioventricular septal defect
    (B) Hypoplastic left heart syndrome
    (C) Transposition of the great arteries
    (D) Tricuspid atresia
    (E) Truncus arteriosus

49. A 2-week-old male is brought for a routine checkup. The mother complains that he nurses every hour, but vomits after every time he eats. He has only had three bowel movements since he has been home. On examination, the infant has not gained any weight since leaving the hospital, and the clinician notes gastric peristaltic waves. Which of the following is the treatment of choice for this patient?

    (A) Laparotomy
    (B) Metoclopramide (Reglan)
    (C) Omeprazole (Prilosec)
    (D) Pyloromyotomy
    (E) Ranitidine (Zantac)

50. An infant is brought by her parents for her 6-month checkup. Her father mentions that they started solid foods after her 4-month checkup. She has had foul-smelling diarrhea off and on for the first month of solids; it now occurs after every meal and looks greasy. They have tried different formulas and different cereals without improvement. What is the diagnostic test of choice for the most likely disorder?

    (A) Gastrin level
    (B) Intestinal biopsy
    (C) Radioallergosorbent assay test (RAST)
    (D) Stool culture for ova and parasites
    (E) Sweat chloride test

51. A 9-year-old child is brought to the clinic with her mother for dark-colored urine. The mother mentions that the child was complaining of sore throat and cold symptoms a few weeks ago. The urine shows gross hematuria without nitrites or leukocytes. Which of the following is the best test to help the clinician confirm the most likely diagnosis?

    (A) Antistreptolysin O titer
    (B) Immunoglobulin electrophoresis
    (C) Monospot
    (D) Renal biopsy
    (E) Renal ultrasound

52. The following findings are found on examination of a newborn patient: widened pulse pressure, paradoxical splitting of S_2, a "machine"-like murmur heard best at the second intercostal space, left sternal border, and inferior to the clavicle. Which of the following is the most likely diagnosis?

    (A) Atrial septal defect
    (B) Patent ductus arteriosus
    (C) Pulmonary stenosis
    (D) Tetralogy of Fallot
    (E) Ventricular septal defect

53. A 15-year-old boy suddenly collapses on the basketball court and basic life support initiated at the scenes is unsuccessful in resuscitation. Upon review of his records, the sports physical conducted at the beginning of the year did not elicit any abnormal findings. Which of the following is the most likely etiology of his sudden death?

   (A) Hypertrophic cardiomyopathy
   (B) Mitral valve prolapse
   (C) Pericarditis
   (D) Rheumatic heart disease
   (E) Surgically corrected aortic stenosis

54. A 7-year-old male is brought to the emergency department for severe dyspnea, dysphagia, drooling, muffled voice, and fever. The pulse oximetry is 91% on room air; lung examination shows stridor and inspiratory retractions. Which of the following is the expected chest radiograph finding for the suspected diagnosis?

   (A) Figure 3 sign
   (B) Scottie dog sign
   (C) Spine sign
   (D) Steeple sign
   (E) Thumbprint sign

55. Which of the following is a characteristic sign or symptom of severe tetralogy of Fallot?

   (A) Blood pressure discrepancy in upper and lower extremities
   (B) Dyspnea and cyanosis with exertion
   (C) Orthopnea
   (D) Paroxysmal nocturnal dyspnea
   (E) Widened pulse pressure

56. Which of the following is the most common cause of childhood gynecomastia?

   (A) Genetic disease
   (B) Idiopathic
   (C) Illicit drug use
   (D) Medications
   (E) Neoplasms

57. A 12-year-old boy presents to the urgent care center complaining of burning pain in his lower extremities with weakness. On examination, the clinician notes symmetric weakness with severely decreased active range of motion of the lower extremities. In addition, there is decreased position and vibratory sensation in the distal portions bilaterally. Upon further questioning, the patient admits to being diagnosed with mononucleosis 2 weeks ago. Which of the following is the most likely diagnosis?

   (A) Botulism
   (B) Guillain–Barré syndrome
   (C) Poliomyelitis
   (D) Tick-bite paralysis
   (E) Transverse myelitis

58. Which thoracic curvature is an indication for treatment with bracing in an adolescent with scoliosis?

   (A) Less than 20 degrees
   (B) 20 to 40 degrees
   (C) 40 to 60 degrees
   (D) 40 degrees with lumbar curvature of 30 degrees
   (E) Greater than 70 degrees

59. A 6-year-old female presents with complaints of chronic hip pain so severe that she has not been able to walk to the school bus. Examination shows severe tenderness at the left hip with markedly decreased active and passive range of motion. Radiologic examination demonstrates joint effusion with widening. Which of the following is the most likely diagnosis?

   (A) Legg–Calvé–Perthes disease
   (B) Osteochondritis dissecans
   (C) Septic hip arthritis
   (D) Slipped capital femoral epiphysis
   (E) Tuberculous arthritis

60. A 16-year-old boy presents to the office with thumb pain. He just returned from a skiing trip. On examination, the practitioner notes a positive ulnar collateral ligament laxity test. What is the most likely diagnosis?

   (A) Boxer fracture
   (B) Gamekeeper thumb
   (C) Jersey finger
   (D) Mallet finger
   (E) Nondisplaced scaphoid fracture

61. A 3-year-old is brought in by her parents to the urgent care center stating that the child "will not bend her arm." They are obviously worried and distraught. The clinician notices the elbow is held in strict pronation and there is tenderness over the radial head. Radiographic examination shows no findings. Which of the following is the treatment of choice for this disorder?

(A) Call child protective services for suspected battery

(B) Immobilization of the elbow in a splint for 2 weeks

(C) Open reduction for epiphyseal fracture

(D) Place elbow in full supination and move from full extension to full flexion

(E) Referral to the orthopedic surgeon for suspected radial head fracture

62. A 7-year-old is brought into the office by her mother who states that the child "is still wetting the bed at night." The child has already decreased liquid intake and uses the bathroom before going to bed. The mother is worried that there is something wrong with the child. Upon examination there is no abnormality. Urinalysis is negative. Which of the following is the treatment of choice for this disorder?

(A) Amitriptyline (Elavil)

(B) Bed-wetting alarm

(C) Desmopressin acetate (DDAVP)

(D) Eliminating fluids 8 hours before bedtime

(E) Imipramine (Tofranil)

63. A 5-year-old girl presents with her mother for a well-child examination. Her mother reports a concern about abdominal weight gain. A smooth, firm mass is palpated in the abdomen and does not cross the midline. Urinalysis reveals microscopic hematuria. Which of the following is the most likely diagnosis?

(A) Constipation

(B) Intussusception

(C) Mesenteric cyst

(D) Nephroblastoma

(E) Volvulus

64. What is the most common cause of type I diabetes in the pediatric patient?

(A) Autoimmune disease

(B) Idiopathic cause

(C) Medication side effects

(D) Obesity

(E) Pancreatic neoplasm

65. A 5-year-old child presents for her kindergarten checkup. The clinician notes that over the past couple of years, her height decreased from the 50th percentile to the 5th percentile. On examination, the clinician also notes truncal adiposity. Her complete blood count and lead levels were normal. Which of the following is the most likely diagnosis?

(A) Congenital adrenal hyperplasia

(B) Congenital hypothyroidism

(C) Cushing disease

(D) Familial short stature

(E) Growth hormone deficiency

66. A 4-year-old boy presents with petechiae and ecchymosis on the lower extremities for 1 day. He did have cold symptoms about a week before and they resolved. His physical examination finds no other abnormalities. Complete blood count is normal except a platelet count of 45,000/uL. Which of the following treatments is appropriate in this case?

(A) Aspirin

(B) Intravenous immunoglobulin

(C) Oral corticosteroids

(D) Platelet transfusion

(E) Watchful waiting

67. A 10-year-old child presents with tachycardia, tachypnea, dyspnea, and bibasilar rales. She denies fever or chest pain. Which of the following disorders is most likely the cause of her symptoms?

(A) Kawasaki disease

(B) Myocarditis

(C) Patent ductus arteriosus

(D) Pericarditis

(E) Ventricular septal defect

68. A 12-year-old girl was treated for a urinary tract infection 3 days ago. She presents today with severe conjunctivitis, target lesions on her trunk, and bullous eruptions in her mouth. Which of the following medications is the likely cause of her symptoms?

(A) Amoxicillin (Amoxil)
(B) Cefdinir (Omnicef)
(C) Ciprofloxacin (Cipro)
(D) Erythromycin (Erythrocin)
(E) Trimethoprim-sulfamethoxazole (Bactrim)

69. Which of the following is a complication of infection with parvovirus B19?

(A) Adrenal crisis
(B) Aplastic crisis
(C) Aseptic meningitis
(D) Leukopenia
(E) Nephritis

70. A 4-year-old female presents with a low-grade fever, malaise, and scattered red macules and vesicles over the face and trunk. She complains of intense pruritus. She is up to date on all of her vaccinations. Which of the following is the most likely diagnosis?

(A) Bullous pemphigus
(B) Herpes simplex
(C) Herpes zoster
(D) Molluscum contagiosum
(E) Varicella

71. According to the DSM-5, symptoms of attention-deficit hyperactivity disorder must be present before what age (years)?

(A) 3
(B) 5
(C) 7
(D) 12
(E) 16

72. A child with an egg allergy that manifests only as hives presents for vaccination. Which of the following vaccines should be avoided?

(A) Diphtheria and tetanus and acellular pertussis (DTaP)
(B) Inactivated poliovirus vaccine (IPV)

(C) Injectable influenza
(D) Live attenuated influenza vaccine (LAIV)
(E) Measles-mumps-rubella vaccine (MMR)

73. A 7-year-old Caucasian female presents to the office with "an itchy head." The child's mother, who is with her, states that this has been bothering her daughter for about a week and she has noticed a lot of "dandruff" in the child's hair that will not come out. She also mentions that several of her daughter's friends are having the same problem. On the basis of the most likely diagnosis, what is the best treatment for this patient?

(A) Ketoconazole cream (Nizoral)
(B) Mayonnaise rinse
(C) Permethrin 1% shampoo (Nix)
(D) Silver sulfadiazine 1% cream (Silvadene)
(E) Tar-based shampoo

74. A young mother brings her 4-year-old son to the clinic for evaluation of a rash on his umbilicus and hands. She has been treating it with an over-the-counter ointment for about a week, without success. She has noticed that he scratches the rash periodically and it seems to bother him the most at night. She noticed this same rash on the hands on one of the other boys at his daycare center. On examination, there are excoriated papules and nodules on his hand and umbilicus. What is the most likely diagnosis?

(A) Herpes simplex
(B) Pediculosis
(C) Papular urticaria
(D) Scabies
(E) Tinea corporis

75. A new mother brings her 3-month-old daughter to the clinic for a rash on the infant's head. On examination, the skin affected by the rash is thickened, yellowish white in color, scaly, and looks waxy. In addition, it involves only the scalp and bilateral postauricular areas. What is the most likely diagnosis?

(A) Contact dermatitis
(B) Keratosis pilaris
(C) Lichen planus
(D) Pityriasis rosea
(E) Seborrheic dermatitis

76. An 8-year-old male presents with brown, nonpruritic, annular lesions on the back of his hands and feet. Intradermal nodules are seen on the extensor surfaces of the elbows and knees that have been present for several months. At today's visit, the lesions are essentially unchanged since his last visit about a month ago. What is the best treatment for this suspected disorder?

    (A) Excision and biopsy
    (B) No treatment
    (C) Topical antifungal
    (D) Topical steroids
    (E) Wet to dry dressings

77. At what age (years) is it appropriate to start seeing children alone for a portion of their examination in order to give the opportunities to share information freely without a parent in the room?

    (A) 4
    (B) 7
    (C) 9
    (D) 12
    (E) 15

78. In a 12-month-old male presenting with acute onset ear pain that is disrupting his sleep, which of the following findings on clinical examination would confirm a diagnosis of acute otitis media?

    (A) Bulging tympanic membrane
    (B) Erythematous external auditory canal
    (C) Erythematous tympanic membrane
    (D) Flat tracing on tympanometry
    (E) Tenderness upon palpation of the tragus

79. Which of the following is an absolute indication for surgical repair of a clavicle fracture in a child?

    (A) Deformity over clavicle
    (B) Failure to control pain with medications
    (C) Fracture located in middle third of bone
    (D) Neurovascular compromise
    (E) Risk of nonunion

80. A 13-year-old boy presents to the clinic for a complaint of right knee pain that he first noticed about a year ago. It started out as mild discomfort in the area just below the kneecap, but has been getting progressively worse. Now, it hurts anytime he uses his leg, even when walking. He does not remember any injury to his knee. On examination of his knee there is swelling and exquisite tenderness over the tibial tubercle. Radiographs are normal. What is the most likely diagnosis?

    (A) Chondromalacia patellae
    (B) Legg–Calvé–Perthes disease
    (C) Osgood–Schlatter disease
    (D) Patellar dislocation
    (E) Patellofemoral overuse syndrome

81. In an infant with highly suspected vitamin K deficiency, which laboratory finding would be expected?

    (A) Decreased activated partial thromboplastin time (aPTT)
    (B) Decreased platelet count
    (C) Elevated fibrinogen
    (D) Elevated hepatic transaminase
    (E) Prolonged PT (prothrombin time)

82. A 13-year-old patient complains of a 2-month history of pain in the knees that is worse in the morning. He denies any injuries but does complain of more fatigue than is usual. His rheumatoid factor is negative and erythrocyte sedimentation rate (ESR) is elevated. Which of the following is the most likely diagnosis?

    (A) Juvenile idiopathic arthritis (JIA)
    (B) Lyme arthritis
    (C) Psoriatic arthritis
    (D) Osgood–Schlatter disease
    (E) Slipped capital femoral epiphysis

83. The complications of Meckel diverticulum occur most frequently in which of the following populations?

    (A) Adolescents
    (B) Breast-fed infants
    (C) Females
    (D) Males
    (E) Toddlers

84. While seeing a 12-week-old girl for her well-child checkup, it is noticed that she has tearing from her left eye. There is a small, reddened area that is swollen and she cries when it is touched. The swollen area is just below the medial inferior eyelid. There is also constant tearing from this same eye. Her mother says it just started about 2 days ago and is getting worse. What is the most likely cause of this problem?

    (A) Anterior uveitis
    (B) Blepharitis
    (C) Chalazion
    (D) Conjunctivitis
    (E) Dacryocystitis

85. A 6-year-old child presents with unilateral purulent nasal drainage in the absence of other upper respiratory symptoms. Which of the following is the most likely diagnosis?

    (A) Acute sinusitis
    (B) Dacryocystitis
    (C) Deviated septum
    (D) Nasal foreign body
    (E) Nasal polyposis

86. Of the following, which is the most frequent cause of epistaxis in children?

    (A) Bleeding disorders
    (B) Choanal atresia
    (C) Digital trauma
    (D) Foreign bodies
    (E) Hypertension

87. A 4-month-old child is brought for evaluation of a fever by her parents. Her temperature measures 39°C rectally. Which of the following scenarios would decrease the risk of serious cause of the fever?

    (A) Associated burning with urination
    (B) Fever began 24 hours after diphtheria–tetanus–pertussis vaccination
    (C) Fever has been present for over 72 hours
    (D) Fever present for 36 hours
    (E) Fever subsided then returned within 24 hours

88. A 10-year-old child is diagnosed with pertussis. Barring medication allergies, what is the recommended treatment for the other family members in the household?

    (A) Azithromycin (Zithromax)
    (B) Ampicillin
    (C) Corticosteroids
    (D) Strict physical isolation from infected child
    (E) Watchful waiting for symptom development

89. Which of the following is indicated for an incarcerated inguinal hernia present for more than 12 hours?

    (A) Bilateral surgical reduction
    (B) Bimanual reduction
    (C) Manual reduction
    (D) Surgical reduction
    (E) Watchful waiting

90. A 2-week-old male is being seen in the clinic for a profuse mucoid discharge from both eyes, with some associated tearing. On examination, both eyes are hyperemic and the eyelids are red and swollen. Which of the following is the most likely cause of this patient's ophthalmia neonatorum?

    (A) Allergic
    (B) Chlamydial
    (C) Gonococcal
    (D) Silver nitrate prophylaxis
    (E) Viral

91. In the process of differentiating the causative etiology of arthritis in a child, which of the following features is more indicative of Lyme disease rather than juvenile rheumatoid arthritis?

    (A) Attacks of symptoms relapsing and remitting
    (B) Elevated erythrocyte sedimentation rate
    (C) Fever
    (D) Joint deformity
    (E) Negative culture of joint fluid

92. A young mother brings her 3-week-old daughter for care of a rash in her mouth. The mother indicates the baby was doing fine until 2 days ago when she noticed white spots in the infant's mouth. On examination, they do not come off easily with a tongue blade. She is bottle-feeding the infant without any problem. Which of the following is the most likely diagnosis of this problem?

    (A) Hand–foot–mouth disease
    (B) Herpangina

(C) Herpes simplex gingivostomatitis

(D) Leukoplakia

(E) Oral candidiasis

93. In a pediatric patient, bipolar disorder predominantly presents as which of the following symptoms?

(A) Delusions

(B) Depression

(C) Hallucinations

(D) Hypomania

(E) Mania

94. A 9-year-old male presents in August with complaints of a red rash on the palms of his hands, soles of his feet, and a little on his legs. His mother states that this rash started about 2 days ago, and just before it appeared her son had been complaining of a severe headache and aching all over. She said he felt "hot to the touch" during that time, as well. The child mentions he was camping in Arkansas about 10 days ago with his dad but did not eat anything abnormal. On the basis of this history, what is the most likely diagnosis?

(A) Endemic typhus

(B) Human ehrlichiosis

(C) Lyme disease

(D) Q fever

(E) Rocky Mountain spotted fever

95. In young children, which of the following is the most common cause of lower respiratory tract infections?

(A) Adenovirus

(B) Human metapneumovirus

(C) Human parvovirus

(D) Parainfluenza virus

(E) Respiratory syncytial virus

96. A 3-year-old male child presents to the clinic for a cough that occurs only after he has been running, according to his mother. She says she first noticed this about 6 months ago, after he had one of his usual winter colds, and his cough persisted for about a week. On the basis of this history, what is the most likely diagnosis?

(A) Airway foreign body

(B) Asthma

(C) Cystic fibrosis

(D) Laryngomalacia

(E) Vocal cord dysfunction

97. A 12-month-old male presents with his mother's concerns that he does not seem to play with other children as his brother and sister did at this age. She indicates she has noticed that he does not seem to respond when she or other children call him by name, he is indifferent to other children or adults when they are present, and he does not seem to know any and "just grunts." On the basis of this history, the most likely diagnosis for this problem is which of the following?

(A) Attention-deficit/hyperactivity disorder (ADHD)

(B) Autism

(C) Fragile X syndrome

(D) Plumbism

(E) Schizophrenia

98. When evaluating a newborn, the inability to pass a small catheter through the nasal cavity is most indicative of which of the following conditions?

(A) Choanal atresia

(B) Cystic fibrosis

(C) Meconium ileus

(D) Nasal infection

(E) Nasal polyps

99. Which of the following is considered a long-term complication associated with anorexia nervosa?

(A) Constipation

(B) Loss of brain tissue

(C) Osteoarthritis

(D) Pericardial effusion

(E) Superior mesenteric artery syndrome

100. For the pediatric population, obesity is defined as which of the following?

(A) BMI of >25

(B) BMI for age in 85th to 95th percentile

(C) BMI of >35

(D) BMI for age >95th percentile

(E) Weight of >10% change in 1 month

Answers and Explanations

1. **(B)** All of the symptoms mentioned in this question can manifest in children exposed to lead, however convulsions are found later in the disease. Of note, small and repeated exposures of lead are more dangerous to children than large, single exposures. *(Wang et al., 2014, p. 377)*

2. **(A)** α-Thalassemia manifests in one of four syndromes depending on the number of mutations on the a-globin chains, but in the majority of cases, Bart's hemoglobin is seen on electrophoresis. β-Thalassemia minor manifests typically as a mild anemia 6 to 12 months after birth and neonatal screen is often normal. β-Thalassemia major manifests as a severe microcytic anemia at birth and electrophoresis shows absent hemoglobin A on neonatal screen. Sickle cell trait demonstrates an FAS pattern (the presence and/or amounts of hemoglobin F, A, and S) on electrophoresis and hemophilia A does not manifest with abnormalities in hemoglobin; hemophilia A is a disorder of factor VIII and is usually identified after patients have difficulties with spontaneous bleeding or hemarthroses. *(Ambruso et al., 2014, pp. 947–950, 952–953, 968–971)*

3. **(A)** In children who present with symptoms of sore throat and fever, approximately 50% to 70% of these cases are due to a viral infection. Adenovirus is one of the most common etiologic viral agents. Epstein–Barr virus is the etiologic agent for mononucleosis and while very common in the United States it is still less than rhinoviruses and coronaviruses. The three remaining choices are bacterial pathogens of which group A beta-hemolytic streptococcus (GAS) is the most common followed by the less common pathogens (group C *Streptococcus*, *Arcanobacterium haemolyticus*, and *Streptococcus pneumoniae*). As a single agent, GAS is the most common etiology of acute tonsillitis and pharyngitis. Early infection with *Corynebacterium diphtheriae* can resemble acute tonsillitis. This is rarely seen in the United States. *Mycoplasma pneumoniae* is a common cause of symptomatic pneumonia in children. *(Friedman et al., 2014, pp. 523–525; Kronman & Smith, 2015, pp. 347–349; Ogle & Anderson, 2014, pp. 1313–1314)*

4. **(E)** Children born with trisomy 21 have congenital heart disease one-third to one-half of the time. The most common of these disorders is an atrial septal canal disorder or ventricular septal defect. Although tetralogy of Fallot can occur in trisomy 21, it is less frequent. *(Saenz et al., 2014, pp. 1151–1153)*

5. **(A)** Acute lymphocytic leukemia (ALL) is the most common malignancy of childhood and accounts for about 25% of all malignancies in children under the age of 15. Astrocytoma, Hodgkin lymphoma, and osteosarcoma are the most common variety of malignancy in their large categories, but do not exceed the incidence of ALL. Nephroblastoma (Wilms tumor) is a second to neuroblastoma in occurrence of abdominal tumors in children and occurs in about 5% children less than 15. *(Graham et al., 2014, pp. 990–993, 997–1003, 1008–1011)*

6. **(E)** Despite the increase in vaccination of infants in the United States, *Streptococcus pneumoniae* remains the most common etiologic agent for bacterial meningitis in the pediatric population. *Haemophilus influenzae* type B is the second most common, but has gone down significantly due to the widespread vaccination of children. *Neisseria meningitidis* has approximately 2,400 to 3,000 cases a year. Meningitis due to *Listeria monocytogenes* is typically seen in the neonatal period due to transmission from the mother. It is present in normal

fecal matter in around 10% of the population. Its rates have gone down due to strict guidelines for the food industry, resulting in less than 1,000 cases per year. *Staphylococcus aureus* may be responsible in patients with recent head injury, surgery, or a shunt. *(Kronman & Smith, 2015, pp. 342–344; Ogle, 2014, pp. 1217–1218)*

7. **(C)** This young patient has acute rheumatic fever. This is confirmed by the presence of two of the major (modified) Jones criteria (carditis, polyarthritis) and in this case, two of the minor criteria (arthralgia and evidence of streptococcal infection). Long-acting benzathine penicillin given via intramuscular injection is the drug of choice for this patient because he does not have a penicillin allergy. The remaining drug choices would be acceptable for first-line treatment if the patient had a penicillin allergy. *(Darst et al., 2014, pp. 626–628)*

8. **(D)** This patient presents with a bleeding disorder causing hemarthrosis and easy bruising. Hemophilia A, a genetic disorder that results in a decrease of factor XIII, will result in a prolonged aPTT due to its effect on the intrinsic pathway. The PT remains normal because factor XIII is not involved in the extrinsic pathway. Both DIC and vitamin K deficiency can cause bleeding, but both affect the intrinsic and extrinsic pathways, which results in prolonged aPTT and prolonged PT. DIC usually presents in conjunction with severe trauma, infection, or shock. Factor V deficiency and antiphospholipid antibody syndrome are thrombotic disorders and usually present with a venous thrombotic event. *(Ambruso et al., 2014, pp. 963, 968–971, 973–975, 977–978)*

9. **(C)** Tanner stages of sexual maturation categorize the progression of pubertal development in girls according to pubic hair and breast development. Menarche usually occurs 18 to 24 months following the onset of breast development. In female breast development, Tanner stage I is an absence of breast development; stage II is a small, raised breast bud; stage III shows further enlargement/elevation of breast and alveolar tissue; stage IV is the areola and papilla forming a secondary mound on breast contour; and stage V is the mature breast with alveolar area as part of the breast contour. For the stages of pubic hair development, stage I is prepubertal, an absence of hair; stage II shows sparse, fine hair,

primarily on the border of labia; stage III is pigmented and curly and increases in quantity on the mons pubis; stage IV is increased quantity of coarser texture with labia and mons pubis well covered; and stage V is mature adult distribution with spreading to medial thighs. *(Blake & Allen, 2015, pp. 237–240; Sass & Kaplan, 2014, pp. 125–127)*

10. **(C)** During the first year of life the average, expected increase in weight of a full-term infant is to regain the birth weight by 2 weeks of age, double the birth weight by 4 months of age, and triple the birth weight by 1 year of age. *(Levine, 2015, p. 10)*

11. **(D)** Subluxation of the radial head occurs mechanistically from being pulled in the upward direction by the hand. This may occur inadvertently but can be seen with abuse, especially when recurrent. Dislocation of the patella occurs in patients with patellar malalignment and is not associated with abuse. Slipped capital femoral epiphysis is not associated with trauma. A nontraumatic knee effusion in a child could be the sign of rheumatoid disease or patellar pathology. *(Erickson & Caprio, 2014, pp. 868–869, 872–873)*

12. **(E)** Rotavirus is a common cause of diarrhea in children, especially in those who have not been vaccinated. The viral infection is usually treated conservatively with oral rehydration solutions as needed to replace fluids and electrolytes that occur due to the vomiting and watery diarrhea. Clear liquids are not recommended for more than 48 hours in a child. Because of the decrease in intestinal lactase levels in the gut during an active infection, lactose-free diets are recommended in the first few days of refeeding. Loperamide or other antidiarrheals could potentially be dangerous to the patients and should be avoided. Immunoglobulin is a treatment option but is reserved for those patients who are immunocompromised. *(Hoffenberg et al., 2014, pp. 678–679)*

13. **(C)** Osteochondroma is the most common benign bone tumor in the pediatric population and usually presents as a pain-free mass. Chondroblastoma is also benign and chondral in nature. It affects the epiphyseal plates of long bones and is associated with pathologic fracture. Ewing sarcoma is a malignant lesion that is associated with pain, tenderness, and limping or difficulty walking. Osteosarcoma is

also an aggressive malignant lesion, which mainly affects the long bones. Osteoid osteoma is a benign bone-forming lesion of unknown etiology that is more rare than osteochondroma. *(Erickson & Caprio, 2014, pp. 880–881)*

14. **(E)** The first sign of pubertal development in boys is the enlargement of testicular size and occurs at the mean age of 11.6 years. Genital stages accelerate before pubic hair development, which occurs, on average, at 13.4 years of age. The deepening of the voice and the development of chest and axillary hair usually occur in midpuberty or 2 years after the growth of pubic hair. Growth of facial hair occurs later at approximately 16 to 17 years of age. *(Blake & Allen, 2015, pp. 239–240; Sass & Kaplan, 2014, pp. 125–127)*

15. **(A)** Huntington disease is an autosomal dominant hereditary disease. Its occurrence is between 1:5,000 and 1:20,000. It is caused by a defect on chromosome 4p16.3 that results in a repeat of "CAG" in the "Huntington" protein gene. *(Kedia et al., 2014, p. 823; Levy & Marion, 2015a, p. 147)*

16. **(D)** Rizatriptan is the only FDA-approved medication for this patient. It is approved for abortive therapy in children ages 6 to 17 years old. Almotriptan is approved for ages 12 to 17 years old. Neither dihydroergotamine, coenzyme Q10, nor topiramate is used for treatment of acute migraine and currently, there are no FDA-approved medications for prevention of migraine in children. *(Kedia et al., 2014, pp. 803–804)*

17. **(D)** Still's murmur is the most common innocent murmur of early childhood and is usually appreciated in children from 3 to 6 years of age. It is a grade I–III/VI early systolic ejection murmur of musical or vibratory quality heard best between the apex and left lower sternal border. It is loudest when the patient is in a supine position. The murmur may diminish or disappear with inspiration, during the Valsalva maneuver, or when the patient is standing or seated. A physiologic peripheral pulmonic stenosis murmur is a soft, short, high-pitched, grade I–II/VI systolic ejection murmur. Typically, it is auscultated with equal intensity at the left upper sternal border, along the back, and in both axillae. It is usually found in newborns and generally disappears

by 3 to 6 months of age. A pulmonary ejection murmur is the most common innocent murmur of later childhood and is usually seen in children 8 to 14 years of age. It is a soft, early to midsystolic ejection, grade I–III/VI murmur heard best along the left upper sternal border. It is louder when the patient is supine or with increased cardiac output. It diminishes with standing or during the Valsalva maneuver. A venous hum is a continuous musical, grade I–II/VI murmur heard at the right or left superior infraclavicular area. The murmur is obliterated when the patient is in a supine position, with head rotation, and with compression of the jugular vein. It is usually auscultated in children from 3 to 6 years of age. A patent ductus arteriosus is a continuous, machine-like murmur that represents an open pathway between the pulmonary artery and aorta. This is necessary when the fetus is in utero but should close spontaneously after birth. They represent approximately 5% to 10% of congenital heart disease. If the opening is large enough to cause significant left to right shunting, then the patient will be symptomatic. A small patent ductus arteriosus may be asymptomatic. *(Darst et al., 2014, pp. 589–590, 605–607; Schneider, 2015, pp. 484, 492–493)*

18. **(E)** Sudden infant death syndrome (SIDS) is defined as the sudden, unexplained death of an apparently healthy infant that is unexpected and not adequately explained by a comprehensive medical history, a postmortem physical, and investigation of the death scene. SIDS is a leading cause of death in infants between the ages of 1 month and 1 year, second only to congenital anomalies. The exact etiology of SIDS is unclear. Prevention of SIDS has become a focus of public health measures. In 1994, The American Academy of Pediatrics initiated a campaign called "back to sleep," which recommended placing infants in the supine position for sleep. Following the institution of this campaign in the United States, the annual death rate decreased from 1.3 per 1,000 to 0.7 per 1,000. *(Federico et al., 2014, pp. 586–587; Ong et al., 2015, pp. 462–463)*

19. **(D)** Because of the weighted end, the straight pin will migrate through the GI system of a child without concern as long as the child remains asymptomatic. Button batteries must be removed from the esophagus due to possible damage to tissue. Open safety pins and toothpicks carry a high risk of

perforation and should be removed via endoscope. A single magnet may pass, but more than one magnet ingested increases the chance for trapping of intestinal tissue and must also be removed. (*Hoffenberg et al., 2014, pp. 657–658*)

20. **(E)** A urinalysis should be performed because renal disease is the most common etiology of hypertension in children. Renal ultrasonography is performed if initial laboratory studies point to underlying renal disease as the cause. Electrocardiograms and chest radiography should be considered as part of the evaluation for end-organ disease as well as an initial basic metabolic panel to include serum creatinine. Although rare, elevated uric acid has also been shown to cause essential hypertension in children. (*Lum, 2014, pp. 767–769; Mahan & Patel, 2015, pp. 563–564*)

21. **(A)** Cytomegalovirus (CMV) is one of the congenital neonatal TORCH infections (toxoplasmosis, other [syphilis, varicella-zoster, parvovirus], rubella, CMV, herpes simplex/hepatitis/HIV). CMV is the most common congenital infection and includes the symptoms described in this question in addition to intrauterine growth retardation, thrombocytopenia, purpura, and sensorineural hearing loss. Congenital rubella is now rare in industrialized nations but causes encephalopathy, microcephaly, and cardiac defects in addition to many others. Congenital varicella is rare and causes limb hypoplasia, microcephaly, and cataracts. Toxoplasmosis manifests asymptomatically in the mother and child initially then leads to mental retardation, visual impairment, and learning disabilities. Parvovirus can lead to fetal hydrops and death in utero in 3% to 6% of cases. If the fetus survives the maternal infection in utero, there are no lasting effects in life. (*Rosenberg & Grover, 2014, pp. 62–63*)

22. **(A)** The most common injuries of child abuse are abdominal injuries, bruises in locations not consistent with mobility or mechanism, burns, fractures, and head trauma. The absence of a red reflex in a 4-month-old child is concerning for ocular disease, but not trauma or abuse. A dry, scaly rash on the cheeks is more likely eczematous rather than due to neglect or burn injury. A single weight in the 25th percentile does not imply anything, but height and weight that shows decline over time could be a sign

of neglect. Children at 4 months of age cry frequently when they are hungry or need to have their diaper changed, and crying alone, is not a sign of child abuse. (*Chiesa & Sirotnak, 2014, Ch. 8*)

23. **(C)** A febrile seizure is a brief (less than 15 minutes), generalized, symmetric, tonic–clonic seizure associated with a febrile illness (temperature greater than 38.8°C) without any central nervous system infection or neurologic cause. An absence (petit mal) seizure is a brief (2 to 25 seconds) loss of consciousness that can occur multiple times per day. There is no loss of tone, and frequently the only observable behaviors are staring or minor movements such as lip smacking and semipurposeful movements of the hands. There is no postictal period. Complex partial seizures (psychomotor) have varied symptoms including alterations in consciousness, unresponsiveness, and repetitive complex motor activities that are purposeless. Often, at the beginning of the attack, there is a psychoillusory phenomenon such as hallucinations, visual distortions, visceral sensations, or feelings of intense emotions. Simple partial seizures include focal motor, adversive, and somatosensory seizures. Manifestations of these seizures are varied including hallucinatory, psychoillusory, or complex emotional phenomena. Children will interact normally with their environment, with the exception of those limitations imposed by the seizure. Following the seizure (minutes to hours), there may be transient paralysis of the affected body part. Psychogenic nonepileptic seizures are manifestations of conversion disorders or malingering. These episodes can be difficult to distinguish from epileptic seizures. Generally the eyes are closed and the physical activity is more of a thrashing nature than tonic–clonic activity. Urinary and bowel function are often preserved. (*Kedia et al., 2014, pp. 786–789, 792; Schiller & Shellhaas, 2015, pp. 618–621*)

24. **(B)** Urinary tract infections (UTIs) are one of the most common infections in children. Clinical features of a UTI vary depending upon the age and sex of the child. In newborns, the most common symptom is failure to thrive associated with poor feeding, diarrhea, and vomiting. In infants, the symptoms may be relatively nonspecific, such as poor feeding, failure to gain weight, vomiting, fever, strong-smelling urine, and irritability. As children grow older,

the initial signs and symptoms become more specific to the urinary tract. In early infancy, males are two times more likely than girls to have a UTI. Also, uncircumcised males are 10 times more likely to be affected than circumcised males. *Escherichia coli* is the most common pathogen for the first UTI (80%) and of recurrent infections (75%). Other organisms that cause infections include *Pseudomonas aeruginosa*, Proteus species, Enterobacter species, *Klebsiella pneumoniae*, and *Enterococcus faecalis*. An infection with *Staphylococcus saprophyticus*, a coagulase-negative staphylococcus, is primarily seen in adolescents with a UTI. *(Kronman & Smith, 2015, pp. 372–374; Lum, 2014, pp. 773–775)*

25. **(E)** Unintentional injury (motor vehicle crashes and unintentional poisoning) is the leading cause of adolescent death in the United States. Unintentional poisoning includes prescription drug overdose and this category has continued to rise over the past decade. Homicide (majority from firearms) and suicide (from firearms and suffocation) account for a smaller percentage of deaths, but are followed by cancer and heart disease. *(Sass & Kaplan, 2014, p. 117)*

26. **(D)** Intussusception is the most common cause of intestinal obstruction between 3 months and 6 years of age. It is twice as common in males than females. It is caused by intestinal invagination, usually around the ileocecal valve. The classic presentation is intermittent severe colicky abdominal pain with legs drawn up, followed by periods of comfort or falling asleep. Vomiting usually occurs in the early phase, which later becomes bilious. A passage of blood and mucus in the stool ("currant jelly stools") occurs in 60% of the cases. Palpation of the abdomen usually reveals a sausage-shaped mass in the right upper quadrant. The classic presentation of pyloric stenosis is in first-born males of 3 to 6 weeks of age, presenting with nonbilious projectile vomiting leading to dehydration with hypochloremia, hypokalemia, and metabolic alkalosis. A firm, movable, 2-cm olive-shaped mass ("olive") is palpable superior and to the right of the umbilicus in the midepigastrium. In addition, peristaltic waves may be visible on the physical examination. The classic presentation of appendicitis presents with a period of anorexia followed by steady periumbilical pain shifting to the right lower quadrant; nausea and vomiting is followed by a low-grade fever. Diarrhea

(nonbloody and nonmucous), if it occurs, is infrequent. Peritoneal signs are present. The incidence increases with age and peaks during adolescence. Infective enteritis usually begins with emesis followed by crampy abdominal pain of hyperperistalsis. This sequence of symptoms with emesis preceding pain is an important factor in distinguishing it from intussusception. Masses are not palpated with infective enteritis. Celiac disease is an immune-mediated injury to the small intestine when gluten is ingested. Symptoms can begin at any age and directly correlate with gluten ingestion. Symptoms include abdominal pain, bloating, and diarrhea. Vomiting typically does not occur. No masses are palpated. *(Bishop & Ebach, 2015, pp. 435–436, 442–444; Hoffenberg et al., 2014, pp. 658–659, 665–666, 668–669, 678–679, 688)*

27. **(D)** Children should have assistance in brushing and flossing until the age of 8 years. At that point, their manual dexterity is developed enough for proper technique. From the time teeth erupt until the age of 8 years, an adult should assist the child in brushing and flossing twice daily. *(Klein, 2014, Ch. 17)*

28. **(C)** The most common etiologic organisms for bacterial meningitis in children are *Streptococcus pneumoniae, Neisseria meningitidis,* and *Haemophilus influenzae.* Because of an increase in resistant *S. pneumoniae,* coverage with vancomycin and a third-generation cephalosporin such as cefotaxime or ceftriaxone is needed for best coverage. Gentamicin can be used but, as with all aminoglycosides, caution is needed regarding toxicity. Ampicillin, rifampin, chloramphenicol, and dexamethasone are alternative treatments if necessary. These are considered on a case-by-case basis. *(Kedia et al., 2014, pp. 836–837)*

29. **(B)** Congenital hypothyroidism is one of the most common disorders tested for in newborn screening tests, revealing an elevated TSH (thyroid stimulating hormone) and a decreased T_4 (thyroxine). Symptoms suggestive of congenital hypothyroidism in the neonate include hypotonia, coarse facial features, hirsute forehead, large fontanels (anterior and posterior), widely open sutures, umbilical hernia, protruding/large tongue, hoarse cry, distended abdomen, and prolonged jaundice. Signs of congenital hypothyroidism include lethargy or hypoactivity,

poor feeding, constipation, mottling, and hypothermia. Congenital adrenal hyperplasia (CAH) is not universally screened for in the newborn screening test, as it is included in 14 of the 50 states. In females with CAH, there may be virilization with abnormalities of the external genitalia varying from mild enlargement of the clitoris to complete fusion of the labioscrotal folds. Signs of adrenal insufficiency (salt loss) may present in the first few days of life. Crigler–Najjar syndrome is not one of the disorders tested for in the standard newborn screening tests. It is an inherited disease producing congenital nonobstructive, nonhemolytic, unconjugated severe hyperbilirubinemia. The physical findings in this infant do not correlate with Crigler–Najjar syndrome. Galactosemia is tested for in the newborn screening test in nearly all 50 states. The infant may have symptoms of cataract, hepatomegaly, and prolonged jaundice. Often, these neonates have *Escherichia coli* sepsis, leading to death in the first 2 weeks of life if not treated promptly. Gilbert syndrome is a familial hyperbilirubinemia secondary to reduced enzymatic activity. It is not tested for in the standard newborn screening. Other than jaundice, there are no physical findings associated with Gilbert syndrome. *(Sokol et al., 2014, p. 707; Thomas & Van Hove, 2014, pp. 1112–1113; Zeitler et al., 2014, pp. 1065–1067, 1089–1091)*

30. **(A)** Caput succedaneum is a result of fluid and blood accumulation in the occipitoparietal region of the newborn's scalp due to the vacuum effect of membrane rupture. A cephalohematoma is a firm, tense external swelling of the cranium that does *not* extend across suture lines because it is limited to the surface of one cranial bone. It occurs most often in the parietal area. This subperiosteal hemorrhage usually is not present at birth, but develops within the first 24 hours of life. Craniotabes is a condition caused by the osteoporosis of the outer table of the involved membranous bone, generally over the temporoparietal or parieto-occipital areas, creating a "ping-pong ball" sensation when gentle pressure is applied. A subgaleal hemorrhage is a firm, fluctuant external swelling of the cranium that does extend across suture lines and increases in size over time. Skull fractures are usually linear. They rarely occur as a result of birth trauma. Treatment is observation. *(Gowen, 2015, pp. 198–199, 202–203; Rosenberg & Grover, 2014, p. 14)*

31. **(C)** Foreign-body aspiration into the respiratory tract is associated with an acute choking or coughing episode with expiratory wheezing (indicative of a lower airway obstruction) in children aged 6 months to 4 years of age. Often, there is a history of the child playing with small toys that are commonly aspirated. Asymmetrical physical findings of decreased breath sounds and localized wheezing are present with foreign-body aspiration. A positive forced expiratory chest x-ray shows a mediastinal shift away from the affected side. Radiolucent foreign bodies such as plastic toys may not appear on an x-ray, but there will be evidence of this mediastinal shift. Asthma is generally characterized by wheezing, but it is neither unilateral nor is of sudden onset. A chest x-ray reveals bilateral hyperinflation with flattening of the diaphragm. Epiglottitis is a life-threatening upper airway obstructive condition that presents with a sudden onset of fever, dysphagia, drooling, and inspiratory retractions with stridor. A lateral neck x-ray reveals an enlarged, indistinct epiglottis ("thumb sign"); however, the chest x-ray is normal. Pulmonary embolism, rare in children, presents clinically with acute dyspnea, tachypnea, and tachycardia. There may be mild hypoxemia, rales, and focal wheezing. Chest x-rays may be normal, or there may be a peripheral infiltrate, small pleural effusion, or elevated hemidiaphragm. Tracheomalacia is a loss of rigidity in the trachea due to a problem with the cartilaginous rings that give the trachea its structure. The cartilage may be absent, damaged, or shortened. This allows the trachea to collapse during exhalation, presenting as expiratory wheezes or barky cough. Inspiratory effort is normal. Viral infections exacerbate tracheomalacia. Imaging is not necessary. *(Chiu, 2015a, pp. 273–282; Kronman & Smith, 2015, p. 354; Ong et al., 2015, pp. 470–471, 474–475)*

32. **(C)** An acute salicylate overdose (greater than 150 mg/kg) will produce symptoms of salicylate intoxication in children this age within a few hours of ingestion. Chronic salicylate intoxication occurs with ingestion of greater than 100 mg/kg/day for at least 2 days. Salicylates affect most organ systems, leading to various metabolic abnormalities. Because salicylates are a gastric irritant, symptoms of vomiting and diarrhea occur soon after the overdose, which may contribute to the development of dehydration. Salicylates stimulate the respiratory center

leading to hyperventilation and hyperpnea resulting in respiratory alkalosis and compensatory alkaluria and evidence is seen of this at its peak 12 to 24 hours after ingestion. Enteric-coated aspirin can cause effects to manifest less predictably. A characteristic feature of salicylate intoxication is the coexistence of a respiratory alkalosis with a widened anion gap metabolic acidosis. *(Greenbaum & Bou-Matar, 2015, p. 121; Wang et al., 2014, pp. 382–383)*

33. **(C)** Generalized tetanus (lockjaw) is a neurologic disease caused by *Clostridium tetani.* Although any open wound is a potential source for contamination with *C. tetani,* those with dirt, soil, feces, or saliva are at increased risk. Tetanus-prone wounds contain devitalized tissue, especially those caused by punctures, frostbite, crush injury, or burns. Recommendations for tetanus prophylaxis in a child with a laceration or abrasion depend upon the number of previous vaccinations, occurrence of last booster, type of wound (clean or tetanus-prone), and age of child. In this case, the patient is older than 7 years and had all of his previous immunizations; however, his most recent booster was greater than 10 years ago. Thus, he should receive an adult-type diphtheria and tetanus toxoid with acellular pertussis. In most cases, when tetanus toxoid is required for wound prophylaxis in a child older than 7 years, the Td instead of tetanus toxoid alone is recommended so that diphtheria immunity is maintained. If tetanus immunization is not up to date at the time of wound treatment, then the immunization series should be completed according to the primary immunization schedule. If a child is younger than 7 years, then the diphtheria, tetanus, acellular pertussis (DTaP) booster is indicated, unless there is a contraindication for pertussis, in which case the diphtheria and tetanus (DT) booster should be administered. Tetanus immune globulin (TIG) is recommended for treatment of tetanus. Under special circumstances, a patient infected with the human immunodeficiency virus (HIV) with a tetanus-prone wound should also receive TIG in addition to the prophylactic vaccine. *(Daley et al., 2014, pp. 282–284)*

34. **(C)** Normally, primitive reflexes are present at birth and should not persist beyond the age of 6 months. However, the parachute reflex is a postural response that normally appears around 7 months of age to coincide with volitional movement and persists for life. It occurs when an infant is held prone by the waist over a surface and lowered with the head downward and extends the arms and legs as a form of protection. The rooting reflex (when the cheek is stroked on the infant and they turn his/her head to feed) and Galant (trunk incurvation upon stroking the back) reflexes disappear by the age of 4 months. The placing (when dorsum of foot comes into contact with a surface the infant places foot onto surface) and Moro (when light drop of head leads to sudden extension then immediate flexion of extremities) reflexes disappear at 6 months. *(Schiller & Shellhaas, 2015, p. 613)*

35. **(B)** Gonococcal ophthalmia neonatorum presents as a unilateral or bilateral serosanguineous discharge and then within 24 hours the discharge becomes mucopurulent, followed by conjunctival injection and edema of the eyelids. The usual incubation period for *Neisseria gonorrhoeae* is 2 to 5 days; however, the infection may be present at birth or delayed greater than 5 days if there has been instillation of silver nitrate prophylaxis. A presumptive diagnosis is made by the demonstration of gram-negative intracellular diplococci on gram stain. Definitive diagnosis is made by culture. Following a positive gram stain and pending culture results, treatment should be promptly initiated with ceftriaxone (50 mg/kg/24 hours IV or IM for one dose not to exceed 125 mg), a third-generation cephalosporin with good coverage for gram-negative bacteria. An alternate drug is cefotaxime (100 mg/kg/24 hours IV or IM every 12 hours for 7 days or 100 mg/kg as a single dose), which is also a third-generation cephalosporin. Although erythromycin drops (0.5%) are used prophylactically for *N. gonorrhoeae,* this is not an effective treatment. Gentamicin would be used for Pseudomonas and Chlamydia is treated with erythromycin. Acyclovir is an antiviral used to treat herpes viral infections, which is a cause of neonatal conjunctivitis. Cephalexin as a first-generation cephalosporin does not have coverage for gram-negative bacteria. *(Kronman & Smith, 2015, pp. 386–389; Rosenberg & Grover, 2014, p. 61)*

36. **(B)** The most likely diagnosis in this patient is mumps. It is endemic in most unvaccinated populations, though increasing in incidence in the United States due to the antivaccination movement. Cranial

nerve palsies are a complication that may be transient or permanent and can lead to deafness. The onset of mumps is characterized by pain and swelling in one or both parotid glands. The pain can be exacerbated by tasting sour liquids such as lemon juice. An elevated serum amylase level is common and coincides with the parotid swelling. Other complications include meningoencephalomyelitis, orchitis, epididymitis, pancreatitis, arthritis, and rarely thyroiditis and myocarditis. *(Levin & Weinberg, 2014, pp. 1264–1265)*

37. **(A)** Café au lait spots are brown patches that may be found on any part of the body. The presentation of six or more spots greater than 1.5 cm is a sign of neurofibromatosis, a genetic disorder that results in neurofibromas that can develop in any organ/tissue system. Miliaria are blocked sweat gland ducts that are commonly found on the face, scalp, or intertriginous areas. Vernix caseosa is a normal finding in newborns and is a whitish, greasy layering on the body—it decreases as an infant comes to full term. Subconjunctival hemorrhages are a common finding in infants secondary to birth trauma. Hemangiomas are commonly noted on newborn examination. These benign tumors will resolve spontaneously over 3 to 10 years. They can lead to functional problems depending on their location. *(Chiu, 2015b, pp. 659–662; Gowen, 2015, pp. 197–199; Schiller & Shellhaas, 2015, pp. 645–646)*

38. **(C)** The Apgar score assesses the newborn at 1-minute and 5-minute intervals to determine the need for resuscitative care. The infant is evaluated by heart rate, respiratory effort, muscle tone, response to catheter in nostril, and color, and each is rated on a scale of 0, 1, or 2 for a total score of 10. The heart rate is scaled 0 to 2 for absent, less than 100 bpm (slow), and greater than 100 bpm; respiratory effort of absent, slow/irregular, and good crying. Muscle tone scale (0–2) consists of limp, some flexion, and active motion; response to catheter stimulation (0–2) is scaled no response, grimace, and cough/sneeze. Finally, color is scored 0 to 2 for blue/pale, body pink with blue extremities, and completely pink. *(Gowen, 2015, p. 194; Rosenberg & Grover, 2014, pp. 12–13)*

39. **(E)** Ventricular septal defect, a hole between the two ventricles, can be cyanotic or acyanotic based on the size of the defect, and accounts for 30% of cases of congenital heart disease. Atrial septal defect occurs in approximately 10% of congenital heart disease cases. Transposition of great vessels is an embryonic malformation resulting in the aorta arising from the right ventricle and the pulmonary artery arising from the left ventricle. It is responsible for about 10% of all congenital malformations. Tetralogy of Fallot, consisting of a ventricular septal defect, overriding aorta, pulmonic/subpulmonic stenosis, and right ventricular hypertrophy, accounts for 10% of congenital heart disease. Atrioventricular septal defect is an incomplete fusion of the embryonic endocardial cushions that form the lower atrial septum and membranous portions of the ventricular septum. It accounts for 4% of congenital heart disease but has a higher incidence in children with Down syndrome. *(Darst et al., 2014, pp. 601–605, 616–617, 621–623; Schneider, 2015, pp. 491–493, 495–497)*

40. **(E)** The immunization schedule is developed biannually by the Centers for Disease Control and Prevention. Assuming that the child has had the appropriate immunizations at the regularly scheduled examinations, the recommended immunizations at the 4- to 6-year-old range are the DTaP (diphtheria, tetanus, acellular pertussis), IPV (inactivated polio), MMR (measles, mumps, and rubella) and varicella. The hepatitis series should have been completed by the age of 6 months and the *Haemophilus influenzae* type B (Hib) should be completed by the age of 12 to 15 months; the PCV (pneumococcal) should be finished by 12 to 15 months. *(Centers for Disease Control and Prevention, 2015)*

41. **(E)** There are only two known absolute contraindications to breastfeeding: active tuberculosis of the mother and galactosemia of the infant. The highly contagious nature of tuberculosis makes the risk greater than the benefit, and infants with galactosemia are unable to digest any lactose due to an enzyme deficiency. Infants of mothers in a methadone program may be breastfed as long as the mother's dose is less than 40 mg. While nicotine is transmitted in breast milk and is therefore strongly discouraged, it is not an absolute contraindication. As long as a breast-fed infant with cystic fibrosis is maintaining normal growth with supplemented

pancreatic enzymes, breastfeeding is encouraged. Maternal HIV infection is not an absolute contraindication to breastfeeding. In developed countries, it is not recommended as safe alternatives are available; however in developing countries the benefits outweigh the risks. *(Buchanan & Marquez, 2015, pp. 87–88; Haemer et al., 2014, pp. 311–313)*

42. **(C)** Failure to thrive is diagnosed in infants younger than the age of 6 months with a decrease in growth velocity that results in a decrease in two major percentile lines on the growth chart. In the case of this patient, she was initially in the 50th percentile and crossed the 25th and 10th percentile and fell into the fifth percentile. Failure to thrive is also known as growth deficiency and may also be diagnosed if the child is younger than 6 months and has not grown for 2 consecutive months or if a child is older than 6 months and has not grown for 3 consecutive months. Growth hormone deficiency/dwarfism may present with decreased growth velocity later in childhood; the drop in percentiles is grossly below the fifth percentile mark. Lactose intolerance presents with varying gastrointestinal symptoms without the marked decrease in weight. Beckwith–Wiedemann syndrome consists of macrosomia, macroglossia, and omphalocele and they are at increased risk for malignancies, hypoglycemia, and dysmorphism (usually of the ears). Laron syndrome is a rare cause of growth hormone deficiency by mutations of the growth hormone receptor. It is an autosomal recessive disorder and has associated dysmorphic features. *(Christian & Blum, 2015, pp. 67–69; Palma Sisto & Heneghan, 2015, p. 588; Saenz et al., 2014, p. 1161; Treitz et al., 2014, pp. 269–270)*

43. **(E)** This patient has presented with classical findings of Reye syndrome—upper respiratory infection followed by unresponsiveness. Reye syndrome is usually preceded by an upper respiratory tract illness, which progresses into vomiting, strange behavior, stupor, and coma. Liver function tests (LFTs) and ammonia levels will be markedly elevated (without jaundice); however, the serum bilirubin and alkaline phosphatase are normal. Unresponsive patients who have a spinal tap will show no cells in the CSF and glucose may be low with increased CSF pressure. Treatment for patients with Reye syndrome is largely supportive—specifically decreasing cerebral edema. There is no place

for antibiotics or steroids. The liver will fully recover if the cerebral edema is decreased. *(Kedia et al., 2014, p. 839; Stone, 2011, Ch. 37)*

44. **(E)** Physiologic jaundice of the newborn, which occurs in up to 60% of newborns in the first week, is due to the breakdown of heme in the presence of decrease intestinal motility and the lack of normal gut flora. It is not due to the digestion of breast milk, rather it is due to the insufficient amounts of breast milk in the early feeding timeframe. Rh-incompatibility is a cause of jaundice but is rare and pathologic, not physiologic. The liver itself is not diseased in physiologic jaundice of the newborn and the red blood cells are normal. *(Rosenberg & Grover, 2014, pp. 19–22)*

45. **(E)** The patient's presentation is consistent with findings of coarctation of the aorta. The pathognomonic finding in coarctation is decreased or absent femoral pulses. However, the majority of children show no signs of coarctation in infancy and develop signs and symptoms during childhood, most notably unequal pulses and blood pressure between arms and legs (arms lower than legs). In addition, a grade II/VI systolic ejection murmur is heard at the aortic area and left sternal border that radiates into the left axilla and left back. Chest x-ray shows a normal-sized heart, a prominent aorta, indents at the level of the coarctation, and a dilated poststenotic segment resulting in the "figure 3" sign. Scalloping or notching of the ribs is due to enlargement of the intercostal arteries. Echocardiography is used to directly visualize the coarctation and estimate the obstruction. Asymptomatic infants and children are encouraged to have corrective surgery prior to age 5, after which they are at increased risk for myocardial dysfunction and hypertension, and require exercise testing prior to participation in aerobic activities. The boot-shaped heart is seen in patients with tetralogy of Fallot secondary to right ventricular hypertrophy; the narrowed mediastinum finding with "egg on a string" is typically seen in patients with transposition of the great vessels. *(Darst et al., 2014, pp. 610–611, 616–617, 621–622; Schneider, 2015, pp. 494–496)*

46. **(A)** Viral croup usually presents with cough that may sound like a dog or a seal barking. The patients are usually afebrile and also present with stridor

either at rest, in severe cases, or when agitated, in mild cases. In addition, the patient may be cyanotic and have retractions and acute shortness of breath. Radiologic examination of the neck shows subglottic narrowing with a normal epiglottis, "steeple sign." However, x-rays are usually not indicated in patients with the common presenting symptoms. Treatment for viral croup is mainly symptomatic, especially in mild cases consisting of oral hydration and mist therapy. Severe cases (stridor at rest) call for oxygen in patients who have desaturated, and nebulized racemic epinephrine and glucocorticoids. Dexamethasone as an intramuscular injection or oral as an one-time dose is effective in alleviating symptoms, decreasing the need for intubation, and decreasing hospital stays. Inhaled budesonide is also effective in decreasing hospital stays and improving symptoms, but dexamethasone is more cost-effective. Patients who are unable to be stabilized need airway maintenance either by intubation with endotracheal tube or by tracheostomy if intubation fails. Because it is a self-limiting disorder, unless there is a secondary infection most children recover in a few days. *(Federico et al., 2014, pp. 545–547; Kronman & Smith, 2015, pp. 354–356)*

47. **(A)** Cystic fibrosis (CF) is a major cause of gastrointestinal and pulmonary morbidity in children due to mutations in the CF genes. The mutations lead to a deficiency in cystic fibrosis transmembrane conductance regulator protein that controls movement of salt and water into and out of epithelial cells and results in production of abnormally thick mucus. About 15% of patients with CF present with meconium ileus at birth. This is typically treated with enema for disimpaction and rarely surgery. Approximately half of the infants with CF will present with failure to thrive, which is diagnosed by lack of growth for 2 consecutive months in patients younger than 6 months of age. They may also present with respiratory compromise. However, not all patients present in childhood. Diagnosis of CF is confirmed by a sweat chloride level above 60 mEq/L or with genetic testing. Treatment for patients with CF is mainly symptomatic therapy for obstructions of the digestive and respiratory tract. In addition, there is pancreatic enzyme supplementation to aid in digestion and vitamin and calorie supplementation for deficiencies in the diet. Gene therapy is now being looked at for future treatment.

Intussusception (telescoping of the small intestine) typically presents in an infant with paroxysmal abdominal pain, vomiting, and diarrhea that may progress into bloody stools. Volvulus is normally the result of intestinal malrotation that causes occlusion of the superior mesenteric artery and eventual bowel necrosis. Infants typically present within 3 weeks of life with bile-stained vomiting and bowel obstruction. Wilson disease is the defect in the ability to excrete copper in the bile that results in accumulation of copper in the liver. Distal intestinal obstruction syndrome is intestinal obstruction that occurs secondary to inspissated mucus. *(Federico et al., 2014, pp. 551–552; Hoffenberg et al., 2014, pp. 665–666; Ong et al., 2015, pp. 475–478; Sokol et al., 2014, pp. 720–721)*

48. **(A)** Cyanotic heart lesions are a result of a right-to-left shunt. These include tetralogy of Fallot, pulmonary atresia with and without ventricular septal defect, tricuspid atresia, truncus arteriosus, hypoplastic left heart syndrome, and transposition of the great arteries. The right-to-left shunt results in deoxygenated blood reaching the left ventricle, aorta, and systemic arteries. The decreased oxygen in the blood results in decreased oxygen to the tissue and subsequently causes cyanosis. Atrial septal defect, ventricular septal defect, atrioventricular septal defect, and patent ductus arteriosus most commonly present with a left-to-right shunt and are acyanotic in nature. *(Darst et al., 2014, pp. 616–626; Schneider, 2015, pp. 495–499)*

49. **(D)** This infant is presenting with signs and symptoms of pyloric stenosis. Infants typically have vomiting (projectile at times) after every feeding and it normally starts between the age of 2 and 4 weeks. The infant nurses fervently and is hungry. In addition, there may be dehydration, constipation, weight loss, and apathy. Abdomen may be distended with gastric peristaltic waves. Occasionally, an olive-sized mass can be felt in the right upper quadrant with deep palpation after the child has vomited. Vomitus is typically nonbilious. Diagnosis is confirmed by an upper gastrointestinal series with delayed gastric emptying, enlarged pyloric muscle, and characteristic semilunar impressions on the gastric antrum. In addition, an ultrasound is needed to verify the hypertrophic muscle. The treatment of choice for these patients is pyloromyotomy, which

can be done laparoscopically. These patients make full recoveries and have an excellent prognosis. *(Bishop & Ebach, 2015, pp. 435–436; Hoffenberg et al., 2014, pp. 658–659)*

50. **(B)** Celiac disease or gluten enteropathy typically presents with diarrhea episodes in the first 6 to 12 months of life—when whole grains are first fed. Therefore, in strictly breast-fed babies, symptoms may not be noticed until solid foods are begun. The diarrhea is usually intermittent at first and then typically progresses into pale, greasy, foul-smelling, frothy stools. Additional symptoms may be constipation, vomiting, and abdominal pain, which may lead the clinician to think of intestinal obstruction. Other findings may be failure to thrive, anemia, and vitamin deficiencies. Stool sample demonstrates excessive fecal fat excretion. Blood tests show hypoproteinemia and impaired carbohydrate absorption. Intestinal biopsy is the diagnostic test of choice for celiac disease. Results show shortened celiac mucosa, absent villi, lengthened crypts of Lieberkü hn, plasma cell infiltration of the lamina propria, and intraepithelial lymphocytes. Treatment consists of dietary restriction of gluten—wheat, rye, and barley. Steroids are given on as needed basis. Sweat chloride testing is utilized in patients suspected of cystic fibrosis. Gastrin level is taken in patients suspected of Zollinger–Ellison syndrome, and RAST (radioallergosorbent assay test) is used in patients to determine different environmental-type allergens. Stool ova and parasites is ordered when there is suspicion of a parasitic infection. *(Bishop & Ebach, 2015, p. 442; Chiu, 2015a, pp. 272–273; Hoffenberg et al., 2014, pp. 688–689; Kronman & Smith, 2015, pp. 404–407)*

51. **(A)** The most likely diagnosis for this patient is poststreptococcal glomerulonephritis. The diagnosis is supported by a documented culture of group A beta-hemolytic streptococcus infection. If a culture is not available, like of the patient in this scenario, the clinician can order an antistreptolysin O titer. Antistreptolysin is an enzyme released by group A streptococcus and is elevated for up to 1 month after strep infection. Glomerulonephritis presents with gross hematuria with or without edema. Hypertension, proteinuria, ascites, and headache may also be present. Treatment with antibiotics is useful if infection is still present, and, if necessary, symptomatic treatment for renal failure is done with

hemodialysis. Symptoms typically resolve within a few weeks. The monospot is used to diagnose infectious mononucleosis. Renal biopsy could be performed on extreme cases of glomerulonephritis but is not typically necessary. Immunoglobulin electrophoresis would be utilized in patients suspected of having immunoglobulinopathies or IgA-mediated glomerulonephritis. Renal ultrasound is done to assess structural abnormalities or renal blood flow. *(Lum, 2014, pp. 755,757–759; Mahan & Patel, 2015, pp. 556, 558–560)*

52. **(B)** Patent ductus arteriosus (PDA) is an isolated abnormality that occurs in infants. The ductus arteriosus is a normal fetal vessel that joins the aorta and pulmonary artery and spontaneously closes after 3 to 5 days. Lack of closure results in the audible murmur that is "machine-like" and maximal at the second intercostal space (ICS), at the left sternal border (LSB), and inferior to the clavicle. It is typically a pansystolic murmur with bounding pulses and a widened pulse pressure. There is also a paradoxical splitting of S_1 and S_2. Echocardiography confirms the PDA, direction and degree of shunting, and presence of lesions for which the PDA is needed to keep. If there are no other cardiac malformations requiring the PDA, then if the PDA is large, surgery should be completed before 1 year of age. Symptomatic PDAs that are relatively small may be closed with indomethacin in preterm infants. The murmur heard in atrial septal defect (ASD) usually is an ejection type, systolic murmur heard best at the LSB, second ICS with a wide, fixed S_2 and normal pulses. Ventricular septal defect (VSD) presents with a harsh, pansystolic murmur heard best at the third and fourth ICS. With increasing size of the VSD, heaves, thrills, and lifts are present along with radiation throughout the chest. Tetralogy of Fallot presents with a rough, ejection, systolic murmur heard best at the LSB and the third ICS with radiation to the back. The clinical presentation of pulmonary stenosis varies according to severity. It can range from asymptomatic with mild disease to cyanotic in severe disease. A systolic ejection murmur at the second ICS with radiation to the back is characteristic. *(Darst et al., 2014, pp. 601–608, 616–617; Schneider, 2015, pp. 491–496)*

53. **(A)** Hypertrophic cardiomyopathy in adolescence is typically due to familial hypertrophic cardiomyopathy

with an incidence of 1:500. Many patients are asymptomatic until a sporting event, which may cause symptoms, specifically sudden cardiac death. Examination may demonstrate a palpable or audible S_4, a left ventricular heave, systolic ejection murmur (may need to stimulate cardiac activity), and/or a left precordial bulge. Echocardiography is the gold standard for diagnosis but family history should be assessed. Stress testing is indicated to assess for ischemia and arrhythmias. Strenuous activities are prohibited for these patients. The other cardiomyopathies (dilated and restrictive) are next but are not as common. Congenital structural abnormalities of the coronary arteries are the next most common cause. Valvular disorders, including surgically repaired aortic stenosis, are typically not causes of sudden death, but these patients should be screened for symptoms and stress tested as necessary. Pericarditis is an inflammation of the pericardium. It presents with sharp pain in the chest, neck, or shoulder that is worsened with deep inspiration. Death can occur if an effusion develops leading to restriction of the heart's contractility. *(Darst et al., 2014, pp. 611–613, 626–628, 631–634; Schneider, 2015, pp. 494, 501–505)*

54. **(E)** This patient presentation describes epiglottitis. Although there is a decreased incidence of epiglottitis secondary to the introduction of the vaccine for *Haemophilus influenzae* type B (Hib), patients still present with sudden onset of fever, dysphagia, muffled voice, drooling, cyanosis, inspiratory retractions, and soft stridor. The patients are usually sitting in a tripod position to aid their breathing. Recognition of the classic symptoms needs to be immediate to stabilize the patient's airway, as these patients will decompensate into respiratory failure quickly. In the event that there is time, a lateral neck x-ray will show the "thumb sign," which is an enlarged, undistinguished epiglottis. Treatment for the patient requires intubation for airway stabilization, blood cultures and throat/epiglottis cultures, and antibiotic coverage for *H. influenzae*. The steeple sign is seen in patients with croup and is due to a subglottic narrowing. The "figure 3" sign is seen in patients with coarctation of the aorta. The "Scottie dog" sign is seen in oblique lumbar films and is a normal finding representing the pars interarticularis. Its absence signifies spondylolysis. The "spine sign" refers to a disruption of progressive lucency of the thoracic vertebral bodies on a lateral chest radiograph when going down the spine. This is indicative of lower lobe pneumonia. *(Darst et al., 2014, p. 610; Kronman & Smith, 2015, p. 354)*

55. **(B)** Tetralogy of Fallot is a congenital heart lesion that causes episodic dyspnea, cyanosis, syncope, and decrease murmur with exercise in children and feeding or crying in infants. The four components are pulmonary outflow obstruction, VSD, RV hypertrophy, and overriding aorta, and these contribute to the symptoms described above. Blood pressure discrepancy is seen with coarctation of the aorta. Orthopnea and PND are associated with pulmonary artery congestion and widened pulse pressure is associated with peripheral vascular resistance. *(Darst et al., 2014, pp. 616–617)*

56. **(B)** The most common etiology of gynecomastia is idiopathic. Occurring in 50% to 60% of adolescent males, idiopathic gynecomastia typically is self-limited. Additional uncommon etiologies of gynecomastia include liver disease, hyperthyroidism, illicit drugs (marijuana, heroin), neoplasms (adrenal, testicular), genetic disease (Klinefelter syndrome, cystic fibrosis), and medications (e.g., antacids, chemotherapy). *(Palma Sisto & Heneghan, 2015, p. 596; Sass & Kaplan, 2014, pp. 138–139)*

57. **(B)** Guillain–Barré syndrome is most likely due to a delayed hypersensitivity with T-cell–mediated antibodies to mycoplasma and viral infections (CMV, EBV, hepatitis B, *Campylobacter jejuni*). The patients may mention a nonspecific respiratory or gastrointestinal infection 1 to 2 weeks prior to symptoms. Complaints may be paresthesias, weakness in bilateral lower extremities with occasional ascension into the arms, trunk, and face, and rarely ataxia and ophthalmoplegia in the Miller Fisher variant. Examination findings demonstrate symmetric flaccid weakness, with impairment of position, vibration, and touch in the distal portions of the extremities. If a spinal tap is performed, it may show few polymorphonuclear neutrophils with high protein and normal glucose. EMG is positive for decreased nerve conduction. Laboratory tests may show high titers of suspected infections or active infection of hepatitis/bacterial pathogens. Guillain–Barré is normally a self-limiting disorder within a few weeks, unless there are issues with respiratory

depression. Poliomyelitis is secondary to polioviruses and presents with fever, paralysis, meningeal signs, and asymmetrical weakness. Botulism secondary to infection with *Clostridium botulinum* in older children presents with blurred vision, diplopia, ptosis, choking, and weakness. In infants, botulism presents as constipation, poor suck and cry, apnea, lethargy, and choking. Tick-bite paralysis presents with rapid onset with ascending flaccid paralysis reaching upper extremities in a couple of days of onset and patients often present with paresthesias and pain. Finding of a tick is usually confirmatory for these patients. Transverse myelitis typically occurs after a viral infection. Early presentation is paraplegia and areflexia with possible hyperreflexia later. Fever is noted in about 50% of cases. *(Kedia et al., 2014, pp. 842–843; Schiller & Shelhaas, 2015, pp. 625–627)*

58. **(B)** Scoliosis is defined by lateral curvature of the spine with rotation of vertebrae and is typically located in the thoracic or lumbar spine in the right or left directions. Idiopathic scoliosis most commonly presents as a right thoracic curve in females from 8 to 10 years of age. Scoliosis is typically asymptomatic unless curvatures are so severe that there is pulmonary dysfunction or there is an underlying disorder (bone or spinal tumor) that is causing the scoliosis. X-rays need to be taken of the entire spine to help determine the degree of curvature. Treatment modalities are based on the degree of curvature: 20 degrees or less does not normally require treatment; 20 to 40 degrees is an indication for bracing in an immature child; and 40 degrees and greater is resistant to bracing and requires surgical fixation with spinal fusion, which is best done at special centers. A greater than 70-degree curvature is associated with poor respiratory function in adulthood. *(Erickson & Caprio, 2014, pp. 867–868; Walter & Tassone, 2015, pp. 685–686)*

59. **(A)** Legg–Calvé–Perthes disease is also known as avascular necrosis of the proximal femur. It typically occurs in children between 4 and 8 years old and persistent hip pain is the main symptom. On examination, the clinician notices a limp and/or limitation of motion of the affected hip. Radiologic examination demonstrates the necrosis with effusion and joint space widening with a negative aspirate. Treatment involves surgical hip replacement.

Slipped capital femoral epiphysis (SCFE) is due to the displacement of the proximal femoral epiphysis owing to disruption of the growth plate. The head is normally displaced medially and posteriorly relative to the femoral neck. It typically occurs in adolescence, specifically obese males, and can also be associated with hypothyroidism. SCFE usually occurs after direct trauma to the hip or a fall. Patients complain of vague symptoms at first that progress into pain of the hip or knee. On examination, there is decreased internal rotation of the hip that can be confirmed by lateral x-ray of the hip. Septic hip arthritis is not common in children between the age of 5 and 12 years. The legs are held in external rotation to minimize pain and will have a positive aspirate. Osteochondritis dissecans typically presents in the knee, elbow, and talus and is characterized by a wedge-shaped necrosis of bone. Tuberculosis arthritis is rare in the United States and commonly affects the intervertebral disks. *(Erickson & Caprio, 2014, pp. 877–879; Kronman & Smith, 2015, pp. 384–386; Walter & Tassone, 2015, pp. 685–686)*

60. **(B)** Gamekeeper thumb is a result of damage to the ulnar collateral ligament during forced abduction of the metacarpophalangeal joint, an injury that is most commonly seen in skiers. An avulsed fragment may or may not be seen on radiologic examination. If the fragment is smaller than 2 mm, a thumb spica cast can be used. If no fragment or joint space opening is seen, a spica cast is indicated for 4 to 6 weeks. If the fragment is larger than 2 mm, surgery is required. Mallet finger is an avulsion of the extensor tendon and occurs in ball-handling sports. Boxer fracture is a distal neck fracture of the fifth metacarpal. Scaphoid fractures are due to hyperextension of the wrist injuries and present with pain in the anatomic snuffbox and swelling. Jersey finger is a flexor tendon avulsion, usually a result of contact sports. *(Coel et al., 2014, p. 908)*

61. **(D)** Nursemaid elbow is the subluxation of the radial head due to a child or infant being lifted or pulled by the hand. The patient will present with the elbow pronated and painful and he or she will not bend the elbow. During the radiologic examination, the dislocation is usually reduced by placing the elbow in full supination and moving it slowly from full extension to full flexion. This typically provides

immediate relief of pain and a sling may be given for comfort for a couple of days. Otherwise, x-rays are normal. Child protective services should be considered if this is a recurrent problem or if there are other associated signs and symptoms of battery. There is no need for orthopedic referral unless reduction is not commonly done in the practice. Immobilization of the elbow is not recommended, because the patient then may have to recover from frozen shoulder. *(Erickson & Caprio, 2014, p. 873; Walter & Tassone, 2015, pp. 685–686)*

62. **(B)** This patient is presenting with signs and symptoms of primary nocturnal enuresis, which is the wetting only at night during sleep without any sustained period of dryness. It is mainly considered a parasomnia occurring in deep sleep. The incidence of enuresis is higher in boys, is typically related to a developmental delay, and most children become continent by adolescence. Patients need to be tested for structural abnormalities and infections, in addition to neurologic diseases, diabetes mellitus and insipidus, and seizure disorders. Treatment includes limiting liquids at bedtime and routine bathroom training during the day. If these are unsuccessful, the next option is a bed-wetting alarm. This device is attached to the child's undergarment and vibrates when the child is wet to arouse the child to be aware of his/her need to urinate. If the alarm is unsuccessful, then the next step is medication—DDAVP (desmopressin acetate) or imipramine. It is important to avoid judgment and shame during treatment, so a punitive disciplinary approach is ineffective. *(Goldson & Reynolds, 2014, pp. 94–95; Mahan & Patel, 2015, pp. 567–568)*

63. **(D)** Nephroblastoma also known as Wilms tumor typically presents with an asymptomatic abdominal mass noticed by the parent or an increasing size of the abdomen. On examination, the mass feels smooth and firm, is well defined, and usually does not cross the midline. Gross hematuria may be present, but rare, and some patients have microscopic hematuria when tested. Wilms tumor accounts for approximately 5% of cancers in children younger than 15 years. Wilms tumor arises from the kidney and the average age at diagnosis is 4 years. Ultrasound and CT of the abdomen can be used to confirm the presence of an intra-abdominal mass. Treatment includes exploratory abdominal surgery

for removal and staging with a mixture of chemotherapy. A mesenteric cyst typically presents as an asymptomatic intra-abdominal mass but are rare. When present, they are often found incidentally in the small bowel mesentery. Microscopic hematuria is not associated with mesenteric cysts. Intussusception (telescoping of the small intestine) typically presents in an infant with paroxysmal abdominal pain, vomiting, and diarrhea that may progress into bloody stools. Volvulus is normally the result of intestinal malrotation that causes occlusion of the superior mesenteric artery and eventual bowel necrosis. Infants typically present within 3 weeks of life with bile-stained vomiting and bowel obstruction. Constipation often begins in infancy and can persist into childhood. It results from either a voluntary or involuntary retentive behavior. Associated gastrointestinal symptoms are common, including involuntary fecal leakage, which occurs in more than 60% of children with constipation. *(Bishop & Ebach, 2015, pp. 437–438, 442–443; Graham et al., 2014, pp. 1008–1009; Hoffenberg et al., 2014, pp. 663–666, 670–671, 677; McLean & Wofford, 2015, pp. 550–551)*

64. **(A)** Most type I diabetes in the pediatric population is due to an autoimmune cause and in the course of the workup, autoantibody testing is positive. Idiopathic type I diabetes is possible, but is much less common. Obesity is not a factor in type I diabetes; it is implicated in type II diabetes, but this is rare before the age of 10 years old. Medication side effects and pancreatic disease do not cause type I diabetes in the pediatric population. *(Rewers & Chase, 2014, p. 1097)*

65. **(E)** Growth hormone (GH) deficiency is defined as a decreased growth velocity, delay in skeletal maturation, absence of other explanations for poor growth (lack of intake), and laboratory tests demonstrating decreased GH secretion. Etiology of GH deficiency can be congenital, genetic, acquired, or idiopathic, which is the most common. Infants usually have a normal birth weight and may have a slightly decreased length. In addition, most infants present with other endocrine deficiencies like hypoglycemia, hypothyroidism, and/or adrenal insufficiency. Children may present with truncal adiposity because growth hormone promotes lipolysis. Serum GH or intrinsic growth factor levels may or may not

be decreased. In patients who do not have a demonstrated decrease in these hormones, a trial period with GH is indicated. These patients and positive GH-deficient patients receive a once-daily subcutaneous injection of recombinant human GH. Congenital hypothyroidism typically presents with short stature (typically noted after the 4-month newborn visit), delayed epiphyseal development, delayed closure of fontanelles, and retarded dental eruption in addition to other signs of hypothyroidism. Cushing disease typically presents with truncal adiposity with thin extremities, muscle wasting, decreased growth rate, and moon facies. Laboratory results show elevated adrenocorticosteroids both in urine and serum, hypokalemia, eosinopenia, and lymphocytopenia. Typically, in patients younger than the age of 12, Cushing disease is secondary to administration of ACTH or glucocorticoids. Congenital adrenal hyperplasia typically presents with pseudohermaphroditism in females or salt-losing crisis in males with or without isosexual precocity. There is an increased linear growth and advanced skeletal maturation. In familial short stature, birth weight and length is typically normal. Growth deceleration is seen in the first 2 years of life until reaching the genetically determined target percentile. Then the child's growth follows the curve at that percentile. *(Palma Sisto & Heneghan, 2015, pp. 583–588, 598–599, 611; Zeitler et al., 2014, pp. 1057–1062)*

66. **(E)** This patient has idiopathic thrombocytopenic purpura and in the absence of active bleeding, can be managed conservatively by watchful waiting. Aspirin therapy is contraindicated due to the influence on platelet activity. IVIG is used in the presence of severe bleeding when corticosteroids fail. *(Ambruso et al., 2014, pp. 964–966)*

67. **(B)** Heart failure in a 10-year-old child is most likely due to an acquired cause rather than a congenital lesion. Both Kawasaki disease and pericarditis can cause heart failure but are usually associated with fever and chest pain, respectively. Myocarditis can be due to viral or bacterial causes and is the most likely cause in this list presented. *(Darst et al., 2014, pp. 628–629, 631, 634–635)*

68. **(E)** This patient has the classic presentation of erythema multiforme major or Stevens–Johnson syndrome. The most common causes in children of erythema multiforme are medications and *Mycoplasma pneumoniae*. Of the antibiotics listed, the one most commonly causing Stevens–Johnson syndrome is sulfonamide followed by penicillin and tetracycline. The most common medications causing SJS in children are nonsteroidal anti-inflammatory drugs. *(Chiu, 2015a, pp. 662–664; Levin & Weinberg, 2014, pp. 1231–1232; Morelli & Prok, 2014, p. 445)*

69. **(B)** Infection with human parvovirus B19 (also known as fifth disease) resulting in the slapped cheek appearance, can also cause aplastic anemia. This is because the virus infects the precursors of erythrocytes and halts erythropoiesis. Recovery is typically spontaneous with an occasional transfusion for severe anemias. *(Levin & Weinberg, 2014, p. 1232; Panepinto et al., 2015, p. 516)*

70. **(E)** Even though this patient was immunized, her clinical findings are consistent with varicella. Up to 15% of children with varicella vaccination can experience the disease. Herpes zoster presents unilaterally and is associated more with pain in the dermatome than itching. Molluscum contagiosum manifests as an umbilicated papule, not a vesicle. Bullous pemphigoid manifests as large vesicles and does not itch. *(Levin & Wineberg, 2014, pp. 1246–1249)*

71. **(D)** The DSM-V describes criteria for ADHD that must be present before the age of 12 years old. This is a change from age 7, as was in the DSMIV-TR. *(Goldson & Reynolds, 2014, pp. 105–107)*

72. **(D)** Children with a sensitivity to egg that causes only hives can still receive the injectable influenza vaccine as long as they are monitored for 30 minutes after the injection. They cannot, however, receive the live attenuated influenza vaccine. Children with egg allergy that cause angioedema or anaphylaxis may be eligible for injectable influenza vaccine but should be administered under the care of an allergist. The DTaP and IPV vaccines do not contain egg product. It was previously believed children with egg allergy could not receive the MMR vaccine, but this is no longer the case. *(Daley et al., 2014, pp. 289–292)*

73. **(C)** The most likely diagnosis is pediculosis. This parasitic infestation is most commonly seen in the

young school-aged child, and more often in female and Caucasian children. The pediculosis louse lives in the hair and on the scalp and intermittently "bites" into the skin to feed. Discrete urticarial papules or erosions may arise at the bite site. By visualizing the live louse on the scalp, or in the hair, one can easily make the diagnosis. However, the louse may be difficult to see, as it is only 1 to 3 mm in size. Otherwise, nits, or the casings of the eggs laid by the louse, can often be seen on the proximal portion of the hair shaft. The nit adheres to the hair shaft and is often difficult to remove. Brown nits are representative of current infestations and white nits past infestations. Treatment of head lice can be difficult due to the increasing resistance to some of the current treatment options. First-line treatment includes permethrin-based products. Secondary treatment options for resistant infestations may include malathion (0.5%). Mayonnaise is a common traditional remedy but not the preferred treatment. Regardless of treatment, visible ova should be removed by combing the patient's wetted hair with a finely toothed comb until all are removed. Ketoconazole cream and tar-based shampoos are utilized in fungal and seborrheic dermatitis infections. Silver sulfadiazine cream is a topical antibiotic. *(Chiu, 2015, pp. 665–666; Morelli & Prok, 2014, p. 439)*

74. **(D)** Scabies, *Sarcoptes scabiei*, is the most common arthropod infestation of children and it is highly contagious. However, its presentation varies widely and is dependent on the child's age, duration of the infestation, and immune status. Most often, the presenting complaint is severe intermittent itching. The linear papule or burrow commonly associated with scabies is often difficult to identify. Instead, most children will present with eczematous eruptions of red, excoriated papules and nodules. Usually, the distribution of the papules is the most diagnostic finding, and may include the web spaces of the fingers and toes, axillae, umbilicus, groin, penis, and the instep of the feet. Usually, in older children and adults, the face and scalp are spared. The treatment for scabies is a 12-hour application of permethrin 5% lotion. In addition, the parents and all caregivers should be treated at the same time. Clothing and bedding should be washed and dried (heat kills scabies). The family should also be educated in the treatment and prevention of future infestations. Moreover, they should be advised that the itching

associated with scabies could persist for 7 to 14 days after successful treatment. Pediculosis is an infestation of louse in the hair. Tinea corporis is a fungal infection of the torso or "ring worm" and presents with annual scaly plaques with central clearing and pustules. Herpes simplex typically presents with grouped vesicles on erythematous base and is painful. It typically is located in the lips, eyes, cheeks, or hands of children. Papular urticaria is generally distributed over shoulders, upper arms, buttocks, and legs. These grouped erythematous papules with urticarial flare result from a delayed hypersensitivity reaction to insect bites or stings. The hypersensitivity is transient (4–6 months). Symptoms are controlled with oral antihistamines and topical steroids. *(Chiu, 2015b, pp. 664–666; Kronman & Smith, 2015, pp. 336–338; Morelli & Prok, 2014, pp. 438–439)*

75. **(E)** Seborrheic dermatitis is common in all age groups. In infants, this inflammatory skin disease is often manifested as thickened, yellowish white, scaly, waxy appearing skin of the scalp and commonly involves the postauricular areas and the forehead. The more common name is "cradle cap." Cradle cap is a self-limiting disease of infants and resolves by the child's first birthday. In all ages, the scalp scale can be treated by shampooing with zinc pyrithione (Head and Shoulders), selenium sulfide 1% to 2.5%, salicylic acid (Tsal), or ketoconazole (Nizoral). The primary lesion in lichen planus presents on the flexor surfaces and is characterized by pruritic papules that are polygonal and flat-topped. Pityriasis rosea typically presents with the "herald patch" that is a solitary pink, round patch with some central clearing typically found on the torso. The rest of the eruption is described as papulovesicular and develops a Christmas tree pattern. Contact dermatitis usually presents with red patches and plaques with scales and is localized to the area exposed to the irritant. Keratoses pilaris are follicular papules with white scale and typically present on extensor surfaces of proximal extremities. *(Berger, 2014; Chiu, 2015a, pp. 656–658; Morelli & Prok, 2014, pp. 441–442)*

76. **(B)** This presentation is typical for granuloma annulare, which is a benign skin disorder, and treatment is not warranted. It is most commonly seen in children aged 6 to 10 years. The red to brown lesions are annular or circinate. These asymptomatic lesions are often confused with tinea corporis. The lesions will disappear on their own over a couple of years. (*Morelli & Prok, 2014, p. 442*)

77. **(D)** Children should be examined alone starting in adolescence between 11 and 12 years. This allows them to share information freely with the provider that they may want to avoid sharing with a parent. (*Sass & Kaplan, 2014, p. 120*)

78. **(A)** The diagnosis of otitis media requires the presence of middle ear effusion, acute onset of symptoms, and signs and symptoms of middle ear inflammation. Presence of the middle ear effusion can be determined by the bulging of the tympanic membrane, air–fluid levels, impaired visibility of ossicular landmarks, absent mobility of the tympanic membrane by pneumatic otoscopy, or otorrhea from perforation. Office tympanometry can be performed to confirm a diagnosis of effusion. Tenderness on palpation of the tragus and erythema of the external auditory canal typically are signs of otitis externa. (*Friedman et al., 2014, pp. 503–509; Kronman & Smith, 2015, pp. 351–352*)

79. **(D)** The only absolute indications for surgical repair of a fractured clavicle are open-fracture and neurovascular compromise. Most clavicular fractures occur in the middle third of the bone and are at a low risk of nonunion. Failure to control pain medically and deformity over the clavicle are not indications for surgery. (*Coel et al., 2014, p. 904*)

80. **(C)** Osgood–Schlatter disease is caused by microfractures of the patellar ligament where it inserts into the tibial tubercle. This condition usually occurs in the preteen and adolescent years, and is more common in males than females. The history of injury can be vague and the patient may not remember a specific injury that precipitated the pain. Often, the pain progresses to the point of interference of even routine physical activities. X-rays may or may not show any abnormalities. Upon x-ray, type I disease appears normal, but type II will reveal fragmentation of the tibial tubercle. Often, after healing there will be enlargement of the tibial tubercle. Generally, treatment consists of rest, limitation of activities, and isometric exercises. Chondromalacia patellae can only be diagnosed under an arthroscopic

examination, not on the basis of clinical features. Patellofemoral overuse syndrome presents with medial knee pain and subpatellar pain. Additional signs are swelling and crepitus in the knee and it is more common in females than males. It is diagnosed by increased Q-angles (anterosuperior iliac spine through center of patella to tibial tubercle). Subluxation of the patella or dislocation is more common in adolescent girls and the patient presents with acute knee pain. The knee is in flexion with a mass lateral to the knee and with absence of the bony prominence of the patella (flat). X-ray confirms the dislocation. Legg–Calvé–Perthes disease is avascular necrosis of the proximal femur and usually presents between 4 and 8 years of age. (*Coel et al., 2014, pp. 912–913; Erikson & Caprio, 2014, p. 878; Walter & Tassone, 2015, p. 680*)

81. **(E)** Vitamin K deficiency causes vitamin K deficiency bleeding. Vitamin K is one of the compounds required for conversion of prothrombin (PT), factors VII, IX, and X of the coagulation cascade. In addition, proteins C and S are also vitamin K dependent. Therefore, the result is an increased PT time out of proportion to the increased aPTT. A prolonged thrombin time occurs late in the course of illness. There is no effect on platelets, fibrinogen, or hepatic transaminase. (*Ambruso et al., 2014, p. 975; Buchanan & Marquez, 2015, pp. 102–103; Gowen, 2015, p. 222*)

82. **(A)** JIA typically presents with arthritis in one or more joints for at least 6 weeks. It presents most commonly in the oligoarticular form, which manifests as arthritis in four or fewer joints. There is no diagnostic test for JIA, and RF is positive in only 5% of cases. ESR is often elevated. Lyme arthritis usually presents in a monoarticular presentation without morning stiffness. Psoriatic arthritis is usually present along with psoriasis. SCFE and Osgood–Schlatter disease can cause knee pain in the teenage boy, but do not have associated elevated ESR and fatigue. (*Soep, 2014, pp. 927–930*)

83. **(D)** Meckel diverticulum may be asymptomatic except when causing complications such as pain, bleeding, ileal ulceration, and obstruction. It is three times more likely to occur in males than females and 50% more likely to occur in children less than 2-year-old. (*Hoffenberg et al., 2014, pp. 667–668*)

84. **(E)** Dacryocystitis, whether acute or chronic, is usually secondary to bacterial infections. It presents as an acutely inflamed swelling and tender area over the lacrimal sac just medial and inferior to the inner canthus of the eye. Because the lacrimal sac is inflamed and blocked there is tearing and usually purulent discharge from the eye. There may also be an orbital cellulitis. Treatment consists of oral and topical antibiotics and warm compresses, and surgical drainage may also be indicated. After the acute episode and for chronic cases, surgical correction of the nasolacrimal obstruction is required. Anterior uveitis typically presents with pain, photophobia, blurred vision, and injection without exudates. Blepharitis is an inflammation of the lid margin that presents with crusty debris along the lashes. Unless there is a concomitant conjunctival infection, there is typically no injection noted. A chalazion results from inflammation of the meibomian glands but is not associated with increased tearing. *(Braverman, 2014, pp. 459–460, 464–467; Kronman & Smith, 2015, pp. 386–389)*

85. **(D)** In a young child with unilateral nasal drainage without evidence of other symptoms, retained foreign body should be suspected. Seeds and beads are the most common objects found in similar situations. Acute sinusitis and nasal polyposis are rare in children this age. Dacryocystitis is an infection of the lacrimal apparatus and would present with localized swelling rather than nasal drainage. Deviated septum may cause recurrent infection, but would rarely present in this way. *(Friedman et al., 2014, p. 522)*

86. **(C)** Most cases of epistaxis in the anterior portion of the nose are caused by digital trauma (nose picking) or some other mechanical cause such as nose blowing or repeated nose rubbing. Other causes may include incorrect use of steroid nasal sprays. Examination of the anterior nose will usually reveal irritation of the Kiesselbach area. Less than 5% of recurrent nosebleeds are caused by bleeding disorders. Choanal atresia, unilateral, usually appears as a chronic nasal discharge that may be mistaken for chronic sinusitis. Foreign bodies typically present with purulent discharge instead of bleeding. Hypertension predisposes children to prolonged epistaxis, but it remains relatively uncommon. *(Friedman et al., 2014, p. 521)*

87. **(B)** In children who present with fever, there are several characteristics that are cause for urgent evaluation based on the potential of serious consequence. A fever within 48 hours of the DTaP vaccination is, however, one exception and the child does not need to be evaluated urgently. The remainder of the scenarios in this list are indications of potentially serious infectious causes of fever and should prompt evaluation within 24 hours. *(Treitz et al., 2014, pp. 267–269)*

88. **(A)** Chemoprophylaxis is recommended for family members of patients diagnosed with pertussis and should be azithromycin unless contraindicated for patient specific reasons. Corticosteroids are helpful in adjuvant therapy for the infected child, but not for prevention. Strict physical isolation is not necessary. *(Ogle & Anderson, 2014, pp. 1331–1333)*

89. **(D)** Surgical reduction is the treatment of choice for incarcerated hernias over 12 hours. At that point the likelihood that the hernia will manually reduce is very small and the bowel is becoming necrotic and needs to be removed as soon as possible. Bilateral surgical reduction is required only in the event of two hernias, and there is no place for prophylaxis surgery for inguinal hernia repairs. *(Hoffenberg et al., 2014, pp. 666–667)*

90. **(B)** Chlamydial infections are the most common cause of conjunctivitis in newborns in developed countries. Other causes of ophthalmia neonatorum include reactions to silver nitrate prophylaxis, other bacterial infections such as gonococcal or staphylococcal, or viral organisms such as adenovirus or echovirus. *Chlamydia trachomatis* causes conjunctivitis and pneumonia in neonates. Treatment for chlamydial conjunctivitis should be with systemic erythromycin to treat the conjunctivitis and as prophylaxis against pneumonia. *(Braverman, 2014, p. 465; Kronman & Smith, 2015, pp. 386–389, Rosenberg & Grover, 2014, p. 61)*

91. **(A)** Arthritis in a child, especially in the knees, leads to a differential diagnosis that includes both Lyme disease and rheumatoid disease. Arthritis symptoms that relapse and remit are characteristic of Lyme arthritis; JIA is characterized by a 6-week duration of symptoms. The remainder of the symptoms in this list—joint deformity, negative joint fluid analysis, elevated ESR, and fever can be found in both disorders. *(Ogle & Anderson, 2014, pp. 1350–1352; Soep, 2014, pp. 927–930)*

92. **(E)** Oral candidiasis (thrush) is very common in the first few weeks of infancy. The diagnosis is usually done by visual inspection and does not usually require further laboratory testing. On visual examination, white, creamy plaques are found on the buccal mucosa and occasionally the gingival and lingual mucosa. For this age group, direct topical application of nystatin in oral suspension to the lesions should suffice. If the lesions are resistant to treatment or if they occur in older children, consideration should be given to the possibility of the patient being immunocompromised. All sources of candida, such as toys and bottle nipples, should be sterilized daily. Herpangina and hand–foot–mouth disease are ulcerating lesions of the oral cavity due to viruses and are self-limiting, but can be very painful. Leukoplakia is a precursor lesion to oral cancer, seen most commonly in oral tobacco users. Herpes simplex gingivostomatitis presents as multiple ulcerations on the mucosa. Associated symptoms include fever and cervical adenopathy. *(Bishop & Ebach, 2015, p. 433; Friedman et al., 2014, p. 523; Lustig & Schindler, 2014, Ch. 8; Messacar et al., 2014, pp. 1386–1389)*

93. **(B)** Depression is the presenting symptom in 70% of children with bipolar disorder. Mania (bipolar type I) and hypomania (bipolar type II) are clearly associated with bipolar disorder because they may not be the presenting symptoms, clinicians should evaluate children with depressive symptoms for bipolar disorder. Delusions and hallucinations can accompany dramatic behavior in a bipolar patient, but do not represent symptoms manifested in the majority of initial presentations of the disorder. *(Burstein et al., 2014, pp. 221–226)*

94. **(E)** Rocky Mountain spotted fever (RMSF) is the most common rickettsial infection in the United States, especially in the eastern, southeastern, and western states, and it is very common in 5- to 9-year-old children. A known tick exposure may or may not be documented. Most exposures to ticks carrying *Rickettsia rickettsii*, the causative organism of this disease, occur in the warmer months of April to September when victims are most likely to participate in outdoor activities in wooded areas. The incubation period of RMSF is 3 to 12 days (mean 7) after a tick exposure. The tick must be attached for 6 hours or greater in order to transmit the disease. Clinical presentation includes fever, often 40°C, myalgias, headache, and less characteristic, red-rose macular or maculopapular rash. The rash usually appears within 2 to 6 days, after the fever. The rash is especially prevalent on the palms, soles, and extremities. After several days, the rash, which starts peripherally and spreads centrally, becomes petechial. Conjunctivitis, edema, splenomegaly, meningismus, and confusion may occur. Up to 5% to 7% of patients with RSMF will die, and therefore, delays in treatment should be avoided. Treatment for children is doxycycline, regardless of age and the possible side effect of stained teeth. In endemic areas, treatment should be started early and is often based on suspicion alone, and prior to the appearance of the rash. Endemic typhus (murine typhus) is not transmitted by ticks but instead by the fleas from infected rodents. The rash of endemic typhus differs from that of RMSF in that it does *not* involve the palms and soles. Q fever is spread by inhalation instead of ticks. The cause of this rickettsial disease is *Coxiella burnetii* hosted by domestic animals including dogs, cats, cattle, and sheep. Unpasteurized milk from infected animals may also be a source of this infection. One form of human monocytic ehrlichiosis is carried by ticks that have fed on infected hosts that may include deer, wild rodents, and sheep, most commonly in the southeast, north, and south central United States. The presentation is usually a viral syndrome without any rash. Although this is usually a self-limiting disease, deaths do occur in children; therefore, treatment should be carried out with the antibiotic of choice, doxycycline, regardless of side effects. Lyme disease can manifest with its characteristic rash, erythema migrans, or be asymptomatic. Low-grade fever, myalgias and headache may occur. *(Kronman & Smith, 2015, pp. 399–401; Levin & Weinberg, 2014, pp. 1267–1270; Ogle & Anderson, 2014, pp. 1350–1352)*

95. **(E)** In young children, respiratory syncytial virus (RSV) accounts for more than 70% of bronchiolitis, approximately 40% of the cases of pneumonia, and about 10% of cases of croup. This seasonal disease occurs in the winter and early spring months of the year. More than 50% of children have been infected with RSV by age 1, and by the age of 2, almost all

children have been infected. Reinfection commonly occurs but is mild. Adenovirus infections, though common in early childhood, only account for approximately up to 10% of all respiratory diseases. The peak incidence of adenovirus respiratory infections occurs in the spring, summer, and early winter. Human parvovirus infection is typically seen in school-aged children. This disease is characterized by the "slapped-cheek" appearing rash on the face that appears about 10 to 17 days following the infection. About 2 days after the appearance of this facial rash, a similar rash appears on the extremities, trunk, neck, and buttocks. The rash often persists for a few days to a few weeks (average of 10 days) and often will recur with exposure to bathing in warm water, exercise, sunlight, and stress. Parainfluenza viruses fall into four categories and are responsible for the majority of cases of croup (65%), laryngitis (50%), and tracheobronchitis (25%). Types 1 to 3 occur as seasonal outbreaks with types 1 and 2 in the fall and type 3 in the spring and summer. Type 4 is an endemic virus. Clinical symptoms of these viruses include laryngotracheitis (croup), laryngitis, bronchiolitis, and less commonly pneumonia (especially in immunocompromised children). Human metapneumovirus is the 2nd leading cause of respiratory infections in children and can cause cough, bronchiolitis, and pneumonia. *(Federico et al., 2014, p. 565; Kronman & Smith, 2015, pp. 357–358; Levin & Weinberg, 2014, pp. 1227–1228)*

96. **(B)** Asthma, in this case exercise induced, is the most likely cause of this problem. The symptoms commonly associated with acute exacerbations of asthma include wheezing, cough, dyspnea, and chest pain. Some symptoms that might be suggestive of asthma include exercise-induced cough, nighttime cough, cough after cold air exposure, and cough after laughing. Airway foreign bodies, though not common, are an acute problem that may present as sudden cough, choking, and wheezing. Cystic fibrosis (CF) is the most common, lethal, genetic disease affecting the Caucasian population. Up to 50% of patients with CF are diagnosed in infancy, but others may not be diagnosed until adolescence or adulthood. Chronic or recurrent cough should be an indicator for consideration of CF as a differential diagnosis. Laryngomalacia is the most common cause of stridor in infants. It is the incomplete development of the cartilaginous support of

the laryngoglottic structures. This congenital condition is usually self-limiting and occurs most commonly in infants at or just after birth. The inspiratory collapse of the epiglottis or arytenoid cartilages is heard as stridor. Vocal cord dysfunction is the paradoxical spasm of vocal cords leading to dyspnea and wheezing. It often is misdiagnosed as asthma but can exist concomitantly with asthma. Direct visualization of vocal cords is necessary for diagnosis. *(Chiu, 2015a, pp. 273–282; Covar et al., 2014, pp. 1171–1186; Federico et al., 2012, pp. 548–552; Ong et al., 2015, pp. 467, 470–471, 475–478)*

97. **(B)** Autism is the most likely diagnosis for this child. The signs of autism often present before the second year of life such as the child's failure to respond to their name, failed speech development, and appearing self-absorbed and withdrawn in the presence of other children or adults. Often in childhood, autistic children may develop ritualistic behaviors and intense interests that if interrupted may cause tantrums and rages. When speech does begin to develop, it may be nonsensical: reversal of speech patterns, echolocation, and other abnormal patterns. Goals of treatment include early intervention to address behavior and communication skills. ADHD is characterized by easy distractibility, inattention, and overactivity. Estimates for the presence of ADHD in school-aged children range from 2% to 20%. Fragile X syndrome is the most common cause of functional mental retardation. This syndrome, affecting approximately 1 in 1,250 males, is caused by a trinucleotide expansion (CGG-repeated sequence) in the fragile X mental retardation I (*FMR1*) gene. Fragile X syndrome is characterized by a wide range of symptoms, which may include language delay, hyperactivity, autistic behavior, and variable levels of mental retardation. Schizophrenia is usually detected in adolescence, with prepubertal onset occurring rarely. Patients may initially present with somatic or social behavior problems. Schizophrenic children and adolescents often have the same symptoms as adults, such as hallucinations, bizarre thought processes, and rambling speech. Plumbism, otherwise known as lead poisoning, manifests in early stages with multiple symptoms; these can include irritability, ataxia, and personality changes. Retarded development is a late symptom. *(Gahagan et al., 2015, pp. 41–42; Goldson & Reynolds, 2014, pp. 105–111, 114–115;*

Levy & Marion, 2015b, p. 153; Scheffer & Tripathi, 2015, pp. 63–66; Wang et al., 2014, pp. 377–378)

98. **(A)** Choanal atresia, whether unilateral or bilateral, is a nasal obstruction that occurs relatively rarely in newborns. If bilateral choanal atresia occurs at birth, it causes a respiratory distress that requires immediate treatment (due to infants being obligate nose breathers) by placing an oral airway and subsequent surgical correction. Unilateral choanal atresia can present as a chronic, single-sided, nasal discharge that may not appear until later in childhood. Meconium ileus, intestinal obstruction secondary to inspissated meconium, occurs in approximately 10% of newborns with cystic fibrosis. Cystic fibrosis affects approximately 1 in 2,500 live Caucasian births, and is a leading cause of death in young adults. Nasal infections may occur secondary to a furuncle (infected hair follicle) in the anterior nares or as a nasal septal abscess following spread of a furuncle. Common causes of nasal infections include picking at the nose and pulling out nose hair. Nasal polyps are uncommon in children younger than age 10, and when they do occur it is usually in older children and adults with allergic rhinitis. *(Chiu, 2015a, p. 284; Federico et al., 2014, pp. 551–552; Friedman et al., 2014, pp. 520–521; Rosenberg & Grover, 2014, p. 14)*

99. **(B)** Changes to brain tissue due to severe malnutrition are a long-term complication of anorexia nervosa. Constipation (due to loss of gastrocolic reflex and muscle tone), pericardial effusion (due to malnutrition), and superior mesenteric artery syndrome (due to shrinking fat pad between the superior mesenteric artery and duodenum) are all complications of anorexia but are considered short-term and resolve when refeeding and weight gain return. Osteoarthritis is not associated with anorexia, but osteoporosis is. *(Sigel, 2014, pp. 174–177)*

100. **(D)** Obesity in pediatric patients is defined as BMI for age >95th percentile. BMI for age in 85th to 95th percentile is classified as overweight and >99th is considered severely obese. BMI must be calculated with reference to age in the pediatric population and is not associated with a percent change in any one given time period. *(Haemer et al., 2014, pp. 323–326)*

REFERENCES

Ambruso DR, Nuss R, Wang M. Hematologic disorders. In: Hay WW Jr, Levin MJ, Deterding RR, Abzug MJ, eds. *Current Diagnosis & Treatment: Pediatrics.* 22nd ed. New York, NY: McGraw-Hill; 2014.

Berger TG. Dermatologic disorders. In: Papadakis MA, McPhee SJ, Rabow MW, eds. *Current Medical Diagnosis & Treatment 2014.* New York, NY: McGraw-Hill; 2014.

Bishop WP, Ebach DR. The digestive system. In: Marcdante KJ, Kleigman RM, eds. *Nelson Essentials of Pediatrics.* 7th ed. Philadelphia, PA: Elsevier Saunders; 2015.

Blake K, Allen LM. Adolescent medicine. In: Marcdante KJ, Kleigman RM, eds. *Nelson Essentials of Pediatrics.* 7th ed. Philadelphia, PA: Elsevier Saunders; 2015.

Braverman R. Eye. In: Hay WW Jr, Levin MJ, Deterding RR, Abzug MJ, eds. *Current Diagnosis & Treatment: Pediatrics.* 22nd ed. New York, NY: McGraw-Hill; 2014.

Buchanan AO, Marquez ML. Pediatric nutrition and nutritional disorders. In: Marcdante KJ, Kleigman RM, eds. *Nelson Essentials of Pediatrics.* 7th ed. Philadelphia, PA: Elsevier Saunders; 2015.

Burstein A, Talmi A, Stafford B, Kelsay K. Child & adolescent psychiatric disorders & psychosocial aspects of pediatrics. In: Hay WW, Jr, Levin MJ, Deterding RR, Abzug MJ, eds. *Current Diagnosis & Treatment: Pediatrics.* 22nd ed. New York, NY: McGraw-Hill; 2014.

Centers for Disease Control and Prevention. Childhood & adolescent immunization schedule; 2015, http://www.cdc.gov/vaccines/schedules/hcp/child-adolescent.html. Accessed January 31, 2015.

Chiesa A, Sirotnak AP. Child abuse & neglect. In: Hay WW, Jr, Levin MJ, Deterding RR, Abzug MJ, eds. *Current Diagnosis & Treatment: Pediatrics.* 22nd ed. New York, NY: McGraw-Hill; 2014. http://accessmedicine.mhmedical.com. Accessed February 02, 2015.

Chiu AM. Allergy. In: Marcdante KJ, Kleigman RM, eds. *Nelson Essentials of Pediatrics.* 7th ed. Philadelphia, PA: Elsevier Saunders; 2015a.

Chiu YE. Dermatology. In: Marcdante KJ, Kleigman RM, eds. *Nelson Essentials of Pediatrics.* 7th ed. Philadelphia, PA: Elsevier Saunders; 2015b.

Christian CW, Blum NJ. Psychosocial issues. In: Marcdante KJ, Kleigman RM, eds. *Nelson Essentials of Pediatrics*. 7th ed. Philadelphia, PA: Elsevier Saunders; 2015.

Coel RA, Hoang QB, Vidal A. Sports medicine. In: Hay WW Jr, Levin MJ, Deterding RR, Abzug MJ, eds. *Current Diagnosis & Treatment: Pediatrics*. 22nd ed. New York, NY: McGraw-Hill; 2014.

Covar RA, Fleischer DM, Cho C, Boguniewicz M. Allergic disorders. In: Hay WW Jr, Levin MJ, Deterding RR, Abzug MJ, eds. *Current Diagnosis & Treatment: Pediatrics*. 22nd ed. New York, NY: McGraw-Hill; 2014.

Daley MF, O'Leary ST, Nyquist AC. Immunizations. In: Hay WW Jr, Levin MJ, Deterding RR, Abzug MJ, eds. *Current Diagnosis & Treatment: Pediatrics*. 22nd ed. New York, NY: McGraw-Hill; 2014.

Darst JR, Collins KK, Miyamoto SD. Cardiovascular diseases. In: Hay WW Jr, Levin MJ, Deterding RR, Abzug MJ, eds. *Current Diagnosis & Treatment: Pediatrics*. 22nd ed. New York, NY: McGraw-Hill; 2014.

Erickson MA, Caprio B. Orthopedics. In: Hay WW Jr, Levin MJ, Deterding RR, Abzug MJ, eds. *Current Diagnosis & Treatment: Pediatrics*. 22nd ed. New York, NY: McGraw-Hill; 2014.

Federico MJ, Baker CD, Balasubramaniam V, et al. Respiratory tract & mediastinum. In: Hay WW Jr, Levin MJ, Deterding RR, Abzug MJ, eds. *Current Diagnosis & Treatment: Pediatrics*. 22nd ed. New York, NY: McGraw-Hill; 2014.

Friedman NR, Scholes MA, Yoon PJ. Ear, nose, & throat. In: Hay WW Jr, Levin MJ, Deterding RR, Abzug MJ, eds. *Current Diagnosis & Treatment: Pediatrics*. 22nd ed. New York, NY: McGraw-Hill; 2014.

Gahagan S, Hui Liu Y, Brown SJ. Behavioral disorders. In: Marcdante KJ, Kleigman RM, eds. *Nelson Essentials of Pediatrics*. 7th ed. Philadelphia, PA: Elsevier Saunders; 2015.

Goldson E, Reynolds A. Child development & behavior. In: Hay WW Jr, Levin MJ, Deterding RR, Abzug MJ, eds. *Current Diagnosis & Treatment: Pediatrics*. 22nd ed. New York, NY: McGraw-Hill; 2014.

Gowen CW. Fetal and neonatal medicine. In: Marcdante KJ, Kleigman RM, eds. *Nelson Essentials of Pediatrics*. 7th ed. Philadelphia, PA: Elsevier Saunders; 2015.

Graham DK, Craddock JA, Quinones RR, et al. Neoplastic disease. In: Hay WW Jr, Levin MJ, Deterding RR, Abzug MJ, eds. *Current Diagnosis & Treatment: Pediatrics*. 22nd ed. New York, NY: McGraw-Hill; 2014.

Greenbaum LA, Bou-Matar R. Fluids and electrolytes. In: Marcdante KJ, Kleigman RM, eds. *Nelson Essentials of Pediatrics*. 7th ed. Philadelphia, PA: Elsevier Saunders; 2015.

Haemer MA, Primak LE, Krebs NF. Normal childhood nutrition & its disorders. In: Hay WW Jr, Levin MJ, Deterding RR, Abzug MJ, eds. *Current Diagnosis & Treatment: Pediatrics*. 22nd ed. New York, NY: McGraw-Hill; 2014.

Hoffenberg EJ, Brumbaugh D, Furuta GT, et al. Gastrointestinal tract. In: Hay WW Jr, Levin MJ, Deterding RR, Abzug MJ,

eds. *Current Diagnosis & Treatment: Pediatrics*. 22nd ed. New York, NY: McGraw-Hill; 2014.

Kedia S, Knupp K, Schreiner T, Yang ML, Levisohn PM, Moe PG. Neurologic & muscular disorders. In: Hay WW Jr, Levin MJ, Deterding RR, Abzug MJ, eds. *Current Diagnosis & Treatment: Pediatrics*. 22nd ed. New York, NY: McGraw-Hill; 2014.

Klein U. Oral medicine & dentistry. In: Hay WW, Jr, Levin MJ, Deterding RR, Abzug MJ, eds. *Current Diagnosis & Treatment: Pediatrics*. 22nd ed. New York, NY: McGraw-Hill; 2014. http://accessmedicine.mhmedical.com. Accessed February 03, 2015.

Kronman MP, Smith S. Infectious diseases. In: Marcdante KJ, Kleigman RM, eds. *Nelson Essentials of Pediatrics*. 7th ed. Philadelphia, PA: Elsevier Saunders; 2015.

Levin MJ, Weinberg A. Infections: viral & rickettsial. In: Hay WW Jr, Levin MJ, Deterding RR, Abzug MJ, eds. *Current Diagnosis & Treatment: Pediatrics*. 22nd ed. New York, NY: McGraw-Hill; 2014.

Levine DA. Growth and development. In: Marcdante KJ, Kleigman RM, eds. *Nelson Essentials of Pediatrics*. 7th ed. Philadelphia, PA: Elsevier Saunders; 2015.

Levy PA, Marion RW. Human genetics and dysmorphology. In: Marcdante KJ, Kleigman RM, eds. *Nelson Essentials of Pediatrics*. 7th ed. Philadelphia, PA: Elsevier Saunders; 2015a.

Levy PA, Marion RW. Patterns of inheritance. In: Marcdante KJ, Kleigman RM, eds. *Nelson Essentials of Pediatrics*. 7th ed. Philadelphia, PA: Elsevier Saunders; 2015b.

Lum GM. Kidney & urinary tract. In: Hay WW Jr, Levin MJ, Deterding RR, Abzug MJ, eds. *Current Diagnosis & Treatment: Pediatrics*. 22nd ed. New York, NY: McGraw-Hill; 2014.

Lustig LR, Schindler JS. Ear, nose, & throat disorders. In: Papadakis MA, McPhee SJ, Rabow MW, eds. *Current Medical Diagnosis & Treatment 2014*. New York, NY: McGraw-Hill; 2014. http://accessmedicine.mhmedical.com. Accessed July 08, 2014.

Mahan JD, Patel HP. Nephrology and urology. In: Marcdante KJ, Kleigman RM, eds. *Nelson Essentials of Pediatrics*. 7th ed. Philadelphia, PA: Elsevier Saunders; 2015.

McLean TW, Wofford MM. Oncology. In: Marcdante KJ, Kleigman RM, eds. *Nelson Essentials of Pediatrics*. 7th ed. Philadelphia, PA: Elsevier Saunders; 2015.

Messacar K, Dominguez SR, Levin MJ. Infections: parasitic & mycotic. In: Hay WW Jr, Levin MJ, Deterding RR, Abzug MJ, eds. *Current Diagnosis & Treatment: Pediatrics*. 22nd ed. New York, NY: McGraw-Hill; 2014.

Morelli JG, Prok LD. Skin. In: Hay WW Jr, Levin MJ, Deterding RR, Abzug MJ, eds. *Current Diagnosis & Treatment: Pediatrics*. 22nd ed. New York, NY: McGraw-Hill; 2014.

Ogle JW. Antimicrobial therapy. In: Hay WW Jr, Levin MJ, Deterding RR, Abzug MJ, eds. *Current Diagnosis & Treatment: Pediatrics*. 22nd ed. New York, NY: McGraw-Hill; 2014.

Ogle JW, Anderson MS. Infections: bacterial & spirochetal. In: Hay WW Jr, Levin MJ, Deterding RR, Abzug MJ, Sondheimer JM, eds. *Current Diagnosis & Treatment: Pediatrics*. 22nd ed. New York, NY: McGraw-Hill; 2014.

Ong T, Striegl A, Marshall SA. The respiratory system. In: Marcdante KJ, Kleigman RM, eds. *Nelson Essentials of Pediatrics.* 7th ed. Philadelphia, PA: Elsevier Saunders; 2015.

Palma Sisto PA, Heneghan MK. Endocrinology. In: Marcdante KJ, Kleigman RM, eds. *Nelson Essentials of Pediatrics.* 7th ed. Philadelphia, PA: Elsevier Saunders; 2015.

Panepinto JA, Punzalan RC, Scott JP. Hematology. In: Marcdante KJ, Kleigman RM, eds. *Nelson Essentials of Pediatrics.* 7th ed. Philadelphia, PA: Elsevier Saunders; 2015.

Rewers M, Chase H. Diabetes mellitus. In: Hay WW, Jr, Levin MJ, Deterding RR, Abzug MJ, eds. *Current Diagnosis & Treatment: Pediatrics.* 22nd ed. New York, NY: McGraw-Hill; 2014.

Rosenberg AA, Grover T. The newborn infant. In: Hay WW Jr, Levin MJ, Deterding RR, Abzug MJ, eds. *Current Diagnosis & Treatment: Pediatrics.* 22nd ed. New York, NY: McGraw-Hill; 2014.

Saenz M, Chun-Hui Tsai A, Manchester DK, Elias ER. Genetics & dysmorphology. In: Hay WW Jr, Levin MJ, Deterding RR, Abzug MJ, eds. *Current Diagnosis & Treatment: Pediatrics.* 22nd ed. New York, NY: McGraw-Hill; 2014.

Sass AE, Kaplan DW. Adolescence. In: Hay WW Jr, Levin MJ, Deterding RR, Abzug MJ, eds. *Current Diagnosis & Treatment: Pediatrics.* 22nd ed. New York, NY: McGraw-Hill; 2014.

Scheffer R, Tripathi A. Psychiatric disorders. In: Marcdante KJ, Kleigman RM, eds. *Nelson Essentials of Pediatrics.* 7th ed. Philadelphia, PA: Elsevier Saunders; 2015.

Schiller JH, Shelhaas RA. Neurology. In: Marcdante KJ, Kleigman RM, eds. *Nelson Essentials of Pediatrics.* 7th ed. Philadelphia, PA: Elsevier Saunders; 2015.

Schneider DS. The cardiovascular system. In: Marcdante KJ, Kleigman RM, eds. *Nelson Essentials of Pediatrics.* 7th ed. Philadelphia, PA: Elsevier Saunders; 2015.

Sigel EJ. Eating disorders. In: Hay WW, Jr, Levin MJ, Deterding RR, Abzug MJ, eds. *Current Diagnosis & Treatment: Pediatrics.* 22nd ed. New York, NY: McGraw-Hill; 2014.

Soep JB. Rheumatic diseases. In: Hay WW, Jr, Levin MJ, Deterding RR, Abzug MJ, eds. *Current Diagnosis & Treatment: Pediatrics.* 22nd ed. New York, NY: McGraw-Hill; 2014.

Sokol RJ, Narkewicz MR, Sundaram SS, Mack CL. Liver & pancreas. In: Hay WW Jr, Levin MJ, Deterding RR, Abzug MJ, eds. *Current Diagnosis & Treatment: Pediatrics.* 22nd ed. New York, NY: McGraw-Hill; 2014.

Stone C. Chapter 37: Neurologic emergencies. In: Stone C, Humphries RL, eds. *Current Diagnosis & Treatment Emergency Medicine.* 7th ed. New York, NY: McGraw-Hill; 2011. http://accessmedicine.mhmedical.com. Accessed March 23, 2015.

Thomas JA, Van Hove JLK. Inborn errors of metabolism. In: Hay WW Jr, Levin MJ, Deterding RR, Abzug MJ, eds. *Current Diagnosis & Treatment: Pediatrics.* 22nd ed. New York, NY: McGraw-Hill; 2014.

Treitz M, Bunik M, Fox D. Ambulatory & office pediatrics. In: Hay WW Jr, Levin MJ, Deterding RR, Abzug MJ, eds. *Current Diagnosis & Treatment: Pediatrics.* 22nd ed. New York, NY: McGraw-Hill; 2014.

Walter KD, Tassone JC. Orthopedics. In: Marcdante KJ, Kleigman RM, eds. *Nelson Essentials of Pediatrics.* 7th ed. Philadelphia, PA: Elsevier Saunders; 2015.

Wang GS, Rumack BH, Dart RC. Poisoning. In: Hay WW Jr, Levin MJ, Deterding RR, Abzug MJ, eds. *Current Diagnosis & Treatment: Pediatrics.* 22nd ed. New York, NY: McGraw-Hill; 2014.

Zeitler PS, Travers SH, Nadeau K, Barker JM, Kelsey MM, Kappy MS. Endocrine disorders. In: Hay WW Jr, Levin MJ, Deterding RR, Abzug MJ, eds. *Current Diagnosis & Treatment: Pediatrics.* 22nd ed. New York, NY: McGraw-Hill; 2014.

CHAPTER 13

Pharmacology and Therapeutics

Raymond J. Pavlick Jr., PhD

DIRECTIONS: Each of the numbered questions or incomplete statements is followed by possible answers or completions of the statement. Select the ONE-lettered answer or completion that is BEST in each case.

1. A history of which of the following warrants special consideration when initially prescribing levothyroxine?

   (A) Coronary heart disease
   (B) Obesity
   (C) Parkinson disease
   (D) Peptic ulcer disease
   (E) Rheumatoid arthritis

2. Which of the following medications is capable of causing agranulocytosis?

   (A) Desmopressin
   (B) Insulin
   (C) Metformin
   (D) Methimazole
   (E) Prednisone

3. A 50-year-old male undergoes a physical examination during which time his blood pressure is determined to be 150/98. An electrocardiogram reveals the presence of atrial fibrillation. No other abnormalities are noted, and otherwise, the patient appears to be in good health. He is not currently taking any medications. Which of the following would be most appropriate to prescribe to the patient at this time?

   (A) Candesartan
   (B) Doxazosin
   (C) Hydrochlorothiazide
   (D) Lisinopril
   (E) Verapamil

4. A 4-year-old male swallows several tablets of a medication that he found in his parent's bathroom cabinet underneath the sink. Approximately 4 to 5 hours after ingesting the tablets, there were no symptoms other than nausea and vomiting. Forty-eight hours after ingesting the tablets, elevated aminotransferase levels were detected followed by jaundice, hepatic encephalopathy, renal failure, and death. What did the child most likely swallow?

   (A) Acetaminophen
   (B) Aspirin
   (C) Diazepam
   (D) Oxycodone
   (E) Phenobarbital

5. Which of the following requires drug-free periods to avoid tolerance when used as prophylaxis for chronic stable angina?

   (A) Digoxin
   (B) Diltiazem
   (C) Metoprolol
   (D) Isosorbide dinitrate
   (E) Propranolol

6. Which of the following induces atrophy of the adrenal glands and, if discontinued, must be tapered following chronic administration?

   (A) Atorvastatin
   (B) Dabigatran
   (C) Metformin
   (D) Omeprazole
   (E) Prednisone

7. A 66-year-old male is diagnosed with idiopathic Parkinson disease (IPD) and is suffering from tremor and bradykinesia that has become troublesome in his job-related activities as a teacher. The patient has expressed that he would like to continue working for another 3 to 4 years and is seeking the most effective medication to control his symptoms. Which of the following would be most appropriate to prescribe to this patient?

(A) Amantadine
(B) Benztropine
(C) Entacapone
(D) Levodopa/carbidopa
(E) Selegiline

8. Of the following choices, which regimen is considered first-line therapy for *Helicobacter pylori*–positive individuals with peptic ulcer disease (PUD) and no known drug allergies?

(A) Misoprostol, clarithromycin, and metronidazole
(B) Omeprazole, clarithromycin, and amoxicillin
(C) Omeprazole, ranitidine, and clarithromycin
(D) Ranitidine, amoxicillin, and bismuth subsalicylate
(E) Ranitidine, ciprofloxacin, and metronidazole

9. Following a gunshot wound to the lower abdomen, a 29-year-old male is hospitalized and treated with clindamycin for a potential anaerobic infection. After 3 days of clindamycin therapy, while recuperating in the hospital, he develops severe diarrhea, dehydration, and lower abdominal cramping. A stool culture is ordered and later discovered to contain *Clostridium difficile*. After discontinuing the clindamycin and assuming no known drug allergies, which of the following would be the most appropriate treatment?

(A) Amoxicillin
(B) Cephalexin
(C) Ciprofloxacin
(D) Doxycycline
(E) Metronidazole

10. A 17-year-old female attempts suicide by swallowing several tablets of acetaminophen. Which of the following is considered the most effective antidote to administer to this patient?

(A) Diazepam
(B) Flumazenil
(C) N-acetylcysteine
(D) Sodium bicarbonate
(E) Sodium nitroprusside

11. Assuming no contraindications, which of the following class of medications is considered the preferred long-term control therapy in adult patients with mild persistent asthma?

(A) Inhaled corticosteroids
(B) Leukotriene antagonists
(C) Long-acting β_2-agonists
(D) Methylxanthines
(E) Muscarinic antagonists

12. Which of the following type 2 diabetes mellitus medications is correctly paired with its mechanism of action?

(A) Glipizide; enhancement of insulin secretion
(B) Metformin; reduction of postprandial glucagon secretion
(C) Miglitol; enhancement of insulin sensitivity at skeletal muscle
(D) Rosiglitazone; inhibition of intestinal sucrase and glucoamylase
(E) Sitagliptin; enhancement of hepatic insulin sensitivity

13. Along with diuretic therapy, which of the following agents is considered appropriate therapy in a 52-year-old male with hypertension who develops systolic heart failure with an ejection fraction of 30%?

(A) Diazoxide
(B) Lisinopril
(C) Prazosin
(D) Salmeterol
(E) Verapamil

14. A 61-year-old male arrives at the emergency department (ED) and is determined to be suffering from an ischemic stroke. Which of the following agents should be administered as quickly as possible to induce thrombolysis?

(A) Alteplase

(B) Clopidogrel

(C) Eptifibatide

(D) Heparin

(E) Warfarin

15. A 64-year-old female who underwent total knee arthroplasty is to begin a 10- to 14-day regimen of oxycodone for pain control. Which of the following would be most appropriate to administer to the patient during this time?

(A) Antidiarrheal agent

(B) Benzodiazepine

(C) Laxative

(D) Proton pump inhibitor

(E) Sulfonylurea

16. A 45-year-old male with recently diagnosed elevation of low-density lipoprotein (LDL-C) is to begin treatment with atorvastatin. Which of the following would be most appropriate to perform or order prior to the initiation of atorvastatin?

(A) Arterial blood gas (ABG) and urinalysis

(B) Chest radiography and serum lipase/amylase

(C) Electrocardiogram (ECG) and serum creatinine

(D) Glycated hemoglobin (A1C) and serum ketones

(E) Serum creatine kinase (CK) and serum aminotransferases

17. One of the most common adverse effects with centrally acting skeletal muscle relaxants such as carisoprodol and cyclobenzaprine is their tendency to cause which of the following?

(A) Hyperglycemia

(B) Hypertension

(C) Myalgia

(D) Rash

(E) Sedation

18. A 68-year-old male is recently diagnosed with depression associated with the loss of his close sister to an automobile accident. He is currently taking oxybutynin for overactive bladder disease and lisinopril for hypertension. He has no known drug allergies. Which of the following medications would be most appropriate to prescribe for this patient?

(A) Alprazolam

(B) Amitriptyline

(C) Buspirone

(D) Desipramine

(E) Sertraline

19. Which of the following acts as a direct thrombin inhibitor to inactivate circulating and clot-bound thrombin?

(A) Clopidogrel

(B) Dabigatran

(C) Heparin

(D) Rivaroxaban

(E) Warfarin

20. A 27-year-old female with Sjögren's syndrome suffers from dry mouth, but continues to have residual salivary gland activity. Which of the following agents would be most appropriate to administer to potentially alleviate the patient's dry mouth?

(A) Atropine

(B) Diphenhydramine

(C) Oxybutynin

(D) Pilocarpine

(E) Salmeterol

21. A 24-year-old male presenting to the clinic 4 days ago was diagnosed with depression and subsequently prescribed 10 mg/day of fluoxetine. He unexpectedly shows up today and states that he is not experiencing any improvement since starting the medication. What is the best treatment option at this time?

(A) Discontinue the fluoxetine and start amitriptyline

(B) Discontinue the fluoxetine and start sertraline

(C) Double the dose of fluoxetine to 20 mg/day and assure the patient that he will experience improvement in the next 48 hours

(D) Maintain the current dose of fluoxetine and add phenelzine to the medication regimen

(E) Maintain the current dose of fluoxetine and comfort the patient that the medication may still take several weeks to have its full effect

22. Assuming no contraindications to their use, which of following antihypertensives are most appropriate for treating hypertension in the type 2 diabetic patient with early signs of diabetic nephropathy?

    (A) Angiotensin converting enzyme inhibitors (AECIs)
    (B) α-Receptor blockers
    (C) β-Blockers
    (D) Calcium channel blockers
    (E) Thiazide diuretics

23. Which of the following medications would be most appropriate for an otherwise healthy 57-year-old man seeking relatively quick relief from urinary obstructive symptoms with slight prostatic enlargement due to benign prostatic hyperplasia (BPH)?

    (A) Atropine
    (B) Desmopressin
    (C) Finasteride
    (D) Tamsulosin
    (E) Testosterone

24. Chronic therapy with which of the following medications can potentially lead to abrupt, unpredictable, and transient motor fluctuations (from mobility to immobility) often referred to as the "wearing-off phenomenon"?

    (A) Carbamazepine
    (B) Cyclobenzaprine
    (C) Diazepam
    (D) Levodopa/carbidopa
    (E) Methotrexate

25. A 1-year-old male with no known drug allergies is diagnosed in your clinic with bilateral acute otitis media. Which of the following is the initial antibiotic of choice?

    (A) Amoxicillin
    (B) Doxycycline
    (C) Gentamicin
    (D) Levofloxacin
    (E) Nitrofurantoin

26. Which of the following medications is indicated for the treatment of anemia associated with chronic kidney disease?

    (A) Dabigatran
    (B) Deferoxamine
    (C) Erythropoietin
    (D) Protamine sulfate
    (E) Warfarin

27. A 57-year-old female with a 10-year history of hypertension presents for her quarterly check-up. She has been treated with amlodipine and her blood pressure has been in control with this medication. However, her current blood pressure is 156/94 mm Hg with a pulse of 54 beats/min. She otherwise appears in good health and has made several lifestyle changes to reduce her blood pressure. Which of the following is the most appropriate approach to managing the patient at this time?

    (A) Add benazepril to the current medication regimen
    (B) Add diltiazem to the current medication regimen
    (C) Discontinue the amlodipine and start hydrochlorothiazide
    (D) Discontinue the amlodipine and start metoprolol
    (E) Remain with the current regimen of amlodipine

28. Which of the following is considered an osmotic laxative?

    (A) Docusate sodium
    (B) Loperamide
    (C) Methylcellulose
    (D) Polyethylene glycol
    (E) Senna

29. A 48-year-old male is brought to the emergency department (ED) by his sister after suffering from loss of consciousness, followed by muscle rigidity and rhythmic contractions, and then a return to a normal state. When asked about medication use, the patient states he is currently being treated with a drug for depression but cannot remember the name. He claims that he has never had a seizure or seizure-like activity prior to this event. Approximately three hours after the first episode, the patient suffers a second one while still in the ED. Which of the following medications is the patient most likely taking?

(A) Bupropion

(B) Duloxetine

(C) Fluoxetine

(D) Mirtazapine

(E) Nortriptyline

30. A 27-year-old male visits the clinic for a preemployment physical. He has a 15-year history of intermittent asthma that is currently being managed prn with a metered-dose inhaler of albuterol. The patient tells you he has been using it daily for the past 6 to 8 weeks due to increased shortness of breath and that it does not seem to be working too well. Which of the following is the most rationale approach to managing the patient at this time?

(A) Add fluticasone for use on a daily basis and continue albuterol prn

(B) Add ipratropium bromide for use on a daily basis and continue albuterol prn

(C) Add methylprednisolone for use on a daily basis and continue albuterol prn

(D) Discontinue the albuterol and prescribe fluticasone for use on a daily basis

(E) Increase the dose of albuterol and keep using prn

31. A progestin-only contraceptive, or "minipill," would be most appropriate for which of the following female patients?

(A) 25-year-old in excellent overall health

(B) 28-year-old with a 20-year history of epilepsy

(C) 32-year-old with a past episode of pelvic inflammatory disease

(D) 36-year-old who smokes 2 packs cigarettes per day and has a 2-year history of adequately controlled hypertension

(E) 38-year-old with a 25-year history of asthma and bronchitis

32. Which of the following most accurately describes the mechanism of action of sildenafil?

(A) Antagonizes nitric oxide receptors

(B) Increases cyclic AMP levels by competitively inhibiting acetylcholinesterase

(C) Increases cyclic GMP levels by competitively inhibiting phosphodiesterase-5

(D) Stimulates the release of acetylcholine

(E) Stimulates the release of norepinephrine

33. Which of the following is the drug of choice for treating a primary herpes simplex virus (HSV) infection?

(A) Acyclovir

(B) Amantadine

(C) Nystatin

(D) Zanamivir

(E) Zidovudine

34. Serotonin 1b/1d agonists, or triptans, are most effective for the acute treatment of which of the following?

(A) Absence seizures

(B) Acute migraine

(C) Chemotherapy-induced nausea and vomiting (CINV)

(D) Myoclonic seizures

(E) Nocturia

35. A 35-year-old male is brought to the emergency department with unremitting, generalized convulsive status epilepticus. The initial, preferred treatment is intravenous administration of which of the following?

(A) Donepezil

(B) Lorazepam

(C) Phenobarbital

(D) Phenytoin

(E) Valproate

36. Abrupt cessation of which of the following antihypertensives can produce significant rebound hypertension, tachycardia, and exacerbation of ischemic symptoms?

(A) Angiotensin converting enzyme inhibitors (ACEIs)

(B) Angiotensin receptor blockers (ARBs)

(C) β-Blockers

(D) Potassium-sparing diuretics

(E) Thiazide diuretics

37. A 54-year-old male with chronic stable angina is being treated with daily doses of metoprolol and sublingual nitroglycerin prn to control occasional angina attacks. Approximately 45 minutes after taking sildenafil, the patient suffers a severe attack and takes several nitroglycerin tablets within a short time frame that ultimately leads to his death. Which of the following best explains what occurred?

    (A) Metoprolol/sildenafil combination led to severe bronchospasm
    (B) Metoprolol/sildenafil combination triggered a fatal coronary vasospasm
    (C) Nitroglycerin/sildenafil combination led to a fatal arrhythmia
    (D) Nitroglycerin/sildenafil interaction led to severe hypotension
    (E) Nitroglycerin/sildenafil interaction triggered acute arterial thromboembolism

38. A patient with myasthenia gravis would most likely experience symptomatic benefit with which of the following?

    (A) Acetylcholinesterase inhibitors
    (B) α_1-Blockers
    (C) β-Blockers
    (D) Dopamine agonists
    (E) Muscarinic antagonists

39. From the choices given below, which medication is considered the safest for use during pregnancy?

    (A) Esomeprazole
    (B) Isotretinoin
    (C) Lisinopril
    (D) Misoprostol
    (E) Warfarin

40. The risk of extrapyramidal side effects (pseudoparkinsonism) and tardive dyskinesia is associated with which class of medications?

    (A) Amphetamines
    (B) Benzodiazepines
    (C) Monoamine oxidase inhibitors (MAOIs)
    (D) Tricyclic antidepressants (TCAs)
    (E) Typical (first-generation) antipsychotics

41. Drug X is an antiseizure medication that is labeled as a "CYP2D6 inducer." CYP2D6 enzymes do not metabolize drug X. Drug Y is an antihypertensive medication that is typically metabolized to inactive products by CYP2D6 enzymes. Assuming the patient has been taking drug Y for the last 3 months and now begins taking drug X simultaneously, the patient will

    (A) be at greater risk for having a seizure.
    (B) likely experience an increase in blood pressure.
    (C) likely experience a decrease in blood pressure.
    (D) likely experience a decrease in blood pressure and be at greater risk for having a seizure.
    (E) likely experience an increase in blood pressure and be at greater risk for having a seizure.

42. A 50-year-old male presents to the emergency department with an episode of paroxysmal supraventricular tachycardia (PSVT). He is hypotensive (88/58 mm Hg), does not feel faint, nor is complaining of any chest pain. His electrocardiogram (ECG) shows a regular arrhythmia with no P waves, narrow QRS complexes, and a heart rate of 172 beats/min. Successive Valsalva maneuvers fail to terminate the PSVT. Which of the following intravenous treatments would be most appropriate for the patient at this time?

    (A) Adenosine
    (B) Amiodarone
    (C) Atenolol
    (D) Digoxin
    (E) Morphine

43. Which of the following is the primary site of action for warfarin?

    (A) Blood
    (B) Kidneys
    (C) Liver
    (D) Red bone marrow
    (E) Small intestine

44. Disulfiram increases the level of which of the following to produce flushing, throbbing headache, vomiting, and palpitations during alcohol intake?

    (A) Acetic acid
    (B) Acetaldehyde
    (C) Alcohol dehydrogenase
    (D) Creatinine
    (E) Glucuronic acid

45. Which of the following exerts its action by inhibiting cell wall synthesis?

    (A) Amoxicillin
    (B) Ciprofloxacin
    (C) Doxycycline
    (D) Erythromycin
    (E) Gentamicin

46. Nasal formulations of which vitamin can be used to successfully treat pernicious anemia?

    (A) B_{12} (cobalamin)
    (B) D
    (C) K
    (D) Folate
    (E) Niacin

47. A single dose of 1.5-mg levonorgestrel or two 0.75-mg tablets of levonorgestrel taken 12 hours apart are effective as _____

    (A) a method to increase the chances of becoming pregnant by inducing ovulation.
    (B) a method for preventing hot flashes in postmenopausal women.
    (C) a method of protection against HIV transmission.
    (D) analgesia for pain associated with endometriosis.
    (E) emergency contraception following unprotected intercourse.

48. Which drug can potentially lead to oropharyngeal candidiasis, and which agent can be used to treat this type of infection?

    (A) Albuterol; ketoconazole
    (B) Cromolyn sodium; levofloxacin
    (C) Flunisolide; metronidazole
    (D) Fluticasone; amantadine
    (E) Triamcinolone; fluconazole

49. A 19-year-old female presents to the clinic with complaints of nausea, diarrhea, flatulence, stomach cramps, and bloating. A stool sample provided while at the clinic has frothy and greasy characteristics but is free of any visible blood. She explains that she just returned from a 2-week camping trip where she did a great deal of lake swimming. Which of the following medications would be most appropriate for this patient?

    (A) Doxycycline
    (B) Erythromycin
    (C) Metronidazole
    (D) Nystatin
    (E) Trimethoprim–sulfamethoxazole

50. A 34-year-old female presents to the clinic with complaints of intermittent flushing and blushing that started 3 to 4 weeks ago. Since then, she has noticed several inflammatory papules on the cheeks, nose, and chin. Upon examination, you notice an overall rosy hue to the face and the absence of any comedones. Which of the following would be the best course of topical therapy at this time?

    (A) Hydrocortisone 1% cream
    (B) Metronidazole gel
    (C) Permethrin cream
    (D) Mupirocin ointment
    (E) Tretinoin gel

51. A 25-year-old female complains of chest pain, shortness of breath, sweating, and trembling. After an extensive negative work-up, the patient is diagnosed with panic disorder. Which of the following would be most appropriate for sustained treatment?

    (A) Buspirone
    (B) Clomipramine
    (C) Clorazepate
    (D) Paroxetine
    (E) Ramelteon

52. A 39-year-old female suffering from palpitations, tachycardia, tremulousness, anxiety and heat intolerance is diagnosed with Graves' disease. She decides to begin a course of thionamide therapy to treat her condition. Which of the following medications would be appropriate to also prescribe at the initiation of thionamide therapy?

    (A) Atenolol
    (B) Diazepam
    (C) Ethinyl estradiol
    (D) Sertraline
    (E) Verapamil

53. A 55-year-old female with a 3-month history of rheumatoid arthritis presents to the clinic with complaints of painful bilateral swelling of her ankles and hands, morning stiffness, loss of appetite, and fatigue. She has taking naproxen sodium 500 mg twice per day since diagnosed. Which medication(s) would be most appropriate to add to this patient's medication regimen?

    (A) Acetaminophen
    (B) Allopurinol
    (C) Cyclosporine
    (D) Oxycodone
    (E) Methotrexate

54. When used for advanced carcinoma of the prostate, chronic administration of leuprolide inhibits the synthesis of androgens by _____

    (A) blocking gonadotropin-releasing hormone (GnRH) receptors at the anterior pituitary.
    (B) blocking luteinizing hormone (LH) receptors on interstitial (Leydig) cells of the testes.
    (C) increasing the secretion of GnRH from the hypothalamus.
    (D) inhibiting pulsatile secretion of gonadotropins from the anterior pituitary.
    (E) upregulation of the number of GnRH receptors at the anterior pituitary.

55. Vinca alkaloids such as vincristine and vinblastine are classified as chemotherapeutic agents because they _____

    (A) block hormone receptors.
    (B) crosslink or alkylate DNA.

    (C) inhibit the function of microtubules.
    (D) inhibit the synthesis of RNA.
    (E) inhibit topoisomerase.

56. A 35-year-old female diagnosed with depression 3 weeks ago has been taking a medication prescribed by her clinician. Recently, she reports complaints of dry mouth, constipation, and visual sensitivity to bright light. Which of the following medications was the patient most likely prescribed?

    (A) Bupropion
    (B) Nortriptyline
    (C) Phenelzine
    (D) Sertraline
    (E) Venlafaxine

57. Which of the following is a common adverse effect associated with the use of stimulants such as methylphenidate for attention-deficit hyperactivity disorder (ADHD) in adults?

    (A) Diarrhea
    (B) Hypoglycemia
    (C) Hypotension
    (D) Paresthesias
    (E) Reduced appetite

58. A 28-year-old female in the emergency department is administered an intravenous paralytic agent prior to endotracheal intubation. The agent produces transient muscle fasciculations, particularly over the thorax and abdomen, prior to paralysis. Which of the following was the patient most likely administered?

    (A) Carbamazepine
    (B) Pyridostigmine
    (C) Rocuronium
    (D) Succinylcholine
    (E) Tubocurarine

59. A 50-year-old female is diagnosed with primary adrenal insufficiency (Addison's disease), and treatment with hydrocortisone and fludrocortisone is started. One month later, she still complains of weakness and fatigue. Which of the following would suggest that the dose of fludrocortisone be increased?

(A) Bilateral ankle edema

(B) Elevation in blood pressure

(C) Hyperkalemia

(D) Hypernatremia

(E) Increased darkening of the skin

60. Which of the following are common adverse effects associated with aminoglycosides?

(A) Blurred vision and hyperglycemia

(B) Diarrhea and bone marrow depression

(C) Headache and hypoglycemia

(D) Ototoxicity and nephrotoxicity

(E) Rash and dyspepsia

61. In the treatment of asthma, long-acting β_2-agonists are _____

(A) an effective substitute for inhaled corticosteroids as monotherapy for long-term control of mild persistent asthma.

(B) effectively used as an adjunct to inhaled corticosteroid therapy for providing long-term control of moderate persistent asthma.

(C) of limited use due to their low therapeutic index, risk of life-threatening toxicity, and numerous drug interactions.

(D) the drugs of choice for providing prompt relief of bronchoconstriction and its accompanying acute symptoms such as cough, chest tightness, and wheezing.

(E) the most effective at reducing inflammation of bronchial airways.

62. A 67-year old male has signs and symptoms of moderate congestive heart failure that includes a modest degree of left ventricular systolic dysfunction, shortness of breath, fatigue, reduced exercise tolerance, and ankle edema. Which of the following drug combinations would be the most appropriate choice for initial treatment?

(A) Digoxin and hydrochlorothiazide

(B) Enalapril and furosemide

(C) Isosorbide dinitrate and furosemide

(D) Metoprolol and enalapril

(E) Metoprolol and triamterene

63. Which of the following inhibits bone resorption and can be used for the treatment of Paget disease in patients who are symptomatic?

(A) Adalimumab

(B) Alendronate

(C) Anakinra

(D) Probenecid

(E) Sulfasalazine

64. Constipation, abdominal distention, bloating, and flatulence are common adverse effects associated with which class of drugs?

(A) Bile acid sequestrants

(B) Fibrates

(C) Proton pump inhibitors

(D) Statins

(E) Triptans

65. A 25-year-old male is hospitalized with symptoms of delusion, paranoia, rambling statements coupled with disorganized thought, and flattened affect. The companion who brings him to the hospital claims this is the first time she has ever witnessed any of these symptoms and is not aware of any medication he is currently taking. Which of the following medications is most appropriate for this patient?

(A) Clomipramine

(B) Risperidone

(C) Sertraline

(D) Thioridazine

(E) Topiramate

66. Which of the following is the primary mechanism by which benzodiazepines exert their sedative and anxiolytic effects?

(A) Acting as dopamine receptor agonists

(B) Acting as NMDA receptor antagonists

(C) Acting as serotonin receptor antagonists

(D) Decreasing reuptake of serotonin and norepinephrine

(E) Increasing $GABA_A$ receptor–mediated chloride conductance

67. Which of the following lists the common adverse effects caused by nitroglycerin when administered sublingually at high doses?

    (A) Constipation, blurred vision, tinnitus
    (B) Dyspepsia, abdominal distention, vomiting
    (C) Facial flushing, headache, lightheadedness
    (D) Photophobia, excessive salivation, excessive tearing
    (E) Wheezing, cough, heartburn

68. Hyperkalemia is a contraindication to the use of which of the following medications?

    (A) Amiloride
    (B) Cimetidine
    (C) Glipizide
    (D) Metformin
    (E) Verapamil

69. Which of the following drugs block the actions of leukotrienes and can be used for long-term control of mild persistent asthma?

    (A) Cromolyn sodium
    (B) Ipratropium bromide
    (C) Omalizumab
    (D) Nedocromil sodium
    (E) Zafirlukast

70. Which of the following has the potential for causing cyanide toxicity?

    (A) Clonidine
    (B) Diazoxide
    (C) Hydralazine
    (D) Reserpine
    (E) Sodium nitroprusside

71. Which of the following therapeutic regimens is most appropriate for a 17-year-old female diagnosed with chlamydial urethritis?

    (A) Amoxicillin–clavulanate
    (B) Azithromycin
    (C) Ceftaroline
    (D) Metronidazole
    (E) Trimethoprim–sulfamethoxazole

72. A 47-year-old female with moderately active and refractory Crohn disease has repeatedly suffered relapses after achieving remission with first-line agents. Assuming no contraindications or barriers to treatment, which of the following is the most appropriate pharmacologic therapy to attempt in this patient?

    (A) Abatacept
    (B) Anakinra
    (C) Infliximab
    (D) Oxycodone
    (E) Tocilizumab

73. Which of the following is a potential adverse effect associated with unfractionated or low–molecular weight heparin?

    (A) Excessive cough
    (B) Hyperglycemia
    (C) Hypothyroidism
    (D) Muscle cramps
    (E) Thrombocytopenia

74. A 26-year-old female in her 31st week of pregnancy is diagnosed with acute cystitis. Which of the following would be the most appropriate empiric treatment for this patient?

    (A) Doxycycline
    (B) Erythromycin
    (C) Levofloxacin
    (D) Metronidazole
    (E) Nitrofurantoin

75. A 43-year-old male employed as an airline pilot is interested in quitting his 20-year habit of smoking. His medical history includes type 2 diabetes mellitus diagnosed 6 years ago for which he is currently taking metformin. Which of the following would be most appropriate to recommend to this patient?

    (A) Alprazolam
    (B) Clonidine
    (C) Nicotine replacement therapy
    (D) Nortriptyline
    (E) Varenicline

76. A 33-year-old female treated with a first-generation antipsychotic for the past 2 weeks is seen in the

emergency department because of recent-onset fever, stiffness and tremor, as reported by her accompanying sister. The patient also appears to be mildly confused when asked about location, day, and time. Her temperature is 104.5°F, and her serum creatine kinase (CK) level is markedly elevated. Which of the following has most likely occurred?

(A) Delayed allergic reaction

(B) Malignant hyperthermia

(C) Neuroleptic malignant syndrome

(D) Rhabdomyolysis

(E) Serotonin syndrome

77. Which of the following, when combined with chemotherapy, can be effective in treating Philadelphia chromosome positive acute lymphoblastic leukemia in adults?

(A) Adalimumab

(B) Imatinib

(C) Methotrexate

(D) Raloxifene

(E) Tamoxifen

78. Which of the following antineoplastic medications is most likely to cause cardiac toxicity and precipitate heart failure?

(A) Cisplatin

(B) Cyclophosphamide

(C) Doxorubicin

(D) Tamoxifen

(E) 6-Mercaptopurine

79. A type 1 diabetic patient who does not experience many of the normal warning signs of hypoglycemia when her blood glucose is 57 mg/dL is most likely receiving which of the following antihypertensive medications?

(A) Diltiazem

(B) Enalapril

(C) Hydrochlorothiazide

(D) Losartan

(E) Propranolol

80. Which of the following medications used for the treatment of insomnia in not a scheduled substance?

(A) Eszopiclone

(B) Quazepam

(C) Ramelteon

(D) Zaleplon

(E) Zolpidem

81. Which of the following agents is most appropriate to help manage a known acute opioid overdose?

(A) Activated charcoal

(B) Butorphanol

(C) Methadone

(D) Nalbuphine

(E) Naloxone

82. Which compound can be applied topically and acts as a keratolytic to remove corns, calluses, and common warts?

(A) Acetaminophen

(B) Colchicine

(C) Hydrocortisone

(D) Hydroxychloroquine

(E) Salicylic acid

83. A 50-year-old male with asymptomatic hyperuricemia is to begin therapy for newly diagnosed hypertension. Which of the following is most likely to increase his serum uric acid levels further and possibly precipitate a gout attack?

(A) Amlodipine

(B) Candesartan

(C) Hydrochlorothiazide

(D) Ramipril

(E) Verapamil

84. In addition to insulin and fluid replacement with 0.9% saline, which electrolyte is commonly infused in the type 2 diabetic patient who arrives in the emergency department in a hyperglycemic, hyperosmolar, nonketotic state?

(A) Bicarbonate

(B) Calcium

(C) Magnesium

(D) Potassium

(E) Sulfate

85. Both rifampin and certain antiepileptics such as phenytoin and carbamazepine have been shown to reduce the effectiveness of which of the following?

    (A) Combined oral hormonal contraceptives
    (B) Nicotine replacement therapy
    (C) Nonsteroidal anti-inflammatory drugs
    (D) Proton pump inhibitors
    (E) Statins

86. Which of the following pairs of medications are antiepileptics approved by the Food and Drug Administration (FDA) for the treatment of neuropathic pain?

    (A) Aripiprazole and topiramate
    (B) Duloxetine and venlafaxine
    (C) Gabapentin and pregabalin
    (D) Modafinil and tolterodine
    (E) Quetiapine and risperidone

87. Drugs such as donepezil and rivastigmine that are used for Alzheimer disease exert their effects by which of the following mechanisms?

    (A) Acetylcholinesterase inhibitors
    (B) Muscarinic agonists
    (C) Muscarinic antagonists
    (D) Serotonin agonists
    (E) Serotonin antagonists

88. A 46-year-old male with a history of nephrolithiasis presents to the clinic with a red, swollen joint at the base of the great toe and is diagnosed with gouty arthritis. Assuming no contraindications, which of the following would be most appropriate for resolution of his acute attack of gout?

    (A) Allopurinol
    (B) Cyclosporine
    (C) Naproxen
    (D) Probenecid
    (E) Sulfasalazine

89. Which agent is most appropriate for the treatment of allergic rhinitis in a 32-year-old male taxi driver?

    (A) Diphenhydramine
    (B) Ergotamine
    (C) Flunisolide

    (D) Hydroxyzine
    (E) Promethazine

90. Which of the following is active against influenza A and B and can shorten the duration of influenza symptoms when initiated promptly?

    (A) Amantadine
    (B) Atazanavir
    (C) Efavirenz
    (D) Oseltamivir
    (E) Rimantadine

91. In general, the bioavailability of a drug will be the greatest when it is administered by which of the following routes?

    (A) Intramuscular
    (B) Intravenous
    (C) Oral
    (D) Respiratory
    (E) Subcutaneous

92. Which of the following is the primary emergency treatment for anaphylaxis?

    (A) Aminophylline
    (B) Antihistamines
    (C) Atropine
    (D) Dopamine
    (E) Epinephrine

93. A 9-year-old male reaches under his friend's porch to retrieve a baseball and suffers a small puncture wound to his left hand as a result of a bite by the friend's cat. Which of the following would be most appropriate to give prophylactically to this patient to reduce the risk of infection?

    (A) Amoxicillin–clavulanate
    (B) Cephalexin
    (C) Ciprofloxacin
    (D) Dicloxacillin
    (E) Erythromycin

94. A 62-year-old male is recently diagnosed with colorectal cancer and is to begin a course of chemotherapy that is highly emetic (i.e., >90% risk of emesis). Which of the following regimens would be most appropriate to use prophylactically for treating his potential acute nausea and vomiting?

(A) Lorazepam + diphenhydramine

(B) Metoclopramide + dexamethasone

(C) Metoclopramide + prochlorperazine

(D) Ondansetron + dexamethasone

(E) Prochlorperazine + diphenhydramine

95. A 52-year-old male is brought to the emergency department by his daughter because she recently notices that he gets extremely tired, has periodic tremors in his hands, and suffers from increasing memory lapses. Initial laboratory work shows a serum creatinine of 2.2 mg/dL. His medical history is significant for bipolar disorder, for which he has been taking the same drug for the past 32 months. Which of the following is most likely responsible for the patient's symptoms?

(A) Carbamazepine

(B) Lithium carbonate

(C) Olanzapine

(D) Risperidone

(E) Valproate

96. Angiotensin receptor blockers (ARBs) are not as likely to produce cough compared to angiotensin converting enzyme inhibitors (ACEIs) because they do not _____

(A) cause hyperkalemia.

(B) cause hyponatremia.

(C) cross the blood–brain barrier.

(D) increase bradykinin levels.

(E) undergo a first-pass effect.

97. A 56-year-old female is currently being treated with daily warfarin for thrombophlebitis. She has contracted a serious lower respiratory tract infection and is admitted to the hospital. The patient is started on ciprofloxacin upon admission, and after 3 days of treatment, her INR increases from 2.7 to 7.4. She also reports a nosebleed on the third night in the hospital. Her lower respiratory function has improved slightly, but the infection has still not resolved. Which of the following is the most likely explanation for the increase in the patient's INR?

(A) Decreased warfarin absorption in the small intestine

(B) Decreased warfarin metabolism by the liver

(C) Increased plasma protein binding of warfarin

(D) Increased warfarin absorption in the small intestine

(E) Increased warfarin metabolism by the liver

98. Which of the following medications increases the risk of developing Reye syndrome in the pediatric patient when used to treat influenza and other viral illnesses?

(A) Acetaminophen

(B) Aspirin

(C) Ibuprofen

(D) Naproxen

(E) Oseltamivir

99. Which of the following is most appropriate for prophylactic treatment of variant (Prinzmetal) angina?

(A) Atenolol

(B) Diltiazem

(C) Isosorbide dinitrate

(D) Lisinopril

(E) Propranolol

100. A 24-year-old male is on a two-injection regimen for his type 1 diabetes mellitus that includes NPH and regular insulin taken before breakfast and then again before dinner. One evening, he has an abnormally light dinner and in the middle of the night, he awakens in a cold sweat with his heart pounding. He obtains a glucometer reading and discovers that his blood glucose is 44 mg/dL. He eats some candy and then goes back to sleep. Immediately after awakening the next morning, his blood glucose is 297 mg/dL. Which of the following would most appropriate to do at this time?

(A) Decrease the morning NPH dose and leave the morning regular insulin dose unchanged

(B) Leave the morning NPH dose unchanged and increase the morning regular insulin dose

(C) Increase both the morning NPH and regular doses

(D) Increase the morning NPH dose and leave the morning regular insulin dose unchanged

(E) Take the usual morning insulin regimen after breakfast instead of before breakfast

Answers and Explanations

1. **(A)** Multiple factors influence the initial dose of levothyroxine when used for thyroid replacement therapy, including age, the duration and severity of hypothyroidism, and the presence of certain underlying conditions. Thyroid hormone increases myocardial oxygen demand, which is associated with a small risk of inducing cardiac arrhythmias, angina pectoris, or myocardial infarction in older patients. In hypothyroid patients with a history of coronary heart disease, initial levothyroxine doses are typically smaller and then titrated upward. This regimen prevents a more immediate increase on the heart's workload that could occur with usual doses and minimizes the chances of an exacerbation of angina. *(Ross, 2014a)*

2. **(D)** Methimazole is an antithyroid agent known as a thionamide. It decreases the synthesis of thyroid hormone by inhibiting the oxidation of iodide and the coupling of iodotyrosines. Minor adverse reactions include skin rash, nausea, vomiting, and drowsiness. Agranulocytosis is a rare but serious complication of thionamide therapy, with a prevalence of 0.1% to 0.5%, and usually occurs within the first 2 months of treatment. Patients who receive methimazole should be closely supervised and cautioned to report immediately any evidence of illness, including sore throat, skin eruptions, fever, headache, or general malaise. In such cases, methimazole should be discontinued and white blood cell and differential counts should be made to determine whether agranulocytosis has developed. *(Ross, 2013)*

3. **(E)** In this particular patient, the atrial fibrillation is a compelling indication for a calcium channel blocker. A nondihydropyridine calcium channel blocker is effective for rate control in patients with atrial fibrillation, and is considered one of the major options for treating hypertension, along with thiazide diuretics, angiotensin converting enzyme (ACE) inhibitors, and angiotensin receptor blockers (ARBs). These other options, however, are not effective for rate control in patients with atrial fibrillation. *(Mann, 2014)*

4. **(A)** Acetaminophen toxicity may result from a single toxic dose (at least 150 mg/kg for a child), from repeated ingestion of large doses of acetaminophen (greater than 12 g in a 24-hour period), or from chronic ingestion of the drug. Dose-dependent hepatic necrosis is the most serious acute toxic effect associated with overdose and is potentially fatal. The patient's progression of sign and symptoms is consistent with acetaminophen toxicity. *(Heard & Dart, 2014)*

5. **(D)** Long-acting nitrates are often added to β-blockers for prophylactic control of chronic (exertional) stable angina. β-Blockers are typically recommended as first-line therapy to reduce anginal episodes and improve exercise tolerance. However, when used in combination with β-blockers, nitrates can often produce greater antianginal and anti-ischemic effects. The development of tolerance is a major limiting step in the efficacy of nitrates when used long term. The degree of tolerance can be limited by utilizing a regimen that includes a minimum 8- to 14-hour period per day without nitrates no matter the route of delivery (oral or transdermal). *(Kannam & Gersh, 2014)*

6. **(E)** Chronic therapy with systemic corticosteroids can induce atrophy of the adrenal glands, which significantly depresses the adrenal response to adrenocorticotropic hormone (ACTH). Stopping prednisone suddenly would leave the body without a source of glucocorticoids, because the hypothalamic–

pituitary–adrenal axis needs time to reestablish its normal functioning. As a result, an acute adrenal crisis (Addisonian crisis) that is marked by dehydration with severe vomiting and diarrhea, hypotension, shock, and loss of consciousness can develop and potentially lead to a fatality. *(Furst & Sagg, 2014)*

7. **(D)** Levodopa/carbidopa is the most effective symptomatic therapy for Parkinson disease (PD) and should be prescribed when the patient feels that life quality is substantially compromised. It is particularly effective for the management of bradykinetic symptoms, which appears to be an issue in this particular patient. While the other choices are indeed used for the treatment of PD in various situations, they are not as effective as monotherapy in controlling symptoms compared to levodopa/carbidopa. *(Tarsey, 2014)*

8. **(B)** Triple-therapy regimens consisting of a proton pump inhibitor (PPI) and two antibiotics are considered first-line therapy for the eradication of *H. pylori*. PPI-based regimens that combine clarithromycin and amoxicillin or clarithromycin and metronidazole have been shown to have the most effective eradication rates. There are also 4-drug (quadruple) regimens that include a PPI, two antibiotics, and bismuth subsalicylate that have been shown to be effective as well. Histamine receptor antagonists like ranitidine have been shown to be less effective than PPIs in controlling acid secretion. Misoprostol is used for reducing the risk of nonsteroidal anti-inflammatory agent (NSAIA)-induced gastric ulcer in patients at high risk of developing complications from these ulcers and in patients at high risk of developing gastric ulceration. It has no effect on *H. pylori* eradication. *(Crowe, 2014)*

9. **(E)** *C. difficile* is a gram-positive, anaerobic, spore-forming bacillus that is responsible for the development of antibiotic-associated diarrhea and colitis. *C. difficile* colitis results from a disturbance of the normal bacterial flora of the colon, colonization with *C. difficile*, and release of toxins that cause mucosal inflammation and damage. Antibiotic therapy is the key factor that alters the colonic flora. Specific therapy aimed at eradicating *C. difficile* is indicated if symptoms are persistent or severe. The drugs of choice are oral metronidazole or oral vancomycin. *(Kelly & Lamont, 2014)*

10. **(C)** N-acetylcysteine is the accepted antidote for acetaminophen poisoning and should be administered to all patients at significant risk for hepatotoxicity. *(Heard & Dart, 2014)*

11. **(A)** Inhaled corticosteroids (e.g., beclomethasone, fluticasone, triamcinolone, etc.) are the preferred long-term control therapy for persistent asthma in all patients because of their potency and consistent effectiveness. Low- to medium-dose inhaled corticosteroids offer several advantages over other medications, including the ability to reduce bronchial hyperresponsiveness, improve overall lung function, and reduce severe exacerbations that often lead to emergency department visits and hospitalizations. *(Fanta, 2014b)*

12. **(A)** Glipizide is an example of a sulfonylurea, which, as a class of medications, enhances the secretion of insulin from pancreatic β-cells. Hence, sulfonylureas are sometimes known as insulin secretagogues. Metformin, a biguanide, enhances insulin sensitivity of both hepatocytes and skeletal muscle cells, by decreasing gluconeogenesis. Miglitol, an α-glucosidase inhibitor, inhibits intestinal enzymes that degrade carbohydrates. Thiazolidinediones (TZDs) or glitazones, such as rosiglitazone, also enhance insulin sensitivity in hepatic and skeletal muscle tissues. Sitagliptin belongs to a relatively new class of type 2 diabetes medications known as DPP-IV (dipeptidyl peptidase 4) inhibitors, which stabilize blood levels of an incretin called glucagon-like peptide-1 (GLP-1). During hyperglycemia, incretins stimulate insulin secretion and inhibit glucagon secretion. DPP-IV metabolizes incretins. Hence, DPP-IV inhibitors block this enzyme, thereby increasing the level of incretins. *(Kester et al., 2012)*

13. **(B)** The goals of antihypertensive therapy in the setting of reduced ejection fraction are to reduce both preload (by using diuretics) and afterload (by using antagonists of the renin-angiotensin-aldosterone system). When administered to patients with mild to advanced systolic heart failure, ACE inhibitors increase cardiac output, diminish congestive symptoms, reduce the rate of progressive cardiac dysfunction, and decrease cardiovascular mortality. *(Kaplan, 2014b)*

14. **(A)** Both warfarin and heparin are anticoagulants that are indicated for the prevention of thrombi.

They do not actively lyse clots, but are capable of preventing further thrombogenesis. Both eptifibatide and clopidogrel are considered antiplatelet agents. Eptifibatide is a glycoprotein (GP) IIb/IIIa inhibitor, which inhibits the final common pathway of platelet aggregation, the crossbridging of platelets secondary to fibrinogen binding to the activated GP IIb/IIIa receptor. Clopidogrel blocks the adenosine diphosphate receptor P2Y12 on platelets. The binding of ADP to these receptors is an important cellular mechanism in stimulating platelet aggregation. Alteplase converts plasminogen to plasmin, which then actively dissolves the fibrin threads associated with a thrombus. Alteplase therapy should be initiated within three hours of clearly defined symptom onset in order to achieve most favorable outcomes. *(Samuels et al., 2014; Simons, 2014)*

15. **(C)** Patients treated with opioids, either for short-term use or chronic administration, can experience a variety of unpleasant side effects including nausea and vomiting, abdominal cramping, pruritus, sedation, and constipation. The use of a laxative regimen, along with increased fluid and fiber consumption, can help prevent and alleviate opioid-induced constipation. *(Rosenquist, 2014)*

16. **(E)** Hepatic dysfunction and myopathy are two side effects that can occur with use of statins. It is useful to obtain baseline serum creatine kinase (CK) and aminotransferase levels prior to starting statin therapy should these side effects develop. Patients treated with statins should always be alerted to immediately report any new onset of myalgias or weakness. *(Rosenson, 2014a)*

17. **(E)** Centrally acting skeletal muscle relaxants are indicated as an adjunct to rest and physical therapy for relief of muscle spasm associated with acute and painful musculoskeletal conditions (e.g., low back pain). The primary adverse effects of centrally acting skeletal muscle relaxants are sedation and dizziness and are common to all drugs within this class. Patients should be advised not to use these drugs with alcohol or other central nervous system (CNS) depressants, as these combinations can cause significant sedation. Operating machinery or driving a motor vehicle should be avoided while taking carisoprodol or cyclobenzaprine. *(Knight et al., 2014)*

18. **(E)** Selective serotonin reuptake inhibitors (SSRIs) such as sertraline are usually considered first-line antidepressants due to their relative safeness in overdose and their minimal affinity for muscarinic, α-adrenergic, and histamine receptors, thereby causing fewer side effects. Tricyclic antidepressants such as amitriptyline and desipramine produce several adverse effects associated with their antimuscarinic properties (e.g., dry mouth, constipation, blurred vision, urinary retention, etc.). The patient is already taking the antimuscarinic agent oxybutynin, so a tricyclic antidepressant could attenuate these adverse effects. Orthostatic hypotension is also common with tricyclic antidepressants, and because the patient is taking lisinopril for hypertension, the risk for a significant drop in blood pressure is high. Buspirone and alprazolam are not indicated for depression. *(Katon & Ciechanowski, 2014)*

19. **(B)** Dabigatran is an oral direct thrombin inhibitor (DTI). Rivaroxaban is a direct factor Xa inhibitor that inactivates circulating and clot-bound factor Xa. Clopidogrel is an antiplatelet agent. Warfarin interferes with the actions of vitamin K in the liver in producing vitamin K-dependent clotting factors (II, VII, IX, and X). Heparin is an indirect thrombin inhibitor that binds to antithrombin, converting it from a slow to a more rapid inactivator of thrombin. *(Leung, 2014)*

20. **(D)** Pilocarpine is a muscarinic agonist that stimulates all muscarinic receptors (M1, M2, and M3) and can significantly increase aqueous secretions in patients with residual salivary gland function. Atropine and oxybutynin are muscarinic antagonists and would worsen dry mouth, as would the antihistamine diphenhydramine due to its anticholinergic properties. Salmeterol is a β_2-agonist and can also potentially cause dry mouth. *(Fox, 2013)*

21. **(E)** Alleviation of symptoms associated with depression is typically slow in onset following initiation with SSRIs. Fluoxetine, for instance, can take anywhere between 2 and 6 weeks to achieve substantial benefit when used for depression. After just 4 days of therapy, there is little justification to increase the current dose or switch to another SSRI such as sertraline. Switching the patient to a TCA such as amitriptyline at this point would further delay symptom relief, as TCAs can take several

weeks to produce improvement. Compared to SSRIs, TCAs are also more likely to create unwanted side effects such as weight gain, orthostatic hypotension, and constipation. Combining an SSRI with a monoamine oxidase inhibitor (MAOI) such as phenelzine can cause serotonin syndrome that can be lethal. In order to avoid interaction between SSRIs and MAOIs, it is recommended that at least 4 to 5 weeks pass after discontinuing one and starting the other. *(Hirsch & Birnbaum, 2014b)*

22. **(A)** In patients with diabetic nephropathy, ACE inhibitors and angiotensin receptor blockers (ARBs) may slow kidney disease progression more effectively than other antihypertensive drugs. *(Bakris, 2014)*

23. **(D)** α_1-Adrenergic antagonists (blockers) such as tamsulosin cause relaxation of the internal urethral sphincter and also decrease prostatic smooth muscle tone. As a result, urinary outflow from the bladder is enhanced and the patient is less likely to experience obstructive symptoms such as weak urine flow, straining to initiate urine flow, dribbling after urination, and the constant feeling of a full bladder. 5α-Reductase inhibitors such as finasteride and dutasteride decrease the production of intraprostatic dihydrotestosterone (DHT) by inhibiting the enzyme type II 5α-reductase. Within the prostate, this enzyme converts testosterone into DHT, which causes prostatic enlargement and growth. As a result, 5α-reductase inhibitors shrink the prostate, which subsequently can provide relief of obstructive symptoms. α_1-Adrenergic antagonists are faster acting in providing symptom relief compared to the 5α-reductase inhibitors, which often take up to 6 months to maximally shrink an enlarged prostate gland. Hence, patients with troublesome symptoms seeking quick relief generally do not prefer 5α-reductase inhibitors. The use of testosterone would not be indicated as this could raise DHT levels and cause further prostatic enlargement. Desmopressin is a synthetic analog of antidiuretic hormone (ADH) and would cause urinary retention, thus exacerbating symptoms. Atropine is a muscarinic antagonist and would also worsen symptoms. *(Cunningham & Kadmon, 2014)*

24. **(D)** One of the drug therapies used to manage the symptoms of Parkinson disease is the combination of levodopa (L-DOPA) and carbidopa. Levodopa is the precursor to dopamine, which is the neurotransmitter whose decreased concentrations in the substantia nigra lead to symptoms of tremor, rigidity, bradykinesia, and postural instability. Levodopa is converted into dopamine by dopa decarboxylase, an enzyme found within the nervous tissue and also the peripheral circulation. Levodopa is used instead of dopamine because it can cross the blood–brain barrier. While levodopa can improve symptoms, it does not halt progression of the disease. Carbidopa inhibits peripheral dopa decarboxylase, which allows more levodopa to cross the blood–brain barrier instead of being converted into dopamine within the circulation. Carbidopa itself does not cross the blood–brain barrier. A complication that can potentially develop over time with this therapy is the "wearing-off phenomenon," which is characterized by abrupt, unpredictable, and transient fluctuations in motor symptoms. *(Tarsey, 2014)*

25. **(A)** First-choice antibiotic treatment for acute otitis media is amoxicillin (80–90 mg/kg/day in two divided doses). *(Klein & Pelton, 2014)*

26. **(C)** Erythropoietin (EPO) is a naturally occurring hormone synthesized and secreted by the kidneys. Recombinant human erythropoietin and other erythropoiesis-stimulating agents (ESAs) have become the standard of care for the treatment of the anemia that occurs in most patients with advanced chronic kidney disease (CKD) and end-stage renal disease (ESRD). In patients with CKD and ESRD, EPO production is usually impaired, and this EPO deficiency leads to anemia. Deferoxamine is an iron-chelating compound that can be given systemically in situations of iron overdose. Warfarin and argatroban are both anticoagulants and do not typically affect red cell count. Protamine sulfate is a heparin-chelating compound that can be given in cases of heparin overdose. *(Berns, 2013)*

27. **(A)** Based upon the results of the ACCOMPLISH trial and the choices given, the most appropriate step is to initiate combination therapy consisting of her current long-acting dihydropyridine calcium channel blocker (amlodipine) plus a long-acting ACE inhibitor (benazepril). The elevated blood pressure warrants the addition of a second medication, plus there is no reason given in the vignette to discontinue the amlodipine for monotherapy from a different class of antihypertensive. For patients

requiring combination therapy, the ACCOMPLISH trial demonstrated that benazepril plus amlodipine was more effective than benazepril plus hydrochlorothiazide at reducing cardiovascular events in hypertensive patients at risk for such events. *(Mann, 2014)*

28. **(D)** Polyethylene glycol (PEG) is an example of an osmotic laxative that leads to water retention in the bowel. It is often used when complete colonic cleansing is required prior to gastrointestinal endoscopic procedures or colorectal surgeries. Senna is a plant derivative found in preparations such as Senokot and Ex-Lax. While the exact mechanism is unknown, it is believed that Senna induces peristalsis by directly stimulating the enteric nervous system of the bowel. Docusate is a typical ingredient found in stool softeners, whereas methylcellulose is a plant product used in bulk-forming laxatives. Loperamide is not a laxative, but rather an antidiarrheal agent. *(A-Rahim & Falchuk, 2014)*

29. **(A)** Bupropion has been shown in some patients to cause seizures in a dose-dependent fashion, particularly in those with a history of head trauma or electrolyte abnormalities. Tricyclic antidepressants (e.g., nortriptyline), selective serotonin reuptake inhibitors (e.g., fluoxetine), serotonin–norepinephrine reuptake inhibitors (e.g., duloxetine) and mirtazapine are typically associated with seizures. *(Hirsch & Birnbaum, 2014a)*

30. **(A)** The patient is likely in need of long-term control therapy due to his worsening symptoms. Whenever increased use of a quick-relief medication such as a β_2-agonist (albuterol) occurs, it is usually indicative of needing to add a long-term control agent to the therapeutic regimen or to increase the dose of an already prescribed long-term control medication. Inhaled corticosteroids like fluticasone are considered first-line long-term control medications for patients with mild persistent asthma. *(Fanta, 2014a)*

31. **(D)** In the majority of cases, a combined hormonal contraceptive (i.e., one that contains both an estrogen and progestin) is the preferred method of oral contraception because of its efficacy when used perfectly (>99%). However, for women older than 35 years of age who are smokers or are obese, or who have a history of hypertension or vascular dis-

ease, progesterone only contraceptives are recommended. Progestin-only contraceptives, however, tend to be less effective than the combined hormonal contraceptives. *(Kaunitz, 2014)*

32. **(C)** Sildenafil is classified as a phosphodiesterase-5 (PDE-5) inhibitor and is used for the treatment of erectile dysfunction. The rationale for the use of PDE-5 inhibitors is based upon the role of nitric oxide-induced vasodilation, which is mediated by cyclic guanosine monophosphate (GMP) in initiating and maintaining an erection; detumescence is associated with catabolism of cyclic GMP by the PDE-5 enzyme. PDE-5 inhibitors act by increasing intracavernosal cyclic GMP levels by competitively inhibiting the PDE-5 enzyme, and as a result, increase both the number and duration of erections in men with ED. *(Cunningham & Seftel, 2014)*

33. **(A)** Acyclovir is the treatment of choice for primary HSV infection, typically in oral doses of 200 mg five times daily or 400 mg three times daily. Famciclovir and valacyclovir are also first-line treatments. *(Albrecht, 2014)*

34. **(B)** The serotonin 1b/1d agonists (triptans) are effective for the acute treatment of migraine. The triptans are considered to be specific therapies for acute migraine since, in contrast to analgesics, they act at the pathophysiologic mechanism of the headache. *(Bajwa & Sabahat, 2014)*

35. **(B)** In most patients suffering from generalized convulsive status epilepticus (GCSE), benzodiazepines such as lorazepam and diazepam are effective initial therapies due to their relatively high lipid solubility. As a result, they are able to cross the blood–brain barrier easily, which gives them the potential to stop seizures quickly. Lorazepam's lipid solubility is less compared to diazepam, and it also redistributes to fat more slowly. Hence, lorazepam tends to have a longer duration of action (12–24 hours) than diazepam (20–30 minutes). *(Drislane, 2014)*

36. **(C)** Gradual tapering of β-blockers over a period of 1 to 2 weeks is advised before discontinuation to avoid rebound hypertension, tachycardia, and exacerbation of ischemic symptoms. Abrupt cessation of β-blockers has also been shown to cause unstable angina, myocardial infarction, and even death in the

hypertensive patient with coronary artery disease. *(Podrid, 2014)*

37. **(D)** Sildenafil and other selective phosphodiesterase (PDE) inhibitors (e.g., tadalafil, vardenafil) profoundly potentiate the vasodilatory effects (e.g., a greater than 25 mm Hg decrease in systolic blood pressure) of organic nitrates and potentially life-threatening hypotension or hemodynamic collapse can result. Nitrates promote the formation of cyclic guanosine monophosphate (cGMP) by stimulating guanylate cyclase. Sildenafil acts to decrease the degradation of cGMP by inhibiting the enzyme that degrades it (PDE type 5). Together, these combined effects of the nitrate and PED-5 inhibitor result in increased accumulation of cGMP, which causes more pronounced smooth muscle relaxation and vasodilation than with either drug alone. In this scenario, the profound hypotension led to a significant decrease in coronary blood flow, thereby worsening the patient's ischemia that he was experiencing during his angina attack. Because of the serious risk of concomitant use of organic nitrates and selective PDE inhibitors, such combined use is contraindicated. *(Cunningham & Seftel, 2014)*

38. **(A)** Myasthenia gravis is characterized by autoantibodies directed against nicotinic cholinergic receptors at neuromuscular junctions. By inhibiting the enzyme responsible for metabolizing acetylcholine (acetylcholinesterase), the synaptic concentration of acetylcholine increases and can bind more frequently to functional nicotinic receptors yet to be affected by the disease. This can alleviate the symptoms such as limb weakness, difficulty swallowing, and difficulty chewing associated with the disease. Examples of acetylcholinesterase inhibitors include neostigmine and pyridostigmine. *(Bird, 2014)*

39. **(A)** Warfarin is contraindicated in all trimesters and is listed as category X by the FDA, because it has been shown to induce fetal bleeding and cause several teratogenic effects including CNS malformations, structural deformities of the nose, and bone dysplasias. ACEIs (e.g., captopril) should not be used due to their increased risk of causing fetal hypotension, fetal renal damage, and major congenital malformations. Isotretinoin is also listed as category X and is a known teratogen that causes malformations of the CNS, face, and ears.

Misoprostol is a synthetic prostaglandin analog indicated for reducing the risk of NSAID-induced gastric ulcers in patients at high risk of complications from gastric ulcer. It also has oxytocic properties, meaning that it can induce uterine contractions that may endanger pregnancy. The drug comes with a black box warning stating that administration to women who are pregnant can cause abortion, premature birth, or birth defects. Esomeprazole is category B and has not been shown to cause birth defects or threaten pregnancy. *(Lockwood & Magriples, 2014)*

40. **(E)** Typical antipsychotics (e.g., haloperidol, chlorpromazine, fluphenazine) can produce extrapyramidal symptoms (EPS) via blockade of dopamine (D_2) receptors in the nigrostriatum. Symptoms can include akinesia, bradykinesia, mask-like facial expression, tremor, cogwheel rigidity, and postural abnormalities. Tardive dyskinesia may also occur. *(Jibson, 2014)*

41. **(B)** As a CYP2D6 inducer, the antiepileptic medication will stimulate or increase the activity of the enzymes responsible for metabolizing the antihypertensive medication into harmless by-products. As a result, the patient is more susceptible to having his/her blood pressure elevate, because the dose of the antihypertensive drug is being cleared from the body more quickly. *(Larson, 2014a)*

42. **(A)** This patient only has mild symptoms resulting from his PSVT. In these situations, nonpharmacologic measures that increase vagal activity (e.g., Valsalva maneuver) to the heart can be attempted to help restore a sinus rhythm. Because this failed in this patient, drug therapy is the best option. Adenosine is often the drug of first choice in patients with PSVT, as it slows conduction and interrupts the reentry pathways through the AV node. *(Ganz, 2014)*

43. **(C)** Warfarin interferes with the actions of vitamin K in the liver. Within hepatocytes, vitamin K is a cofactor required for the activation of clotting factors II (prothrombin), VII, IX, and X. By disrupting the actions of vitamin K, warfarin indirectly results in a slower rate of synthesis of these four clotting factors, thereby creating the anticoagulant effect. *(Valentine & Hull, 2014)*

44. (B) Disulfiram inhibits the hepatic enzyme aldehyde dehydrogenase in the biochemical pathway for alcohol degradation. This effect causes acetaldehyde to accumulate which produces severe facial flushing, throbbing headache, nausea and vomiting, palpitations, weakness, dizziness, blurred vision, and confusion. This reaction only occurs if the patient drinks alcohol while taking disulfiram. In the absence of alcohol, disulfiram has little or no effect. *(Johnson, 2014)*

45. (A) All β-lactam antibiotics, including the penicillins (e.g., amoxicillin) and cephalosporins, prevent bacterial growth by inhibiting cell wall synthesis. Fluoroquinolones (e.g., ciprofloxacin) block bacterial DNA synthesis. Erythromycin, doxycycline, and gentamicin all inhibit protein synthesis but via different mechanisms. *(Calderwood, 2014)*

46. (A) The primary problem in pernicious anemia is a lack of intrinsic factor that is required for vitamin B_{12} absorption in the ileum. Parental forms of vitamin B_{12} can be used to circumvent the problem created by a lack of intrinsic factor. *(Schrier, 2014)*

47. (E) Levonorgestrel is available as a single dose emergency contraceptive containing 1.5 mg in a single tablet and as a pack that contains two 0.75 mg tablets to be taken 12 hours apart. *(Zieman, 2014)*

48. (E) If they coat the mouth and throat, inhaled corticosteroids (e.g., triamcinolone, fluticasone, flunisolide) can alter the local bacteria and fungal population, thereby enhancing fungal growth. In cases of oropharyngeal candidiasis (thrush), white spots on the tongue and hard palate can be visualized, and the patient usually has pain on swallowing. In the asthma patient, the utilization of a spacer with a metered dose inhaler (MDI) can help minimize the chances of oropharyngeal candidiasis, as can routine gargling and rinsing following each inhaled treatment. Fluconazole is an antifungal agent that is effective in treating oropharyngeal candidiasis. *(Kauffman, 2014)*

49. (C) The patient is most likely suffering from giardiasis that could have been contracted on her camping trip. While swimming, she may have inadvertently swallowed water contaminated with *Giardia lamblia*, whose incubation period is generally 1 to 3 weeks, after which symptoms develop. An effective treatment is metronidazole. *(Munoz, 2013)*

50. (B) Metronidazole is the topical treatment of choice for papulopustular rosacea, which is consistent with the clinical findings in this 34-year-old female patient. *(Maier, 2014)*

51. (D) For sustained treatment of panic disorder, SSRIs are the initial drugs of choice, based on their efficacy and propensity for minimal side effects. *(Roy-Byrne, 2013)*

52. (A) Thionamides inhibit the synthesis of newly synthesized thyroid hormones. Because of the thyroid gland's ability to store significant amounts of thyroid hormone, hyperthyroid symptoms can persist for a time until this stored hormone is released and metabolized. During the period, β-blockers like atenolol are beneficial for symptom control until the patient reaches a euthyroid state with thionamide therapy. *(Ross, 2014b)*

53. (E) Whereas NSAIDs such as naproxen provide some symptomatic relief in rheumatoid arthritis, they do not alter disease progression like DMARDs (disease-modifying antirheumatic drugs). Support for an early aggressive approach with a DMARD is based upon evidence that joint damage, which may ultimately result in disability, begins early in the course of disease and that, the longer active disease persists, the less likely the patient is to respond to therapy. Hence, her NSAID would best be used in conjunction with a DMARD as she was just diagnosed 3 months ago. Methotrexate is one of several DMARDs available for the treatment of rheumatoid arthritis. *(Schur & Cohen, 2014)*

54. (D) Leuprolide is a GnRH (LHRH) agonist that suppresses the pulsatile secretion of follicle-stimulating hormone (FSH) and LH (gonadotropins) from the anterior pituitary when given chronically. Continuous administration of a GnRH agonist causes downregulation of GnRH receptors on gonadotropes, which, in turn suppresses gonadotropin release and gonadal function. Decreased amounts of LH, in particular, lead to diminished production of androgens by the testes which support prostate growth. It is believed that by using this form of androgen deprivation therapy (ADT), tumor development and metastasis is slowed. *(Lee & Smith, 2014)*

55. **(C)** Vinca alkaloids (e.g., vincristine, vinblastine) bind to tubulin, the structural protein that forms the microtubules, which comprise the mitotic spindle. Through this binding, the microtubules are unable to assemble to form the mitotic spindle, which results in a cell's (both normal and cancerous) inability to divide. *(Lee & Wen, 2014)*

56. **(B)** Tricyclic antidepressants (e.g., nortriptyline) produce anticholinergic side effects not seen with other types of antidepressants such as SSRIs, SNRIs, and MAOIs. Anticholinergic side effects include dry mouth, constipation, photophobia, blurred vision, urinary retention, and tachycardia. *(Hirsch & Birnbaum, 2014a)*

57. **(E)** Stimulants (e.g., amphetamines, methylphenidate) are considered first-line therapy in the majority of cases of ADHD in adults. Both amphetamines and methylphenidate block dopamine and norepinephrine reuptake, while amphetamines also stimulate norepinephrine release. Elevated levels of CNS norepinephrine have been associated with an anorexigenic effect, leading to reduce caloric intake and potential weight loss. *(Bukstein, 2014)*

58. **(D)** Tubocurarine and rocuronium are classified as nondepolarizing neuromuscular blocking drugs, whereas succinylcholine is depolarizing. Nondepolarizing agents competitively block nicotinic receptors on skeletal muscle, which leads to flaccid muscle paralysis. Depolarizing agents, on the other hand, activate nicotinic receptors on skeletal muscle cells leading to membrane depolarization, initial fasciculations, and intense contractions. Succinylcholine is not metabolized efficiently at neuromuscular junctions; hence, the cells remain depolarized and are unable to repolarize or recover back to a resting state. This failure to repolarize then leads to a flaccid muscle paralysis. Pyridostigmine in an acetylcholinesterase inhibitor indicated for myasthenia gravis and causes an increase in skeletal muscle activity. *(Caro, 2014)*

59. **(C)** Most patients with primary adrenal insufficiency eventually require mineralocorticoid replacement to prevent sodium loss, intravascular volume depletion, and hyperkalemia. Oral fludrocortisone is a potent synthetic mineralocorticoid. Physiologically, mineralocorticoids cause renal sodium retention and potassium excretion. Hypertension, edema, and hypokalemia are signs of excessive mineralocorticoid replacement. Hyperkalemia is a sign of inadequate mineralocorticoid replacement. *(Lieman, 2014)*

60. **(D)** All aminoglycosides are ototoxic and nephrotoxic. The likelihood of experiencing these toxicities occurs when treatment lasts beyond 5 days, at higher doses, in elderly patients, and those suffering from renal insufficiency. Other agents that produce either of these toxicities should not be used concurrently. *(Drew, 2014)*

61. **(B)** Long-acting β_2-agonists are the preferred adjunctive therapy to inhaled corticosteroids in the long-term treatment of moderate persistent asthma. A combination of an inhaled corticosteroid and long-acting β_2-agonist provides greater asthma control than increasing the dose of the inhaled corticosteroid alone. Because they lack anti-inflammatory properties, long-acting β_2-agonists should not be used as monotherapy for long-term control of asthma. *(Fanta, 2014a)*

62. **(B)** A combination of a loop diuretic and an ACE inhibitor is typically the initial treatment in patients with volume overload and left ventricular systolic heart failure. ACE inhibitors improve survival in patients with left ventricular systolic dysfunction. Loop diuretics offer the best option to reduce the congestive symptoms in the lungs and fluid retention in the ankles. *(Colucii, 2014)*

63. **(B)** Bisphosphonates, such as alendronate, inhibit bone resorption with relatively few side effects. They have been widely used for the prevention and treatment of postmenopausal osteoporosis, but are also primary agents used in the initial treatment of Paget disease. *(Seton, 2013)*

64. **(A)** Bile acid sequestrants (e.g., cholestyramine, colestipol, colesevelam) are used for lowering LDL-C. They bind bile acids in the intestinal lumen, thereby preventing them from carrying out their normal functions of emulsification and micelle formation. Emulsification is an important process for

lipid digestion, while the formation of micelles is required for lipid absorption. These actions not only inhibit lipid digestion and absorption from the intestinal lumen, but they also deplete the hepatic pool of cholesterol as a result of increased bile acid synthesis. Normally, bile acids are recirculated (enterohepatic circulation) from the intestine and back to the liver for reincorporation into the bile. Resins cause the bile acids to be excreted with the feces, so the liver needs to continually synthesize new bile acids from endogenous cholesterol. Constipation, abdominal distention, bloating, and flatulence result from the increased lipid content of the stool, because lipids are not being absorbed across the intestinal wall. These adverse effects can often be managed by increasing fluid and fiber intake and also using stool softeners. *(Rosenson, 2014a)*

65. **(B)** The patient is showing signs and symptoms of schizophrenia for which antipsychotic agents are the treatment of choice. Risperidone is an atypical antipsychotic (e.g., second-generation) that has less risk of causing extrapyramidal side effects (EPS) compared to typical antipsychotics (e.g., first-generation) such as thioridazine. Because of the risk of EPS, typical or first-generation antipsychotics are not considered first-line treatments. Even though both typical and atypical antipsychotics appear to have similar efficacy, the atypical agents also tend to be better tolerated, which enhances compliance. *(Stroup & Marder, 2014)*

66. **(E)** Benzodiazepines bind to $GABA_A$ receptors, which consist of many peripheral subunits that form chloride channels at their core. GABA is one of the major inhibitory neurotransmitters in the brain; hence, benzodiazepines enhance this inhibitory influence to produce sedation and calm. *(Bystritsky, 2014)*

67. **(C)** Nitroglycerin produces venodilation and vasodilation, which causes secondary responses of flushing and headache. Lightheadedness can also occur with the drop in blood pressure produced by the vasodilation. *(Kannam & Gersh, 2014)*

68. **(A)** Amiloride is a K^+-sparing diuretic based on its mechanism of action. In the kidneys, it will lead to less K^+ excretion in the urine and hence retention of plasma K^+. In patients with elevated plasma K^+, amiloride can cause further hyperkalemia, which

can impact neuromuscular and cardiac function. *(Brater, 2013)*

69. **(E)** Leukotrienes are inflammatory mediators that are generated within the lungs. When they bind to specific receptors, they induce a variety of responses, including bronchospasm and mucus production. Zafirlukast (and also montelukast) are leukotriene receptor antagonists that block these effects in the lungs and improve asthma symptoms. Zafirlukast is considered an alternative therapy for long-term control of asthma, as it has been shown to be less effective than inhaled corticosteroids. Both cromolyn and nedocromil are mast cell stabilizers and can also be used as an alternative treatment to inhaled corticosteroids. Omalizumab is an anti-IgE antibody, whereas ipratropium bromide is a muscarinic receptor antagonist. *(Fanta, 2014b)*

70. **(E)** Intravenous nitroprusside is a medication used for hypertensive emergencies. It is metabolized to cyanide and then to thiocyanate, which is excreted in the urine. Risk factors for nitroprusside-induced cyanide poisoning include a prolonged treatment period (>24–48 hours), underlying renal impairment, and the use of doses that exceed the capacity of the body to detoxify cyanide (i.e., more than 2 µg/kg per minute). *(Elliot & Varon, 2014)*

71. **(B)** In general, *C. trachomatis* is highly susceptible to tetracyclines and macrolides. Within these two classes, first-line agents include doxycycline and azithromycin, respectively. The CDC recommends either agent as first-line therapy for the treatment of chlamydial infection. Sulfonamides and cephalosporins have limited activity and should not be used. *(Marrazzo, 2014)*

72. **(C)** First-line agents for Crohn disease include glucocorticoids, 5-aminosalicylic acids and antibiotics. Patients are considered refractory if they repeatedly relapse after achieving remission with first-line agents, or if they remain symptomatic despite adequate doses of first-line agents. Antitumor necrosis factor (anti-TNF) therapies are approved for treatment of Crohn disease, including infliximab. *(Farrell & Peppercorn, 2014)*

73. **(E)** Heparin-induced thrombocytopenia (HIT) is a potentially serious complication of unfractionated

heparin therapy and has been reported in up to 5% of patients exposed to heparin for more than 4 days. *(Coutre, 2014)*

74. **(E)** Nitrofurantoin has been shown to be a safe and effective drug during pregnancy for treating acute cystitis. Tetracyclines and fluoroquinolones are not recommended for use in pregnancy because of the various risks they pose on the fetus. *(Hooton & Gupta, 2014)*

75. **(C)** Nicotine replacement therapy is relatively safe in the majority of patients and comes in many forms (transdermal patches, gums, sprays, and inhalers). Both clonidine and nortriptyline are considered second-line smoking cessation agents because of their many side effects. Neither has been approved by the FDA for smoking cessation. Alprazolam is also not indicated, and there is currently no evidence that it aids in smoking cessation. Varenicline is a partial agonist to α_4–β_2 nicotinic acetylcholine receptors. It has been approved by the FDA; however, varenicline is banned from use by pilots and air traffic controllers as per the Federal Aviation Administration (FAA). *(Rennard et al., 2014)*

76. **(C)** Neuroleptic malignant syndrome is an uncommon but serious complication with therapeutic doses of antipsychotic drug therapy, particularly the first-generation (typical) class. Cardinal signs and symptoms include a body temperature above 100.4°F, altered state of consciousness, autonomic dysfunction, and rigidity. *(Wijdicks, 2014)*

77. **(B)** A key component of Philadelphia chromosome positive acute lymphoblastic leukemia therapy is the use of a BCR-ABL tyrosine kinase inhibitor (TKI), which is directed against the protein product of the Philadelphia chromosome. The TKI must be combined with other therapy since remissions induced by TKI therapy alone are short-lived. The largest experience has been with imatinib combined with conventional acute lymphoblastic leukemia chemotherapy regimens. *(Larson, 2014b)*

78. **(C)** Doxorubicin is a common antineoplastic drug used for a variety of cancers, including breast, bladder, ovarian, and endometrial, among many others. It has well-established, dose-dependent cardiotoxic effects. *(Floyd & Morgan, 2014)*

79. **(E)** Nonselective β-blockers can mask many of the signs and symptoms of hypoglycemia in patients who tightly regulate their blood glucose levels. This is due to the fact that many of the symptoms are mediated through the sympathetic nervous system and β-receptors, including tachycardia, palpitations, and tremor. Sweating is another warning sign of hypoglycemia, but should still occur with β-blocker therapy, because it is mediated via cholinergic receptors. *(Podrid, 2014)*

80. **(C)** Ramelteon is a melatonin receptor agonist and is not a scheduled substance. Quazepam is a benzodiazepine and is a schedule IV drug (C-IV). Eszopiclone, zaleplon, and zolpidem are nonbenzodiazepine receptor agonists and are all C-IV. *(Bonnet & Arand, 2014)*

81. **(E)** Naloxone is a specific opioid antagonist administered intravenously in cases of opioid overdose. *(Stolbach & Hoffman, 2014)*

82. **(E)** Salicylic acid is a commonly used over-the-counter keratolytic that is typically applied as a lotion, gel, or plasters to corn pads. *(Goldstein & Goldstein, 2014)*

83. **(C)** Thiazide diuretics can raise plasma levels of uric acid, which can be problematic in patients who already have hyperuricemia or a previous history of gout. *(Kaplan, 2014c)*

84. **(D)** Insulin not only causes cellular uptake of glucose but also of potassium. Hypokalemia may develop when insulin is infused to correct either a hyperglycemic hyperosmolar state or a diabetic ketoacidosis. Hence, in order to avoid hypokalemia or correct an ongoing hypokalemia, potassium chloride can be administered. *(Kitabchi et al., 2014)*

85. **(A)** Certain medications have been implicated in decreasing the efficacy of oral contraceptives, including rifampin and some of the antiepileptics (AEDs). A back-up method of contraception is suggested for females taking rifampin and combined hormonal contraceptives concomitantly on a short-term basis. For those patients taking either phenytoin or carbamazepine for seizure disorder, an alternative method of contraception is highly recommended. *(Martin & Barbieri, 2014)*

86. **(C)** Gabapentin and pregabalin are both antiepileptics that have proven efficacy versus placebo in several neuropathic pain conditions. Gabapentin is particularly effective for the treatment of postherpetic neuralgia and painful diabetic neuropathy. Pregabalin has been show to effective in patients with postherpetic neuralgia, painful diabetic neuropathy, central neuropathic pain, and fibromyalgia. *(Rosenquist, 2014)*

87. **(A)** Acetylcholinesterase inhibitors for Alzheimer disease were designed around the "cholinergic hypothesis," which stated that the replenishment of acetylcholine could help restore memory and cognitive ability, both of which are lost as the disease progresses. While numerous cholinergic pathways are destroyed during Alzheimer disease, many others are also lost. Even though these acetylcholinesterase inhibitors are indicated for Alzheimer disease, they are not curative and do not restore function. *(Press & Alexander, 2014)*

88. **(C)** NSAIDs, colchicine, and glucocorticoids have all been used successfully to treat acute attacks of gout. Probenecid is classified as a uricosuric drug, meaning it increases the renal clearance of uric acid. Allopurinol is an inhibitor of xanthine oxidase, a key enzyme necessary for the production of uric acid. Both probenecid and allopurinol are used for prevention of recurrent attacks of gout, not for ongoing attacks. Cyclosporine and sulfasalazine are not indicated for acute management of gout or for prophylactic therapy. *(Becker, 2014)*

89. **(C)** Because the patient is employed as a taxi driver, remaining alert is of prime importance. Intranasal corticosteroids are nonsedating and are presently the most effective single maintenance therapy for allergic rhinitis. First-generation antihistamines (e.g., diphenhydramine, hydroxyzine) have a much higher potential for causing sedation and should be avoided in this particular patient. *(deShazo & Kemp, 2014)*

90. **(D)** Oseltamivir is a neuraminidase inhibitor active against both influenza A and B. Amantadine and rimantadine are only active against influenza A. *(Zachary, 2014)*

91. **(B)** Bioavailability represents the fraction of an administered drug that reaches the systemic circulation. Because the intravenous route represents direct administration of a drug into the circulation, the bioavailability would be 100%. All of the other routes listed as choices possess biologic barriers to a drug before it can be absorbed into the vasculature. These barriers can often impede a percentage of the drug dose from reaching the blood. In addition, some drugs (particularly when given orally) can also be metabolized by enzymes or influenced by the first-pass effect through the liver before reaching the circulation. *(Kester et al., 2012)*

92. **(E)** Intramuscular administration of epinephrine is the drug of choice to quickly reverse the considerable vasodilation (and subsequent drop in blood pressure) and bronchoconstriction that often occurs with anaphylaxis. Several adjunctive therapies (e.g., intravenous fluids, antihistamines, corticosteroids) may also be necessary to help maintain blood pressure, reduce inflammation, and prevent bronchospasm. However, epinephrine should be the first drug administered. *(Simons & Carmargo, 2014)*

93. **(A)** *Pasteurella multocida* is the typical cause (approximately 75%) of an early infection (within 24 hours) due to a cat bite. Amoxicillin–clavulanate offers the best coverage for *P. multocida*, compared to other antibiotics. *(Baddour, 2014)*

94. **(D)** Chemotherapy-induced nausea and vomiting (CINV) is a common problem for cancer patients that can often be avoided if treated prophylactically. Patients who receive chemotherapeutic regimens that are classified as being of high emetic risk should receive a serotonin (5-HT3) receptor antagonist (e.g., ondansetron, granisetron, dolasetron) and dexamethasone. Single-agent 5-HT3 receptor antagonists are more effective than less-specific agents such as high-dose metoclopramide and as effective as the combination of high-dose metoclopramide and dexamethasone. When 5-HT3 antagonists are used in combination with dexamethasone, they are more effective than high-dose metoclopramide plus dexamethasone. Other agents that have been used in the treatment or prevention of CINV include phenothiazines (e.g., prochlorperazine), butyrophenones, and cannabinoids. These agents have a lower therapeutic index than the 5-HT3 receptor antagonists and glucocorticoids for highly or moderately emetogenic chemotherapy regimens. *(Hesketh, 2014)*

95. **(B)** The patient's symptoms are consistent with long-term lithium therapy, which can cause a variety of neuropsychiatric side effects (e.g., tremor, ataxia, mental confusion, fatigue, poor concentration). Lithium is also known to produce adverse effects on the kidneys that can lead to nephrogenic diabetes insipidus and increased serum creatinine concentrations. *(Janicak, 2014)*

96. **(D)** ACEIs not only inhibit the conversion of angiotensin I to angiotensin II, but they also block the metabolism of bradykinin, thus elevating bradykinin levels. Cough and other side effects of ACEIs are believed to be due to increased bradykinin. ARBs do not appear to inhibit bradykinin metabolism and hence, they have limited, if any, potential in causing cough. *(Kaplan, 2014a)*

97. **(B)** There are several clinically important warfarin drug interactions, with most of them causing an increase in the drug's anticoagulant effect (i.e., increasing the INR). Warfarin metabolism occurs via hepatic cytochrome P450 enzymes that can be inhibited by a large number of drugs, including the fluoroquinolones. When this inhibition occurs, plasma levels of warfarin rise, thereby enhancing the anticoagulant effect. *(Valentine & Hull, 2014)*

98. **(B)** The pathogenesis of Reye syndrome is unknown, but there is an association between aspirin use and the development of the disease. Reye syndrome is marked by hepatic failure and encephalopathy and has a poor prognosis. *(Chiriboga, 2014)*

99. **(B)** Both long-acting nitrates and calcium channel blockers are effective prophylactically for spasm of coronary arteries. Calcium channels blockers are generally preferred over nitrates because of the need for a nitrate-free interval to avoid tolerance. The use of β-blockers is not advised because the use of these drugs can cause unopposed α_1-mediated vasoconstriction of coronary arteries, thereby worsening the ischemia. ACE inhibitors do not have a role in the treatment of variant angina. *(Pinto et al., 2014)*

100. **(B)** Regular insulin is a short-acting insulin that starts working 30 to 60 minutes after administration. Increasing the dose by a few units can help quickly restore a normoglycemic state. NPH is an intermediate-acting insulin, which has an onset of action of 2 to 4 hours. Therefore, adjusting the NPH dose at breakfast time will not correct the morning hyperglycemia. If the NPH dose was increased, it could cause him to experience hypoglycemia in the middle of the day once it starts to work. *(McCulloch, 2014)*

REFERENCES

A-Rahim YI, Falchuk M. Bowel preparation for colonoscopy and flexible sigmoidoscopy in adults. In: *UpToDate*, 2014.

Albrecht, MA. Treatment of genital herpes simplex virus infection. In: *UpToDate*, 2014.

Baddour LM. Soft tissue infections due to dog and cat bites. In: *UpToDate*, 2014.

Bajwa ZH, Sabahat A. Acute treatment of migraine in adults. In: *UpToDate*, 2014.

Bakris GL. Treatment of hypertension in patients with diabetes mellitus. In: *UpToDate*, 2014.

Becker MA. Treatment of acute gout. In: *UpToDate*, 2014.

Berns JS. Anemia of chronic kidney disease: Target hemoglobin/hematocrit for patients treated with erythropoietic agents. In: *UpToDate*, 2013.

Bird SJ. Treatment of myasthenia gravis. In: *UpToDate*, 2014.

Bonnet MH, Arand DL. Treatment of insomnia. In: *UpToDate*, 2014.

Brater DC. Mechanism of action of diuretics. In: *UpToDate*, 2013.

Bukstein O. Pharmacotherapy for adult attention deficit hyperactivity disorder. In: *UpToDate*, 2014.

Bystritsky A. Pharmacotherapy for generalized anxiety disorder. In: *UpToDate*, 2014.

Calderwood SB. Beta-lactam antibiotics: Mechanisms of action and resistance and adverse effects. In: *UpToDate*, 2014.

Caro D. Neuromuscular blocking agents (NMBA) for rapid sequence intubation in adults. In: *UpToDate*, 2014.

Chiriboga CA. Acute toxic-metabolic encephalopathy in children. In: *UpToDate*, 2014.

Colucii WS. Overview of the therapy of heart failure due to systolic dysfunction. In: *UpToDate*, 2014.

Coutre S. Clinical presentation and diagnosis of heparin-induced thrombocytopenia. In: *UpToDate*, 2014.

Crowe SE. Treatment regimens for Helicobacter pylori. In: *UpToDate*, 2014.

Cunningham GR, Kadmon D. Medical treatment of benign prostatic hyperplasia. In: *UpToDate*, 2014.

Cunningham GR, Seftel AD. Treatment of male sexual dysfunction. In: *UpToDate*, 2014.

deShazo RD, Kemp SF. Pharmacotherapy of allergic rhinitis. In: *UpToDate*, 2014.

Drew RH. Dosing and administration of parenteral aminoglycosides. In: *UpToDate*, 2014.

Drislane FW. Convulsive status epilepticus in adults: Treatment and prognosis. In: *UpToDate*, 2014.

Elliot WJ, Varon J. Drugs used for the treatment of hypertensive emergencies. In: *UpToDate*, 2014.

Fanta CH. An overview of asthma management. In: *UpToDate*, 2014a.

Fanta CH. Treatment of intermittent and mild persistent asthma in adolescents and adults. In: *UpToDate*, 2014b.

Farrell RJ, Peppercorn MA. Overview of the medical management of severe or refractory Crohn disease in adults. In: *UpToDate*, 2014.

Floyd, J, Morgan, JP. Cardiotoxicity of anthracycline-like chemotherapy agents. In: *UpToDate*, 2014.

Fox R. Treatment of dry mouth and other non-ocular sicca symptoms in Sjögren's syndrome. In: *UpToDate*, 2013.

Furst DE, Sagg KG. Glucocorticoid withdrawal. In: *UpToDate*, 2014.

Ganz LI. Clinical manifestations, diagnosis, and evaluation of narrow QRS complex tachycardias. In: *UpToDate*, 2014.

Goldstein BG, Goldstein AO. Overview of benign lesions of the skin. In: *UpToDate*, 2014.

Heard K, Dart R. Clinical manifestations and diagnosis of acetaminophen (paracetamol) poisoning in children and adolescents. In: *UpToDate*, 2014.

Hesketh PJ. Prevention and treatment of chemotherapy-induced nausea and vomiting. In: *UpToDate*, 2014.

Hirsch M, Birnbaum RJ. Atypical antidepressants: Pharmacology, administration, and side effects. In: *UpToDate*, 2014a.

Hirsch M, Birnbaum RJ. Selective serotonin reuptake inhibitors: Pharmacology, administration, and side effects. In: *UpToDate*, 2014b.

Hirsch M, Birnbaum RJ. Tricyclic and tetracyclic drugs: Pharmacology, administration, and side effects. In: *UpToDate*, 2014c.

Hooton TM, Gupta K. Urinary tract infections and asymptomatic bacteriuria in pregnancy. In: *UpToDate*, 2014.

Janicak PG. Bipolar disorder in adults and lithium: Pharmacology, administration, and side effects. In: *UpToDate*, 2014.

Jibson MD. First-generation antipsychotic medications: Pharmacology, administration, and comparative side effects. In: *UpToDate*, 2014.

Johnson BA. Pharmacotherapy for alcohol use disorder. In: *UpToDate*, 2014.

Kannam JP, Gersh BJ. Nitrates in the management of stable angina pectoris. In: *UpToDate*, 2014.

Kaplan NM. Major side effects of angiotensin-converting enzyme inhibitors and angiotensin II receptor blockers. In: *UpToDate*, 2014a.

Kaplan NM. Treatment of hypertension in patients with heart failure. In: *UpToDate*, 2014b.

Kaplan NM. Use of thiazide diuretics in patients with primary (essential) hypertension. In: *UpToDate*, 2014c.

Katon W, Ciechanowski P. Unipolar major depression in adults: Choosing initial treatment. In: *UpToDate*, 2014.

Kauffman CA. Treatment of oropharyngeal and esophageal candidiasis. In: *UpToDate*, 2014.

Kaunitz AM. Progestin-only pills (POPs) for contraception. In: *UpToDate*, 2014.

Kelly CP, Lamont JT. Clostridium difficile in adults: Treatment. In: *UpToDate*, 2014.

Kester M, Karpa KD, Vrana KE. *Elsevier's Integrated Review Pharmacology*. 2nd ed. Philadelphia, PA: Elsevier Saunders; 2012.

Kitabchi AE, Hirsch IB, Emmett M. Diabetic ketoacidosis and hyperosmolar hyperglycemic state in adults: Treatment. In: *UpToDate*, 2014.

Klein JO, Pelton S. Acute otitis media in children: Treatment. In: *UpToDate*, 2014.

Knight CL, Deyo RA, Staiger TO, Wipf JE. Treatment of acute low back pain. In: *UpToDate*, 2014.

Larson AM. Drugs and the liver: Metabolism and mechanisms of injury. In: *UpToDate*, 2014a.

Larson RA. Induction therapy for Philadelphia chromosome positive acute lymphoblastic leukemia in adults. In: *UpToDate*, 2014b.

Lee EQ, Wen PY. Overview of neurologic complications of non-platinum cancer chemotherapy. In: *UpToDate*, 2014.

Lee RJ, Smith MR. Initial therapy for castration sensitive metastatic prostate cancer. In: *UpToDate*, 2014.

Leung LK. Anticoagulation with direct thrombin inhibitors and direct factor Xa inhibitors. In: *UpToDate*, 2014.

Lieman LK. Treatment of adrenal insufficiency in adults. In: *UpToDate*, 2014.

Lockwood CJ, Magriples U. Initial prenatal assessment and first trimester prenatal care. In: *UpToDate*, 2014.

Maier LE. Management of rosacea. In: *UpToDate*, 2014.

Mann JFE. Choice of drug therapy in primary (essential) hypertension: Recommendations. In: *UpToDate*, 2014.

Marrazzo J. Treatment of Chlamydia trachomatis infection. In: *UpToDate*, 2014.

Martin KA, Barbieri RL. Overview of the use of estrogen-progestin contraceptives. In: *UpToDate*, 2014.

McCulloch DK. Management of blood glucose in adults with type 1 diabetes mellitus. In: *UpToDate*, 2014.

Munoz FM. Treatment and prevention of giardiasis. In: *UpToDate*, 2013.

Pinto DS, Beltrame JF, Crea F. Variant angina. In: *UpToDate*, 2014.

Podrid PJ. Major side effects of beta blockers. In: *UpToDate*, 2014.

Press D, Alexander M. Cholinesterase inhibitors in the treatment of dementia. In: *UpToDate*, 2014.

Rennard SI, Rigotti NA, Daughton DM. Pharmacotherapy for smoking cessation in adults. In: *UpToDate*, 2014.

Rosenquist EWK. Overview of the treatment of chronic pain. In: *UpToDate*, 2014.

Rosenson RS. Lipid lowering with drugs other than statins and fibrates. In: *UpToDate*, 2014a.

Rosenson RS. Statins: Actions, side effects, and administration. In: *UpToDate*, 2014b.

Ross DS. Pharmacology and toxicity of thionamides. In: *UpToDate*, 2013.

Ross DS. Treatment of hypothyroidism. In: *UpToDate*, 2014a.

Ross DS. Treatment of Graves' hyperthyroidism in adults. In: *UpToDate*, 2014b.

Roy-Byrne PP. Pharmacotherapy for panic disorder. In: *UpToDate*, 2013.

Samuels OB. Intravenous fibrinolytic (thrombolytic) therapy in acute ischemic stroke: Therapeutic use. In: *UpToDate*, 2014.

Schrier SL. Diagnosis and treatment of vitamin B12 and folate deficiency. In: *UpToDate*, 2014.

Schur PH, Cohen S. Initial treatment of moderately to severely active rheumatoid arthritis in adults. In: *UpToDate*, 2014.

Seton M. Treatment of Paget disease of bone. In: *UpToDate*, 2013.

Simons FER, Carmargo CE, Jr. Anaphylaxis: Rapid recognition and treatment. In: *UpToDate*, 2014.

Simons M, Cutlip D, Lincoff AM. Antiplatelet agents in acute non-ST elevation acute coronary syndromes. In: *UpToDate*, 2014.

Stolbach A, Hoffman RS. Acute opioid intoxication in adults. In: *UpToDate*, 2014.

Stroup TS, Marder S. Pharmacotherapy for schizophrenia: Acute and maintenance phase treatment. In: *UpToDate*, 2014.

Tarsy D. Pharmacologic treatment of Parkinson disease. In: *UpToDate*, 2014.

Valentine KA, Hull RD. Therapeutic use of warfarin and other vitamin K antagonists. In: *UpToDate*, 2014.

Wijdicks EFM. Neuroleptic malignant syndrome. In: *UpToDate*, 2014.

Zachary KC. Treatment of seasonal influenza in adults. In: *UpToDate*, 2014.

Zieman M. Emergency contraception. In: *UpToDate*, 2014.

CHAPTER 14

Psychiatry

Daniel S. Cervonka, PA-C, CAS, DHSc

DIRECTIONS: Each of the numbered questions or incomplete statements is followed by possible answers or completions of the statement. Select the ONE-lettered answer or completion that is BEST in each case.

1. While interviewing a 29-year-old computer programmer, you find that he denies any close friends or prior sexual relationships and has no interest in developing them. He describes little enjoyment in any activities except role play video games. He denies past emotional difficulties or stressors. His examination reveals a flat affect throughout the visit but is otherwise normal. Which is the most likely diagnosis in this scenario?

   (A) Antisocial personality disorder
   (B) Adjustment disorder
   (C) Seasonal affective disorder
   (D) Schizoid personality disorder

2. What is another name for multiple personalities?

   (A) Dissociative amnesia
   (B) Dissociative fugue
   (C) Depersonalization
   (D) Dissociative disorder not otherwise specified
   (E) Dissociative identity disorder

3. Which medication when coadministered with lithium may cause a potential fatal neurotoxicity?

   (A) Calcium channel inhibitors
   (B) Potassium-sparing diuretics
   (C) Loop diuretics
   (D) ACE inhibitors

4. What is the most common personality disorder in prison populations?

   (A) Paranoid
   (B) Antisocial
   (C) Borderline
   (D) Avoidant

5. What diagnosis should be given to a patient who has nonbizarre delusions for at least a month and no other symptoms?

   (A) Schizoaffective disorder
   (B) Delusional disorder
   (C) Brief psychotic disorder
   (D) Schizophreniform disorder

6. A patient presented to your office with multiple somatic complaints. During the mental status examination, you notice that the patient loses the thread of conversation and discusses irrelevant topics based on an external stimulus. The patient never gets back to the main point he or she was trying to express. What is this thought process called?

   (A) Tangentiality
   (B) Circumstantiality
   (C) Looseness of association
   (D) Word salad
   (E) Neologisms

7. A colleague is frustrated with one of his patients. He describes her as being extremely dramatic and overly provocative in her dress and behavior. She uses rapidly shifting emotions to maintain her position as the center of attention. He is concerned that she believes that their provider–patient relationship is much more than it actually is. Which of the following is the most likely diagnosis you might suggest to him?

   (A) Narcissistic personality disorder

   (B) Dependent personality disorder

   (C) Histrionic personality disorder

   (D) Schizotypal personality disorder

8. Mr. Smith leaves home. He recently lost his job of 30 years and filed for bankruptcy. Recently, he was notified that his home is now in foreclosure. A friend of Mr. Smith sees him in another state while on vacation. When he approaches Mr. Smith, he does not recognize him and has a total different demeanor. What type of disorder does Mr. Smith have?

   (A) Amnesia

   (B) Dissociative fugue

   (C) Schizophrenia

   (D) Dissociative identity disorder

   (E) Depersonalization

9. This disorder develops within 3 months of an identified stressor such as finances, going to school, divorce, or illness in their life. The stressor often causes impairment in their job and relationships, but typically symptoms resolve within 6 months. What is the most likely disorder?

   (A) Depression

   (B) Bereavement

   (C) Posttraumatic stress disorder

   (D) Personality disorder

   (E) Adjustment disorder

10. This finding would be necessary to determine if a child has shaken baby syndrome.

   (A) Poor feeding

   (B) Lethargy

   (C) Retinal hemorrhages

   (D) Irritability

   (E) Vomiting

11. A 9-year-old male is reported by his mother to be excessively and deliberately annoying to her and others at home and school, most always to those he knows well. She states that over the last year he frequently loses his temper, argues with adults, is easily annoyed by others and consistently blames others for his mistakes. She admits that he is not violent and really does not do anything out of the social norm. There have been no changes in his surroundings, exposures, or life events. Which of the following is the most likely diagnosis based on the information presented?

   (A) Tourette disorder

   (B) Adjustment disorder

   (C) Disruptive behavior disorder

   (D) Oppositional defiant disorder

12. Generally, patients who are malingering:

   (A) Use illness to attain a goal

   (B) Have avoidant personalities

   (C) Follow prescribed treatment regimens

   (D) Have a history that agrees with their physical symptoms

13. A patient presents to your office claiming that the FBI is trying to poison him. What would these types of beliefs be called?

   (A) Somatic delusion

   (B) Delusion of persecution

   (C) Illusion

   (D) Delusion of grandeur

   (E) Hallucination

14. A phobia is an excessive fear of an object or place that leads to or can be preceded by:

   (A) Panic attack

   (B) Depression

   (C) Hallucinations

   (D) Delusions

   (E) Confabulations

15. A 33-year-old woman presents with a 3-year history of a persistent, unfluctuating depressed mood. She also notes persistent insomnia, poor concentration, and very little appetite. She denies previous similar symptoms, substance abuse, current prescriptive

drug use, and has had no change in her overall life circumstances. She remains functional at work and in most relationships. On the basis of the information presented, what is the most likely diagnosis?

(A) Dysthymic disorder

(B) Premenstrual dysphoric disorder

(C) Major depressive disorder

(D) Cyclothymic disorder

16. Of the following, which is the one criterion that differentiates a manic versus a hypomanic episode?

(A) Duration of symptoms

(B) Presence of pressured speech

(C) Involvement in high-risk activities

(D) Exhibiting decreased need for sleep

17. Ms. Smith is diagnosed with a panic disorder. On the basis of the history gathered from the patient, you decide to treat her with an MAOI. Which side effect is considered common for this medication?

(A) Orthostatic hypotension

(B) Paresthesias

(C) Muscle pain

(D) Myoclonus

(E) Inducing mania in a bipolar patient

18. Ms. Jones wakes up from a deep sleep after having a nightmare. The nightmare caused her to re-experience the time she received third-degree burns on her arms. The next day at work, she was very jumpy and had difficulty concentrating. What diagnosis would be made in the case of Ms. Jones?

(A) Adjustment disorder

(B) Posttraumatic stress disorder

(C) Personality disorder

(D) Anxiety

(E) Schizophrenia

19. In which of the following conditions would electro-convulsive therapy (ECT) be effective?

(A) Somatization

(B) Anxiety disorders

(C) Major depressive disorder refractory to pharmacologic treatment

(D) Personality disorders

(E) Geriatric patients who can't take antidepressants

20. Which statement is true regarding vascular dementia?

(A) Occurs more frequently in females

(B) Patients with a stroke are at increased risk

(C) Has a chronic onset

(D) Patients have a normal funduscopic examination

(E) Cardiac chambers are normal size

21. A 24-year-old presents with difficulty sleeping and jumpiness since returning from his tour of duty in Iraq 1 year ago. He also notes poor concentration, fatigue, and having no emotions. He avoids leaving his home, has lost three jobs in the last few months, and has numerous speeding tickets. He remains distant from his family but finds some comfort talking to his surviving friends at the local bar. Based on the information, what is the most likely diagnosis?

(A) Bipolar I disorder

(B) Major depressive disorder

(C) Posttraumatic stress disorder

(D) Social phobia disorder

22. Which of the following indicates a poor prognosis for someone diagnosed with schizophrenia?

(A) Acute onset

(B) Comorbid mood disorder

(C) Obvious precipitating event

(D) Younger age at diagnosis

23. You are asked to see a patient who was admitted to the hospital. As you attempt to obtain a history, you notice the patient states words that sound similar, but do not have the same meaning. He also does some rhyming of his words. What type of thought process would this be?

(A) Flight of ideas

(B) Circumstantiality

(C) Looseness of association

(D) Word salad

(E) Clanging

24. A patient presents to the clinic with a family member. Upon obtaining history from the patient, he responds with excessive details of his symptoms and the reason for his visit. He is unable to answer a question directly without signification elaboration. What problem does this patient have?

    (A) Circumstantiality
    (B) Derailment
    (C) Incoherence
    (D) Tangentiality

25. What primitive, or immature, defense mechanism is demonstrated by a patient who attributes their own, unacknowledged, feelings onto others while they search for perceived wrongdoings, no matter how small?

    (A) Acting out
    (B) Isolation
    (C) Projection
    (D) Splitting

26. A mother brings her 5-year-old child to the hospital after the child collapses at home. The mother states the child has been having diarrhea for the last 3 days. She has tried to get him to drink fluids. Upon further questioning, the mother states the child has had 12 loose stools a day for the last 3 days. Examination reveals the child to be responsive, but lethargic and dehydrated. The child is admitted to the hospital and mom is very involved in the child's care. While mom is there, the child is improving slightly, but still having multiple loose stools. When the mother had to leave to go to work, the child responded well to treatment without any further episodes of diarrhea. What is the most likely diagnosis?

    (A) Munchausen syndrome
    (B) Schizophrenia
    (C) Malingering
    (D) Munchausen by proxy
    (E) Factitious disorder

27. QT interval delay may occur in which antipsychotic medication?

    (A) Risperidone
    (B) Olanzapine
    (C) Ziprasidone
    (D) Quetiapine
    (E) Aripiprazole

28. A patient describes a desire for close relationships and to be more successful at work. However, she views herself as being undesirable and inferior. Because of these feelings she avoids social activities and extra occupational projects out of fear of criticism, rejection, and embarrassment. Which diagnosis would best fit this description?

    (A) Avoidant personality disorder
    (B) Borderline personality disorder
    (C) Histrionic personality disorder
    (D) Schizoid personality disorder

29. Which disorder is characterized by episodes of hypomania and depression for greater than 2 years?

    (A) Dysthymia
    (B) Major depressive disorder
    (C) Cyclothymia
    (D) Bipolar
    (E) Mood disorder

30. A 32-year-old male presents to your office with the complaint of low back pain for 7 months. The patient states he was initially injured on the job while trying to lift a 50-lb barrel off a truck. He denies any paresthesias or bowel/bladder problems associated with the low back pain. The patient states that he had been given NSAIDs and a muscle relaxer, followed by physical therapy treatments. X-rays that were taken 5 months ago were reported as normal. He was placed on light duty at that time. The patient has seen many practitioners who have "not helped him." Another person who works with this patient was at the clinic and stated the patient has had problems with one of his other coworkers. You consider trying the patient on an antidepressant first and then possibly sending him to a pain clinic if there is no success. What is the most likely diagnosis?

    (A) Factitious disorder
    (B) Hypochondriasis
    (C) Drug addiction
    (D) Somatoform pain disorder
    (E) Schizophreniform

31. A child who has oppositional defiant disorder is at high risk for developing which of the following?

    (A) Mood disorder
    (B) Personality disorder
    (C) Conduct disorder
    (D) ADHD
    (E) Developmental disorder

32. A 24-year-old woman comes to your office complaining of anxiety. The patient had witnessed a traumatic event 3 days earlier that made her feel fearful. She has not been able to tell her family about this experience. She now feels like she is numb and in a dazed, dream-like state with poor concentration, and difficulty sleeping. She experienced a flashback of the event yesterday. What is the most likely diagnosis?

    (A) Posttraumatic stress disorder
    (B) Dissociative fugue
    (C) Psychosis
    (D) Acute stress disorder
    (E) Depersonalization

33. Sleepwalking disorders occur during what part of the night?

    (A) First one-third
    (B) Second half
    (C) Second one-third
    (D) Last third
    (E) First half

34. Which pharmacologic agent most frequently causes postural hypotension?

    (A) Quetiapine
    (B) Risperidone
    (C) Olanzapine
    (D) Ziprasidone

35. What sleep changes occur in patients older than 65 years?

    (A) Redistribution of REM sleep
    (B) Less REM episodes

    (C) Longer REM episodes
    (D) More total REM sleep

36. Which of the following do the majority of patients with dissociative identity disorder also meet diagnostic criteria for?

    (A) Schizophrenia
    (B) Posttraumatic stress disorder
    (C) Bipolar II disorder
    (D) Major depressive disorder

37. When admitting a patient for anorexia nervosa, what laboratory finding would you expect to see?

    (A) Metabolic acidosis
    (B) Hyperkalemia
    (C) Decreased serum bicarbonate level
    (D) Leukopenia

38. A 40-year-old female presents to the emergency department after what appears to be an overdose of her lorazepam. Her respiratory rate is 6 breath per minute. The team is supporting her airway via AMBU bag, her airway is clear and her pulse is 70. The best choice to counteract the effects of the suspected ingestion is:

    (A) Flumazenil (Romazicon)
    (B) Naloxone (Narcan)
    (C) Chlordiazepoxide (Librium)
    (D) Clonidine (Catapres)

39. A 37-year-old female presents to the emergency department for complaints of cold symptoms and multiple other complaints. She is dramatic, emotional, and sexually provocative in her interaction and dress. She seems to overemphasize the severity of her current cold. You suspect what personality disorder?

    (A) Histrionic
    (B) Borderline
    (C) Narcissistic
    (D) Antisocial

40. A 47-year-old male presents to the emergency department intoxicated. He becomes violent and combative with staff and is given haloperidol (haldol) IM. While he subsequently becomes manageable, several hours later he develops confusion, an inability to open his mouth, and a temperature of 105°F. Initial treatment should consist of which of the following?

    (A) Additional haldol
    (B) Corticosteroid
    (C) Benzodiazepine
    (D) Dantrolene

41. A 20-year-old female presents to the emergency room via ambulance. She was found by the police walking naked in the woods behind her home. Her speech displays minimal thoughts and is disorganized and she appears to be responding to internal stimuli. Further questioning reveals she feels that she is being watched by aliens. Her family provided further history that she has been acting bizarre for 2 months now. What is the most likely diagnosis?

    (A) Schizophrenia
    (B) Schizophreniform disorder
    (C) Schizoaffective disorder
    (D) Schizotypal personality disorder

42. A 50-year-old male is being considered for a course of clozapine (clozaril). The physician assistant must review and monitor which laboratory regularly to guard against this uncommon but concerning side effect of the medication?

    (A) Thyroid stimulation hormone
    (B) White blood cell count
    (C) Platelet count
    (D) Aspartate aminotransferase

43. A 35-year-old female presents to the office with the complaint of worry which she cannot control for the last year. She tells you that her symptoms daily consisting of sleep disturbances, difficulty concentrating, and irritability. She reports her symptoms started around age 17 but have worsened. What is the most likely diagnosis?

    (A) Panic disorder
    (B) Generalized anxiety disorder

    (C) Posttraumatic stress disorder
    (D) Obsessive-compulsive disorder

44. A 29-year-old female patient presents with her first episode of major depression. She has no medical problems and there is no family history of psychiatric disorders. In addition to psychotherapy, which class of drugs should be your first choice for the treatment of this patient?

    (A) Monoamine oxidase inhibitors (MAOIs)
    (B) Tricyclic antidepressants (TCAs)
    (C) Selective serotonin reuptake inhibitors (SSRIs)
    (D) Benzodiazepines

45. A 43-year-old female with a history of hypertension and bipolar disorder presents to her physician assistant for routine blood work after 6 months on hydrochlorothiazide and lithium to treat her conditions. What laboratory is most important to obtain considering the patients current medication?

    (A) Complete blood count
    (B) Calcium
    (C) Potassium
    (D) Lithium level

46. Higher doses of SSRIs are usually required in which of the following conditions?

    (A) Obsessive-compulsive disorders
    (B) Depression
    (C) Manic depression
    (D) Panic disorder

47. A 36-year-old man has a 30 pack-year history of smoking cigarettes and wants to quit. He is otherwise healthy at this time. Which of the following drugs would be appropriate for him?

    (A) Amitriptyline (Elavil)
    (B) Bupropion (Wellbutrin)
    (C) Fluoxetine (Prozac)
    (D) Venlafaxine (Effexor)

48. Which of the following drugs is first-line therapy for schizophrenia?

(A)   Chlorpromazine (Thorazine)

(B)   Clozapine (Clozaril)

(C)   Haloperidol (Haldol)

(D)   Olanzapine (Zyprexa)

49. A 42-year-old female patient returns to the clinic for a follow-up after starting fluoxetine 20 mg (prozac) for depression. She reports that her depression has not improved in a way that she feels significantly better. She denies suicidal or homicidal ideation. The next step in the treatment of this patient should be:

(A)   Add a tricyclic antidepressant to her regimen

(B)   Increase the dose of fluoxetine

(C)   Provide a mood stabilizer to her current regimen

(D)   Admit the patient to the hospital for ECT

50. A mother brings her 4-year-old to the clinic. She is considering prekindergarten and needs a physical examination. She is worried because the child seems distant, does not make eye contact, and does not like to interact with other children. She reports that the child does not respond to his name or use gestures to communicate in any way. Which of the following is the most likely diagnosis?

(A)   Normal 4-year-old

(B)   Social phobia

(C)   Autism

(D)   Avoidant personality

51. A 26-year-old male graduate engineering student presents to the student health center for the fourth time in 1 week to be sure he does not have chlamydia. Despite having one sex partners, he learned there is an increase in the incidence of the STDs on campus. He reports that he has only had sex once but learned that chlamydia is hard to culture. He reports he may have dysuria intermittently but is not sure. He has been evaluated at each visit, and physical examination has been completely normal each time. Which of the following is the most likely diagnosis?

(A)   Conversion disorder

(B)   Hypochondriasis

(C)   Malingering

(D)   Somatization disorder

52. A 26-year-old male brought to you by family because he was found in front of a department store handing out $100 bills to all passers-by. His mother noted that he had been depressed lately, and was prescribed citalopram (celexa) but now seems completely euphoric. Which of the following is the most appropriate treatment?

(A)   Inpatient olanzapine (Zyprexa) therapy

(B)   Inpatient electroconvulsive therapy

(C)   Outpatient paroxetine (Paxil) therapy

(D)   Inpatient treatment and start of valproic acid (Depakote)

53. What laboratory test should be closely monitored in patients on long-term lithium treatment for bipolar disorder?

(A)   ALT

(B)   Calcium

(C)   Lipase

(D)   TSH

54. A father brings his 24-year-old son in for a sore throat as an aside the father explains that the son is withdrawn, indifferent to praise or criticism and generally, appears unfeeling toward his family and essentially a loner. This diagnosis most likely is:

(A)   Schizophrenia

(B)   Schizotypal personality

(C)   Depression

(D)   Schizoid personality disorder

55. A 30-year-old female who is overweight presents with signs and symptoms of depression. She does not have any other known medical problems. What diagnostic study is indicated in the initial evaluation of this patient?

(A)   Thyroid stimulating hormone (TSH)

(B)   Prolactin

(C)   Growth hormone (GH)

(D)   Cortisol

56. A 24-year-old male presents to the practice with complaints of fear of abandonment and a lack of ability to care for his daily needs. His family reports he can do very little without their agreement or involvement in his decisions. What is the most likely personality disorder?

(A) Narcissistic

(B) Borderline

(C) Dependent

(D) Obsessive-compulsive

57. A 52-year-old male presents with an exaggerated sense of self-importance and sense of entitlement. He is described as being arrogant, envious, exploitative, and lacking in empathy. He is prone to mood swings and though he has a productive career in business he has few meaningful personal relationships. His history includes rejection from medical school after college graduation and seeking multiple degrees at the doctoral level to compensate. Which of the following is the most appropriate management for this patient?

(A) Alprazolam (Xanax)

(B) Clozaril (Clozapine)

(C) Lithium (Lithobid)

(D) Olanzapine (Zyprexa)

58. A 52-year-old male is admitted to the hospital for acute cholecystitis. During the history the wife reports that the patient drinks daily. While the patient disagrees with the wife, she is adamant that this is the case. In the interest of the patient your admission orders should include which drug to ensure the patient does not have withdrawal from alcohol?

(A) Antipsychotics

(B) Benzodiazepines

(C) Melatonin agonists

(D) Selective serotonin reuptake inhibitors

59. A 30-year-old female is seen who has a history of eating large amounts of food at lunch. The patient would often disappear after her lunch break for an hour. When she reappeared she would appear withdrawn, tired, and difficult to engage. She is a hard worker and expects a lot of herself. Her physical examination is normal except for what appears to be an erosion of the enamel of her teeth. What is the best initial intervention for this patient?

(A) Begin an anxiolytic

(B) Immediate hospitalization

(C) Start an antidepressant

(D) Test for substance abuse

60. What are the most effective agents in treating somatoform spectrum pain disorder?

(A) Analgesics

(B) Antidepressants

(C) Antipsychotics

(D) Anxiolytics

61. A patient with obsessive-compulsive disorder would most likely have which of the following findings?

(A) Raw, red hands

(B) Priapism

(C) Memory impairment

(D) Abdominal pain

62. A 48-year-old female reports that she cannot sleep. She reports a long-standing problem with sleep through most of her life and recently it has worsened. She reports feelings of anxiety throughout most of her life. She worries every day and often feels that life is out of control for her. She becomes sweaty and dry mouth when she begins worrying. She has never sought treatment but feels that she can no longer handle the nervousness every day. The best treatment option is:

(A) Alprazolam (Xanax)

(B) Haloperidol (Haldol)

(C) Paroxetine (Paxil)

(D) Diphenhydramine (Benadryl)

63. A 43-year-old male presents with an episode of an expansive, elevated mood during which he cleaned his garage, barn, and all of his cars without sleeping. Which of the following is the most likely diagnosis?

(A) Major depressive disorder

(B) Bipolar disorder

(C) Schizoaffective disorder

(D) Dysthymic disorder

64. A patient tells you that he is receiving special messages from the TV. This is an example of which of the following?

    (A) Delusions
    (B) Ideas of reference
    (C) Paranoia
    (D) Suicidal ideation

65. A 45-year-old female became confused and collapsed at home. Medical history is significant for hypertension treated with an ACE inhibitor. She was diagnosed a year ago with a mood disorder and since has been treated with several medications. Her symptoms today consist of nausea, vomiting, fatigue, tremor, and hyperreflexia. Laboratory results show an elevated BUN and creatinine, low sodium, and elevated drug levels. All other results are normal. Which of the following medications is most likely the cause of her symptoms?

    (A) Lithium (Lithobid)
    (B) Lorazepam (Ativan)
    (C) Carbamazepine (Tegretol)
    (D) Risperidone (Risperdal)

66. Which of the following classes of antidepressants is associated with anticholinergic side effects, including cardiac dysrhythmias, dry mouth, sedation, and orthostatic hypotension?

    (A) Selective serotonin reuptake inhibitors
    (B) Monoamine oxidase inhibitors
    (C) Tricyclic antidepressants
    (D) Atypical antidepressants

67. Which of the following is the drug of choice for the prevention of Wernicke's encephalopathy?

    (A) Folic acid
    (B) Calcium gluconate
    (C) Vitamin B_{12}
    (D) Thiamine

68. Which of the following laboratory tests would differentiate seizure from pseudoseizure?

    (A) Urine cortisol
    (B) Serum prolactin
    (C) Dexamethasone suppression
    (D) Fasting blood sugar

69. A 30-year-old male patient presents to the service with a history of abuse of heroin and multiple convictions for robbery and assault. He is described by family members as difficult and violent at times with both neighbors and family. He is well known to express harmful behaviors to the neighborhood animals. Which of the following is the most likely personality disorder in this patient?

    (A) Borderline
    (B) Antisocial
    (C) Avoidant
    (D) Narcissistic

70. A 60-year-old male with mental status changes presents with his wife reporting his cognitive decline that has worsened over the last several months. Examination reveals that he is alert and oriented × 2, has a shuffling gait, a reduced arm swing, and masked facies. He has no delusions but is reacting to visual hallucinations. His affect is flat, thought process reveals blocking. He has deficits in short- and long-term memory and confabulates when answering questions. A previous medical provider gave the patient an antipsychotic medication which caused catatonia. Which of the following is the most likely etiology of his symptoms?

    (A) Alzheimer's dementia
    (B) Pick's disease
    (C) Vascular dementia
    (D) Lewy body dementia

Answers and Explanations

1. **(D)** A patient with ambivalence toward sexual relationships, no close contacts, and no desire for either, along with anhedonism and flat affect are typical for this disorder. The preference for solitary activities and use of fantasy furthers this picture. The lack of aggressiveness and risk-taking behavior lessons the antisocial diagnosis. The patient denied any precipitating event that would lend the problem to an adjustment disorder and the lack of variance, seasonal or otherwise, lessens the seasonal affective disorder diagnosis. *(Eisendrath & Lichtmacher, 2009, pp. 925–926; Sadock & Sadock, 2008, p. 378)*

2. **(E)** Dissociative identity disorder is also called multiple personality disorder. There are usually at least two personalities both distinct in their own rights. The dominant personality at the time determines the behavior and attitudes. *(Eisendrath & Lichtmacher, 2009, pp. 914–918; Sadock & Sadock, 2008, p. 299)*

3. **(A)** The combination of taking a calcium channel inhibitor with lithium can potentially cause a fatal neurotoxicity. The potassium-sparing diuretics may increase serum lithium levels while loop diuretics do not affect the lithium levels. Patients taking ACE inhibitors require a 50% to 75% reduction in lithium to maintain therapeutic levels. *(Sadock & Sadock, 2008, p. 518)*

4. **(B)** It is estimated that as many as three-quarters of the prison population have antisocial personality disorder. It has been found to be more common in males especially those from large families in poor urban areas. Although they may appear charming, they are otherwise known for their failure to conform to social norms and having a lack of remorse for their actions. Substance abuse, theft, lying, and aggressiveness are all common features as well. *(Sadock & Sadock, 2008, p. 380)*

5. **(B)** A delusional disorder presents with nonbizarre delusions for at least a month. The disorder does not present with any other symptoms related to schizophrenia or a mood disorder. A brief psychotic disorder has symptoms that last for 1 day to 1 month. Schizophreniform has symptoms that last at least a month, but no longer than 6 months. In schizoaffective disorders, depression or mania develops along with schizophrenic symptoms. *(Sadock & Sadock, 2008, p. 171)*

6. **(A)** Tangentiality is a disturbance in thought causing the person to start a train of thought, but never getting to the point. Circumstantiality is seen in someone who eventually gets to the point after a delay in the thought process. Word salad is a mixture of words and phrases that are incoherent. Looseness of association is when the ideas shift between subjects that are totally unrelated to each other. Neologisms are the creation of new words. *(Nurcombe & Ebert, 2008, p. 48)*

7. **(C)** Patients with this diagnosis will resort to any means to remain the center of attention. They are commonly seen as emotionally shallow and obsessed with their physical appearance. Impressionistic speech, tantrums, and accusations are commonly employed. They commonly believe relationships to be much deeper and more solid than they actually are even after limited contact and interaction. *(Eisendrath & Lichtmacher, 2009, pp. 925–926; Sadock & Sadock, 2008, p. 383)*

8. **(B)** Dissociative or psychogenic fugue is precipitated by a stressful event that causes the patient to

develop amnesia, leave home, and assume another identity. *(Eisendrath & Lichtmacher, 2009, p. 915; Sadock & Sadock, 2008, p. 297)*

9. **(E)** A response to a stressor that disturbs the mood of the patient causes impairment in function. The symptoms occur within 3 months of the stressor and last no longer than 6 months. Anxiety, depression, or combination is associated with adjustment disorders. *(Eisendrath & Lichtmacher, 2009, p. 912; Sadock & Sadock, 2008, p. 371)*

10. **(C)** It is sometimes difficult to tell if shaken baby syndrome has occurred or a child is having a viral illness unless identifiable signs of fractures, traumatic brain injury, optic nerve edema, retinal hemorrhages, or subdural hemorrhage can be found. The presentation can also include irritability, change in mental status, emesis, and cardiac arrest. *(Braverman, 2009, p. 404)*

11. **(D)** The diagnosis is indicated in this case due to the age of the patient, age of onset, and the deliberate and frequent attempts to counter well-known adult authority. It is differentiated from adjustment disorder because there is no reported precipitating change in his environment or life circumstances. Disruptive behavior disorder is made less likely in that his indifference is primarily applied to adults and that he is not violating the rights of others and not completely parting from age-appropriate societal norms. *(Sadock & Sadock, 2008, p. 623)*

12. **(A)** Patients who are malingerers do not want to improve until their goal is met. Goals may be financial, occupational, or legal. These patients will act differently when they think they are not being observed. They may fake their symptoms in order to be admitted to a hospital or to obtain drugs. These patients have an antisocial personality disorder. *(Ford, 2008, p. 417; Sadock & Sadock, 2008, pp. 421–422)*

13. **(B)** Patients who have delusions of persecution often feel that people are taking pictures and tape recording them. Patients often believe that external agencies or relatives are attempting to harm them. *(Sadock & Sadock, 2008, p. 185; Shelton, 2008, p. 294)*

14. **(A)** Patients who have a phobia realize it is an irrational fear and try to avoid whatever they have the

fear of. In attempts to avoid the "problem," patients can develop anxiety or panic attacks. *(Sadock & Sadock, 2008, p. 250; Shelton, 2008, p. 361)*

15. **(A)** The main historical component that points to this diagnosis is the long-term (equal to or greater than 2 years), unfluctuating symptoms without mention of manic or hypomanic symptoms that would be typical of cyclothymic disorders. No variances with menstrual cycles are mentioned. Major depressive disorder is generally associated with more intense symptoms, including suicidal ideation, and only requires a 2-week duration of symptoms to diagnose. *(Loosen & Shelton, 2008, p. 328; Sadock & Sadock, 2008, p. 226)*

16. **(A)** The two differentiating factors between mania and hypomania are the duration of symptoms (mania: at least a week or longer; hypomania: at least 4 days) and their severity. Manic episodes cause a marked disturbance in function, generally resulting in hospitalization, while hypomania results in noticeable but functional changes in behavior and lacks any psychotic attributes. *(Sadock & Sadock, 2008, p. 206)*

17. **(A)** Orthostatic hypotension is the most frequent side effect with MAOIs. Weight gain, edema, insomnia, and sexual dysfunction can also occur. *(Sadock & Sadock, 2008, p. 522)*

18. **(B)** Posttraumatic stress disorder is a type of anxiety disorder characterized by re-experiencing a traumatic event. Patients have difficulty concentrating, insomnia, illusions, nightmares about the event, and startle reactions. Treatment needs to begin as soon as possible, though sometimes the symptoms do not occur until quite a while after the initial traumatic event. *(Johnson et al., 2008, p. 367; Sadock & Sadock, 2008, p. 258)*

19. **(C)** ECT is used for treating major depressive disorder. ECT can also be used in patients who do not respond to medication, have severe psychotic symptoms, or stupor, or are homicidal or suicidal. Severe bouts of depression with psychotic episodes do not respond as well to ECT. *(Sadock & Sadock, 2008, p. 562)*

20. **(B)** Vascular dementia is an abrupt onset in comparison to Alzheimer, which is slower in onset. Vascular

dementia can be prevented by reduction of risk factors such as hypertension and diabetes. The disease typically occurs in males. Carotid bruits, cardiac chamber enlargement, and abnormalities on funduscopic examination may be found. *(Johnson & Yaffe, 2008, pp. 280–286)*

21. **(C)** The recent combat exposure and implied loss of comrades qualifies as a significant traumatic event. Combat exposures are not the only such event, as rape, sexual abuse, and assault can also be precipitating events. Hyperarousal and avoidance are typical along with insomnia, anhedonia, poor concentration, and problem-solving skills. Feelings of isolation from even close friends and family is common as the patient feels they would not be able to understand or that they do not share a common ground. The lack of structure and the need to avoid aggressive responses can be difficult for service members to adjust to upon their return. Onset of symptoms may not develop for many months after the event or return to the civilian world. Whether an introverted or extroverted response occurs, family, relationship, occupational, and sometimes legal issues arise. *(Eisendrath & Lichtmacher, 2009, p. 913; Sadock & Sadock, 2008, p. 260)*

22. **(D)** A younger age of onset/diagnosis along with an insidious onset, social isolation, family history of schizophrenia, and negative symptoms (affective flattening, alogia, apathy, anhedonia) all portend a poor prognosis. To the contrary, acute onset, late diagnosis, positive symptoms (hallucinations, delusions, disordered thought processes, etc.), and a concomitant mood disorder actually lend to a better prognosis. *(Sadock & Sadock, 2008, p. 163)*

23. **(E)** Clanging is a disturbance in thought in which the person selects words that are similar by sound, but do not mean the same. Sometimes the person will rhyme the words. Flight of ideas is rapid transitioning between subjects, but tends to be connected. Looseness of association is when a person changes subjects, but there is no connection between the subjects. Circumstantiality is where the person has a point and eventually gets to that point, but with delay in the thought process. Word salad is a mixture of words that have no sense. *(Sadock & Sadock, 2008, pp. 23–32)*

24. **(A)** Circumstantiality is seen in someone who eventually gets to the point after a delay in the thought process. Tangentiality is a disturbance in thought causing the person to start a train of thought, but never getting to the point. Derailment is when a patient skips to another subject. This mainly occurs if a topic is brought up that the patient does not wish to discuss. *(Nurcombe & Ebert, 2008, p. 48)*

25. **(C)** These patients are sensitive to any criticism and are constantly searching for any insult or mistreatments, no matter how small or unintentional they may be. Confrontation is to be avoided as it is only counterproductive and will reinforce their beliefs. This is commonly seen in paranoid personality disorders. *(Sadock & Sadock, 2008, p. 30)*

26. **(D)** Munchausen by proxy is when a parent, usually the mother, exaggerates, induces, or creates an illness in their child. The parent remains very involved in the child's care. The problem seems to originate when the parent is around and disappears if the parent is away from the child for a period of time. *(Eisendrath & Lichtmacher, 2009, p. 919)*

27. **(C)** Ziprasidone has been found to induce a QT-interval delay in some patients. It is important to screen patients for cardiac risk factors. *(Eisendrath& Lichtmacher, 2009, p. 931)*

28. **(A)** An individual with avoidant personality disorder differs from schizoid in that they desire interaction and closeness but are unable to overcome their deep seated self-beliefs and fears. They tend to be less impulsive and more stable than borderline personality disorder patients and have less of a need to be the center of attention than those with histrionic personality disorders. *(Sadock & Sadock, 2008, p. 385)*

29. **(C)** Cyclothymia is characterized by symptoms of depression and hypomania for at least 2 years. Symptoms are milder than a regular depressive or manic episode. Occasionally, patients will have regular depressive or manic symptoms at which time they need to be reclassified as bipolar. *(Loosen & Shelton, 2008, p. 326)*

30. **(D)** Somatoform pain disorder is a focus on pain for greater than 6 months. The subjective findings outweigh the objective findings. Pain in the neck,

pelvic, or low back areas are frequent sites, as well as headaches. The disorder may be precipitated by an injury. The patient will have a history of seeing multiple providers and possibly many medical and surgical treatments. The patient is unresponsive to treatment. Stressors can aggravate or precipitate the pain. There may be an expectation of secondary gains. Age of onset is around 30s and 40s. Treatment consists of placing the patient on an antidepressant and sending the patient to a pain clinic. *(Ford, 2008, pp. 407–408; Sadock & Sadock, 2008, pp. 284–285)*

31. **(C)** Oppositional defiant disorder is a less intense form of conduct disorder. Children who continue with the chronic behavior are at risk of developing conduct disorder. This disorder is most often seen in boys, with problems being worse at school. The behavior can occur at home and with peers. *(Sadock & Sadock, 2008, p. 622)*

32. **(D)** Acute stress disorder is characterized by experiencing or witnessing a traumatic event where the person felt threatened by death or injury or the people they witnessed. The person feels fearful and helpless. Symptoms usually occur within a month of the event, last 2 days, and resolve in a month. The person feels numb, has lack of awareness of surroundings, and sees everything in a dream-like state. Sometimes, they develop amnesia. Flashbacks or recurrent images can occur with acute stress disorder. Difficulty sleeping, poor concentration, anhedonia, irritability, and despair are associated with this disorder. If not treated at the early stages, the patient is at risk of developing PTSD. *(Johnson et al., 2008, pp. 377–378; Sadock & Sadock, 2008, p. 260)*

33. **(E)** Sleepwalking disorders occur in the first half of the night. Nightmare disorders occur in the last third, sleep terrors in the first third, and REM sleep behavior disorders in the second half of the night. *(Eisendrath & Lichtmacher, 2009, p. 950)*

34. **(A)** Quetiapine is more frequently associated with postural hypotension as well as somnolence and dizziness. Ziprasidone has side effects that include nausea, lightheadedness, headache, dizziness, and somnolence. Weight gain is more prevalent in olanzapine. Risperidone is associated with anxiety, nausea, vomiting, erectile dysfunction, orgasmic dysfunction, increased pigmentation, and rhinitis. *(Sadock & Sadock, 2008, pp. 543–544)*

35. **(A)** People older than the age of 65 have a redistribution of REM sleep. They also have more REM episodes, shorter REM episodes, and less total REM sleep. *(Sadock & Sadock, 2008, p. 696)*

36. **(B)** Dissociative identity disorder (DID), formerly known as multiple personality disorder, is classified as a trauma spectrum disorder due to the strong link with early childhood trauma and/or maltreatment. As such, approximately 70% of DID patients also meet criteria for PTSD. *(Sadock & Sadock, 2008, pp. 299–300)*

37. **(D)** Leukopenia is seen in anorexia nervosa. Other laboratory values include an abnormal LH release, elevated liver function tests, serum bicarbonate, and cortisol. There are also hypercarotenemia, hypochloremia, hypokalemia, hypozincemia, and hypercholesterolemia along with low estrogen in females, low normal T_3, and low T_4. *(Gwirtsman et al., 2008, p. 458)*

38. **(A)** Flumazenil is the treatment of choice for benzodiazepine intoxication. *(Seger, 2004, pp. 209–216)*

39. **(A)** Patients who are histrionic tend to be attention seeking, dramatic, and provocative. They often seek approval and work hard to draw you into their story. They exaggerate on most instances where they are the center of conflict. *(Young, 2008, Ch. 26)*

40. **(D)** In addition to supportive treatment, the most commonly used medications for neuroleptic malignant syndrome are dantrolene (dantrium) and bromocriptine (parlodel). However, these medications are not well studied regarding efficacy. *(Rosenberg & Green, 1989, pp. 1927–1931)*

41. **(B)** Schizophreniform disorder is characterized by the same features as schizophrenia except the total duration of the illness is at least 1 month and less than 6 months in contrast to schizophrenia where symptom duration is greater than 6 months. *(American Psychiatric Association, 2000)*

42. **(B)** Leukopenia, granulocytopenia, and agranulocytosis occur in approximately 1% of patients on this

medication, clozapine should not be dispensed without proof of monitoring. *(Meyer, 2011, Ch. 16)*

43. **(B)** A patient needs to have symptoms for 6 months or more, and needs three of six symptoms to diagnose generalized anxiety disorder. *(Longo et al., 2012, Ch. 391)*

44. **(C)** SSRIs are the first-line treatment for depression because of ease of use, safety, and broad spectrum of treatment. MAOIs and TCAs are not first-line treatments for depression. MAOIs have significant side effect potential. *(DeBattista et al., 2014)*

45. **(D)** Thiazide and loop diuretics compete for elimination and can precipitate elevated lithium levels. *(Labbate et al., 2010, p. 110)*

46. **(A)** Higher doses of SSRIs are needed in the treatment of OCD for a beneficial effect. *(Hewlett, 2008, Ch. 21)*

47. **(B)** The only two approved drugs for aiding smoking cessation are nicotine and bupropion. *(DeBattista, 2012, Ch. 30)*

48. **(D)** The "atypical" antipsychotic drugs, such as olanzapine, risperidone, quetiapine, ziprasidone, and clozapine because their side effect profile is significantly better than the older drugs, and they may be more effective for negative psychotic symptoms. However, haldol is still the first-line treatment in psychotic patients who are pregnant. *(Leucht et al., 2009, pp. 31–41)*

49. **(D)** Attention deficit hyperactivity disorder is characterized by inattention, distractibility, and difficulty sustaining attention; poor impulse control and decreased self-inhibitory capacity; and motor over activity and motor restlessness, which are pervasive and interfere with the individual's ability to function under normal circumstances. *(Szymanski et al., 2008, Ch. 31)*

50. **(C)** Children with autism do not tend to make eye contact, and even avoid it. They do not accept comfort when hurt and stiffen up when hugged. They do not tend to play with others, and do not tend to imitate grown-ups in play. They approach play in a more mechanical way, using others as props rather than interacting with them. *(Goldson & Reynolds, 2013, Ch. 3)*

51. **(B)** Hypochondriasis is the chronic preoccupation with the idea of having a serious disease, which is usually not amenable to reassurance or redirection. *(Ford, 2008, Ch. 22)*

52. **(A)** Treatment of the manic phase is usually done in the hospital to protect patients from behaviors associated with grandiosity (spending inordinate amounts of money, making embarrassing speeches, etc.). Lithium, valproate, and olanzapine are considered effective in the manic stage; the depressive stage is treated with antidepressants. *(Meyer, 2011, Ch. 16)*

53. **(D)** Patients with bipolar disorder and those on long-term lithium therapy are prone to hypothyroidism severe enough to require treatment. Liver and pancreatic complications are not a common concern. Electrolyte/renal issues can arise with poor fluid intake and severe vomiting and diarrhea or diuretics, calcium does not require routine monitoring. *(Labbate et al., 2010, p. 110)*

54. **(D)** Persons with schizoid personalities are very withdrawn and do not seek or enjoy relationships and are indifferent to praise or criticism. They generally appear cold and unfeeling to others. *(Young, 2008, Ch. 26)*

55. **(A)** Patients who are presenting with symptoms of depression should be evaluated with a TSH because 10% of patients evaluated for depression have previously undetected thyroid dysfunction. *(Cole et al., 2008, Ch. 22)*

56. **(C)** These patients are constantly seeking external support and will do even unpleasant things for others to gain approval and nurturing. Narcissistic patients are egotistic and would not seek the opinion of others. Patients with borderline disorder can share some of these traits as they make aggressive efforts to avoid abandonment but the suicidal tendencies, impulsivity, and self-mutilation differentiate it. Obsessive-compulsive patients do not rely on external support and obey very strict personal rules of perfection and efficiency and choose not to rely on others. *(Young, 2008, Ch. 26)*

57. **(C)** The diagnosis of narcissistic personality disorder is indicated in this scenario. Since it is clear he is successful antipsychotic medications are not useful. Lithium will help with mood stability and even a mood stabilizer such as valproate would be useful. *(Young, 2008, Ch. 26)*

58. **(B)** It is prudent for the clinician to take the report of the wife seriously and prescribe a benzodiazepine to prevent withdrawal from alcohol. Considering the patient is admitted with cholecystitis and may have a long history of alcoholism and consequent liver impairment, a shorter acting benzodiazepine like ativan is likely the best choice. *(Amato et al., 2010)*

59. **(C)** Bulimia can manifest in many ways to the clinician including serious electrolyte, metabolic, and cardiac abnormalities. However in a patient without these complications an antidepressant may be useful in addition to therapy by an expert in eating disorders to help the patient gain control over the clinical issue. *(Romano, 2008, Ch. 20)*

60. **(B)** Antidepressants, especially SSRIs and TCAs are the main pharmacologic treatments used in somatoform spectrum pain disorder. *(Ford, 2008, Ch. 22)*

61. **(A)** Common manifestations of obsessive-compulsive disorder include phobias of germ and contaminants which results in frequent hand washing leading to chafed and reddened hands. *(Hewlett, 2008, Ch. 21)*

62. **(C)** SSRIs, specifically paxil, are the mainstay for treatment of generalized anxiety disorder. While benzodiazepines are a viable option for short-term management, they are not good long-term. Antihistamines are useful but not for long term and may have a paradoxical affect when treating generalized anxiety. *(Clark et al., 2008, Ch. 27)*

63. **(B)** Bipolar disorder is characterized by episodic mood shifts from depression to manic-type moods which is often rapid with depression lasting longer than manic episodes. Bipolar disorder may initially present with a manic episode. Dysthymia has no elevated moods or manic-type behaviors. *(Brent & Pan, 2008, Ch. 39)*

64. **(B)** Ideas of reference are fixed beliefs that people are referring to you and about you through media. *(Nurcombe & Ebert, 2008, Ch. 4)*

65. **(A)** Any sodium loss results in increased lithium levels. Signs and symptoms include vomiting and diarrhea which exacerbate the problem. Tremors, muscle weakness, confusion, vertigo, ataxia, hyperreflexia, rigidity, seizures, and coma may also be present. *(Waring, 2006, pp. 221–230)*

66. **(C)** TCAs have well-known anticholinergic effects. *(Young, 2008, Ch. 26)*

67. **(D)** Wernicke's encephalopathy, also called alcoholic encephalopathy, is an acute neurological disorder of thiamine deficiency. Patients are given 100 mg po BID to TID for 1 to 2 weeks or parenterally 100 mg in each liter of glucose. *(Galvin et al., 2010, pp. 1408–1418)*

68. **(B)** The serum prolactin level can rise briefly after a seizure and therefore may assist in the determination between true seizure activity and pseudo seizure activity. *(Wroe et al., 1989, pp. 248–252)*

69. **(B)** Antisocial personality disorder is characterized by behaviors that illustrate a blatant disregard for the rights of others (i.e., theft, assault, and harmful behaviors toward other beings). Patients with this disorder have no regard for right and wrong. Lying is the norm and substance abuse common. They can be labile and show difficulty with impulse control. While Substance abuse may be a co-occurring issue it is not the reason for the above behaviors. *(Janowsky, 2008, Ch. 30)*

70. **(D)** Lewy body disease (LBD) is a dementia similar to Alzheimer's and is characterized by hallucinations, parkinsonian features, and extrapyramidal signs. Patients with LBD lose cholinergic neurons which cause a loss in cognitive functioning and a loss in dopaminergic neurons causes the loss in motor control. Patients with LBD are very sensitive to neuroleptic and antiemetic medications that effect dopaminergic and cholinergic systems. They respond with catatonia, loss of cognitive function, and/or develop life-threatening muscle rigidity. *(Kwentus & Kirshner, 2008, Ch. 14)*

REFERENCES

Amato L, Minozzi S, Vecchi S, Davoli M. Benzodiazepines for alcohol withdrawal. *Cochrane Database Syst Rev.* 2010; 17(3):CD005063. doi:10.1002/14651858.cd005063.pub3.

American Psychiatric Association. *Diagnostic and Statistical Manual of Mental Disorders.* 4th ed. Text Revision (DSM-IV-TR). Washington, DC: American Psychiatric Association; 2000.

Braverman RS. Eye. In: Hay W, Levin M, Deterding R, Sondheimer J, eds. *Current Diagnosis and Treatment in Pediatrics.* New York, NY: McGraw-Hill; 2009.

Brent DA, Pan RJ. Chapter 39: Bipolar disorder. In: Ebert MH, Loosen PT, Nurcombe B, Leckman JF, eds. *CURRENT Diagnosis & Treatment: Psychiatry.* 2nd ed. New York, NY: McGraw-Hill; 2008.

Clark CP, Moore PJ, Gillin J. Chapter 27: Sleep disorders. In: Ebert MH, Loosen PT, Nurcombe B, Leckman JF, eds. *Current Diagnosis & Treatment: Psychiatry.* 2nd ed. New York, NY: McGraw-Hill; 2008.

Cole SA, Christensen JF, Raju Cole M, Cohen H, Feldman MD. Chapter 22: Depression. In: Feldman MD, Christensen JF, eds. *Behavioral Medicine: A Guide for Clinical Practice.* 3rd ed. New York, NY: McGraw-Hill; 2008.

DeBattista C. Chapter 30: Antidepressant agents. In: Katzung BG, Masters SB, Trevor AJ, eds. *Basic & Clinical Pharmacology.* 12th ed. New York, NY: McGraw-Hill; 2012.

DeBattista C, Eisendrath SJ, Lichtmacher JE. Psychiatric disorders. In: Papadakis MA, McPhee SJ, Rabow MW, eds. *Current Medical Diagnosis & Treatment 2015.* New York, NY: McGraw-Hill; 2014.

Eisendrath SJ, Lichtmacher JE. Psychiatric disorders. In: McPhee SJ, Papadakis MA, eds. *Current Medical Diagnosis and Treatment.* 48th ed. New York, NY: McGraw-Hill; 2009:4252.

Ford CV. Chapter 22: Somatoform disorders. In: Ebert MH, Loosen PT, Nurcombe B, Leckman JF, eds. *Current Diagnosis & Treatment: Psychiatry.* 2nd ed. New York, NY: McGraw-Hill; 2008.

Galvin R, Bråthen G, Ivashynka A, Hillbom M, Tanasescu R, Leone M. EFNS guidelines for diagnosis, therapy and prevention of Wernicke encephalopathy. *European Journal of Neurology.* 2010;17(12):1408–1418.

Goldson E, Reynolds A. Chapter 3: Child development & behavior. In: Hay WW Jr., Levin MJ, Deterding RR, Abzug MJ, eds. *Current Diagnosis & Treatment: Pediatrics.* 22nd ed. New York, NY: McGraw-Hill; 2013.

Gwirtsman HE, Mitchell JE, Ebert MH. Eating disorders. In: Ebert MH, Loosen PT, Nurcombe B, Leckman JF, eds. *Current Diagnosis and Treatment in Psychiatry.* New York, NY: McGraw-Hill; 2008.

Hewlett WA. Chapter 21: Obsessive–compulsive disorder. In: Ebert MH, Loosen PT, Nurcombe B, Leckman JF, eds. *Current Diagnosis & Treatment: Psychiatry.* 2nd ed. New York, NY: McGraw-Hill; 2008.

Janowsky D. Chapter 30: Personality Disorders. In: Ebert MH, Loosen PT, Nurcombe B, Leckman JF, eds, *CURRENT Diagnosis & Treatment: Psychiatry.* 2nd ed. New York, NY: McGraw-Hill; 2008.

Johnson B, Yaffee K. Dementia & delirium. In: Feldman MD, Christensen JF, eds. *Behavioral Medicine in Primary Care: A Practical Guide.* 3rd ed. New York, NY: McGraw-Hill; 2008.

Johnson DC, Krystal JH, Southwick SM. Posttraumatic stress disorder and acute stress disorder. In: Ebert MH, Loosen PT, Nurcombe B, Leckman JF, eds. *Current Diagnosis and Treatment in Psychiatry.* New York, NY: McGraw-Hill; 2008.

Kwentus JA, Kirshner HS. Chapter 14: Delirium, dementia, and amnestic syndromes. In: Ebert MH, Loosen PT, Nurcombe B, Leckman JF, eds. *Current Diagnosis & Treatment: Psychiatry.* 2nd ed. New York, NY: McGraw-Hill; 2008.

Labbate LA, Fava M, Rosenbaum JF, et al. Drugs for treatment of bipolar disorders. In: *Handbook of Psychiatric Drug Therapy.* 6th ed. Philadelphia, PA: Lippincott Williams & Wilkins; 2010:110.

Leucht S, Corves C, Arbter D, Engel R, Li C, Davis J. Second-generation versus first-generation antipsychotic drugs for schizophrenia: a meta-analysis. *The Lancet.* 2009;373 (9657):31–41.

Longo DL, Fauci AS, Kasper DL, et al., eds. Chapter 391: Mental disorders. *Harrison's Principles of Internal Medicine.* 18th ed. New York, NY: McGraw-Hill; 2012.

Loosen PT, Shelton RC. Chapter 18: Mood disorders. In: Ebert MH, Loosen PT, Nurcombe B, Leckman JF, eds. *Current Diagnosis & Treatment: Psychiatry.* 2nd ed. New York, NY: McGraw-Hill; 2008.

Meyer JM. Chapter 16: Pharmacotherapy of psychosis and mania. In: Brunton LL, Chabner BA, Knollmann BC, et al., eds. *Goodman & Gilman's The Pharmacological Basis of Therapeutics.* 12th ed. New York, NY: McGraw-Hill; 2011.

Nurcombe B. Chapter 36: Oppositional defiant disorder and conduct disorder. In: Ebert MH, Loosen PT, Nurcombe B, Leckman JF, eds. *Current Diagnosis & Treatment: Psychiatry.* 2nd ed. New York, NY: McGraw-Hill; 2008.

Nurcombe B, Ebert MH. Chapter 4: The psychiatric interview. In: Ebert MH, Loosen PT, Nurcombe B, Leckman JF, eds. *Current Diagnosis & Treatment: Psychiatry.* 2nd ed. New York, NY: McGraw-Hill; 2008.

Romano SJ. Chapter 20: Eating disorders. In: Feldman MD, Christensen JF, eds. *Behavioral Medicine: A Guide for Clinical Practice.* 3rd ed. New York, NY: McGraw-Hill; 2008.

Rosenberg MR, Green M. Neuroleptic malignant syndrome. Review of response to therapy. *Arch Intern Med.* 1989;149(9): 1927–1931.

Sadock BJ, Sadock VA. *Concise Textbook of Clinical Psychiatry.* 3rd ed. Philadelphia, PA: Lippincott Williams & Wilkins; 2008.

Salomon RM, Salomon L. Chapter 29: Adjustment disorders. In: Ebert MH, Loosen PT, Nurcombe B, Leckman JF, eds. *Current Diagnosis & Treatment: Psychiatry.* 2nd ed. New York, NY: McGraw-Hill; 2008.

Satterfield JM, Feldman MD. Anxiety. In: Feldman MD, Christensen JF, Satterfield JM, eds. *Behavioral Medicine: A Guide for Clinical Practice.* 4th ed. New York, NY: McGraw-Hill; 2014.

Seger D. Flumazenil—treatment or toxin. *Clinical Toxicology.* 2004;42(2):209–216.

Shelton RC. Other psychotic disorders. In: Ebert MH, Loosen PT, Nurcombe B, Leckman JF, eds. *Current Diagnosis and Treatment in Psychiatry.* New York, NY: McGraw-Hill; 2008.

Szymanski LS, Friedman SL, Leonard EL. Chapter 31: Intellectual disability. In: Ebert MH, Loosen PT, Nurcombe B, Leckman JF, eds. *Current Diagnosis & Treatment: Psychiatry.* 2nd ed. New York, NY: McGraw-Hill; 2008.

Waring S. Management of lithium toxicity. *Toxicological Reviews.* 2006;25(4):221–230.

Wroe SJ, Henley R, John R, Richens A. The clinical value of serum prolactin measurement in the differential diagnosis of complex partial seizures. *Epilepsy Research.* 1989;3(3):248–252.

Young JQ. Chapter 26: Personality disorders. In: Feldman MD, Christensen JF, eds. *Behavioral Medicine: A Guide for Clinical Practice.* 3rd ed. New York, NY: McGraw-Hill; 2008.

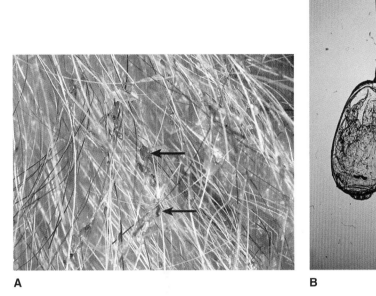

A   B

Figure 3-1. Reproduced with permission from Fitzpatrick, Johnson, Wolff, et al. *Dermatology in General Medicine*. 4th ed. New York, NY: McGraw-Hill, 1993.

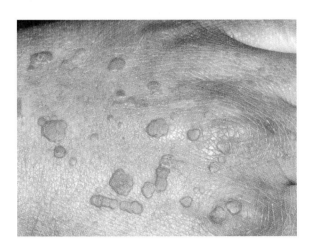

Figure 3-2. Reproduced, with permission, from Goldsmith LA, Katz SI, Gilchrest BA, et al. *Fitzpatrick's Dermatology in General Medicine*. 8th ed. New York, NY: McGraw-Hill Education, 2012. Figure 196–8.

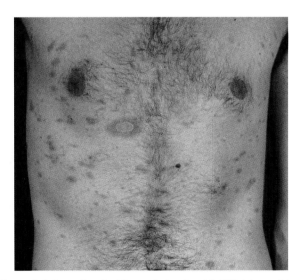

Figure 3-3. Reproduced, with permission, from Wolff K, Johnson RA, Suurmond D. *Fitzpatrick's Color Atlas & Synopsis of Clinical Dermatology*. 5th ed. New York, NY: McGraw-Hill Education, 2005:119.

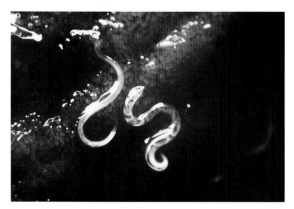

Figure 7-1. Centers for Disease Control and Prevention, National Center for Infectious Diseases, Division of Parasitic Diseases.

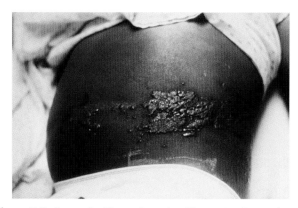

Figure 7-2. Centers for Disease Control and Prevention, National Immunization Program.

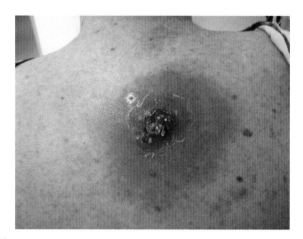

Figure 7-3. National Center for Emerging and Zoonotic Infectious Diseases, Centers for Disease Control and Prevention. Photographer: Gregory Moran, MD.

CHAPTER 15

Emergency Medicine
Ariel S. McGarry, MSPAS, PA-C
Michael A. Mastroleo, BA, BS, PA-C

DIRECTIONS: Each of the numbered questions or incomplete statements is followed by possible answers or completions of the statement. Select the ONE-lettered answer or completion that is BEST in each case.

1. A 45-year-old male is brought to the ED having an active grand mal seizure that has lasted greater than 15 minutes. The patient has a known history of seizure disorder. No treatment has been initiated up to this point, and the patient is still actively seizing. What is the best immediate treatment choice for the patient in this scenario?

   (A) Emergent bedside EEG
   (B) IV lorazepam
   (C) IV midazolam
   (D) IV phenobarbital
   (E) IV phenytoin

2. A 30-year-old male presents to the ED with headache, fever, nuchal rigidity, and altered mental status. Lumbar puncture reveals: an opening pressure of 25 mm H_2O, CSF protein of 400, CSF glucose of 25, and pleocytes of 4,000 (mostly neutrophilic). Appropriate IV antibiotics have been started immediately. What adjunct treatment in addition to the antibiotics has been shown to reduce mortality and improve overall outcomes?

   (A) Acyclovir
   (B) Dexamethasone
   (C) Mannitol
   (D) Phenytoin
   (E) Solumedrol

3. A 70-year-old ill-appearing female presents to the ED complaining of shortness of breath, tachycardia, and tachypnea. Lab values: ABG: pH: 7.10, PCO_2: 80, HCO_3^-: 36. Which of the following is the most likely diagnosis?

   (A) Uncompensated respiratory acidosis
   (B) Partially compensated respiratory alkalosis
   (C) Partially compensated metabolic acidosis
   (D) Uncompensated metabolic acidosis
   (E) Partially compensated respiratory acidosis

4. A 64-year-old woman presents to the ED with dyspnea and exertional fatigue. There is a high clinical suspicion for pulmonary embolism. Of the following, which would be the most appropriate next step?

   (A) Obtain a CT chest angiography
   (B) Obtain D-dimer
   (C) Send the patient home for further outpatient work-up the next day
   (D) Obtain an echocardiogram

5. Which of the following is the most reliable clinical assessment tool to confirm endotracheal intubation?

   (A) Endotracheal tube condensation
   (B) Symmetrical chest expansion
   (C) Breath sounds auscultated equally over the chest
   (D) No breath sounds auscultated over the stomach
   (E) Use of a carbon dioxide (CO_2) detection device

6. A 76-year-old woman (60 kg) with organic brain syndrome presents to the ED with a serum sodium level of 180 mg/dL. What is the approximate calculation of the water deficit in this hypernatremic patient?

   (A) 4 L
   (B) 6 L
   (C) 8 L
   (D) 11 L
   (E) 14 L

7. A 65-year-old man with chronic obstructive pulmonary disease taking daily theophylline therapy presents to the ED with palpitations, chest pain, and the feeling that his heart is beating irregularly after starting erythromycin for bronchitis. What is the most likely dysrhythmia?

   (A) Atrial fibrillation
   (B) Atrial flutter
   (C) Mobitz type II AV heart block
   (D) Multifocal atrial tachycardia
   (E) Sinus bradycardia

8. A 58-year-old man with multiple myeloma presents to the ED with altered mental status, hypertension, back pain, and constipation. These findings are suggestive of which of the following medical conditions?

   (A) Hypercalcemia
   (B) Hyperkalemia
   (C) Hypoglycemia
   (D) Hypomagnesemia
   (E) Hyponatremia

9. A 22-year-old female presents to the ED with complaints of dizziness and palpitations. Cardiac examination reveals tachycardia. The EKG shows a narrow complex tachycardia with a PR interval of 0.08 second and a delta wave. What is the dysrhythmia associated in this scenario?

   (A) Atrial fibrillation
   (B) Multifocal atrial tachycardia
   (C) Supraventricular tachycardia
   (D) Ventricular tachycardia
   (E) Wolff–Parkinson–White

10. A 68-year-old man with a medical history of coronary artery disease presents to the ED with a 2-day history of intermittent chest tightness. The pain was not relieved with three nitroglycerin sublingual tablets. What would be the initial assessment if the electrocardiogram demonstrated 2-mm ST-segment elevations in leads II, III, and aVF?

    (A) Acute anterior wall myocardial infarction
    (B) Acute inferior wall myocardial injury
    (C) Acute lateral wall myocardial injury
    (D) Subendocardial anterior wall myocardial ischemia
    (E) Subendocardial inferior wall myocardial infarction

11. A 64-year-old woman presents to the ED with complaints of left-sided headache, low-grade fever, malaise, pain with chewing, and decreased vision in her left eye. Which of the following would be the most appropriate measure in managing this patient?

    (A) Aspirin therapy
    (B) Intravenous steroids
    (C) Lumbar puncture
    (D) Muscle relaxants
    (E) Oxygen (O_2) therapy

12. What maneuver is used to help diagnose benign paroxysmal positional vertigo in an otherwise healthy individual?

    (A) Dix–Hallpike
    (B) Epley
    (C) Lachmann
    (D) Semont
    (E) Tilt table

13. Cardiac enzymes in a patient with a 2-hour history of chest pain secondary to an acute myocardial infarction would commonly demonstrate which of the following findings?

    (A) Normal creatinine kinase (CK-MB) and troponin I levels
    (B) Elevated troponin I and normal CK-MB levels
    (C) Elevated CK-MB and normal troponin I levels

(D) Normal myoglobin with elevated CK-MB levels

(E) Elevated myoglobin, troponin I, and CK-MB levels

14. Which of the following is the most appropriate indication for IV thrombolytic therapy in a patient with acute coronary syndrome?

(A) 0.5-mm ST-segment elevation in the inferior wall leads resolving with two sublingual nitroglycerins

(B) Posterior wall myocardial infarction duration of 12 to 14 hours

(C) Right bundle branch block

(D) 2-mm of ST-segment elevation in the anterior/lateral wall

(E) 3-mm of ST-segment depression

15. A 50-year-old male presents to the ED complaining of chest pain, palpitations, and dizziness after a syncopal episode. The patient feels his heart racing. The EKG reveals a narrow complex tachycardia consistent with paroxysmal supraventricular tachycardia (PSVT). Vitals: P: 188 bpm, regular, BP: 78/52 supine. What is the best treatment for this patient in this scenario?

(A) Defibrillation

(B) IV adenosine (Adenocard)

(C) IV diltiazem (Cardizem)

(D) Synchronized cardioversion

(E) Vagal maneuvers

16. A 44-year-old AIDS patient being treated for *Pneumocystis jirovecii* pneumonia presents to the ED with an acute onset of confusion, pallor, diaphoresis, and tachycardia. What is the most likely cause of the patient's symptoms?

(A) Hypoglycemia

(B) Hypoxemia

(C) Meningitis

(D) Mucous plugging

(E) Subarachnoid hemorrhage (SAH)

17. A patient presents to the ED complaining of severe pain, photophobia, excessive tearing, and a foreign body sensation in the right eye after an injury. Examination reveals conjunctival injection, tearing, lid swelling, but no foreign body. After fluorescein instillation, slit lamp evaluation reveals a single superficial irregular corneal defect consistent with a corneal abrasion. The patient wears contacts. The treatment of this patient should include eye drops that will cover what bacterial pathogen?

(A) *Haemophilus influenzae*

(B) *Klebsiella pneumoniae*

(C) Methicillin-resistant *Staphylococcus aureus*

(D) *Pseudomonas aeruginosa*

(E) *Staphylococcus aureus*

18. A 30-year-old male presents to the ED after being rescued from a house fire. The patient complains of a headache, fatigue, confusion, nausea, vomiting, and some shortness of breath. Pulse oximetry is 93% on room air, Respirations: 18/min. Labs: COHb level is 27. What is the immediate treatment for the patient in this scenario?

(A) 100% oxygen via nonrebreather mask

(B) β_2-Adrenergic agonists

(C) Hyperbaric oxygen

(D) Oxygen via nasal cannula 2 L

(E) Solumedrol 125 mg IV

19. What is the most common bacterial pathogen causing pneumonia in alcoholics?

(A) *Chlamydia pneumoniae*

(B) *Haemophilus influenzae*

(C) *Klebsiella pneumoniae*

(D) *Staphylococcus aureus*

(E) *Streptococcus pneumoniae*

20. A patient is diagnosed with a transient ischemic attack. What is the risk of having a stroke within the next 90 days?

(A) 2% to 7%

(B) 10% to 15%

(C) 20% to 25%

(D) 30% to 45%

21. The most immediate management priority in a patient with septic shock is

(A) acid–base status.

(B) empiric antimicrobial therapy.

(C) fluid therapy.

(D) inotropic support.

(E) oxygenation and ventilation.

22. Which of the following drugs represents the most appropriate antidotal agent for benzodiazepine overdose?

(A) Activated charcoal

(B) Flumazenil

(C) Flutamide

(D) Ketamine

(E) Naloxone

23. A 22-year-old female presents to the ED complaining of right knee pain, fever, and chills. Examination reveals a swollen and reddened knee joint that is tender and warm to touch. Patient has limited ROM of the knee. What is the most likely bacteria causing the infection in this scenario?

(A) Group B streptococci

(B) *Haemophilus influenzae*

(C) *Neisseria gonorrhoeae*

(D) *Staphylococcus aureus*

(E) *Streptococcus pyogenes*

24. A 68-year-old male presents to the ED with complaints of weakness and palpitations. The patient has a history of end-stage renal disease and is on hemodialysis. On the cardiac monitor there is evidence of increasing QRS widening and sine wave. Labs reveal potassium of 8.5. If dialysis is unavailable, what is most immediate treatment necessary in this scenario?

(A) 1 ampule of D50 followed by 10 units of regular insulin IV

(B) 10 mL of 10% calcium gluconate IV

(C) β_2-Adrenergic agonist

(D) Sodium bicarbonate IV

(E) Sodium polystyrene sulfonate 30 g orally

25. A 59-year-old cancer patient presents to the ED with fever, pneumonia, hypotension, and tachycardia. Investigative studies demonstrate hyperkalemia, hyponatremia, and hypoglycemia. What is the most likely concomitant diagnosis in this scenario?

(A) Adrenal insufficiency

(B) Cushing syndrome

(C) Hyperparathyroidism

(D) Hypothyroidism

(E) Syndrome of inappropriate antidiuretic hormone (SIADH)

26. An 18-year-old male presents to the ED with a complaint of left testicular pain that started 4 hours ago. The patient also complains of lower abdominal pain, nausea and vomiting. Examination reveals pain with palpation over the left testicle and a higher riding left testicle in relation to the contralateral testicle. The cremasteric reflex is absent. Which of the following is the most likely diagnosis?

(A) Epididymitis

(B) Fournier's gangrene

(C) Hydrocele

(D) Testicular cancer

(E) Testicular torsion

27. Which of the following best defines the peripheral wedge-shaped consolidation on the pleural surface observed on a chest radiograph in a patient with a pulmonary embolism?

(A) Atelectatic lesion

(B) Hampton hump

(C) Pleural effusion

(D) Reticular pattern

(E) Westermark sign

28. A 50-year-old female presents to the ED complaining of fatigue and lethargy. The patient also admits to abdominal pain, muscle spasms, and paresthesias of the fingers, toes, and around the mouth. The examination reveals hyperreflexia and both Chvostek and Trousseau signs are present. Labs: serum calcium: 5.5 mg/dL. Which of the following would most likely be seen on this patient's EKG?

(A) Delta wave

(B) Osborn wave

(C) Prolonged QT interval

(D) Shortened QT interval

(E) Sine wave

29. Which of the following is the drug of choice for treating hypertensive encephalopathy in the non-pregnant patient?

(A) Esmolol

(B) Hydralazine

(C) Labetalol

(D) Nitroglycerin

(E) Sodium nitroprusside

30. An abrupt, severe ripping pain in the chest or between the scapulae that is associated with a feeling of "impending doom" is most indicative of which of the following diagnoses?

(A) Cauda equina syndrome

(B) Dissecting thoracic aortic aneurysm

(C) Myocardial infarction

(D) Pancreatitis

(E) Peptic ulcer disease

31. A 46-year-old patient was diagnosed 8 days ago with a DVT of his right leg. He now presents with a white leg and absent dorsalis pedis and posterior tibial pulses on the right. Which of the following is the most likely diagnosis?

(A) Phlegmasia alba dolens

(B) Phlebitis areta

(C) Phlegmasia cerulea dolens

(D) Phlebitis fulminans

32. An 89-year-old female patient from a nursing home presents to the ED with abdominal pain and distention. The abdominal radiograph demonstrates multiple air–fluid levels and dilated large-bowel loops consistent with a large-bowel obstruction. What is the most likely cause of the obstruction?

(A) Abdominal wall hernias

(B) Adhesions

(C) Carcinoma of the colon

(D) Diverticulitis

(E) Sigmoid volvulus

33. A 26-year-old male presents to the ED after an overdose of an unknown substance. The patient is anxious, agitated, with delirium and psychosis. Examination reveals a patient with tachycardia, hypertension, hyperthermia, diaphoresis, dilated pupils, and muscular hyperactivity. Which drug class is most likely responsible in this scenario?

(A) Anticholinergic

(B) Cocaine

(C) Lithium

(D) Opiate

(E) Salicylate

34. A 20-year-old male who is an IV drug user presents to the ED complaining of fever, cough, chest pain, weakness, and malaise for the last several days. Cardiac examination reveals a heart murmur previously not known to this patient. Which valve is most likely involved?

(A) Aortic

(B) Mitral

(C) Pulmonic

(D) Tricuspid

35. A 26-year-old male presents to the ED after an MVA. The patient is on a backboard with c-collar immobilization. On neurological examination the patient has numbness from the umbilicus down. This finding reveals an injury at which dermatome level?

(A) T4

(B) T7

(C) T10

(D) L3

(E) S1

36. Which of the following extrapulmonary findings is most likely to be associated with *Mycoplasma pneumoniae*?

(A) Bullous myringitis

(B) Conjunctivitis

(C) Guttate psoriasis eruption

(D) Lymphangitis

(E) Otitis externa

37. Which of the following signs and symptoms is most likely to be indicative of acute myocardial ischemia or infarction?

    (A) Dyspnea
    (B) Left arm numbness and tingling
    (C) Referred back pain
    (D) Sternal chest pain
    (E) Substernal chest discomfort

38. A tall, thin, 26-year-old woman presents to the ED with an acute onset of right-sided pleuritic chest pain and dyspnea. What is the most likely diagnosis?

    (A) Right tension pneumothorax
    (B) Left tension pneumothorax
    (C) Right pleural effusion
    (D) Right spontaneous pneumothorax
    (E) Left atelectasis

39. A patient presents with an acute asthmatic attack. Multiple doses of inhaled adrenergic agents are used but the patient continues to have bronchospasms. Which of the following medications is most paramount in this patient?

    (A) Anticholinergics
    (B) Corticosteroids
    (C) Leukotriene modifiers
    (D) Magnesium
    (E) Theophylline

40. A 20-year-old female presents to the ED complaining of a headache. The patient is 26 weeks' pregnant. There have been no complications with this pregnancy up to this point. Examination reveals mild hyperreflexia and 3+ pitting edema of the lower legs. Vitals: P: 88 bpm, regular, BP: 180/110 seated. Urinalysis reveals proteinuria. What is the best IV medicinal agent for the prevention and treatment of seizures in this scenario?

    (A) Enalapril
    (B) Labetalol
    (C) Lorazepam
    (D) Magnesium
    (E) Phenobarbital

41. Which of the following is the most common etiology of upper gastrointestinal (GI) bleeding?

    (A) Diverticulosis
    (B) Erosive gastritis
    (C) Inflammatory bowel disease
    (D) Mallory–Weiss syndrome
    (E) Peptic ulcer disease

42. A 51-year-old man presents to the ED with complains of colicky right upper quadrant and epigastric pain radiating to his back about 3 hours after eating. Which of the following would be the diagnostic study of choice?

    (A) Acute abdominal plain radiographs
    (B) Cardiac stress test with echocardiogram
    (C) Chest CT with IV contrast
    (D) Helical CT with rectal contrast
    (E) Right upper quadrant ultrasound

43. A 26-year-old female presents to the ED complaining of right-sided suprapubic pain. The patient's LMP was 6 weeks prior. She denies any vaginal bleeding. Labs: Rh+, β-hCG quantitative: 4,500. Pelvic U/S reveals a 2-cm right adnexal mass without any evidence of rupture and no evidence of intrauterine pregnancy. Vitals: P: 76 bpm, reg., BP: 124/82. What is the next best step in the treatment for this patient?

    (A) IM methotrexate
    (B) IM-Rhogam
    (C) Laparoscopic left salpingectomy
    (D) Oral mifepristone
    (E) Vaginal prostaglandin

44. A patient presents with a bite to her left arm due to a venomous snake. Which of the following complications is the most likely to develop?

    (A) Compartment syndrome
    (B) Delayed absorption of antivenom
    (C) Delayed serum sickness
    (D) Dislodged teeth contaminating the wound
    (E) Immediate death after venomous snakebite

45. Which of the following is the most common cause of erosive esophagitis?

    (A) Candidiasis
    (B) Gastrointestinal reflux
    (C) Herpes simplex virus
    (D) Pills
    (E) Radiation therapy

46. Which of the following items represents a true medical emergency if swallowed by a toddler and lodged in the esophagus?

    (A) Closed clothespin
    (B) Cotton ball
    (C) Dime
    (D) Disk-shaped battery
    (E) Single magnet

47. A 62-year-old patient presents to the ED with generalized abdominal pain, nausea, vomiting, and abdominal distention. The radiographs demonstrate multiple loops of dilated small bowel, air–fluid levels, and a string of pearls sign. What is the most likely cause of this clinical scenario?

    (A) Adhesions following abdominal surgery
    (B) Bezoars
    (C) Gallstone ileus
    (D) Incarceration of abdominal hernias
    (E) Neoplasm

48. A patient presents to the ED with frequent, mucoid, watery stools, nausea, and lower abdominal pain. The patient has been on a cephalosporin-type antibiotic for about 3 months. Which of the following is the most likely diagnosis?

    (A) Anal fissures
    (B) Anorectal tumor
    (C) Diverticulitis
    (D) Pseudomembranous enterocolitis
    (E) Ulcerative colitis (UC)

49. A 30-year-old female presents to the ED complaining of fever of 104°F, nausea, vomiting, and agitation. Physical examination reveals warm, moist skin throughout, thyromegaly, tachycardia, and a systolic flow murmur. EKG reveals supraventricular tachycardia. Which of the following is the most likely diagnosis?

    (A) Addisonian crisis
    (B) Hashimoto's thyroiditis
    (C) Inappropriate secretion of antidiuretic hormone
    (D) Pheochromocytoma
    (E) Toxic multinodular goiter

50. Which of the following measures is the most beneficial in evaluating a pediatric patient with suspected volume depletion?

    (A) Serial cerebrospinal fluid analyses
    (B) Urinary bladder catheter to measure output
    (C) Serial vital sign measurements
    (D) Serial electrolyte measurements

51. Which of the following is the recommended dosage for nitrous oxide in an adult patient requiring minimal sedation in the ED for reduction of an elbow dislocation?

    (A) 10% nitrous oxide, 90% oxygen
    (B) 40% nitrous oxide, 60% oxygen
    (C) 50% nitrous oxide, 50% oxygen
    (D) 70% nitrous oxide, 30% oxygen
    (E) 95% nitrous oxide, 5% oxygen

52. Which of the following is the most common side effect of antipsychotic medications seen in the ER setting?

    (A) Acute dystonia
    (B) Delirium
    (C) Neuroleptic malignant syndrome
    (D) Parkinsonism
    (E) Seizure

53. Which of the following is the treatment of choice in a 32-year-old pregnant female, at 28 weeks' gestation, with a pulmonary embolism?

    (A) Aspirin
    (B) Embolectomy
    (C) Rivaroxaban (Xarelto)
    (D) Unfractionated heparin (Lovenox)
    (E) Warfarin (Coumadin)

54. A patient presents with anxiety, tremors, palpitations, fatigue, and hemiplegia. Which of the following is the most likely disorder associated with these symptoms?

(A) Euglycemia

(B) Hyperglycemia

(C) Hyperglycemic hyperosmolar nonketotic coma

(D) Hypoglycemia

(E) Ketoacidosis

55. A 45-year-old woman presents to the ED with acute painless loss of vision and photophobia associated with a smaller unilateral pupil on the involved side. Which of the following is the most likely diagnosis?

(A) Central retinal artery occlusion

(B) Central retinal vein occlusion

(C) Hyphema

(D) Iritis/uveitis

(E) Retrobulbar hemorrhage or hematoma

56. Which of the following patient populations is at the greatest risk for an epidural hematoma following head trauma?

(A) Elderly patients

(B) Infants

(C) Young adults

(D) Young children

57. Which of the following patient profiles would be most likely to present with a chronic subdural hematoma?

(A) 12-year-old male gymnast with hemophilia A

(B) 20-year-old male suffering a head injury 2 hours ago

(C) 36-year-old female with head injury 30 minutes ago

(D) 55-year-old female with a cerebral aneurysm

(E) 78-year-old male with long-standing alcoholism

58. Which of the following findings is an independent risk factor for mortality in patients suffering a head injury?

(A) Absence of gag reflex

(B) Hypoxia

(C) Mandibular fracture

(D) Scalp laceration

(E) Unconsciousness

59. A 19-year-old man presents with delirium, dilated pupils, tachycardia, urinary retention, and hyperthermia. Which of the following classes of drugs is suspected to be the offending agent the patient ingested?

(A) Acetaminophen

(B) Anticholinergic

(C) Caffeine

(D) Heroin

(E) Salicylate

60. Which of the following diagnostic studies is the most reliable marker of rhabdomyolysis?

(A) Aldolase

(B) Creatinine kinase (CK)

(C) CK-MB

(D) Lactate dehydrogenase (LDH)

(E) Urine myoglobin

61. Which of the following regions best describes the location of a Le Fort fracture?

(A) Mandible

(B) Midfacial

(C) Occipital

(D) Temporal

(E) Zygoma

62. Which of the following is among the most common location for injuries to abused women and children?

(A) Elbow

(B) Neck

(C) Shin

(D) Thigh

(E) Wrists

63. Which of the following conventional or plain radiographic views of the face is most beneficial for evaluating trauma of the midface?

(A) Caldwell view

(B) Panorex

(C) Submental vertex

(D) Towne view

(E) Waters view

64. Which of the following physical examination findings is most likely present in a patient with extraocular muscle entrapment following facial trauma?

(A) Binocular double vision

(B) Binocular loss of vision

(C) Monocular double vision

(D) Monocular loss of vision

(E) Tear drop-shaped pupil

65. A patient is involved in an MVA and suffered a fractured neck. The fracture lines extend through the pedicles of C2. Which of the following describes this unstable hyperextension fracture to the cervical spine?

(A) Clay-shoveler fracture

(B) Extension teardrop fracture

(C) Hangman fracture

(D) Jefferson fracture

(E) Johnson fracture

66. A 68-year-old woman presents to the ED with an exacerbation of chronic low-back pain. Which of the following indicates the patient has developed cauda equina syndrome?

(A) Anesthesia to entire leg, bilateral leg weakness, and loss of deep tendon reflexes

(B) Bilateral leg pain, saddle anesthesia, urinary incontinence, and fecal incontinence

(C) Bilateral leg weakness, loss of peripheral pulses, and incontinence

(D) Loss of deep tendon reflexes bilaterally and urinary retention

(E) Lower leg weakness, paresthesias to both legs, and incontinence

67. A 78-year-old male presents to the emergency room with sudden onset of left eye pain, nausea, and vomiting. His past medical history is significant for dementia and migraine. Physical examination reveals cloudy cornea bilaterally, left conjunctival injection, and a fixed, midposition pupil on the left. Which of the following is the most likely diagnosis?

(A) Acute angle-closure glaucoma

(B) Dementia exacerbation

(C) Migraine

(D) Optic neuritis

(E) Temporal arteritis

68. A 60-year-old patient presents with new-onset localized headache. The erythrocyte sedimentation rate is 55 mm/h. Which of the following is the most likely diagnosis?

(A) Cluster headache

(B) Migraine

(C) Subarachnoid hemorrhage

(D) Temporal arteritis

(E) Trigeminal neuralgia

69. A 40-year-old man presents to the ED with acute blunt chest and abdominal trauma following a motor vehicle crash. The patient presented with jugular venous distention, decreased BP, and muffled heart tones. Which of the following is the most likely diagnosis?

(A) Aortic rupture

(B) Myocardial contusion

(C) Myocardial rupture

(D) Pericardial tamponade

(E) Tension pneumothorax

70. Spontaneous esophageal rupture following forceful vomiting after overindulging in food and alcohol is known as which of the following?

(A) Bezoar

(B) Boerhaave syndrome

(C) Brudzinski sign

(D) Burger sign

71. A 65-year-old female presents to the ED with the complaint of dysphagia and a feeling that something is stuck in her throat since having dinner one hour ago. Examination reveals nothing visible in the posterior oropharynx. The patient is not drooling, but unable to swallow. Based on the most likely diagnosis and assuming there is no underlying esophageal disease, what is the best treatment choice in this scenario?

(A) Barium swallow

(B) IV calcium chloride

(C) IV depacon

(D) IV glucagon

(E) Meat tenderizer

72. Which of the following diagnoses is best described as a tear of the tunica albuginea and subsequent rupture of the corpus cavernosum?

(A) Balanoposthitis

(B) Hair thread tourniquet syndrome

(C) Penile fracture

(D) Peyronie disease

(E) Phimosis

73. A 41-year-old man injures his index finger while playing basketball. The radiograph shows an avulsion fracture to the proximal dorsal region of the distal phalanx. Figure 15-1 demonstrates the patient attempting to fully extend his index finger DIP joint. What is the most likely diagnosis?

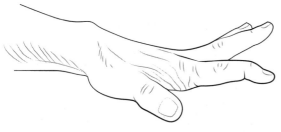

Figure 15-1. Reproduced, with permission, from LaDou J, Harrison RJ. *CURRENT Diagnosis & Treatment: Occupational & Environmental Medicine.* 5th ed. New York, NY: McGraw-Hill Education; 2013. Figure 9-8.

(A) Bennett fracture

(B) Mallet finger fracture

(C) Rolando fracture

(D) Swan neck deformity

74. A child falls on an outstretched hand. Physical examination reveals pain and swelling of the distal radius. The radiograph is depicted in Figure 15-2. Which of the following is the best diagnosis?

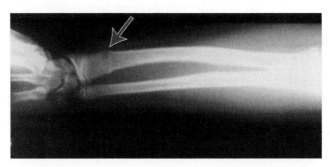

Figure 15-2. Reproduced with permission from Strange GR, Ahrens WR, Lelyveld S, et al. *Pediatric Emergency Medicine.* 2nd ed. New York: McGraw-Hill Education, 2002.

(A) Complete fracture

(B) Greenstick fracture

(C) Plastic deformation

(D) Torus fracture

75. A 40-year-old man slips on the ice, injuring his left arm. He complains of pain and swelling to the mid-shaft humeral region. The physical examination reveals a wrist drop on the injured side. Which nerve is most likely injured?

(A) Axillary

(B) Median

(C) Radial

(D) Subclavian

(E) Ulnar

76. A 70-year-old male presents to the ED with the complaint of sudden, severe, steady mid to lower abdominal pain. The pain is not relieved by narcotics and is out of proportion to findings on physical examination. There is associated nausea and vomiting. Labs: WBC: 18,000, Lactic acid: 3.0. Which is the best diagnostic test for the patient in this scenario?

(A) Abdominal x-rays

(B) Emergent endoscopy

(C) Mesenteric angiography

(D) MRI of abdomen and pelvis

(E) Ultrasound of the abdomen

77. A 7-year-old child presents to the ED with fever, neck pain, and a "duck-like" voice. Which of the following is the most likely diagnosis?

(A) Epiglottitis

(B) Ludwig angina

(C) Peritonsillar abscess

(D) Retropharyngeal abscess

(E) Streptococcus pharyngitis

78. What is the mechanism of injury for an anterior shoulder dislocation?

(A) Shoulder internal rotation and adduction

(B) Shoulder internal rotation with abduction

(C) Shoulder external rotation with adduction

(D) Shoulder external rotation with abduction

(E) Fall on an outstretched hand

79. Which of the following medications is responsible for the most drug-related deaths?

(A) Benzodiazepines

(B) Lithium

(C) Monoamine oxidase inhibitors

(D) Stimulants

(E) Tricyclic antidepressants

80. A 30-year-old male patient presents to the ED with an acute change in mental status. The examination reveals a patient who is sleepy but arouses to loud verbal stimuli. His airway is intact and the vital signs are stable. Investigative studies indicate an alcohol level of 150 mg/dL, an anion gap of 30 mEq/L, a metabolic acidosis, an osmolar gap of 20, and calcium oxalate crystalluria. What is the most likely etiologic agent?

(A) Buspirone

(B) Ethanol

(C) Ethylene glycol

(D) Isopropanol

(E) Methanol

81. A 20-year-old man presents to the ED following a lethal overdose of acetaminophen. What is best medication for his overdose?

(A) Ethanol

(B) Flumazenil

(C) Narcan

(D) N-acetylcysteine

(E) Vitamin K

82. Which of the following clinical findings differentiates periorbital from orbital cellulitis?

(A) Development of a rash on the face

(B) Erythema

(C) Fever

(D) Lid edema

(E) Worsening pain with eye movements

83. A 47-year-old man presents to the ED comatose after ingesting an unknown liquid substance. Investigative studies include the following: pH: 7.45; Na: 140; Cl: 110; HCO_3: 19; glucose: 180; BUN: 30; Cr: 1.5; ETOH: 0.0; high serum ketones; and a measured osmolality of 380. These findings are most consistent with which of the following?

(A) Alcoholic ketoacidosis

(B) Diabetic ketoacidosis

(C) Ethylene glycol

(D) Isopropanol

(E) Methanol

84. A 58-year-old man presents to the ED hypothermic after an environmental exposure to cold weather and snow. The patient's core temperature is 85.5°F. Which of the following is the most accurate statement regarding this scenario?

(A) Shivering is common.

(B) An Osborne (J) wave on EKG is pathognomonic.

(C) Rough handling can produce serious dysrhythmias.

(D) A nasogastric tube should be inserted to protect the airway from regurgitation.

(E) The patient is in an excitation phase of hypothermia.

85. A patient presents to the ED after being bitten by an unknown "insect" while camping. The pain began as a pinprick sensation at the bite site and spread quickly to include the entire bitten extremity. The bite wound became erythematous 45 minutes after the bite. The bite evolved into a target lesion and the patient complains of muscle cramp-like spasms in the large muscle groups. Which of the following is the most likely cause?

(A) Black widow spider
(B) Brown recluse spider
(C) Hobo spider
(D) Scorpion
(E) Tarantula

86. Which of the following is the most important treatment option in a patient with moderate acute mountain sickness?

(A) Acetazolamide
(B) Dexamethasone
(C) Hyperbaric therapy
(D) Immediate descent
(E) Oxygen therapy

87. A patient presents to the ED after being trapped in a house fire. The patient suffered partial thickness burns over the entire anterior chest and abdomen, entire right arm, and the entire right leg. Using the rule of nines, what is the estimated percentage of burn?

(A) 36%
(B) 45%
(C) 48%
(D) 54%
(E) 72%

88. A 45-year-old female presents to the ED complaining of right foot and ankle pain. The patient states that she fell while running and externally rotated her foot with the injury. Examination reveals tenderness and swelling over the medial malleolus and proximal fibular pain. What is the most likely cause of the proximal fibular pain in this scenario?

(A) Compartment syndrome
(B) Lateral meniscus tear
(C) Maisonneuve fracture

(D) Proximal gastrocnemius tear
(E) Quadriceps tendon rupture

89. A 30-year-old male presents to the ED with right knee pain after a basketball injury. There is a palpable defect distal to the patella. Which of the following findings would help confirm the most likely diagnosis?

(A) Inability to extend knee
(B) Low riding patella
(C) Positive straight leg raise
(D) Positive Thompson test

90. A 39-year-old woman presents to the ED with agitation, tremors, visual hallucinations, fever, and tachycardia. The eye examination reveals nystagmus and a sixth cranial nerve palsy. Which of the following conditions best describes this clinical scenario?

(A) Acute cocaine toxicity
(B) Acute dystonia
(C) Korsakoff psychosis
(D) Trigeminal neuralgia
(E) Wernicke encephalopathy

91. In addition to dental referral, which of the following represents the most appropriate standard therapy for a routine periodontal abscess in the ED setting?

(A) Intravenous penicillin and topical analgesics
(B) Intravenous penicillin and incision and drainage (I/D)
(C) Oral penicillin and oral analgesics
(D) Oral penicillin and saline rinses
(E) Oral clindamycin and topical analgesics

92. Which of the following demographic groups below would be most likely to suffer from a primary tuberculosis (TB) infection presenting as extrapulmonary tuberculosis meningitis?

(A) Alcoholics
(B) Children younger than 2 years
(C) Elderly
(D) HIV patients with CD4 counts higher than 350/μL
(E) Young adults

93. Which of the following is most significant in the ED setting for management of a patient with suspected active TB infection?

(A) Discharge home on broad-spectrum oral antibiotic

(B) Respiratory isolation in negative pressure room

(C) Health care providers should wear a surgical mask with face shield

(D) Direct reporting of cases to the World Health Organization

94. Air contrast enema is diagnostic in approximately what percentage of intussusception cases of less than 24 hours of duration?

(A) 1%

(B) 10%

(C) 30%

(D) 70%

(E) 95%

95. A 2-year-old child is brought to the ER by his parents after having a tonic–clonic seizure at home lasting 7 minutes. His parents report he has been sick with a cough and wheezing for the past few days and spiked a fever of 101°F just prior to the episode. His parents deny a previous episode. On physical examination he is well appearing. Which of the following is indicated in the work-up of this patient?

(A) CBC with differential

(B) EEG

(C) Lumbar puncture

(D) Neuroimaging

(E) No work-up is indicated

96. A 3-month-old infant presents in November with low-grade fevers, rhinorrhea, cough, wheezing, mild retractions, and no difficulty feeding for 3 days. The oxygen saturation was greater than 93%. The medical history is noted for 35 weeks' gestation at birth. Immunizations are up to date. Otherwise, the infant has been healthy. Based on the most likely diagnosis, which of the following clinical rationales would most likely warrant hospital admission?

(A) Evaluation for additional coexisting respiratory infections

(B) Intravenous antimicrobial therapy

(C) Intravenous steroid therapy

(D) Monitoring for episodes of apnea or respiratory failure

(E) Parent education

97. A 20-year-old college student presents with fatigue, fever, pharyngitis, and lymphadenopathy. On physical examination of the abdomen, splenomegaly is noted. Which of the following interventions may induce a morbilliform rash?

(A) Delayed treatment with ceftriaxone

(B) Oral corticosteroids

(C) Oral amoxicillin

(D) Oral acyclovir

(E) IV vancomycin

Answers and Explanations

1. **(B)** Status epilepticus traditionally refers to continuous seizure activity lasting greater than 15 minutes in duration or repetitive seizures with impaired consciousness and with little or no recovery in between. A more useful description is to consider any seizure whose duration provokes the acute use of anticonvulsant therapy. This happens typically when seizures last beyond 5 minutes. Status epilepticus is a medical emergency and requires quick but careful medical treatment. If left untreated, it could be fatal. Prolonged seizures can lead to serious cardiorespiratory dysfunction, hyperthermia, metabolic disorders, and permanent brain injury. The drugs most often used in the therapy of status epilepticus are benzodiazepines and anticonvulsants. Benzodiazepines are used as the emergent initial treatment for status epilepticus. IV lorazepam (2–4 mg) and IV diazepam (5–10 mg) have equal capability in controlling status epilepticus. Lorazepam is associated with fewer seizure recurrences than diazepam and is considered the initial agent of choice. Benzodiazepines are followed by longer-acting antiepileptics such as fosphenytoin, valproic acid, and levetiracetam. Phenobarbital may be considered as a third-line drug in patients whose seizures are not controlled despite the use of benzodiazepines and phenytoin. If seizures continue even after benzodiazepine or antieleptics, administration of general anesthesia with medications such as propofol or midazolam is used. *(Lung & Catlett, 2011)*

2. **(B)** Bacterial meningitis should be suspected in a patient presenting with headache fever, nuchal rigidity, and altered mental status. Prompt treatment with empiric antibiotics should be initiated without delay. This should be done before any diagnostic imaging or lumbar puncture because of the high morbidity and mortality associated bacterial meningitis. Specific empiric antibiotics are chosen based upon the patient's age, community setting, immune status, medical history, and recent travel. Some leading causes of bacterial meningitis include *H. influenzae*, *S. pneumoniae*, *Listeria monocytogenes, Neisseria meningitidis,* and group B streptococcus. Glucocorticoids, particularly dexamethasone, when given concomitantly with intravenous antibiotics have shown to reduce mortality in both adults and children. Dexamethasone decreases mortality by reducing cerebral edema and inflammation. The recommended dose for dexamethasone in adults is 10 mg IV and 0.15 mg/kg IV in children. Intravenous mannitol is an osmotic diuretic used in patients with elevated intracranial pressure and cerebral edema, but has not been studied for the treatment of meningitis. IV acyclovir is utilized in the treatment of herpes simplex virus meningitis. *(Loring & Tintinalli, 2011)*

3. **(E)** With a partially compensated respiratory acidosis, the pH is low, $paCO_2$ is high, and HCO_3^- is also high. With an uncompensated respiratory acidosis, the pH is low, $paCO_2$ is high, and HCO_3^- is normal. With a partially compensated respiratory alkalosis, the pH is high, $paCO_2$ is low, and the HCO_3^- is low. With a partially compensated metabolic acidosis, the pH is low, $paCO_2$ is low, and HCO_3^- is low. With an uncompensated metabolic acidosis, the pH is low, $paCO_2$ is normal, and HCO_3^- is low. *(Gomella & Haist, 2007; Levitzky, 2013)*

4. **(A)** Pulmonary thromboembolism (PTE) is primarily the result of clot migration from DVT. In a patient with a high clinical suspicion of PTE, the clinician shoulder order pulmonary vascular imaging, such as a CT chest angiography as the initial step. A D-dimer

is not indicated as the next step in evaluation of a patient with a high clinical suspicion of PTE. Sending the patient home for further outpatient management is incorrect given the potentially deadly missed diagnosis of PTE. An echocardiogram may be part of the work-up in this patient presentation, but would not be the next best step. *(Kline, 2014)*

5. **(E)** Direct visualization of the endotracheal tube passing through the vocal cords is the most reliable indicator for endotracheal tube placement. The next most reliable is an end CO_2 device. Auscultation of the chest and epigastric areas may reveal transmitted sounds from the endotracheal tube in the stomach. Condensation in the tube can be an unreliable indicator of proper endotracheal tube placement. *(Vissers & Danzl, 2011)*

6. **(C)** The definition of hypernatremia is a serum sodium level more than 145 mEq/L. Hypernatremia is classified as isovolemic (diabetes insipidus, skin loss through hyperthermia, and iatrogenic), hypervolemic (administration of hypernatremic solutions, mineralocorticoid excess as in Conn or Cushing syndrome, and salt ingestion), and hypovolemic (renal losses through diuretics or glycosuria, GI, respiratory, or skin losses, and adrenal deficiencies). Water deficit in hypernatremic patients is calculated by the following formula:

Total Body Weight (TBW) deficit = TBW × (serum NA+/140) − 1

TBW/Women = .5 × weight (kg)

Water deficit = 0.5 (60) = 30 [(180/140) − 1]
= 30 (0.2857) = 8.6 L.

(Pfennig & Slovis, 2014)

7. **(D)** Multifocal atrial tachycardia (MAT) is defined as a chaotic, irregular rhythm with atrial rates of 100 to 150 bpm. Typically, there are more than two foci of impulse formation with at least three distinctly different P waves with varying P' R, RR, and P' P' intervals. MAT is commonly associated with COPD, theophylline toxicity, and β-adrenergic agonist therapy. Atrial fibrillation (AF) is a totally chaotic atrial rhythm with multiple microreentry circuits of atrial rates from 300 to 600 impulses/min. The most common causes of AF include ischemic heart disease, valvular heart disease, pericarditis, and hyperthyroidism. Atrial flutter is characterized by regular atrial depolarization rates of 250 to 350 bpm, with varying degrees of atrioventricular block. Common causes of atrial flutter include atherosclerotic heart disease, myocardial infarction, thyrotoxicosis, pulmonary embolism, mitral valve disease, congestive heart failure, and metabolic derangements. Sinus bradycardia is a regular rhythm with atrial and ventricular rates of less than 60 bpm with normal P-wave morphology and PR duration. Sinus bradycardia can be found in healthy adults or it may be associated with pathologic conditions such as hypothermia, excessive parasympathetic tone, carotid sensitivity, or myocardial infarction. A type II second-degree AV block or Mobitz II block is characterized by a sudden interruption of AV conduction without prior prolongation of the PR interval. Mobitz II is often associated with a variety of acute and chronic diseases such as anterior wall ischemia. *(Yealy & Kosowsky, 2014)*

8. **(A)** Hypercalcemia associated with malignancies is commonly due to increased bone resorption through osteoclastic factors, parathyroid hormone (PTH) factors, prostaglandins, peptides, steroids, and direct erosion by tumor cells. Common neoplasms include multiple myeloma, lymphosarcoma, adult T-cell lymphoma, and Burkitt lymphoma. Symptoms of hypercalcemia are variable depending on the degree elevation. Typical symptoms include constipation, anorexia, vomiting, confusion, obtundation, psychosis, nephrolithiasis, renal insufficiency, myopathy, back pain, weakness, and hypertension. Hyperkalemia may produce manifestations of weakness, irritability, paresthesias, paralysis, cardiac arrhythmia, and decreased deep tendon reflexes. Hypomagnesemia symptoms include weakness, fasciculations, tremors, convulsions, delirium, coma, hyperreflexia, and cardiac arrhythmias. Hypoglycemia commonly presents with varying degrees of diaphoresis, anxiety, tremors, tachycardia, palpitations, fatigue, syncope, headache, visual disturbances, hemiplegia, and seizures. Hyponatremia may present as confusion, muscle cramps, anorexia, nausea, lethargy, seizures, and coma depending on the degree and rapidity of onset. *(Pfennig & Slovis, 2014)*

9. **(E)** Wolff–Parkinson–White (WPW) syndrome is a heart disorder in which an abnormal accessory pathway exists between the atria and ventricles providing a pathway for a reentry tachycardia. WPW may be asymptomatic or can lead to recurrent episodes of tachydysrhythmias. The diagnosis of WPW is classically made by 12-lead electrocardiogram (ECG). It is characterized by a short PR interval (<0.12 second), a prolonged QRS complex (>0.12 second) with a slurred upstroke of the QRS complex known as a delta wave. Supraventricular tachycardia is a tachycardia arising above the Bundle of His. Findings on EKG include: regular tachycardia with rate usually between 120 and 240, P waves may be visible or buried in QRS complex. Atrial fibrillation is described as an irregularly irregular rhythm. EKG characteristics include: absent p waves with the presence of fibrillation waves best seen in V1 to V3 and aVF, and a fast ventricular response between 140 and 180 with unequal R-R intervals. Multifocal atrial tachycardia is a tachydysrhythmia caused by multiple sites of competing atrial activity. EKG findings: Rate greater than 100, varying PP, PR, and RR intervals, and three distinct different p wave morphologies seen in the same lead. Ventricular tachycardia originates in the ventricles. ECG findings: Broad QRS complexes (>160 ms), rate greater than 100, typically a regular rhythm. *(Meckler, 2011)*

10. **(B)** An acute inferior wall MI is the correct answer. The following are the anatomical sites of coronary ischemia related to the ECG leads: anterior wall is leads V1 to V4; lateral wall is leads V5, V6, plus I, and aVL; inferior wall are leads II, III, and aVF; posterior wall is leads V1 through V3, V8, and V9; and right ventricular infarction in lead aVR. *(Kurz et al., 2014)*

11. **(B)** The patient in this scenario has clinical signs and symptoms associated with temporal arteritis or giant-cell arteritis. The most appropriate course of action is to treat with intravenous steroids and obtain ophthalmology consultation when patient has visual loss. Lumbar puncture would be an appropriate intervention if meningitis was suspected. Oxygen therapy is a customary intervention for treating cluster headaches. Nonsteroidal anti-inflammatory drugs are indicated for tension headaches. *(Hellmann & Imboden, 2014)*

12. **(A)** Benign positional paroxysmal vertigo (BPPV) is a common disorder of the inner ears vestibular system. It is thought to be caused by problems within the labyrinth system located in the inner ear. BPPV produces a sensation of spinning that is increased by positional change. Other associated symptoms include nausea, vomiting, or loss of balance. It can be diagnosed by history, physical examination or by vestibular tests. The Dix–Hallpike maneuver is a vestibular test in which the patient starts in a sitting position with the head turned 45 degrees; the examiner holds the back of the head and then gently lowers the patient into a supine position with the head extended backward by about 20 degrees. A positive test is seen when the examiner observes nystagmus during the maneuver. BPPV can be treated with repositioning maneuvers such as the Epley and Semont maneuvers. These maneuvers can be performed at the provider's office and also can be taught to the patient for home treatment. The Tilt table test is used in the diagnosis of vasovagal syncope. Lachman test is used to assess any laxity or rupture of the ligaments that support the knee. *(Walker & Daroff, 2012)*

13. **(A)** Two hours after the onset of an acute myocardial infarction, the cardiac enzymes would most commonly demonstrate a normal troponin and CK-MB levels. Cardiac troponin I and CK-MB levels elevate in 3 to 12 hours after the onset of myocardial infarction. Serum myoglobin level elevates 1 to 4 hours after the onset of myocardial infarction. *(Hollander & Diercks, 2011)*

14. **(D)** Indications for IV thrombolytic therapy include acute myocardial infarction less than 6 to 12 hours old, new or presumed new left bundle branch block, and an ECG that has at least 1 mm of ST-segment elevation in two or more contiguous leads. Additional indications include chest pain and ST elevation unresolved with nitroglycerin. ST-segment depression is not an indication for thrombolytic therapy. Known absolute and relative contraindications to use of thrombolytics must always be taken in consideration. *(Hollander & Diercks, 2011)*

15. **(D)** Emergent synchronized cardioversion is indicated in any patient who is found to be clinically unstable with a tachydysrhythmia as the cause. A patient with a tachydysrhythmia is considered

clinically unstable when there is associated chest pain, dyspnea, altered level of consciousness, hypotension, or new-onset congestive heart failure. Dosing for an unstable tachydysrhythmia is dependent on multiple factors including: the specific arrhythmia involved, previous cardiac history, and age. In adults the initial charge is between 50 and 100 J. Cardioversion will be repeated with increasing energy until the tachydysrhythmia is terminated. Conversely, treatment of a hemodynamically stable patient with a tachydysrhythmia is directed at increasing vagal tone either by using vagal maneuvers or drugs. Vagal maneuvers can be accomplished by having the patient bear down, cough, or by unilateral carotid sinus massage. In patients where vagal maneuvers are unsuccessful IV adenosine in increasing doses should be considered. This is followed by the use of either IV calcium channel blockers or IV β-blockers. *(Goshorn et al., 2011)*

16. **(A)** The symptoms described are due to hypoglycemia caused by pentamidine isethionate. Pentamidine is a common treatment for pneumocystis in the AIDS patient. Pentamidine is an antiprotozoal agent that inhibits synthesis of DNA, RNA, phospholipids, and proteins. Common side effects include hypoglycemia, renal impairment, leukopenia, hepatotoxicity, nausea, anorexia, hypotension, fever, and rash. Monitor metabolic parameters such as BUN, creatinine, glucose, CBC, platelet count, liver function tests, and calcium regularly while on pentamidine therapy. *(Takhar & O'Laughlin, 2014)*

17. **(D)** Corneal abrasions commonly present with a foreign body sensation in the affected eye, photophobia, excessive tearing, and eye pain. Treatment is self-limited and is usually aimed at relieving pain and preventing infection. Topical nonsteroidal eye drops or oral narcotics can be used for analgesia. Contact lens-associated abrasions warrant antibiotic treatment due to their propensity for developing corneal ulcers. They are specifically at risk of developing pseudomonas eye infections. These patients should be prescribed antibiotic eye drops that cover pseudomonas species such as ciprofloxacin, ofloxacin, or tobramycin. Patching the affected eye, which has been used in the past, typically does not promote healing and may increase the risk of infections in contact lens wearers. *(Walker & Adhikari, 2011)*

18. **(A)** Carbon monoxide (CO) is a poisonous, tasteless, odorless gas. Carbon monoxide is one of the most common causes of fatal poisoning either through intentional (suicidal) or accidental exposure. With mild CO poisoning symptoms include headache, nausea, and vomiting. Moderate to severe CO poisoning can be associated with an altered level of consciousness, chest pain, syncope, and seizures. If CO poisoning is highly suspected by history, supplemental oxygen in the highest concentrations should be started immediately. A face mask such as a nonrebreather mask is typically used and can deliver up to 80% to 100% oxygen. Concentrated oxygen enables the body to rapidly clear CO from the blood and relieves CO poisoning symptoms. The decision to use hyperbaric oxygen (HBO) therapy is made on a case by case basis. Commonly, HBO therapy is considered in patients with altered mental status, severe neurological deficits, coma, chest pain, seizures, COHb level >25, and pregnancy with COHb level >15. *(Maloney, 2011)*

19. **(E)** *S. pneumoniae* is the most common pathogen causing community acquired pneumonia in alcoholics, but *Klebsiella* and *Haemophilus* species are also commonly reported. The incidence of pneumonia is greater in individuals with a history of alcohol abuse, since they are undernourished; heavy smokers with chronic lung disease; and immunosuppressed secondary to liver disease. Chronic alcohol abuse can cause severe reductions in white blood cells and depress the normal defense mechanisms in the lungs, thereby increasing the risk for pneumonia. Aspiration may be seen with alcoholics because of a diminished level of consciousness seen with heavy drinking or a decreased cough/gag reflex with withdrawal seizures. Alcoholics usually have an overall increased length of hospital stay and mortality rates compared to a nonalcoholic patient with pneumonia. *(Emerman et al., 2011)*

20. **(B)** A transient ischemic attack (TIA) is an episode with stroke symptoms lasting less than 24 hours. The standard definition of duration is <24 hours, but most neurological function is restored within 1 to 2 hours after the onset of symptoms. Clinical features of both TIAs and strokes are similar and can include: weakness or numbness of the face, arm, and leg, especially on one side; slurred speech or trouble speaking; confusion; or trouble seeing or

walking. The causes of TIAs and strokes are also similar and occur when there is a temporary blockage of blood vessels in the brain. TIAs can be caused by emboli traveling from another part of the body to the brain, or from a thrombosis formation in an intracranial vessel. People that have TIAs recover completely from their symptoms, however they have an increased risk of stroke in the near future. The risk of having a stroke within the first 3 months after a TIA is 10% to 15%. Most events will occur in the first several days after a TIA. Therefore, urgent evaluation and appropriate treatment of TIAs are warranted. *(Smith et al., 2012)*

21. **(E)** The first priority in the management of septic shock is assessment of the airway, oxygenation, and ventilation. Oxygen should be administered at 100% via mask or endotracheal tube. Fluid resuscitation is the second priority in the patient with septic shock. Tissue and organ perfusion can be assessed by parameters such as the patient's mental status, blood pressure, respiratory rate, pulse rate, skin color and temperature, central venous pressure, and urine output more than 30 mL/h (1 mL/kg/h in pediatric patients). Other important areas of assessment and management include acid–base status and antimicrobial therapy. *(Jui, 2011)*

22. **(B)** Flumazenil competitively blocks the effects of benzodiazepines on GABAnergic pathway–mediated inhibitors in the central nervous system (CNS). Naloxone HCl (Narcan) is a narcotic antagonist. Ketamine is a rapid-acting general anesthetic. Flutamide is a nonsteroidal, antiandrogenic agent used for prostate carcinoma. *(Quan, 2011)*

23. **(C)** Septic arthritis can be caused by bacterial, viral, and by fungal infections. Bacterial agents are the most common cause. Presenting features can include: fever, redness, and swelling of the joint, severe pain, and immobility of the affected joint. Bacteria can gain entrance to the affected joint by traveling through the blood stream from another source in the body; from infections to the bone and soft tissues around the joint; or directly by trauma, bites, surgery, or injection. Many different bacterial pathogens are capable of causing septic arthritis. They are typically divided into gonococcal and nongonococcal causes. *N. gonorrhoeae* is the most commonly implicated organism found among young adults and adolescents who are sexually active. Women are at greater risk for gonococcal infections than men. Nongonococcal bacterial causes of septic arthritis are *S. aureus* (most common), Streptococcus species, and *H. influenzae*. *(Madoff, 2012)*

24. **(B)** Hyperkalemia should be considered a medical emergency because of the potential effects on the heart and the risk of fatal heart arrhythmias. Hyperkalemia is defined as serum potassium levels >5.5 mEq/L and is diagnosed by a blood sample. The earliest EKG changes reveal tall, peaked T waves which then progress to a lengthening of the PR interval and eventual loss of P waves altogether. With worsening hyperkalemia a widened QRS complex may develop and progress to a sine wave pattern, and death without treatment. With severe hyperkalemia, the initial treatment should be directed at stabilizing the myocardium against potential cardiac toxicity and fatal arrhythmias. Intravenous calcium, either calcium chloride or calcium gluconate, should be given immediately as calcium reverses the depolarization blockade caused by hyperkalemia and serves to protect the heart. It should be repeated if there is no change in the EKG findings or if they recur after initial improvement. Secondly, measures should be taken to correct hyperkalemia. This can be accomplished by giving either intravenous insulin in combination with intravenous 50% dextrose, or nebulized β_2-agonists (albuterol), which both work to move extracellular potassium into cells. Potassium levels can also be lowered by enhancing the excretion of potassium through the gastrointestinal tract. Kayexalate (sodium polystyrene sulfonate) exchanges sodium for potassium in the gastrointestinal tract and eventually excretes the potassium with feces. This is a slow process and should not be used in the treatment of acute hyperkalemia. Intravenous sodium bicarbonate should be only given if there is a metabolic acidosis along with the hyperkalemia. *(Mount, 2012)*

25. **(A)** In primary adrenocortical insufficiency, or Addison disease, low aldosterone leads to laboratory findings of hyperkalemia and hyponatremia, while low cortisol leads to hypoglycemia. There are many causes of adrenal insufficiency, with autoimmune disorders making up the largest group at 70%. Metastasis from cancer is also implicated in causing Addison disease. *(Idrose, 2011)*

26. **(E)** Testicular torsion is a true urological emergency. Any delay in the diagnosis or management of testicular torsion can lead to the loss of the testicle. It is most commonly seen in adolescent males, but may present at any age. Severe pain develops abruptly in the affected testicle and there can be associated nausea and vomiting. The affected testicle is usually swollen, high riding, and might have an abnormal transverse lie. The most sensitive finding seen with testicular torsion is the unilateral absence of the cremasteric reflex. Conversely, the onset of pain and swelling with epididymitis or epididymo-orchitis is usually gradual. Bacterial infections are the most common cause and is typically associated with fever and irritative voiding symptoms. In men <35 years of age, most cases are due to a sexually transmitted pathogen, especially *N. gonorrhoeae* or *Chlamydia trachomatis*. In men >35 years of age, most cases are due to coliforms which are gram-negative bacteria. Relief may be offered by elevation of the scrotum above the pubic symphysis (Prehn sign). Testicular cancer usually presents as a painless, hard, unilateral scrotal mass. Later symptoms may include pain in the abdomen, back, or groin; or a fluid collection in the scrotum. A hydrocele is a painless collection of fluid around one or both of the testicles that can cause the scrotum to swell. Fournier gangrene is a serious, rapidly progressing, infective necrotizing fasciitis that involves the perineal, genital, or perianal areas. Fournier gangrene is caused by many different microorganisms and may be a result from local trauma, operative procedures, or urinary tract disease. *(Nicks & Manthey, 2011)*

27. **(B)** A Hampton hump generally represents a focal area of hemorrhage within the lung or an actual pulmonary infarction. It is a wedge-shaped, dense, consolidated area on the pleural surface of the chest wall. A Westermark sign is a regional area of decreased pulmonary vascularity. Other more common findings of pulmonary embolism on a chest radiograph include atelectasis, elevated hemidiaphragm, patchy consolidation, and pleural effusions. *(Kline, 2014)*

28. **(C)** Hypocalcemia can vary from an asymptomatic presentation to a life-threatening disorder in acute hypocalcemia. Normal serum calcium is between 8.5 to 10.5 mg/dL. Mild symptoms include paresthesias; usually of the fingers, toes, and circumoral regions. Physical findings can reveal spasms of facial muscles in response to tapping the ipsilateral facial nerve anterior to the ear (Chvostek's sign). Trousseau's sign is illicited when carpal spasms are induced after inflation of a blood pressure cuff to the arm. Features of severe hypocalcemia can include: generalized seizures, stridor, wheezing, bronchospasm, laryngospasm, and tetany. EKG findings with hypocalcemia show a prolongation of the QT interval, narrowing of the QRS complex, and a reduced PR interval. EKG findings with hypercalcemia include: a shortened QT interval, bradycardia, and AV block. Therefore, changes in serum calcium can be monitored by following the QT interval. Osborn waves are seen with hypothermia and represent positive defections at the J point on the EKG. They are best seen in the inferior and lateral precordial leads. Delta waves are seen in Wolff–Parkinson–White syndrome and are represented by a slurred upstroke of the QRS complex on an EKG. In severe hyperkalemia there can be a loss of the P wave and progressive widening of the QRS complex resulting in the development of a sine wave. A sine wave suggests impending ventricular fibrillation or asystole. *(Khosla, 2012)*

29. **(E)** Most of the medications listed are a good option for hypertensive emergencies. Sodium nitroprusside is the most widely used/available, is a rapidly acting arterial and venous dilator, and is the drug of choice for most hypertensive emergencies unless there is severe kidney disease. Labetalol is an excellent drug for hypertensive emergencies. It is a competitive, selective α_1-blocker and a competitive, nonselective β-blocker, with the β-blocking action four to eight times that of α-blocking. Esmolol is an ultra-short-acting β_1 selective adrenergic blocker with rapid distribution and elimination. Nitroglycerin causes both arterial and venous dilation, with a greater effect on the venous system. The onset of action with nitroglycerin is almost immediate when given IV, and the half-life is 4 minutes. Hydralazine is a direct arterial dilator, with the onset of action within 10 minutes when given IV and duration of action 4 to 6 hours. *(Cline & Machado, 2011)*

30. **(B)** Severe, abrupt ripping or tearing chest pain that may also be located between the scapulae is common in aortic dissection. In addition, patients may state a feeling of "impending doom" in association with these symptoms. Pancreatitis typically causes pain more in the abdomen, localized to the epigastric region. Pain may radiate to the back with pancreatitis, however there is usually not a feeling of "impending doom." Patients with myocardial infarction may have feelings of "impending doom" and have pain localized to the chest, however the quality of the pain is typically more dull and crushing rather than ripping or tearing. Cauda equina syndrome typically involves the lower spinal roots of the lumbar, sacral, and coccygeal regions. Cauda equina syndrome causes pain in the lower extremities, loss of bowel or bladder function, and saddle anesthesia. Peptic ulcer disease typically presents with a dull or gnawing midepigastric pain. Peptic ulcer disease pain is typically most notable after meals. (Atilla & Oktay, 2011; Baron et al., 2011; Green & Hill, 2011; Hollander & Diercks, 2011; Johnson & Prince, 2011)

31. (A) Phlegmasia alba dolens, "milk leg," is an uncommon presentation of DVT in which there is massive iliofemoral thrombosis. The leg is usually white or pale secondary to associated arterial spasm. When the dorsalis pedis and posterior pulses are diminished or absent, a false diagnosis of arterial occlusion may be made. A patient with phlegmasia cerulea dolens presents with an extensively swollen, cyanotic leg from venous engorgement due to massive iliofemoral thrombosis. This high-grade obstruction can compromise perfusion to the foot from high compartment pressures and lead to venous gangrene. (Chopra & Carr, 2011)

32. (C) Carcinoma of the colon is the most common cause of large bowel obstructions (LBOs) in adults. Diverticulitis can also cause LBOs, and patients often give a history of intermittent left lower quadrant pain. Sigmoid volvulus is a less common cause of LBO. It is seen most often in the elderly with poor bowel habits and chronic constipation. (McQuaid, 2014)

33. (B) Cocaine is a powerful stimulant and the intoxication of cocaine manifests itself as a sympathomimetic toxidrome. Clinical features include: tachycardia, hypertension, diaphoresis, mydriasis, delirium, agitation, paranoia, and hyperthermia. Temperatures can exceed 104°F with cocaine intoxication and are due to increased psychomotor

activity caused by increased anxiety and agitation. The anticholinergic toxidrome is best known by the mnemonic: "hot as a hare, blind as a bat, mad as a hatter, red as a beet, and dry as a bone." The anticholinergic overdose can cause both physical and mental impairment. Features include: dry mucus membranes, hyperthermia, mydriasis, tachycardia, decreased gastrointestinal motility, and urinary retention. If delerium does occur with an anticholinergic overdose, the patient is typically not violent or combative. The classic opioid toxidrome is a clinical triad of altered level of consciousness, respiratory depression, and miosis. Symptoms can range from mild sedation and euphoria to hypotension and coma. Lithium overdose presents early with gastrointestinal symptoms including nausea, vomiting, abdominal pain, and diarrhea. As lithium toxicity progresses, neurologic symptoms manifest as hyperreflexia, ataxia, muscle fasciculation, and confusion. Eventually, the patient may develop seizures and become comatose. Salicylate poisoning presents early with gastrointestinal symptoms such as nausea, vomiting, and abdominal pain. Later symptoms may include: confusion, fever, seizures, metabolic acidosis, rhabdomyolysis, acute renal failure, and respiratory failure. (Williams et al., 2010)

34. (D) Infective endocarditis in the general population most often occurs on the left side of the heart, affecting the aortic or mitral valves. Conversely, infective endocarditis in IV drug users is typically right sided and over 50% involve the tricuspid valve. The frequency of infective endocarditis in injection drug users is much greater compared to the general population. The overall clinical features of endocarditis are nonspecific, but fever is most commonly seen. Other features may include: heart murmur, pleuritic chest pain, malaise, fatigue, cough, and hemoptysis. Any febrile patient with coexistent valvular abnormalities and who is an injection drug user should be suspected to have infective endocarditis. Staphylococcus species are the predominant etiologic agent. Injection of cocaine has been linked with an increased risk of endocarditis because of frequent injections due to the short half-life of the drug. (Baumann & Shepherd, 2011)

35. (C) Innervation of the skin around the umbilicus is supplied by the thoracic spinal nerve T10 (T10 dermatome). T4 gives cutaneous innervation at the

level of the nipples. The dermatome of T7 gives innervation to the inferior projection of the sternum. L2 and L3 provide cutaneous innervation to the anterior, medial, and lateral parts of the thigh. S1 gives cutaneous innervation of the skin overlying fifth digit of the foot and the calcaneus. *(Ropper et al., 2014; Waxman, 2013)*

36. **(A)** *M. pneumoniae* is most prevalent in older children, young adults, and the elderly. Bullous myringitis, rash (erythema multiforme), neurologic symptoms, arthritis, and arthralgia are common extrapulmonary symptoms found in patients with *M. pneumoniae*. *(Emerman et al., 2011)*

37. **(E)** Substernal chest discomfort that is best described as pressure or squeezing as opposed to a pain is most likely to indicate myocardial ischemia or infarction. Dyspnea is often an associated symptom of MI, however dyspnea alone is not as indicative of MI. Left arm numbness and tingling and referred back pain are also often associated with MI, but are more commonly associated with spinal stenosis and pancreatitis, respectively, and therefore not as specific. *(Kurz et al., 2014)*

38. **(D)** Spontaneous pneumothorax most commonly affects tall, thin men, between the ages of 20 and 40 years, who are heavy cigarette smokers. The pain is usually pleuritic and localizes to the affected side. Most patients have decreased breath sounds on the affected side, but few have a significant tachypnea or tachycardia. *(Humphries & Young, 2011)*

39. **(B)** Corticosteroids remain one of the keystones of treatment for asthma. Steroids are thought to decrease airway inflammation and restore β-adrenergic responsiveness. The peak onset of inflammatory effects is delayed at least 4 to 8 hours following oral or intravenous administration. Theophylline is no longer considered a first-line therapy for acute asthma because of its high risk for toxicity, especially when combined with β-adrenergic drugs. Magnesium does have some bronchodilating effects and can be used in the management of acute asthma. Magnesium should be used only after standard therapy has been unsuccessful. Leukotriene modifiers decrease inflammation, edema, mucous secretion, and bronchoconstriction, thereby diminishing the need for short-acting β$_2$ agonists; however, their

role in the ED setting has not proven to be of significant benefit in the setting of acute bronchospasms. *(Cydulka, 2011)*

40. **(D)** Preeclampsia is a serious condition that women can develop during pregnancy. It typically develops after the 20th week of pregnancy and is characterized by high blood pressure and proteinuria. It can range from mild to severe and approximately 5% to 7% of all pregnant women develop preeclampsia. Features of severe preeclampsia may include: marked elevation of blood pressure (>160/110 mm Hg), severe proteinuria (>5 g/24 h), or evidence of central nervous system (CNS) dysfunction such as headaches, blurred vision, seizures, and coma. Magnesium sulfate is the drug of choice for the prevention and treatment of eclamptic seizures. It is indicated for all patients with severe preeclampsia and has been shown to reduce the overall risk of seizures. Patients with severe preeclampsia are usually treated with magnesium sulfate beforehand before delivery. Benzodiazepines (lorazepam) and some antiepileptics (phenytoin) have been utilized as second-line agents for refractory seizures in patients with severe preeclampsia. Intravenous labetalol and hydralazine are most commonly used to manage elevated blood pressure in pregnancy. Angiotensin-converting enzyme (ACE) inhibitors (enalapril) should be avoided in the second and third trimesters of pregnancy because of associated adverse effects on the fetus. *(Barbieri & Repke, 2012)*

41. **(E)** The most common etiology of upper GI bleeding (60%) is peptic ulcer disease. This includes gastric, duodenal, and stomal ulcers. Diverticular bleeding usually results from erosion into a penetrating artery of the diverticulum. The GI bleeding associated with diverticular bleeding is usually painless and profuse. Recurrent episodes of retching can cause longitudinal tears in the cardioesophageal portion of the stomach. GI bleeding associated with this tear is known as Mallory–Weiss syndrome. *(Overton, 2011)*

42. **(E)** Sonography of the right upper quadrant has been established as the most appropriate initial diagnostic imaging study in the ED for suspected biliary tract disease. *(Atilla & Oktay, 2011)*

43. **(A)** An ectopic pregnancy is described as a pregnancy occurring outside the uterus and without

intervention is a life-threatening condition. It typically occurs in one of the fallopian tubes and if not treated can lead to tubal rupture with significant intra-abdominal hemorrhaging. Medical therapy is the preferred treatment of choice if detected early. Only the drug methotrexate has been extensively studied as an alternate to surgical therapy. Methotrexate is given by injection, and works by halting the growth of embryonic, fetal, and early placenta cells. The best prognostic indicators of treatment success with methotrexate therapy include; β-hCG level <5,000; ectopic mass <3.5 cm without tubal rupture or bleeding; U/S with absent fetal heartbeat, and compliant, asymptomatic women. Absolute contraindications for methotrexate use include hemodynamic instability, liver disease, noncompliance with posttherapeutic monitoring, and contraindications to the use of methotrexate. Surgery, with either salpingostomy or salpingectomy, is indicated when there is unsuccessful resolution of the ectopic pregnancy after methotrexate injections. It is also indicated in any hemodynamically unstable patient with internal bleeding. It can be performed at any stage of the pregnancy and is the fastest treatment option of an ectopic pregnancy. Vaginal prostaglandins and mifepristone are indicated for elective medical abortions in early pregnancies, but are not typically used for the treatment of ectopic pregnancies. Rhogam is given to a pregnant woman whose blood type is Rh-negative to keep the baby's blood from interacting with the mother's. *(Hoffman et al., 2012)*

44. **(A)** Venomous poisoning is noted by the following clinical findings: localized pain, the spreading of edema in the affected area, and the presence of at least one fang mark. The development of compartment syndrome of a snake-bitten extremity is a noted complication. The clinical symptoms of the compartment syndrome are noted by severe localized pain that is unrelieved with narcotic medications. Delayed serum sickness after Fab AV antivenom treatment occurs only in 5% of patients and is treated with oral steroids. Dislodged teeth contaminating a wound are often associated with bites from the midwestern gila monsters. Delayed absorption of the antivenom is not an expected complication as intramuscular injection in not recommended in lieu of venom-induced hypovolemia in the snake-bitten patient. Intravenous infusion of the

Fab AV antivenom is the recommended method of therapy. Rapid collapse and death are associated with the bite of the Australian brown snake (elapids) as its venom causes severe cardiovascular depression. *(Dart & Daly, 2011)*

45. **(B)** Gastroesophageal reflux disease (GERD) has been established as the most widespread etiology of inflammation of the esophagus, also known as esophagitis. Additional commonly occurring sources of esophagitis comprise pill esophagitis, esophageal damage and inflammation associated with the effects of alkaline or acidic ingestions, radiation, and infectious agents. It is suspected that the true incidence of pill esophagitis is underreported. Candida is one of the primary infectious pathogens for the infection of the esophagus. As more individuals in immunocompromised immune states receive preventative therapy for opportunistic fungal infections, viral esophagitis has increased in prevalence. Herpes simplex I (HSV) and cytomegalovirus (CMV) have been established as the most common viral agents. *(Hess & Lowell, 2014)*

46. **(D)** Ingestion of a disk-shaped battery, often found in watches, is a true medical emergency. Disk-shaped batteries, or button batteries, if ingested may cause significant complications in as little as 4 to 6 hours due to the rapid action of alkaline in the battery. Severe burns of the esophagus or perforation may occur. A battery lodged in the esophagus should be removed emergently with endoscopy. A surgical consult may be indicated for symptomatic ingestions past the esophagus. Disk-shaped batteries, and sharp objects require more invasive interventions. Most other objects pass spontaneously and do not require emergent intervention. *(Thomas & Goodloe, 2014)*

47. **(A)** Small bowel obstruction (SBO) is most often due to adhesions following surgery. Incarcerated groin hernias are the second most common cause of SBOs. Other hernias that are responsible for SBOs are umbilical, femoral, and obturator foramen. Less common causes of SBOs are polyps, lymphoma, and adenocarcinoma. Bezoars (undigested vegetable matter) represent an intraluminal obstruction in those having undergone prior surgeries such as pyloric resection. Gallstone ileus is an unusual cause of intraluminal SBO. The most common

cause of large bowel obstruction is neoplasm. *(Vicario & Price, 2011)*

48. **(D)** Pseudomembranous enterocolitis is an inflammatory bowel disorder caused by *Clostridium difficile*. The disorder is associated with antibiotic use and is marked by membrane-like plaques of exudates that overlie and replace necrotic intestinal mucosa. The use of broad-spectrum antibiotics, notably clindamycin, cephalosporins, and ampicillin/amoxicillin, is a common cause of *C. difficile* colonization. The treatments of choice include supportive measures and antibiotics such as metronidazole and vancomycin. Inflammation of the diverticulum, or diverticulitis, a common disorder of industrialized nations most commonly presents as pain and may be associated with changes in bowel habits. Ulcerative colitis (UC) is a progressive chronic inflammatory bowel condition that usually affects the colon. UC has a variable presentation and is frequently associated with rectal bleeding. With the exception of pseudomembranous enterocolitis, none of the preceding diseases are precipitated by the use of antimicrobial agents. *(Kman & Werman, 2011)*

49. **(E)** The patient described in this case has findings suggestive of thyroid storm—thyromegaly, agitation, diaphoresis, fever, and tachycardia. Patients may also present with ophthalmopathy, tremor, stare, mental status changes, or even coma. Patients with Graves' disease, toxic multinodular goiter, and toxic adenoma are more likely to be thyrotoxic and are therefore susceptible to thyroid storm. Patients with Hashimoto's thyroiditis, may initially present with mild signs of hyperthyroid before switching over to hypothyroid symptoms. In Addisonian crisis patients will have nausea, vomiting, diarrhea, and mental depression, however they typically do not present with fever, thyromegaly, and tachycardia. Pheochromocytoma is a catecholamine crisis causing palpitations, hypertension, headache, and flushing. Patients with inappropriate secretion of antidiuretic hormone range of asymptomatic in mild disease, to coma in severe hyponatremia. *(Huecker & Danzl, 2011)*

50. **(B)** In a pediatric patient with suspected volume depletion, measuring output via urinary bladder catheter is one of the most important measures.

Urine production of 1 to 2 mL/kg/h suggests adequate core blood flow. Vital signs are generally not specific or sensitive enough to measure the patient's volume status. Cerebrospinal fluid and electrolyte measurements are not specific to volume status and are typically delayed findings and more invasive. *(Stephan et al., 2011)*

51. **(C)** Nitrous oxide, also known as "laughing gas," is an inhalant used to provide analgesia, sedation, and as an adjunct to general anesthesia. Pure nitrous oxide has been shown to cause severe hypoxia and is therefore given with at least 30% oxygen to prevent this from happening. For mild sedation and analgesia a 1:1 ratio of N_2O and O_2 is typically used. Nitrous oxide concentrations of 60% to 70% can result in severe sedation. The amount of available oxygen is insufficient when nitrous oxide concentrations are greater than 80%. *(Miner, 2011; Patel et al., 2011)*

52. **(A)** While restlessness, parkinsonism, seizure, anticholinergic effects, and neuroleptic malignant syndrome can occur as side effects of the atypical class of antipsychotics, acute dystonia is often the most common side effect. *(Martel & Biros, 2011)*

53. **(D)** Unfractionated heparin's chemical composition makes it safe in pregnancy, because the molecule is too large to cross the placental barrier. Warfarin has teratogenic effects on the fetus. Aspirin is not recommended in pregnancy, and rivaroxaban is category C. *(Echevarria & Kuhn, 2011)*

54. **(D)** Hypoglycemia is defined as a plasma glucose level less than 50 mg/dL; however, the criteria for the diagnosis should include the presence of symptoms, low plasma glucose level in a symptomatic patient, and relief of symptoms after ingestion of carbohydrates. Contributing factors to symptoms of hypoglycemia include the rate at which the glucose decreases patient's overall size, underlying health conditions, and previous hypoglycemic reactions. Common symptoms include anxiety, diaphoresis, tremors, tachycardia, palpitations, fatigue, syncope, headache, mental status changes, visual disturbances, and hemiplegia. Patients with ketoacidosis are noted to frequently have Kussmaul respirations, changes in BP, and increased respirations and heart rate. These patients may also have ketone or acetone breath odor. Patients with new-onset hyperglycemia may present with increased thirst, increased urination, and increased appetite. Euglycemia refers to normal blood glucose levels; subsequently, patients should be asymptomatic. Hyperglycemic hyperosmolar nonketotic coma (HHNC) relates to a disorder that affects elderly diabetic patients with findings of increased osmolarity, blood glucose level, and dehydration. These patients have a spectrum of changes in mentation from confusion to frank coma. *(Cydulka & Maloney, 2014)*

55. **(A)** Central retinal artery occlusion is characterized by acute visual loss usually attributed to ischemic or thrombus to the major retinal arterial blood supply. Typically, the patient presents with sudden, painless onset of markedly decreased unilateral loss of vision. Physical examination findings include significant decrease in visual acuity, relative afferent pupillary defect (i.e., Marcus Gunn pupil), and a pale retina with a red spot that is visible on fundoscopic examination. Central retinal vein occlusion (CRVO) is characterized by painless, unilateral vision loss of varying severity, slower onset of decreased vision than with arterial occlusion, retinal hemorrhages, cotton wool spots, and macular edema. Physical examination findings include ciliary flush (i.e., circumcorneal perilimbal injection of the episcleral and scleral vessels), conjunctival injection, and cells may be present in the anterior chamber. The pupil on the affected side is often small and irregular. Direct and consensual light reflex will cause pain on the affected side to increase. Retrobulbar hemorrhage is associated with decreased ocular range of motion, decreased vision, ptosis of the lid, and increased pressure in the globe raising intraocular pressure. The high pressure decreases retinal artery perfusion, which results in retinal ischemia. The patient presents with decreased visual acuity, proptosis, and a dilated nonreactive pupil. A hyphema is caused by bleeding from the vasculature of the iris usually precipitated by trauma. Blood is often visualized in the anterior chamber and can be seen via slit lamp evaluation. Symptoms usually consist of pain, photophobia, and decreased vision. Intraocular pressures may increase as well. The major clinical consideration is the potential of reoccurring bleeding. *(Sharma & Brunette, 2014)*

56. **(C)** Young adults are the population at the greatest risk for epidural hematomas (EDHs) following head trauma. Direct force on the skull's temporal and parietal bones fracture and lead to lacerations of the middle meningeal artery or the dural sinus. These specific vessel lacerations account for 80% of the incidence of EDH. Subsequently, arterial hemorrhage occurs, leading to blood clotting in the space between the skull's inner table and the dura. This specific type of head injury rarely occurs in the elderly population because of the anatomical close attachment of the dura to periosteum of the inner skull's table. The dura is also closely adhered in the pediatric skull with infrequent occurrences of EDH seen in children younger than 2 years. *(Heegaard & Biros, 2014)*

57. **(E)** An elderly patient with long-standing alcoholism is most likely to present with a chronic, asymptomatic subdural hematoma. These patients typically have brain atrophy and more fragile veins that are more likely to tear. *(Humphries, 2011)*

58. **(B)** Hypoxia is an independent risk factor for mortality in patients that have suffered a head injury. There is a 50% greater risk of mortality if hypoxia is present after a head injury. The loss of gag reflex is an indication for intubation. *(Humphries, 2011)*

59. **(B)** Anticholinergic overdose is often characterized by the following: "blind as a bat, hot as hades, red as a beet, dry as a bone, mad as a hatter." Other frequently encountered clinical findings include tachycardia, gastrointestinal ileus, urinary retention, seizures, delirium, and hallucinations. Caffeine at higher doses (1 g) is noted to have symptoms of gastrointestinal disturbance, similar to theophylline toxicity. Additional findings associated with very high levels of caffeine are tachycardia, agitation, tachypnea, and electrolyte disturbances. Heroin overdose is accompanied by findings of respiratory depression, changes in mental status, hypotension, somnolence, nausea, and emesis, urinary retention, and histamine release–related complaints. Salicylate overdose is associated with nausea and vomiting and multiple acid–base disturbances. Acetaminophen overdose initially is associated with minimal clinical signs and symptoms. Later in the course of the drug's effects of toxicity, hepatic failure, coagulation disturbance, metabolic acidosis, renal failure, and GI

symptoms will develop. *(Doyon, 2011; Gresham & Brooks, 2011; Wax & Young, 2011; Yip, 2011)*

60. **(B)** Measuring serum levels of the enzyme creatine phosphokinase (CK or CPK) is the most sensitive marker for evaluating muscle damage as associated with rhabdomyolysis. In rhabdomyolysis, the isoenzyme CK-MB would not be more than 5% of the total CK or CPK. Myoglobin is also associated with muscle injury; however, it is a less sensitive marker than CPK. LDH and aldolase are additional laboratory tests that can be used in evaluating rhabdomyolysis. However, both are less specific than CPK. *(Counselman & Lo, 2011)*

61. **(B)** There are four classifications of Le Fort fractures, all of which describe fracture patterns in the midfacial region. *(Bailitz, 2011)*

62. **(B)** The head, face, and neck are the most common locations for injuries in abused women and children. *(Bailitz, 2011)*

63. **(E)** In evaluating facial trauma of the midface region, the Waters view has been established as the most sensitive of plain radiographs. The Waters view is useful in evaluation of the presence of orbital rim fractures and air–fluid levels in the maxillary sinuses. The most appropriate plain radiograph to evaluate the upper face is the Caldwell or posteroanterior view. To evaluate the base of the skull and zygoma, the submental view is the most appropriate plain radiograph. Although not available at all institutions, when available, the Panorex is the best imaging study for evaluation for suspected fracture of the mandible fractures. To evaluate the mandible ramus and condyles, the Towne view is the best imaging view. *(Bailitz, 2011)*

64. **(A)** Entrapment of extraocular muscles following facial trauma will cause binocular double vision. Monocular double vision is associated with lens dislocation. Loss of vision is associated with an injury to the optic nerve or globe. A tear drop-shaped pupil is found in a globe injury. *(Bailitz, 2011)*

65. **(C)** An unstable, hyperextension fracture through the pedicles of C2 is known as a hangman fracture. Fortunately, cord damage is usually minimal because the anteroposterior diameter of the neural canal is greatest at the C2 level. Furthermore, less neurological damage occurs because bilateral pedicle fractures tend to decompress themselves, allowing more space for the spinal cord. A Jefferson fracture of C1 is produced by an axial loading injury to the cervical spine, transmitting a force through the occipital condyles to the superior articular surfaces of the lateral masses of the atlas. A clay-shoveler fracture is an avulsion fracture of the spinous process of the lower cervical vertebrae. This oblique fracture of the base of the spinous process, classically C7, derived its name in the 1930s when Australian miners lifted a heavy shovelful of clay causing an abrupt flexion of the head, in opposition to the stabilizing force of the strong supraspinous muscle, resulting in an avulsion fracture of the spinous process. An extension teardrop fracture involves a hyperextension injury in which the anterior longitudinal ligament avulses the inferior portion of the anterior vertebral body at its insertion. The second cervical vertebra is the most common location for an extension teardrop fracture. *(Kaji et al., 2014)*

66. **(B)** The most severe neurological dysfunction, as a result of inadequate or delayed treatment of disk herniation, is cauda equina syndrome. The most common presenting symptoms are saddle anesthesia, bilateral leg pain, urinary incontinence or retention, and fecal incontinence or retention. Most cases of cauda equina syndrome and cord compression develop over a matter of hours. If the symptoms are delayed, these patients are at high risk for chronic neurological deficits. *(Perron & Huff, 2014)*

67. **(A)** Acute angle–closure glaucoma is found in patients with sudden-onset eye pain, conjunctival injection, rock hard globe, fixed midposition pupil, and a cloudy cornea. This disease process can be misdiagnosed as migraine, dementia exacerbation, or temporal arteritis. However, the finding of rock hard globe, midposition-fixed pupil, and cloudy cornea together is diagnostic for acute angle-closure glaucoma. In optic neuritis, there is acute vision reduction. *(Walker & Adhikari, 2011)*

68. **(D)** To make the diagnosis of temporal arteritis, three of the following five criteria must be present: age >50 years, new-onset localized headache, temporal artery tenderness or decreased pulse, erythrocyte sedimentation rate >50 mm/h, or abnormal

biopsy findings. If left untreated, temporal arteritis can lead to vision loss. *(Denny & Schull, 2011)*

69. **(D)** Any patient who has sustained a penetrating wound or blunt trauma to the thorax or upper abdomen should be suspected of having a diagnosis of pericardial tamponade. The most common signs of pericardial tamponade are hypotension and tachycardia-associated elevation in central venous pressure. Beck triad of pericardial tamponade consists of hypotension, distended neck veins, and distant heart sounds. A tension pneumothorax is an accumulation of air under pressure within the pleural cavity. The air under pressure shifts the mediastinum to the opposite hemithorax and compresses the contralateral lung and great vessels. A myocardial rupture refers to an acute traumatic perforation of the ventricles and atria. Acute myocardial rupture also includes rupture of the interventricular septum, pericardium, chordae, interatrial septum, and papillary muscles and valves. The most common vessel injured in an acute blunt trauma is the thoracic aorta. Deceleration injuries most commonly injure the thoracic aorta because the descending aorta is relatively fixed by the attachments of the intercostal arteries and ligamentous arteriosum. Myocardial contusion will usually demonstrate direct areas of hemorrhage in the anterior wall of the right ventricle and atria. *(Eckstein & Henderson, 2014)*

70. **(B)** Boerhaave syndrome, postemetic rupture, and spontaneous esophageal rupture are synonymous terms. The most common site of injury is the distal esophagus, which demonstrates a longitudinal tear occurring in the left posterolateral aspect. Most cases occur in middle-aged men after they have overindulged in food and alcohol. Burger sign is defined as a physical examination finding of advanced peripheral vascular disease. Brudzinski sign is a physical examination diagnostic maneuver in which hip flexion occurs with passive flexion of the neck and is interpreted as a positive meningeal sign. Bezoars (undigested vegetable matter) represent an intraluminal obstruction in those having undergone prior surgeries such as pyloric resection. *(Aufderheide, 2014; Vicario & Price, 2011; Zun, 2014)*

71. **(D)** Most food bolus impactions resolve without intervention, either by moving forward into the stomach, or by the patient regurgitating the ingested contents. If symptoms persist patients will seek medical attention. Food bolus impactions are commonly associated with either a mechanical etiology: esophageal stricture, carcinoma, Schatzki ring, eosinophilic esophagitis, or by motility disorders. Preferably all meat boluses should be removed or advanced into the stomach because of the risk for aspiration. A complete esophageal obstruction is implied when a patient is drooling and is unable to swallow secretions. It is an indication for urgent endoscopic intervention and should not be delayed. The administration of intravenous glucagon is often tried prior to endoscopy to promote spontaneous passage. Glucagon has been found to be effective with lower esophageal impactions as it relaxes the smooth muscles of the lower esophageal sphincter, but has little effect on the proximal esophagus. It has been shown to stimulate spontaneous passage of the food bolus in up to 50% of cases. Meat tenderizers were commonly used in the past for treatment of esophageal obstructions, but are now avoided because of the potential for complications. IV Depacon and calcium chloride have no practical use for treatment of esophageal food bolus obstructions. *(Thompson, 2012)*

72. **(C)** A penile rupture (or fracture) is a traumatic rupture of the corpus cavernosum when the tunica albuginea is torn. During vigorous sexual intercourse, a patient commonly will hear a snapping sound followed by localized pain, detumescence, and slowly progressive penile hematoma. Phimosis is when the foreskin and glans penis cannot be retracted. Balanoposthitis is when the glans penis and foreskin are inflamed. Penile hair-tourniquet syndrome leads to constriction of the glans penis, it is often caused by a strand of hair that becomes wrapped around the glans penis in uncircumcised males aged 3 to 5 years. Peyronie disease is defined as curvature of the penis with associated erectile dysfunction. *(Nicks & Manthey, 2011)*

73. **(B)** Mallet finger is a disruption of the distal tendon, resulting in a flexion deformity at the distal interphalangeal joint (DIP). It is the most common zone I injury. Bennett fracture is a combination of a dislocated carpometacarpal joint and the thumb's metacarpophalangeal joint (MCP) that is fractured intra-articularly. Rolando fracture is defined as a

comminuted fracture involving the base of the thumb's MCP. A Boutonniere deformity involves deformity of the index finger. The swan neck deformity does not represent an acute finding but rather is associated with an untreated mallet finger. *(Mailhot & Lyn, 2014)*

74. **(D)** The developing bones of the child are more pliable and flexible than an adult mature bone. In a torus fracture, there is a buckling of the cortex of the bone without complete disruption of the cortical segment. Multiple radiographic views may be necessary to make the diagnosis in small, nondisplaced fractures. *(Williams & Hyung, 2014)*

75. **(C)** The most common nerve injured with a humeral shaft fracture is the radial nerve. The radial nerve runs in close proximity to the posterior midhumeral shaft. A radial nerve injury is evident by a wrist drop. *(Mayer, 2014)*

76. **(C)** The hallmark of acute mesenteric ischemia (AMI) is severe abdominal pain that is out of proportion to the degree of pain on physical examination. Abdominal tenderness is minimal to nonexistent early in the course of ischemia. Symptoms can include nausea, vomiting, and diarrhea. Peritoneal signs along with rectal bleeding tend to develop late, when infarction with necrosis or perforation occurs. Laboratory values may reveal leukocytosis, metabolic acidosis, lactic acidosis, hyperkalemia, and renal impairment. The definitive diagnosis of acute mesenteric vascular disease is made by mesenteric angiography as it is the most specific. Positive findings on plain abdominal radiographs are usually found late and are nonspecific for mesenteric ischemia. However, they may help in excluding other causes of acute abdominal pain such as intestinal obstruction, perforation, or volvulus. Upper endoscopy, colonoscopy, and barium radiography do not provide any beneficial information for the evaluation of acute mesenteric ischemia. Duplex ultrasonography is considered a second-line study for AMI. It is a noninvasive study that can assess the patency of the mesenteric vessels, but is less useful in the presence of dilated loops of small bowel. Finally, MRI/MRA of the abdomen has been promising in providing clear radiographic assessment of the mesenteric vessels. However, they are used less often for the diagnosis AMI because of the cost and time involved. *(Lin et al., 2010)*

77. **(D)** Retropharyngeal abscess is an infected fluid collection in the fascial plane between the posterior pharyngeal muscles and the paraspinous muscles. Primarily, retropharyngeal abscess is a pediatric problem because there are lymph nodes in the retropharyngeal space that can become suppurative. Clinical manifestations include an ill-appearing child with fever, sore throat, neck pain, and voice changes (i.e., "duck-like voice"). A CT scan with IV contrast of the soft tissues of the neck and upper chest is the best diagnostic test. Peritonsillar abscess is an infected fluid collection in the pharyngeal pillar. The most common etiology is β-hemolytic streptococcus. Symptoms include fever, sore throat (unilateral), and odynophagia. In addition, the patient drools and finds it hard to handle his/her own secretions. Streptococcal pharyngitis is an infection of the pharynx and tonsils due to group A β-hemolytic streptococci. Clinical features include sudden onset of fever and sore throat with enlargement of the cervical lymph nodes. Headache, vomiting, abdominal pain, meningismus, and torticollis can occur as well. Epiglottitis is an inflammatory disorder of the supraglottic laryngeal region. Etiologies of epiglottitis include bacterium, viruses, chemical damage (e.g., aspiration of fuel), and mechanical damage (e.g., trauma, burns). Symptoms include sore throat, fever, a muffled voice, dysphagia, and respiratory distress. Clinical features include drooling, dyspnea, tachypnea, inspiratory stridor, tripod position (i.e., patient leans forward, supporting himself/herself with both hands), and toxic appearance. Ludwig angina is an abscess formation of the submaxillary, sublingual, and submental spaces accompanied by elevation of the tongue. The cause is due to an infection of the lower second and third molars usually due to β-hemolytic streptococcus, staphylococcus, and mixed anaerobic and aerobic infections. Patients commonly present with swelling beneath the chin. The tongue is displaced up and posteriorly. Trismus often makes opening the mouth for examination difficult. *(Cukor & Manno, 2014; Melio & Berge, 2014)*

78. **(D)** The most common mechanism of injury for an anterior shoulder dislocation is abduction, extension, and external rotation. The lateral edge of the

acromion process is prominent and the arm is held in slight abduction and external rotation by the opposite extremity. Anterior shoulder dislocations account for 95% to 97% of all glenohumeral dislocations. Falls onto an outstretched hand as mechanism of injury is more common in older patient population. *(Daya & Bengtzen, 2014)*

79. **(E)** The class of prescription medications responsible for the most drug-related deaths is tricyclic antidepressants (TCAs). The clinical toxicity is due to the complex pharmacologic activity, low therapeutic index, and general availability. The clinical toxicity is quite variable, ranging from mild antimuscarinic activity to severe cardiotoxicity. Benzodiazepine related overdoses account for few deaths; however, in combination with other agents, they account for significant deaths and disability due to additive effects. Although not reflected in death rates, monoamine oxidase inhibitors have greater toxicity than the newer antidepressants. The toxic effects of lithium are frequently related to drug interactions. Stimulants are associated with significant side effects, but less likely to result in deaths than TCAs. *(Mills, 2011, Ch. 173; Prosser & Perrone, 2011; Quan, 2011; Schneider & Cobaugh, 2011)*

80. **(C)** Patients with ethylene glycol ingestion usually present with an acute change in mental status, high anion gap metabolic acidosis, osmolar gap, and calcium oxalate crystals in the urine. Ethylene glycol is commercially available as preservatives, glycerine substitutes, and antifreeze. Ethylene glycol may be ingested in suicide attempts, accidentally by children, and by alcoholics as an alcohol substitute. The toxic metabolites formed by ethylene glycol metabolism are primarily formaldehyde, formic acid, and oxalic acid. When noteworthy acidosis is present, ethanol is most likely not the underlying source of intoxication. Isopropyl alcohol ingestion usually has abnormal anion gap. Methanol is noted to have a delay in presentation of toxic-related symptoms. *(Smith & Quan, 2011)*

81. **(D)** Treatment priorities of acetaminophen toxicity consist of supportive care, gastrointestinal decontamination, and the use of the antidote *N*-acetylcysteine (NAC). No additional therapies are recognized for intervention in acetaminophen overdoses. If given early (less than 8 hours after ingestion), NAC can prevent toxicity by inhibiting the binding of the toxic metabolite *N*-acetyl-*p*-benzoquinoneimine to hepatic proteins. In acetaminophen toxicity, more than 24 hours after ingestion, NAC diminishes hepatic necrosis by nonspecific mechanisms. The standard 72-hour oral NAC regimen used in the United States is a loading dose of 140 mg/kg followed by maintenance doses of 70 mg/kg every 4 hours for 17 doses. *(Hung & Nelson, 2011)*

82. **(E)** Periorbital cellulitis is characterized by warmth, redness, swelling, and tenderness over the affected eye, along with conjunctival injection, eyelid swelling, chemosis, and fever. Orbital cellulitis includes all the symptoms of periorbital (preseptal) cellulitis with the addition of ocular pain and limitation of eye movement due to pain. Other physical examination findings may include lid edema, proptosis, marked tenderness to the globe, decreased visual acuity, and pupillary paralysis. *(Pallin & Nassisi, 2014)*

83. **(D)** Isopropyl alcohol (isopropanol), commonly referred to as rubbing alcohol, is a solvent and disinfectant used in many household items such as hair and skin products, antifreeze, and window-cleaning solutions. The toxic dose is 1 mL/kg of a 70% solution. Isopropanol is metabolized to acetone. Mild acidosis may occur because of the formation of acetate and formate. This toxicity is associated with high serum and urine ketone levels. However, a distinguishing factor is that there is no increase in the osmolal gap or anion gap acidosis. Methanol, also referred to as wood alcohol, is commonly used in products such as solvents, antifreeze, windshield washer fluid, and varnishes. The lethal ingested dose is approximately 15 to 30 mL in adults. Methanol is oxidized in the liver to formaldehyde and formate, subsequently a severe lactic acidosis develops. These metabolites concentrate in the vitreous humor and optic nerve, causing ocular toxicity and blindness. This toxicity is associated with an osmolal gap and an anion gap acidosis but no ketosis. Ethylene glycol is frequently implicated in overdoses of antifreeze. Clinical findings include increase in serum potassium level and the presence of a wide anion gap metabolic acidosis. Diabetic ketoacidosis (DKA) is a disorder found in insulin-dependent diabetes patients that is characterized by hyperglycemia, ketonemia, and acidosis. Serum glucose levels are typically higher than 300 mg/dL.

Metabolic acidosis is demonstrated by a serum bicarbonate concentration of less than 15 mEq/L and a pH of less than 7.2. Ketonemia results from β-hydroxybutyrate and acetoacetate. This toxicity results in an anion gap acidosis, a ketotic state, but no osmolal gap. Alcoholic ketoacidosis is typically seen in alcoholic patients who are forced to stop drinking shortly after a drinking binge. β-Hydroxybutyric acid is the predominant ketone formed in alcoholic ketoacidosis. A metabolic acidosis may occur from vomiting, dehydration, and respiratory alkalosis. Therefore, this toxicity is characterized by an anion gap acidosis and a high ketone level but an osmolal gap is not found. *(Cydulka & Maloney, 2014; Finell, 2014; White, 2014)*

84. **(C)** Mild hypothermia is defined as a temperature from 32° to 35°C (89.6°–95°F). In mild hypothermia, the body responds by increasing metabolic activity to produce heat. This is known as the excitation or the responsive phase. When the temperature drops to less than 32°C (89.6°F), bodily functions slow down, giving way to the adynamic phase. As metabolism slows, there is a decrease in both oxygen utilization and carbon dioxide production. As the body temperature falls to less than 30° to 32°C (86°–89.6°F), shivering will cease. Hypothermia may induce life-threatening dysrhythmias and ECG changes. A characteristic, but not pathognomonic, ECG finding in hypothermia is the Osborne (J) wave. This abnormal wave is a slow, positive deflection at the end of the QRS complex. *(Bessen & Ngo, 2011)*

85. **(A)** The black widow spider (*Latrodectus*) is found in many areas of the United States. Its bite produces immediate pain and pinprick sensations that soon encompass the entire extremity. Erythema of the bitten area develops usually within 1 hour and in about half of the cases quickly evolves into a target pattern. Patients frequently complain of cramp-like spasms in the large muscle groups. The physical examination rarely exhibits muscle rigidity, and serum creatine kinase concentrations usually are not elevated significantly. The brown recluse (*Loxosceles*) spider bites are difficult to identify. The bite lesion is usually mildly erythematous and may become firm and heal with little scarring over several days to weeks. Occasionally, the lesion may

become necrotic over 3 to 4 days with subsequent eschar formation. The hobo spider (*Tegenaria*) usually causes a painless local reaction similar to that of the brown recluse spider. Blisters eventually develop that rupture, leaving an encrusted cratered wound. A tarantula bite typically causes pain and local swelling at the site. Treatment consists of local wound care. Scorpions (*Scorpionida*) present with a multitude of local and systemic manifestations. Some of these manifestations include pain, paresthesia, cranial nerve and somatic motor dysfunction, uncontrolled jerking, restlessness, pharyngeal incoordination, and respiratory compromise. *(Scheir, 2011)*

86. **(D)** The three principles of treatment regarding acute mountain sickness (AMS) are (1) to stop the ascent, (2) to descend to lower altitude, and (3) to treat immediately in the presence of change in normal mental status, ataxia, or pulmonary edema. Emergent treatments include oxygen, acetazolamide, nifedipine, dexamethasone, hyperbaric therapy, and continuous positive airway pressure. *(Hackett & Hargrove, 2011)*

87. **(B)** The answer is 45% burn. The rule of nines to estimate percentage of burns is as follows: head 9%, anterior trunk 18%, posterior trunk 18%, each leg 18%, each arm 9%, and perineum 1%. *(Schwartz & Balakrishnam, 2011)*

88. **(C)** A Maisonneuve fracture is a fracture of the proximal third of the fibula resulting from an external rotation force applied to the foot. This injury starts at the medial ankle with either a deltoid ligament rupture or a medial malleolus injury. The force of the injury is led upward and laterally tearing the interosseous membrane resulting in a fracture of the proximal fibula. The fibula may be fractured at its head or as far down as 6 cm above the ankle joint. A Quadriceps tendon rupture occurs when the tendon that connects the quadriceps muscle to the patella is torn. There is significant pain and diffuse swelling with this injury. The patient is unable to extend a flexed knee against mild resistance. A defect may be palpable above the patella. A patient with compartment syndrome will initially complain of severe pain that is often difficult to control even with narcotic pain medications. The symptoms of compartment syndrome traditionally were

associated with the five P's: pain, paresthesia, pallor, pulselessness, and poikilothermia. With a lateral meniscus tear there is pain and tenderness over the lateral joint line of the knee joint. The pain increases with squatting or by rising up from a seated position. *(Glaspy & Steele, 2011; Haller, 2011)*

89. **(A)** A patellar tendon rupture represents a rupture of the tendon that connects the patella to the tibia. It occurs more frequently in patients less than 40 years old. On examination, the patient is unable to extend the affected knee and there is a palpable patellar tendon defect. The patella of the affected knee might be "high riding" on examination. Surgical repair is the treatment of choice. A positive Thompson test is diagnostic for a complete tear of the Achilles tendon. When the Achilles tendon is intact, and the calf is squeezed, the ankle should plantar flex. The test is positive when there is no plantar flexion when the calf is squeezed. Straight-leg tests are done to help find the reason for low back and leg pain. The test stretches the sciatic nerve that runs down the back of the leg and the nerve roots that lead to it. The test is positive when the patient has pain down the back of the leg when the affected leg is raised and the ankle is dorsi-flexed. *(McMahon et al., 2014)*

90. **(E)** Wernicke encephalopathy is a potentially fatal neurologic disorder found in alcoholics with poor nutritional status that is caused by chronic vitamin B_6 deficiency. Alcoholism interferes with gastrointestinal absorption of vitamin B_6 and impairs conversion of vitamin B_6 to its active metabolite. In many patients, concomitant liver disease impairs storage of vitamin B_6. The administration of glucose to an alcoholic patient with an inadequate supply of thiamine may precipitate this disorder. Clinical features include the triad of abnormal mental status, ophthalmoplegia, and gait ataxia. Patients are often disoriented, forgetful, and unable to recognize familiar objects. With prompt therapy, the ophthalmoplegia usually resolves within hours and the coma resolves in hours to days, but the memory deficit may never resolve. Thiamine 100 mg administered intravenously is the treatment of choice. Thiamine 100 mg intravenous administration is continued daily until the patient has achieved proper oral nutritional status. It is essential that thiamine be given prior to the administration of glucose. *(Finell, 2014)*

91. **(C)** In the emergency medicine setting, treatment of small dental abscess or periapical abscess with oral antibiotics is warranted. The most appropriate antimicrobial agents include Penicillin VK 500 mg PO QID, clindamycin 300 mg PO QID, or erythromycin 500 mg QID. Small periodontal abscess may respond to antibiotic therapy along with the application of warm saline rinses. Larger abscesses warrant incision and drainage. It is crucial to provide sufficient analgesic therapy for dental abscesses. Analgesic therapy may include NSAIDs and/or short courses of opioid medications. Definitive therapy for dental abscesses is provided by a dentist. *(Beaudreau, 2011)*

92. **(B)** Six percent of the cases of extrapulmonary TB affect the CNS. The peak incidence of extrapulmonary CNS TB is seen in the pediatric age range of birth to 4 years. Among children younger than 4 years, about 25% will develop extrapulmonary TB manifestations. In recent years, miliary TB (acute disseminated TB) has become more common in the elderly and those with HIV infections; previously this form of TB was more common in children. The multisystem or miliary form of TB is also seen in chronic alcoholics and those with cirrhotic liver disease. *(Sokolove & Derlet, 2014)*

93. **(B)** Suspected active TB warrants hospital admission, and not discharge home. Limiting exposure to these patients, who are likely infectious, is best accomplished by early identification and placement in a negative airflow room (respiratory isolation). Staff working in the ED should be accustomed to using respiratory protective equipment, specifically protective masks, with the more advanced staff using the N-95 particulate respirators. A simple mask and face shield is not adequate. Cases should be reported to the local public health department. *(Sokolove & Derlet, 2014)*

94. **(D)** In evaluating a pediatric patient for suspected intussusception, air contrast enema has proven to be diagnostic and therapeutic in approximately 60% to 80% of cases. Contrast enema utilizing air is preferred to barium because of greater management of colonic pressures when performing the reduction when compared with the barium technique. An

additional benefit in the case of bowel perforation is that there is no risk of spillage of barium contrast into the peritoneum. The patient should be stable and well resuscitated before undergoing the contrast enema procedure. *(Albanese & Sylvester, 2010)*

95. **(E)** The American Academy of Pediatrics (AAP) recommends no blood studies, EEG, lumbar puncture (LP), or neuroimaging is necessary for a simple febrile seizure in a child older than 18 months of age who appears well. The evaluation should focus on the cause of fever. The AAP does strongly recommend an LP in infants <12 months old, and consideration for LP in infants 12 to 18 months old. *(Holsti, 2011)*

96. **(D)** Based on the scenario, the most likely diagnosis is respiratory syncytial virus (RSV). RSV pulmonary infections in young infants can be accompanied by apneic episodes as well as chlamydia and pertussis infections. Mucous plugging results from necrosis of the respiratory epithelium and destruction of ciliated epithelial cells. This and submucosal edema lead to peripheral airway narrowing and variable obstruction mechanism inducing RSV-related apnea in young infants is not completely understood but may be related to hypoxemia and upper airway obstruction. Infants at the highest risk are those younger than 6 weeks and those who have a history of prematurity, apnea of prematurity, and low O_2

saturation on admission. It is difficult to predict apneic events. Steroids are not recommended as studies have failed to prove benefit unless underlying asthma; in addition, they can be administered in the oral formulation. Hospital admission is recommended for children with clinically defined hypoxia and RSV diagnosis; the frequently chosen parameter is pulse oximetry of less than 90% to 93%. Ribavirin (antiviral) is clinically indicated for RSV infections in high-risk patients and comes in oral and aerosol formulations. Educating the parents on the clinical course of RSV infection and signs and symptoms or respiratory distress is critical in disposition of pediatric patients. Children with mild symptoms who are tolerating fluids can be released in the care of capable caregivers with good follow-up. Additional home care options can include home health nursing visits and discharging the patient with nebulizer machines if medically necessary. *(Arnold et al., 2011)*

97. **(C)** Oral ampicillin or amoxicillin in a patient with Epstein–Barr virus often induces a morbilliform rash. Oral corticosteroids are not recommended due to increased risk of complications, unless the patient has severe diseases such as hemolytic anemia, neurologic disease or upper airway obstruction. Oral acyclovir is helpful in patients with hairy leukoplakia. Recommended treatment for Epstein–Barr virus is rest and analgesia. *(Takhar & Moran, 2011)*

REFERENCES

Albanese CT, Sylvester KG. Chapter 43: Pediatric surgery. In: Doherty GM, eds. *Current: Diagnosis and Treatment: Surgery.* 13th ed. New York, NY: McGraw-Hill; 2010.

Arnold DH, Spiro DM, Langhan ML. Chapter 120: Wheezing in infants and children. In: Tintinalli JE, Stapczynski JS, Ma O, Cline DM, Cydulka RK, Meckler GD, eds. *Tintinalli's Emergency Medicine: A Comprehensive Study Guide.* 7th ed. New York, NY: McGraw-Hill; 2011.

Atilla R, Oktay C. Chapter 82: Pancreatitis and cholecystitis. In: Tintinalli JE, Stapczynski J, Ma O, Cline DM, Cydulka RK, Meckler GD, eds. *Tintinalli's Emergency Medicine: A Comprehensive Study Guide.* 7th ed. New York, NY: McGraw-Hill; 2011.

Aufderheide T. Chapter 87: Peripheral arteriovascular disease. In: Marx JA, Hockberger RS, Walls RM, et al., eds. *Rosen's Emergency Medicine: Concepts and Clinical Practice.* 8th ed. Philadelphia, PA: Saunders; 2014.

Bailitz J. Chapter 256: Trauma to the face. In: Tintinalli JE, Stapczynski J, Ma O, Cline DM, Cydulka RK, Meckler GD, eds. *Tintinalli's Emergency Medicine: A Comprehensive Study Guide.* 7th ed. New York, NY: McGraw-Hill; 2011.

Barbieri RL, Repke JT. Chapter 7: Medical disorders during pregnancy. In: Longo DL, Fauci AS, Kasper DL, Hauser SL, Jameson J, Loscalzo J, eds. *Harrison's Principles of Internal Medicine.* 18th ed. New York, NY: McGraw-Hill; 2012.

Baron BJ, McSherry KJ, Larson JL, Jr., Scalea TM. Chapter 255: Spine and spinal cord trauma. In: Tintinalli JE, Stapczynski J, Ma O, Cline DM, Cydulka RK, Meckler GD, eds. *Tintinalli's Emergency Medicine: A Comprehensive Study Guide*, 7th ed. New York, NY: McGraw-Hill; 2011.

Baumann BM, Shepherd SM. Chapter 294: Injection drug users. In: Tintinalli JE, Stapczynski J, Ma O, Cline DM, Cydulka RK, Meckler GD, eds. *Tintinalli's Emergency Medicine: A Comprehensive Study Guide*. 7th ed. New York, NY: McGraw-Hill; 2011.

Beaudreau RW. Chapter 240: Oral and dental emergencies. In: Tintinalli JE, Stapczynski JS, Ma O, Cline DM, Cydulka RK, Meckler GD, eds. *Tintinalli's Emergency Medicine: A Comprehensive Study Guide*. 7th ed. New York, NY: McGraw-Hill; 2011.

Bessen HA, Ngo B. Chapter 203: Hypothermia. In: Tintinalli JE, Stapczynski JS, Ma O, Cline DM, Cydulka RK, Meckler GD, eds. *Tintinalli's Emergency Medicine: A Comprehensive Study Guide*. 7th ed. New York, NY: McGraw-Hill; 2011.

Chopra A, Carr D. Chapter 64: Occlusive arterial disease. In: Tintinalli JE, Stapczynski J, Ma O, Cline DM, Cydulka RK, Meckler GD, eds. *Tintinalli's Emergency Medicine: A Comprehensive Study Guide* 7th ed. New York, NY: McGraw-Hill; 2011.

Cline DM, Machado AJ. Chapter 61: Systemic and pulmonary hypertension. In: Tintinalli JE, Stapczynski J, Ma O, Cline DM, Cydulka RK, Meckler GD, eds. *Tintinalli's Emergency Medicine: A Comprehensive Study Guide* 7th ed. New York, NY: McGraw-Hill; 2011.

Counselman FL., Lo BM. Chapter 92: Rhabdomyolysis. In: Tintinalli JE, Stapczynski J, Ma O, Cline DM, Cydulka RK, Meckler GD, eds. *Tintinalli's Emergency Medicine: A Comprehensive Study Guide*. 7th ed. New York, NY: McGraw-Hill; 2011.

Cukor J, Manno M. Chapter 168: Pediatric respiratory emergencies: upper airway obstruction and infection. In: Marx JA, Hockberger RS, Walls RM, et al., eds. *Rosen's Emergency Medicine: Concepts and Clinical Practice*. 8th ed. Philadelphia, PA: Saunders; 2014.

Cydulka RK. Chapter 72: Acute asthma in adults. In: Tintinalli JE, Stapczynski J, Ma O, Cline DM, Cydulka RK, Meckler GD, eds. *Tintinalli's Emergency Medicine: A Comprehensive Study Guide*. 7th ed. New York, NY: McGraw-Hill; 2011.

Cydulka RK, Maloney GE. Chapter 126: Diabetes mellitus and disorders of glucose homeostasis. In: Marx JA, Hockberger RS, Walls RM, et al., eds. *Rosen's Emergency Medicine: Concepts and Clinical Practice*. 8th ed. Philadelphia, PA: Saunders; 2014.

Dart RC, Daly FS. Chapter 206: Reptile bites. In: Tintinalli JE, Stapczynski JS, Ma O, Cline DM, Cydulka RK, Meckler GD, eds. *Tintinalli's Emergency Medicine: A Comprehensive Study Guide*. 7th ed. New York, NY: McGraw-Hill; 2011.

Daya M, Bengtzen RR. Chapter 53: Shoulder. In: Marx JA, Hockberger RS, Walls RM, et al., eds. *Rosen's Emergency Medicine: Concepts and Clinical Practice*. 8th ed. Philadelphia, PA: Saunders; 2014.

Denny CJ, Schull MJ. Chapter 159: Headache and facial pain. In: Tintinalli JE, Stapczynski J, Ma O, Cline DM, Cydulka RK, Meckler GD, eds. *Tintinalli's Emergency Medicine: A Comprehensive Study Guide*. 7th ed. New York, NY: McGraw-Hill; 2011. (Table 159-3)

Doyon S. Chapter 180: Opioids. In: Tintinalli JE, Stapczynski JS, Ma O, Cline DM, Cydulka RK, Meckler GD, eds. *Tintinalli's Emergency Medicine: A Comprehensive Study Guide*. 7th ed. New York, NY: McGraw-Hill; 2011.

Echevarria MA, Kuhn GJ. Chapter 104: Emergencies after 20 weeks of pregnancy and the postpartum period. In: Tintinalli JE, Stapczynski J, Ma O, Cline DM, Cydulka RK, Meckler GD, eds. *Tintinalli's Emergency Medicine: A Comprehensive Study Guide*. 7th ed. New York, NY: McGraw-Hill; 2011.

Eckstein ME, Henderson SO. Chapter 45: Thoracic trauma. In: Marx JA, Hockberger RS, Walls RM, et al., eds. *Rosen's Emergency Medicine: Concepts and Clinical Practice*. 8th ed. Philadelphia, PA: Saunders; 2014.

Emerman CL, Anderson E, Cline DM. Chapter 68: Community-acquired pneumonia, aspiration pneumonia, and noninfectious pulmonary infiltrates. In: Tintinalli JE, Stapczynski J, Ma O, Cline DM, Cydulka RK, Meckler GD, eds. *Tintinalli's Emergency Medicine: A Comprehensive Study Guide*. 7th ed. New York, NY: McGraw-Hill; 2011.

Finell JT. Chapter 185: Alcohol-related disease. In: Marx JA, Hockberger RS, Walls RM, et al., eds. *Rosen's Emergency Medicine: Concepts and Clinical Practice*. 8th ed. Philadelphia, PA: Saunders; 2014.

Glaspy JN, Steele MT. Chapter 271: Knee injuries. In: Tintinalli JE, Stapczynski JS, Ma O, Cline DM, Cydulka RK, Meckler GD, eds. *Tintinalli's Emergency Medicine: A Comprehensive Study Guide*. 7th ed. New York, NY: McGraw-Hill; 2011.

Gomella LG, Haist SA. Chapter 8: Blood gases and acid–base disorders. In: Gomella LG, Haist SA, eds. *Clinician's Pocket Reference: The Scut Monkey*. 11th ed. New York, NY: McGraw-Hill; 2007.

Goshorn EC, Kan JA, Vicario SJ. Chapter 9: Basic and advanced cardiac life support. In: Stone C, Humphries RL, eds. *Current Diagnosis & Treatment Emergency Medicine*. 7th ed. New York, NY: McGraw-Hill; 2011.

Green GB, Hill PM. Chapter 52: Chest pain: Cardiac or not. In: Tintinalli JE, Stapczynski J, Ma O, Cline DM, Cydulka RK, Meckler GD, eds. *Tintinalli's Emergency Medicine: A Comprehensive Study Guide*. 7th ed. New York, NY: McGraw-Hill; 2011.

Gresham C, Brooks DE. Chapter 186: Methylxanthines and nicotine. In: Tintinalli JE, Stapczynski J, Ma O, Cline DM, Cydulka RK, Meckler GD, eds. *Tintinalli's Emergency Medicine: A Comprehensive Study Guide*. 7th ed. New York, NY: McGraw-Hill; 2011.

Hackett PH, Hargrove J. Chapter 216: High-altitude medical problems. In: Tintinalli JE, Stapczynski JS, Ma O, Cline DM,

Cydulka RK, Meckler GD, eds. *Tintinalli's Emergency Medicine: A Comprehensive Study Guide.* 7th ed. New York, NY: McGraw-Hill; 2011.

Haller PR. Chapter 275: Compartment syndrome. In: Tintinalli JE, Stapczynski J, Ma O, Cline DM, Cydulka RK, Meckler GD, eds. *Tintinalli's Emergency Medicine: A Comprehensive Study Guide.* 7th ed. New York, NY: McGraw-Hill; 2011.

Heegaard WG, Biros MH. Chapter 41: Head injury. In: Marx JA, Hockberger RS, Walls RM, et al., eds. *Rosen's Emergency Medicine: Concepts and Clinical Practice.* 8th ed. Philadelphia, PA: Saunders; 2014.

Hellmann DB, Imboden JB, Jr. Chapter 20: Rheumatologic and immunologic disorders. In: Papadakis MA, McPhee SJ, Rabow MW, eds. *Current Medical Diagnosis & Treatment 2014.* New York, NY: McGraw-Hill; 2014.

Hess JM, Lowell MJ. Chapter 89: Esophagus, stomach and duodenum. In: Marx JA, Hockberger RS, Walls RM, et al., eds. *Rosen's Emergency Medicine: Concepts and Clinical Practice.* 8th ed. Philadelphia, PA: Saunders; 2014.

Hoffman BL, Schorge JO, Schaffer JI, et al. Chapter 7: Ectopic pregnancy. In: Hoffman BL, Schorge JO, Schaffer JI, et al., eds. *Williams Gynecology.* 2th ed. New York, NY: McGraw-Hill; 2012.

Hollander JE, Diercks DB. Chapter 53: Acute coronary syndromes: acute myocardial infarction and unstable angina. In: Tintinalli JE, Stapczynski J, Ma O, Cline DM, Cydulka RK, Meckler GD, eds. *Tintinalli's Emergency Medicine: A Comprehensive Study Guide.* 7th ed. New York, NY: McGraw-Hill; 2011.

Holsti M. Chapter 129: Seizures and status epilepticus in children. In: Tintinalli JE, Stapczynski J, Ma O, Cline DM, Cydulka RK, Meckler GD, eds. *Tintinalli's Emergency Medicine: A Comprehensive Study Guide.* 7th ed. New York, NY: McGraw-Hill; 2011.

Huecker MR, Danzl DF. Chapter 43: Metabolic and endocrine emergencies. In: Stone C, Humphries RL, eds. *Current Diagnosis & Treatment Emergency Medicine.* 7th ed. New York, NY: McGraw-Hill; 2011.

Humphries RL. Chapter 22: Head injuries. In: Stone C, Humphries RL, eds. *Current Diagnosis & Treatment Emergency Medicine.* 7th ed. New York, NY: McGraw-Hill; 2011.

Humphries RL, Young W, Jr. Chapter 71: Spontaneous and iatrogenic pneumothorax. In: Tintinalli JE, Stapczynski J, Ma O, Cline DM, Cydulka RK, Meckler GD, eds. *Tintinalli's Emergency Medicine: A Comprehensive Study Guide.* 7th ed. New York, NY: McGraw-Hill; 2011.

Hung OL, Nelson LS. Chapter 184: Acetaminophen. In: Tintinalli JE, Stapczynski JS, Ma O, Cline DM, Cydulka RK, Meckler GD, eds. *Tintinalli's Emergency Medicine: A Comprehensive Study Guide.* 7th ed. New York, NY: McGraw-Hill; 2011.

Idrose A. Chapter 225: Adrenal insufficiency and adrenal crisis. In: Tintinalli JE, Stapczynski J, Ma O, Cline DM, Cydulka

RK, Meckler GD, eds. *Tintinalli's Emergency Medicine: A Comprehensive Study Guide.* 7th ed. New York, NY: McGraw-Hill; 2011.

Johnson GA, Prince LA. Chapter 62: Aortic dissection and related aortic syndromes. In: Tintinalli JE, Stapczynski J, Ma O, Cline DM, Cydulka RK, Meckler GD, eds. *Tintinalli's Emergency Medicine: A Comprehensive Study Guide.* 7th ed. New York, NY: McGraw-Hill; 2011.

Jui J. Chapter 146: Septic shock. In: Tintinalli JE, Stapczynski J, Ma O, Cline DM, Cydulka RK, Meckler GD, eds. *Tintinalli's Emergency Medicine: A Comprehensive Study Guide.* 7th ed. New York, NY: McGraw-Hill; 2011.

Kaji AH, Newton EJ, Hockberger RS. Chapter 43: Spinal injuries. In: Marx JA, Hockberger RS, Walls RM, et al., eds. *Rosen's Emergency Medicine: Concepts and Clinical Practice.* 8th ed. Philadelphia, PA: Saunders; 2014.

Khosla S. Chapter 46: Hypercalcemia and hypocalcemia. In: Longo DL, Fauci AS, Kasper DL, Hauser SL, Jameson J, Loscalzo J, eds. *Harrison's Principles of Internal Medicine.* 18th ed. New York, NY: McGraw-Hill; 2012.

Kline JA. Chapter 88: Pulmonary embolism and deep venous thrombosis. In: Marx JA, Hockberger RS, Walls RM, et al., eds. *Rosen's Emergency Medicine: Concepts and Clinical Practice.* 8th ed. Philadelphia, PA: Saunders; 2014.

Kman NE, Werman HA. Chapter 76: Disorders presenting primarily with diarrhea. In: Tintinalli JE, Stapczynski JS, Ma O, Cline DM, Cydulka RK, Meckler GD, eds. *Tintinalli's Emergency Medicine: A Comprehensive Study Guide.* 7th ed. New York, NY: McGraw-Hill; 2011.

Kurz MC, Mattu A, Brady WJ. Chapter 78: Acute coronary syndrome. In: Marx JA, Hockberger RS, Walls RM, et al., eds. *Rosen's Emergency Medicine: Concepts and Clinical Practice.* 8th ed. Philadelphia, PA: Saunders; 2014.

Levitzky MG. Chapter 8: Acid-base balance. Table 8-5. In: Levitzky MG, ed. *Pulmonary Physiology.* 8th ed. New York, NY: McGraw-Hill; 2013.

Lin PH, Kougias P, Bechara C, Cagiannos C, Huynh TT, Chen CJ. Chapter 23: Arterial disease. In: Brunicardi F, Andersen DK, Billiar TR, et al., eds. *Schwartz's Principles of Surgery.* 9th ed. New York, NY: McGraw-Hill; 2010.

Loring KE, Tintinalli JE. Chapter 168: Central nervous system and spinal infections. In: Tintinalli JE, Stapczynski J, Ma O, Cline DM, Cydulka RK, Meckler GD, eds. *Tintinalli's Emergency Medicine: A Comprehensive Study Guide.* 7th ed. New York, NY: McGraw-Hill; 2011.

Lung DD, Catlett CL, Tintinalli JE. Chapter 165: Seizures and status epilepticus in adults. In: Tintinalli JE, Stapczynski J, Ma O, Cline DM, Cydulka RK, Meckler GD, eds. *Tintinalli's Emergency Medicine: A Comprehensive Study Guide.* 7th ed. New York, NY: McGraw-Hill; 2011.

Madoff LC. Chapter 334: Infectious arthritis. In: Longo DL, Fauci AS, Kasper DL, Hauser SL, Jameson J, Loscalzo J, eds. *Harrison's Principles of Internal Medicine.* 18th ed. New York, NY: McGraw-Hill; 2012.

Mailhot T, Lyn E. Chapter 50: Hand. In: Marx JA, Hockberger RS, Walls RM, et al., eds. *Rosen's Emergency Medicine: Concepts and Clinical Practice*. 8th ed. Philadelphia, PA: Saunders; 2014.

Maloney G. Chapter 217: Carbon monoxide. In: Tintinalli JE, Stapczynski J, Ma O, Cline DM, Cydulka RK, Meckler GD, eds. *Tintinalli's Emergency Medicine: A Comprehensive Study Guide*. 7th ed. New York, NY: McGraw-Hill; 2011.

Martel ML, Biros MH. Chapter 285: Psychotropic medications and rapid tranquilization. In: Tintinalli JE, Stapczynski J, Ma O, Cline DM, Cydulka RK, Meckler GD, eds. *Tintinalli's Emergency Medicine: A Comprehensive Study Guide*. 7th ed. New York, NY: McGraw-Hill; 2011.

Mayer TA. Chapter 52: Humerus and elbow. In: Marx JA, Hockberger RS, Walls RM, et al., eds. *Rosen's Emergency Medicine: Concepts and Clinical Practice*. 8th ed. Philadelphia, PA: Saunders; 2014.

McMahon PJ, Kaplan LD, Popkin CA. Chapter 3: Sports medicine. In: Skinner HB, McMahon PJ, eds. *Current Diagnosis & Treatment in Orthopedics*. 5th ed. New York, NY: McGraw-Hill; 2014.

McQuaid KR. Chapter 15: Gastrointestinal disorders. In: Papadakis MA, McPhee SJ, Rabow MW, eds. *Current Medical Diagnosis & Treatment 2014*. New York, NY: McGraw-Hill; 2014.

Meckler GD. Chapter 143: Pediatric procedures: electrocardiogram interpretation. In: Tintinalli JE, Stapczynski J, Ma O, Cline DM, Cydulka RK, Meckler GD, eds. *Tintinalli's Emergency Medicine: A Comprehensive Study Guide*. 7th ed. New York, NY: McGraw-Hill; 2011.

Melio FR, Berge LR. Chapter 75: Upper respiratory tract infection. In: Marx JA, Hockberger RS, Walls RM, et al., eds. *Rosen's Emergency Medicine: Concepts and Clinical Practice*. 8th ed. Philadelphia, PA: Saunders; 2014.

Mills KC. Chapter 171: Cyclic antidepressants. In: Tintinalli JE, Stapczynski J, Ma O, Cline DM, Cydulka RK, Meckler GD, eds. *Tintinalli's Emergency Medicine: A Comprehensive Study Guide*. 7th ed. New York, NY: McGraw-Hill; 2011.

Mills KC. Chapter 173: Monoamine oxidase inhibitors. In: Tintinalli JE, Stapczynski JS, Ma O, Cline DM, Cydulka RK, Meckler GD, eds. *Tintinalli's Emergency Medicine: A Comprehensive Study Guide*. 7th ed. New York, NY: McGraw-Hill; 2011.

Miner JR. Chapter 41: Procedural sedation and analgesia. In: Tintinalli JE, Stapczynski J, Ma O, Cline DM, Cydulka RK, Meckler GD, eds. *Tintinalli's Emergency Medicine: A Comprehensive Study Guide*. 7th ed. New York, NY: McGraw-Hill; 2011. (Table 41-9)

Mount DB. Chapter 45: Fluid and electrolyte disturbances. In: Longo DL, Fauci AS, Kasper DL, Hauser SL, Jameson J, Loscalzo J, eds. *Harrison's Principles of Internal Medicine*. 18th ed. New York, NY: McGraw-Hill; 2012.

Nicks BA, Manthey DE. Chapter 96: Male genital problems. In: Tintinalli JE, Stapczynski JS, Ma O, Cline DM, Cydulka RK, Meckler GD, eds. *Tintinalli's Emergency Medicine: A Comprehensive Study Guide*. 6th ed. New York, NY: McGraw-Hill; 2011.

Overton DT. Chapter 78: Upper gastrointestinal bleeding. In: Tintinalli JE, Stapczynski J, Ma O, Cline DM, Cydulka RK, Meckler GD, eds. *Tintinalli's Emergency Medicine: A Comprehensive Study Guide*. 7th ed. New York, NY: McGraw-Hill; 2011.

Pallin DJ, Nassisi D. Chapter 137: Skin and soft tissue infections. In: Marx JA, Hockberger RS, Walls RM, et al., eds. *Rosen's Emergency Medicine: Concepts and Clinical Practice*. 8th ed. Philadelphia, PA: Saunders; 2014.

Patel PM, Patel HH, Roth DM. Chapter 19: General anesthetics and therapeutic gases. In: Brunton LL, Chabner BA, Knollmann BC, eds. *Goodman & Gilman's The Pharmacological Basis of Therapeutics*. 12th ed. New York, NY: McGraw-Hill; 2011.

Perron AD, Huff JS. Chapter 106: Spinal cord disorders. In: Marx JA, Hockberger RS, Walls RM, et al., eds. *Rosen's Emergency Medicine: Concepts and Clinical Practice*. 8th ed. Philadelphia, PA: Saunders; 2014.

Pfennig CL, Slovis CM. Chapter 125: Electrolyte disturbances. In: Marx JA, Hockberger RS, Walls RM, et al., eds. *Rosen's Emergency Medicine: Concepts and Clinical Practice*. 8th ed. Philadelphia, PA: Saunders; 2014.

Prosser JM, Perrone J. Chapter 181: Cocaine, methamphetamine, and other amphetamines. In: Tintinalli JE, Stapczynski JS, Ma O, Cline DM, Cydulka RK, Meckler GD, eds. *Tintinalli's Emergency Medicine: A Comprehensive Study Guide*. 7th ed. New York, NY: McGraw-Hill; 2011.

Quan D. Chapter 177: Benzodiazepines. In: Tintinalli JE, Stapczynski J, Ma O, Cline DM, Cydulka RK, Meckler GD, eds. *Tintinalli's Emergency Medicine: A Comprehensive Study Guide*. 7th ed. New York, NY: McGraw-Hill; 2011.

Ropper AH, Samuels MA, Klein JP. Chapter 9: Figures 9.3 & 9.4. Other somatic sensation. In: Ropper AH, Samuels MA, Klein JP, eds. *Adams & Victor's Principles of Neurology*. 10th ed. New York, NY: McGraw-Hill; 2014.

Scheir AB. Chapter 205: Arthopods bites and stings. In: Tintinalli JE, Stapczynski JS, Ma O, Cline DM, Cydulka RK, Meckler GD, eds. *Tintinalli's Emergency Medicine: A Comprehensive Study Guide*. 7th ed. New York, NY: McGraw-Hill; 2011.

Schneider SM, Cobaugh DJ. Chapter 175: Lithium. In: Tintinalli JE, Stapczynski JS, Ma O, Cline DM, Cydulka RK, Meckler GD, eds. *Tintinalli's Emergency Medicine: A Comprehensive Study Guide*. 7th ed. New York, NY: McGraw-Hill; 2011.

Schwartz LR, Balakrishnam C. Chapter 210: Thermal burns. In: Tintinalli JE, Stapczynski JS, Ma O, Cline DM, Cydulka RK, Meckler GD, eds. *Tintinalli's Emergency Medicine: A Comprehensive Study Guide*. 7th ed. New York, NY: McGraw-Hill; 2011.

Sharma R, Brunette DD. Chapter 71: Ophthalmology. In: Marx JA, Hockberger RS, Walls RM, et al., eds. *Rosen's Emergency Medicine: Concepts and Clinical Practice*. 8th ed. Philadelphia, PA: Saunders; 2014.

Smith JC, Quan D. Chapter 179: Alcohols. In: Tintinalli JE, Stapczynski JS, Ma O, Cline DM, Cydulka RK, Meckler GD, eds. *Tintinalli's Emergency Medicine: A Comprehensive Study Guide*. 7th ed. New York, NY: McGraw-Hill; 2011.

Smith WS, English JD, Johnston S. Chapter 370: Cerebrovascular diseases. In: Longo DL, Fauci AS, Kasper DL, Hauser SL, Jameson J, Loscalzo J, eds. *Harrison's Principles of Internal Medicine*. 18th ed. New York, NY: McGraw-Hill; 2012.

Sokolove PE, Derlet RW. Chapter 135: Tuberculosis. In: Marx JA, Hockberger RS, Walls RM, et al., eds. *Rosen's Emergency Medicine: Concepts and Clinical Practice*. 8th ed. Philadelphia, PA: Saunders; 2014.

Stephan M, Carter C, Ashfaq S. Chapter 50: Pediatric emergencies. In: Stone C, Humphries RL, eds. *Current Diagnosis & Treatment Emergency Medicine*. 7th ed. New York, NY: McGraw-Hill; 2011.

Takhar SS, Moran GJ. Chapter 148: Disseminated viral infections. In: Tintinalli JE, Stapczynski J, Ma O, Cline DM, Cydulka RK, Meckler GD, eds. *Tintinalli's Emergency Medicine: A Comprehensive Study Guide*. 7th ed. New York, NY: McGraw-Hill; 2011.

Takhar SS, O'Laughlin KN. Chapter 132: Viral illnesses. In: Marx JA, Hockberger RS, Walls RM, et al., eds. *Rosen's Emergency Medicine: Concepts and Clinical Practice*. 8th ed. Philadelphia, PA: Saunders; 2014.

Thomas SH, Goodloe JM. Chapter 60: Foreign bodies. In: Marx JA, Hockberger RS, Walls RM, et al., eds. *Rosen's Emergency Medicine: Concepts and Clinical Practice*. 6th ed. Philadelphia, PA: Saunders; 2014.

Thompson CC. Chapter 34: Gastrointestinal foreign bodies. In: Greenberger NJ, Blumberg RS, Burakoff R, eds. *Current Diagnosis & Treatment: Gastroenterology, Hepatology, & Endoscopy*. 2th ed. New York, NY: McGraw-Hill; 2012.

Vicario SJ, Price TG. Chapter 86: Bowel obstruction and volvulus. In: Tintinalli JE, Stapczynski JS, Ma O, Cline DM, Cydulka RK, Meckler GD, eds. *Emergency Medicine: A Comprehensive Study Guide*. 7th ed. New York, NY: McGraw-Hill; 2011.

Vissers RJ, Danzl DF. Chapter 30: Tracheal intubation and mechanical ventilation. In: Tintinalli JE, Stapczynski J, Ma O, Cline DM, Cydulka RK, Meckler GD, eds. *Tintinalli's Emergency Medicine: A Comprehensive Study Guide*. 7th ed. New York, NY: McGraw-Hill; 2011.

Walker MF, Daroff RB. Chapter 21: Dizziness and vertigo. In: Longo DL, Fauci AS, Kasper DL, Hauser SL, Jameson J, Loscalzo J, eds. *Harrison's Principles of Internal Medicine*. 18th ed. New York, NY: McGraw-Hill; 2012.

Walker RA, Adhikari S. Chapter 236: Eye emergencies. In: Tintinalli JE, Stapczynski J, Ma O, Cline DM, Cydulka RK, Meckler GD, eds. *Tintinalli's Emergency Medicine: A Comprehensive Study Guide*. 7th ed. New York, NY: McGraw-Hill; 2011.

Wax PM, Young AC. Chapter 196: Anticholinergics. In: Tintinalli JE, Stapczynski JS, Ma O, Cline DM, Cydulka RK, Meckler GD, eds. *Tintinalli's Emergency Medicine: A Comprehensive Study Guide*. 7th ed. New York, NY: McGraw-Hill; 2011.

Waxman SG. Chapter 5: The spinal cord. In: Waxman SG, eds. *Clinical Neuroanatomy*. 27th ed. New York, NY: McGraw-Hill; 2013. (Figure 5-8)

White SR. Chapter 155: Toxic alcohols. In: Marx JA, Hockberger RS, Walls RM, et al., eds. *Rosen's Emergency Medicine: Concepts and Clinical Practice*. 8th ed. Philadelphia, PA: Saunders; 2014.

Williams DT, Hyung TK. Chapter 51: Wrist and forearm. In: Marx JA, Hockberger RS, Walls RM, et al., eds. *Rosen's Emergency Medicine: Concepts and Clinical Practice*. 8th ed. Philadelphia, PA: Saunders; 2014.

Williams SR, Sztajnkrycer MD, Thurman R. Chapter 17: Toxicological conditions. In: Knoop KJ, Stack LB, Storrow AB, Thurman R, eds. *The Atlas of Emergency Medicine*. 3th ed. New York, NY: McGraw-Hill; 2010.

Yealy DM, Kosowsky JM. Chapter 79: Dysrhythmias. In: Marx JA, Hockberger RS, Walls RM, et al., eds. *Rosen's Emergency Medicine: Concepts and Clinical Practice*. 6th ed. Philadelphia, PA: Saunders; 2014.

Yip L. Chapter 183: Aspirin and salicylates. In: Tintinalli JE, Stapczynski JS, Ma O, Cline DM, Cydulka RK, Meckler GD, eds. *Tintinalli's Emergency Medicine: A Comprehensive Study Guide*. 7th ed. New York, NY: McGraw-Hill; 2011.

Zun LS. Chapter 29: Nausea and vomiting. In: Marx JA, Hockberger RS, Walls RM, et al., eds. *Rosen's Emergency Medicine: Concepts and Clinical Practice*. 8th ed. Philadelphia, PA: Saunders; 2014.

CHAPTER 16

General Surgery

Frank A. Acevedo, PA-C, MS, DFAAPA

DIRECTIONS: Each of the numbered questions or incomplete statements is followed by possible answers or completions of the statement. Select the ONE-lettered answer or completion that is BEST in each case.

1. A paraplegic patient developed a sacral decubitus ulcer secondary to sitting in a wheelchair for prolonged periods of time. Initial treatment included debridement and saline dressing changes. The wound has significant serous drainage without evidence of infection. Which of the following interventions would be recommended to promote rapid closure of the wound?

   (A) Application of platelet-derived growth factor
   (B) Negative pressure wound vacuum device
   (C) Occlusive dressings
   (D) Topical 1% silver nitrate

2. A patient with no known drug allergies is scheduled for a mitral valve replacement. Which of the following pharmacologic agents would be recommended for surgical prophylaxis?

   (A) Cefazolin
   (B) Ciprofloxacin
   (C) Nafcillin
   (D) Vancomycin

3. A 35-year-old man is postoperative day 4 after an exploratory laparotomy for a gunshot wound to the abdomen. At the time of exploration, a perforation to the left colon was found and he underwent repair with proximal colostomy. He now is confused, agitated, and has developed oliguria over the past 8 hours. His vital signs are temperature 104°F, respiratory rate 24/min, heart rate 134/min, blood pressure 85/60 mm Hg. Which of the following types of shock is most likely present?

   (A) Cardiogenic
   (B) Hypovolemic
   (C) Neurogenic
   (D) Septic

4. A 22-year-old man is evaluated in the emergency department after having sustained a single stab wound along the left sternal border at the fourth intercostal space. Upon arrival he is hypotensive and tachycardic. The neck veins are distended and heart sounds are muffled. Which of the following interventions is the most appropriate first-line management?

   (A) Fluid resuscitation
   (B) Immediate intubation
   (C) Left tube thoracostomy
   (D) Pericardiocentesis

5. A 32-year-old lactating female is evaluated for a fluctuant mass of her left breast. The area directly above the lesion is erythematous and tender to touch. You make the diagnosis of a localized breast abscess. Which of the following pathogens is the most likely cause?

   (A) *Escherichia coli*
   (B) *Pseudomonas aeruginosa*
   (C) *Staphylococcus aureus*
   (D) *Viridans streptococcus*

6. A 52-year-old female is evaluated for right upper quadrant pain associated with fever, nausea, and vomiting. Which of the following best describes the underlying pathology associated with her diagnosis?

   (A) Intermittent obstruction of the cystic duct without inflammation
   (B) Obstruction of the common bile duct with inflammation
   (C) Obstruction of the common bile duct without inflammation
   (D) Sustained obstruction of the cystic duct with inflammation

7. A 63-year-old male is evaluated for midepigastric pain, weight loss, and jaundice. On examination, his skin is jaundiced and his sclerae are icteric. On palpation of the abdomen, you find a distended nontender gallbladder. Which of the following is the most likely diagnosis?

   (A) Choledocholithiasis
   (B) Chronic pancreatitis
   (C) Gastric carcinoma
   (D) Pancreatic carcinoma

8. A 48-year-old female presented with the new onset of jaundice and right upper quadrant abdominal pain. Which of the following findings on abdominal ultrasound would be consistent with choledocholithiasis?

   (A) Air in the lumen of the gallbladder
   (B) Dilated hepatic ducts
   (C) Pericholecystic fluid
   (D) Thickened gallbladder wall

9. A 46-year-old male is evaluated for right upper quadrant pain radiating to the right infrascapular area. The pain is colicky and was precipitated by a meal of fried fish and french fries. Which of the following is the diagnostic study of choice?

   (A) Computed tomography (CT)
   (B) Plain abdominal x-ray
   (C) Radionuclide scan (HIDA scan)
   (D) Ultrasonography

10. A 58-year-old male presents with the acute onset of abdominal pain associated with fever and shaking chills. The patient is hypotensive and febrile with a temperature of 102.2°F. He is confused and disoriented and complains of right upper quadrant pain during palpation. His sclerae are icteric. Which of the following is the most likely diagnosis?

    (A) Acute cholecystitis
    (B) Ascending cholangitis
    (C) Acute pancreatitis
    (D) Choledocholithiasis

11. A 54-year-old male with a history of chronic ethanol abuse is evaluated for subjective fever and severe epigastric pain radiating to the back. Pain has been present for the past 8 hours and is associated with nausea and vomiting. Laboratory data reveals a WBC of 14,000/mm^3 and serum amylase of 500 U/L (reference range 0–286 U/L). Plain films of the abdomen were unremarkable. Which of the following is the most likely diagnosis?

    (A) Acute cholecystitis
    (B) Acute pancreatitis
    (C) Mesenteric ischemia
    (D) Perforated duodenal ulcer

12. A 49-year-old male is evaluated for a 3-day history of epigastric pain radiating to the back. He admits to chronic ethanol abuse and upon presentation his serum amylase is 645 U/L (normal range 0–286 U/L) along with a serum lipase of 427 U/L (normal range 10–73 U/L). Which of the following clinical prediction systems can most accurately predict mortality within the first 24 hours of admission?

    (A) Acute physiology and chronic health evaluation II (APACHE II score)
    (B) Atlanta classification
    (C) Bedside index for severity in acute pancreatitis score (BISAP score)
    (D) Ranson criteria

13. A 54-year-old male complains of persistent midepigastric abdominal pain 2 weeks following the diagnosis of acute pancreatitis. The patient also complains of anorexia that was preceded by early satiety. There is a palpable mass in the midepigastrium with normal

bowel sounds in all four quadrants. Which of the following is the most likely diagnosis?

(A) Adynamic ileus

(B) Infected pancreatic necrosis

(C) Pancreatic carcinoma

(D) Pancreatic pseudocyst

14. A 22-year-old obese female is found to have a mass in the upper outer quadrant of her left breast. The lesion is smooth, firm, and freely movable, measuring 3 cm in size. Which of the following is the most likely diagnosis?

(A) Breast cyst

(B) Fibroadenoma

(C) Fibrocystic changes

(D) Lipoma of the breast

15. A 1-year-old girl is brought by her mother for evaluation due to abdominal distention of 1-day duration. She has not had a bowel movement or passed flatus in 72 hours and her mother reports bloody mucoid stools per rectum. Examination reveals markedly diminished bowel sounds with tympany to percussion. There is no history of prior surgery and no hernias are detected on examination. Which of the following is the most likely diagnosis?

(A) Acute appendicitis

(B) Meckel diverticulum

(C) Pyloric stenosis

(D) Regional enteritis

16. Of the following, which are the most common symptoms of Crohn disease?

(A) Abdominal pain, diarrhea, and weight loss

(B) Abdominal pain, rectal bleeding, and fever

(C) Bloody diarrhea, anal fistulas, and fever

(D) Weight loss, fever, and melena

17. A 45-year-old male develops abdominal distention with associated nausea and vomiting 4 days after a small bowel resection. Which of the following findings is consistent with a paralytic ileus?

(A) Crampy abdominal pain

(B) Gas in small intestine only on KUB (kidney, ureter, bladder)

(C) Hyperactive bowel sounds

(D) Obstipation and failure to pass flatus

18. A 56-year-old male is evaluated for abdominal distention associated with protracted nausea and vomiting over the past 4 days. Physical examination reveals abdominal distention with tympany in all four quadrants. Bowel sounds are hyperactive with a metallic quality. Past surgical history (PMH) is positive for an exploratory laparotomy for a ruptured appendix 20 years ago. Which of the following interventions is the most appropriate first-line management?

(A) Correction of fluid and electrolyte abnormalities

(B) Emergency surgery

(C) Obtaining barium radiograph studies

(D) Scheduling a sigmoidoscopy

19. A 64-year-old male has been experiencing intermittent left lower abdominal pain associated with alternating diarrhea and constipation. The pain has been increasing over the past 24 hours and is now associated with a fever. Physical examination reveals rebound tenderness and involuntary guarding. Which of the following is the best diagnostic test for making the diagnosis and detecting the presence of an abscess?

(A) Barium enema

(B) Colonoscopy

(C) Computed tomography (CT)

(D) Sigmoidoscopy

20. Which of the following patients would be recommended for an ELECTIVE surgical repair for treatment of symptoms due to diverticular disease?

(A) Patient with an initial presentation of left lower quadrant pain

(B) Patient who is refractory to medical management of their symptoms

(C) Patient with fever and a 5-cm left lower quadrant abscess

(D) Patient with a rigid abdomen and free air on a KUB

21. Which of the following types of colon polyps should be treated by surgical excision because of a high risk of malignant degeneration?

    (A) Hamartoma
    (B) Hyperplastic
    (C) Inflammatory
    (D) Villous adenoma

22. Which of the following guidelines for screening colonoscopy would be recommended for a 40-year-old female whose father was diagnosed with colon cancer at the age 58?

    (A) She should undergo an air-contrast barium enema at 50 years of age and repeat every 10 years
    (B) She should have a flexible sigmoidoscopy and air-contrast barium enema every 10 years starting at age 50
    (C) She should have a flexible sigmoidoscopy every 1 to 2 years starting at age 30
    (D) She should undergo a screening colonoscopy every 5 years starting at age 48

23. An 82-year-old female is evaluated for right lower quadrant pain, an unintentional 7.5-kg weight loss over the past month, and fatigue. Examination reveals conjunctival pallor, and a palpable 6- × 7-cm mass in the right lower quadrant. Which of the following is the most likely diagnosis?

    (A) Acute appendicitis
    (B) Cecal carcinoma
    (C) Incarcerated hernia
    (D) Sigmoid volvulus

24. A 57-year-old female underwent a left hemicolectomy for adenocarcinoma of the colon. Which of the following recommendations is part of annual postoperative monitoring for a potential recurrence?

    (A) CA 19-9 testing
    (B) Chest radiograph
    (C) Colonoscopy
    (D) Fecal occult blood testing

25. Which of the following pathologic findings is most frequently associated with ulcerative colitis?

    (A) Terminal ileum involvement
    (B) Granulomas
    (C) Rectal involvement
    (D) Transmural inflammation

26. A 55-year-old male has a history of ulcerative colitis for the past 22 years, and colonoscopy has now revealed a low-grade dysplasia in the left colon. Which of the following surgical interventions would be most appropriate at this time?

    (A) Diverting ileostomy
    (B) Left colon resection
    (C) Total colectomy with permanent ileostomy
    (D) Total proctocolectomy ileoanal pull-through

27. A 63-year-old male is evaluated for intestinal obstruction. Plain radiographs of the abdomen reveal dilated loops of large bowel highly suspicious for volvulus. What is the next best imaging study in this patient?

    (A) Computed tomography
    (B) Contrast enema
    (C) Magnetic resonance imaging (MRI)
    (D) Ultrasound

28. A 54-year-old male presents for evaluation due to crampy abdominal pain, nausea, and vomiting. The patient has not passed gas or had a bowel movement for the past 3 days. On examination, the abdomen is distended and there are high-pitched bowel sounds with peristaltic rushes. A plain radiograph of the abdomen reveals cecal distention to 12 cm. What is the most appropriate definitive management?

    (A) Intravenous fluids
    (B) Nasogastric suction
    (C) Observation
    (D) Surgical exploration

29. An 80-year-old male nursing home patient is brought to the emergency department with abdominal distention. A plain film of the abdomen is shown in Figure 16-1. Which of the following is the most likely diagnosis?

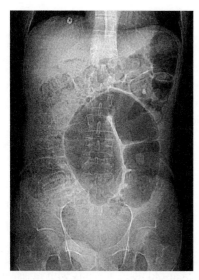

Figure 16-1. (Reproduced, with permission, from Fauci AS, Braunwald E, Kasper DL, et al. Harrison's Principles of Internal Medicine, 17th ed. New York: McGraw-Hill, 2008:1842.)

(A) Cecal volvulus

(B) Sigmoid volvulus

(C) Small bowel obstruction

(D) Toxic megacolon

30. A 34-year-old female presents for evaluation due to bleeding per rectum during bowel movements. Examination reveals a large internal hemorrhoid that required manual manipulation for reduction. Which of the following classifications best describes this type of hemorrhoid?

(A) First degree

(B) Second degree

(C) Third degree

(D) Fourth degree

31. A 10-year-old boy with rectal pain presents with his mother for evaluation of pain during bowel movements. He has noticed bright red blood on the toilet paper after wiping himself. Which of the following is the most likely diagnosis?

(A) Anal fissure

(B) Fistula in ano

(C) Perianal abscess

(D) Pilonidal cyst

32. During a routine lung radiograph a 45-year-old non-smoking female is found to have a 2-cm mass in the periphery of the left. She has no significant medical history, known exposures, or contributory family history. A subsequent biopsy confirms malignancy. Which of the cancers does the lesion represent?

(A) Adenocarcinoma

(B) Bronchoalveolar

(C) Large cell

(D) Squamous cell

33. Which of the following is considered first-line surgical treatment for achalasia?

(A) Esophagectomy

(B) Gastrojejunostomy

(C) Myotomy and partial fundoplication

(D) Vagotomy with pyloroplasty

34. A 49-year-old male is evaluated for pain and swelling of his right lower extremity. Examination is significant for a warm, palpable cord along the posterior aspect of the right calf. Doppler examination reveals superficial venous thrombophlebitis of the greater saphenous vein with extension to the tributaries of the greater saphenous vein in the distal thigh. Which of the following is the most appropriate next step in management?

(A) Antibiotics

(B) Heparin

(C) Nonsteroidal anti-inflammatory drugs

(D) Warfarin

35. A 54-year-old female is evaluated for difficulty breathing after extubation immediately after undergoing parathyroidectomy. Which of the following is the most likely cause?

(A) Cervical hematoma

(B) Hypocalcemia

(C) Recurrent laryngeal nerve injury

(D) Wound infection

36. A 28-year-old female presents for evaluation of a left thyroid lobe nodule. A fine needle aspiration is performed, after ultrasound revealed a 3-cm solid hypoechoic lesion, and the report comes back positive for a follicular neoplasm. A thyroid scan is performed and it reveals the mass to be a "cold" nodule and molecular testing is unavailable. The best management for this patient would be:

(A) Diagnostic lobectomy

(B) Observation

(C) Radioiodine ablation

(D) Total thyroidectomy

37. Which of the following thyroid carcinomas is associated with multiple endocrine neoplasia type 2 (MEN2) syndrome?

(A) Anaplastic

(B) Follicular

(C) Medullary

(D) Papillary

38. A 58-year-old male presented with a history of episodic fluctuations in his blood pressure associated with anxiety, palpitations, and flushing. Urinary tests were positive for elevated metanephrine levels. Which of the following interventions is the first step in preparing the patient for surgical intervention?

(A) α-Blockers to control the blood pressure

(B) β-Blockers to control the heart rate

(C) Cortisol replacement for adrenal insufficiency

(D) Nitrates for vasodilation

39. A 58-year-old male is in the hospital postoperative day 3 after a laparoscopic right colon resection. Your morning labs reveal a serum potassium level of 2.9 mEq/L (normal 3.5–5.0 mEq/L) despite aggressive potassium replacement during the previous shift. At this time you should check which of the following laboratory values?

(A) Calcium

(B) Magnesium

(C) Phosphorous

(D) Sodium

40. A patient with peritonitis secondary to a ruptured appendix was admitted to the intensive care unit with hypotension and tachycardia. Which of the following crystalloid solutions would be recommended for fluid resuscitation?

(A) 5% dextrose water

(B) 5% dextrose water with 0.45% sodium chloride

(C) 0.45% sodium chloride

(D) 0.9% sodium chloride

41. Which of the following treatment options is recommended for a patient with a grade I splenic laceration on CT scan who is otherwise hemodynamically stable?

(A) Exploratory laparotomy and partial splenectomy

(B) Exploratory laparotomy and splenectomy

(C) Exploratory laparotomy and splenorrhaphy

(D) Nonoperative management with splenic preservation

42. A 39-year-old male presents with massive hematemesis. His physical examination reveals slight jaundice, palmar erythema, spider angiomas, and marked ascites. Vitals at the time of presentation are as follows: BP: 85/44 mm Hg, P: 122/min, R: 16/min, oxygen saturation: 96%, and T: 99.8°F. Which of the following is the most likely cause of the hematemesis?

(A) Achalasia

(B) Esophageal varices

(C) Esophageal web

(D) Gastroesophageal reflux disease (GERD)

43. Which of the following interventions is utilized in the treatment of a patient with portal hypertension and associated variceal bleeding?

(A) Distal splenorenal shunt

(B) End-to-side portocaval shunt

(C) Side-to-side portocaval shunt

(D) Transjugular intrahepatic portosystemic shunt

44. Which of the following is the most common indication for a splenectomy?

(A) Hereditary spherocytosis

(B) Myeloproliferative disorders

(C) Sickle cell disease

(D) Traumatic injury

45. What is the most common site of an acute arterial occlusion due to embolic disease?

(A) Aortic bifurcation

(B) Femoral artery

(C) Iliac artery

(D) Mesenteric arteries

46. A 59-year-old female presents with an acute upper gastrointestinal hemorrhage. Her medical history is pertinent for peptic ulcer disease for the past 5 years and hypertension. A nasogastric tube is inserted and bright red blood is seen. Her vital signs are BP: 110/70 mm Hg, P: 94/min, R: 14/min, oxygen saturation: 97%, T: 99°F. Which of the following diagnostic studies would be the most appropriate next step to determine the site of bleeding?

(A) Abdominal ultrasound

(B) Bleeding scan

(C) Endoscopy

(D) Upper barium contrast study

47. A 21-year-old male presents for evaluation of a low-grade fever, anorexia, and right lower abdominal pain that began approximately 24 hours ago. Which of the following etiologies is the most common cause of the patient's symptoms?

(A) Cecal volvulus

(B) Fecalith

(C) Intussusception

(D) Lymphoid hyperplasia

48. Which of the following is the appropriate age for closing an asymptomatic umbilical hernia in a child that is >1.5 cm in size?

(A) 2 years

(B) 5 years

(C) 7 years

(D) 12 months

49. A 45-year-old male presents with progressive painless dysphagia and regurgitation of undigested food. The patient has tried drinking large amounts of fluids with meals in an attempt to wash down his food. What is the most likely diagnosis?

(A) Achalasia

(B) Esophageal carcinoma

(C) Esophageal leiomyoma

(D) Reflux esophagitis

50. A 64-year-old male has been experiencing signs and symptoms compatible with diverticular disease for the past 3 weeks. He now presents malnourished with severe left lower quadrant abdominal pain. Upright chest radiograph reveals free air under the diaphragm. He is resuscitated, given intravenous antibiotics and taken to the operating room where a perforated sigmoid colon is discovered with gross peritoneal contamination. What is the most appropriate surgical intervention at this time?

(A) Abdominoperineal resection

(B) Hartmann procedure

(C) Left colectomy with primary anastomosis

(D) Proctocolectomy

51. A patient has severe pancreatitis. Vitals are: BP 70/50 mm Hg, HR 132/min, RR 24/min, temp 103°F, sat 94%. Laboratory values reveal a WBC count of 28,000 and a serum lactate level of 17.3 mmol/L (normal: 0.5–2.2 mmol/L). What is the most likely diagnosis?

(A) Cardiac tamponade

(B) Congestive heart failure

(C) Septic shock

(D) Pulmonary embolus

52. A 76-year-old patient who has gram-negative pneumonia becomes hypotensive, and resuscitative measures are started. After 4 L of normal saline administration, the following parameters are obtained: BP: 60/0 mm Hg; P: 140/min; central venous pressure: 14 mm Hg (normal 2–6 mm Hg); arterial blood gases: pH 7.33; PO_2 100 mm Hg; PCO_2 35 mm Hg. A decision is made to commence treatment with an adrenergic agent. An intravenous infusion of which of the following drugs should be started?

(A) Dopamine

(B) Norepinephrine

(C) Phenylephrine

(D) Vasopressin

53. A 24-year-old male is brought in for evaluation after a fall from a ladder. His breathing is labored and he is cyanotic. No breath sounds can be heard in the right lung field, which is resonant to percussion. The first step in his management should be:

(A) Cricothyroidotomy

(B) Stat chest radiograph

(C) Tube thoracostomy

(D) CT scan of the thorax

54. A 22-year-old male is brought to the ED after having been involved in a head-on motor vehicle accident as an unrestrained passenger. A chest radiograph performed in the ED reveals multiple segmental rib fractures of ribs 3 to 7 on the left side. His respiratory rate is 26/min (labored) with discordant motion on the left side. The most likely diagnosis is:

(A) Cardiac tamponade

(B) Flail chest

(C) Pulmonary contusion

(D) Tension pneumothorax

55. A 45-year-old male patient is brought to the ED after having been involved in a head-on collision with another vehicle. As part of your initial resuscitation efforts you administer 2,000 mL of normal saline that brings the patient's blood pressure from 80/60 to 105/60 mm Hg. However, this increase in blood pressure is short lived and the patient again becomes hypotensive. The most likely cause of this recurring hypotension is:

(A) Abdominal aorta injury

(B) Hepatic laceration

(C) Renal laceration

(D) Transection of pancreas

56. You are called to evaluate a 65-year-old male who had earlier that day undergone an exploratory laparotomy for resection of a gastric ulcer. When you get to the floor the patient's vital signs are: BP: 125/78, R: 24/min, P: 106/min, T: 101°F. Examination reveals some bronchial breath sounds at the left lung base. The rest of the examination is essentially normal. The MOST likely diagnosis is:

(A) Atelectasis

(B) Pneumonia

(C) Pneumothorax

(D) Pulmonary embolism

57. A 45-year-old male is diagnosed with myasthenia gravis. He complains of some dysphagia and has a CT scan of the chest performed which reveals a large mediastinal mass in the anterior portion of the anterior/superior mediastinum. This mass most likely represents a/an:

(A) Esophageal tumor

(B) Neuroblastoma

(C) Thoracic aneurysm

(D) Thymoma

58. A 65-year-old female develops tall, peaked T waves on her monitor that are confirmed by an electrocardiogram. The most important initial intervention would be:

(A) Calcium gluconate

(B) Bicarbonate

(C) D50 and insulin

(D) Kayexalate

59. A 29-year-obese male presents to the clinic with a complaint of painful swelling at the base of his spine. Examination reveals a large fluctuant mass that is erythematous and extremely painful to the touch. The most likely diagnosis is:

(A) Anal fissure

(B) Anorectal carcinoma

(C) Colorectal polyp

(D) Pilonidal cyst

60. A 42-year-old female presents for evaluation of abdominal pain and distention present for the past 5 days. She has not passed flatus or had a bowel movement in 3 days. Rectal examination reveals an empty rectal vault. There is no obvious hernia and the patient has not had previous surgery. Of note on physical examination, she is found to have some decreased sensation on the medial aspect of her right thigh. The most likely cause of her symptoms is:

(A) Adhesions

(B) Femoral hernia

(C) Incisional hernia

(D) Obturator foramen hernia

61. A 58-year-old male with a 45-year pack history of smoking presents to the office with hoarseness for the past 3 weeks. A radiograph taken in the office reveals a central bulky mediastinal mass with lymph nodes. The most likely diagnosis is:

    (A) Hamartoma
    (B) Mesothelioma
    (C) Small cell carcinoma
    (D) Solitary pulmonary nodule

62. The most common symptom of a primary lung tumor is:

    (A) Cough
    (B) Dyspnea
    (C) Hemoptysis
    (D) Weight loss

63. The best way to determine a solitary pulmonary nodule requires surgical intervention is by:

    (A) Fine needle aspiration
    (B) Comparison with previous imaging
    (C) Positron emission tomography (PET)
    (D) Magnetic resonance imaging (MRI)

64. A 57-year-old male with an 80 pack-year history presents to the clinic with a complaint of cough, hemoptysis, and weakness in his left hand. Physical examination reveals atrophy of the intrinsic muscles of the hand as well as meiosis, ptosis, and anhidrosis of the left eye and face. The most likely diagnosis is:

    (A) Pancoast tumor
    (B) Paraneoplastic syndrome
    (C) Superior vena cava syndrome
    (D) Tumor lysis syndrome

65. A 19-year-old female presents with significant RLQ pain and tenderness. Physical examination reveals positive McBurney's and iliopsoas signs. In order to make the diagnosis in this patient you should depend upon:

    (A) Abdominal ultrasound
    (B) CT scan of the abdomen and pelvis

    (C) Flat plate of the abdomen
    (D) Physical examination

66. A 67-year-old male has a syncopal episode at home and is brought in for evaluation. Physical examination reveals a palpable pulsatile abdominal mass. He is taken to the operating room where a tube graft AAA repair is performed. His blood loss is 1,110 mL and he is not hypotensive during the case. In the recovery room, while you are evaluating him, he has a large bowel movement that is nonbloody and his vital signs remain stable. The most important component of his management would be:

    (A) Abdominal radiography
    (B) Intravenous bicarbonate
    (C) Sigmoidoscopy
    (D) Transfusion

67. The most common type of inguinal hernia in females is:

    (A) Direct inguinal hernia
    (B) Femoral hernia
    (C) Indirect inguinal hernia
    (D) Spigelian hernia

68. Small bowel obstruction in a 6-year-old boy with no history of prior surgery is most likely due to:

    (A) Adhesions
    (B) Colon cancer
    (C) Incarcerated hernia
    (D) Meckel diverticulum

69. A 65-year-old female with a known duodenal ulcer is being treated with diet and H_2-blocker therapy. She is admitted with massive upper gastrointestinal hemorrhage. After blood replacement is begun, the next step in her management should be:

    (A) Beginning bismuth, tetracycline, and metronidazole
    (B) Beginning omeprazole
    (C) Beginning sucralfate
    (D) Endoscopy and coagulation of the bleeding vessel

70. The first-choice diagnostic study for suspected deep venous thrombosis of the lower extremity is:

(A) Helical CT scan

(B) Isotope injection with gamma scintillation scanning

(C) Radioactive-labeled fibrinogen uptake

(D) Real-time Doppler imaging

71. A 33-year-old female develops a pulmonary embolism while appropriately anticoagulated on unfractionated heparin. The next MOST appropriate step would be:

(A) Discontinue heparin and switch to warfarin

(B) Increase the rate of delivery of unfractionated heparin

(C) Insert an inferior vena cava (Greenfield) filter

(D) Keep unfractionated heparin at present dose and do nothing else

72. A 43-year-old female had an abdominal exploration 5 years ago for a gunshot wound. She now is evaluated and found to have marked abdominal distention and hypoactive bowel sounds. An abdominal flat plate reveals air within the intrahepatic radicals with a radiolucency in the right lower quadrant. The MOST likely etiology of these findings is:

(A) Adhesions

(B) Colon cancer

(C) Gallstone

(D) Hernia

73. A 65-year-old male with hypertension, hyperlipidemia, and gastroesophageal reflux disease (GERD) presents to the office complaining of worsening nocturia and postvoid dribbling. Physical examination reveals an enlarged nontender prostate. You make the decision to start him on tamsulosin (Flomax) for his symptomatic benign prostatic hyperplasia. Which of the following medications may result in an adverse reaction in this patient?

(A) Coreg (Carvedilol)

(B) Lipitor (Atorvastatin)

(C) Miglitol (Glyset)

(D) Prilosec (Omeprazole)

74. A 54-year-old male is seen on the fifth postoperative day because of increased serous drainage from his midline incision. Examination reveals intact wound edges without erythema. The lower pole of the wound as well as the midportion is leaking copious amounts of serous fluid. The most likely diagnosis is:

(A) Wound dehiscence

(B) Wound evisceration

(C) Wound hematoma

(D) Wound seroma

75. A 32-year-old female presents to the ED with a history of a single gunshot wound to the left hemithorax. Physical examination reveals a pericardial crunching sound that is not affected by breath holding. The most likely diagnosis is:

(A) Esophageal perforation

(B) Pericarditis

(C) Pneumothorax

(D) Tension pneumothorax

76. A 64-year-old male presents to the ED with dyspnea and tachypnea. A chest radiograph reveals a large left-sided pleural effusion. Thoracocentesis yields a fluid that has a pH <7.2, high proteins, and RBC count $>100,000$ mm^3. The most likely cause of this finding is:

(A) Cirrhosis

(B) Congestive heart failure

(C) Malignancy

(D) Myxedema

77. A 23-year-old female is evaluated for a complaint of difficulty swallowing, fatigue, and night fevers. Computerized tomography (CT) of the neck and chest reveals a 3- × 4-cm mass in the superior mediastinum. The most likely diagnosis is:

(A) Neuroblastoma

(B) Lymphoma

(C) Pericardial cyst

(D) Thymoma

78. A 49-year-old male presents to the ED with jaundice and right upper quadrant pain. An ultrasound reveals a dilated common bile duct with an impacted stone at the ampulla of Vater. The best diagnostic test to order would be:

(A) Biliary scintigraphy

(B) Computed tomography

(C) Endoscopic retrograde cholangiopancreatography

(D) Intravenous cholangiography (IVC)

79. A 77-year-old female has been in the SICU for 15 days where she has been treated for complications associated with a perforated left colon carcinoma. She is now noted to be confused and combative. Vital signs are: BP: 100/60 mm Hg, P: 120/min, R: 32/min, T: 103°F. Her most recent labs reveal a WBC of 23,000 and an ABG of pH: 7.22, PCO_2: 52, PO_2: 78, O_2 sat: 88%, HCO_3: 19 (100% oxygen). The above findings are MOST compatible with:

(A) Acute respiratory distress syndrome (ARDS)

(B) Acute myocardial infarction

(C) Bacteremia

(D) Pancreatitis

80. A 4-year-old boy is brought in by his mother due to increasing irritability and a complaint of abdominal pain. Examination reveals a markedly distended abdomen with hyperactive bowel sounds and an empty rectal vault. Palpation of the lower abdomen detects a "sausage"-shaped lesion. The MOST likely etiology of these findings is:

(A) Adhesions

(B) Intussusception

(C) Meckel diverticulum

(D) Pyloric stenosis

81. A 66-year-old female is evaluated for a complaint of abdominal pain and distention for the past 3 days. Examination reveals a protuberant abdomen with diminished bowel sounds and tympany to percussion. Flat and upright abdominal radiographs reveal distended loops of bowel with prominent haustral markings. The most likely etiology of these findings is:

(A) Colon cancer

(B) Hernia

(C) Small bowel obstruction

(D) Appendicitis

82. A 54-year-old male is admitted to the SICU for the management of gram-negative septicemia. As part of his admission a central venous catheter is inserted in the right subclavian vein. While awaiting a post-procedure chest radiograph the patient becomes acutely dyspneic with decreased breath sounds on the right side and a left sided tracheal shift. The MOST likely diagnosis is:

(A) Air embolism

(B) Cardiac arrhythmia

(C) Pneumothorax

(D) Pulmonary artery rupture

83. A 23-year-old male presents to the ED with a single stab wound to the left chest, fourth ICS, midclavicular line. While being assessed he drops his blood pressure and sustains a cardiac arrest. What is the most appropriate next step in the management of this patient?

(A) Perform immediate open thoracotomy

(B) Perform pericardiocentesis

(C) Perform tube thoracostomy

(D) Take to operating room emergently for thoracotomy

84. A 78-year-old male with a history of coronary artery disease and an asymptomatic reducible inguinal hernia requests an elective hernia repair. Which of the following is a valid reason for delaying the proposed surgery?

(A) CABG within 3 months of surgery

(B) History of cigarette smoking

(C) Hyperlipidemia

(D) Jugular venous distention

85. A patient develops a large milky pleural effusion after an attempt at a left subclavian line. This effusion most likely represents?

(A) Chylothorax secondary to injury of the thoracic duct

(B) Enteral tube feeds

(C) Hemothorax

(D) Hypercholesterolemia

Answers and Explanations

1. **(B)** A negative pressure wound vacuum device or wound VAC (vacuum-assisted closure system, Kinetic Concepts, Inc., San Antonio, TX) is a porous sponge that is packed into the wound cavity and then connected to negative pressure. The negative pressure stimulates rapid wound healing by removing exudates and promoting angiogenesis, new tissue growth, and contraction of the wound. In addition the use of a VAC helps to control odors coming from wounds. *(Ferri, 2013, Pressure Ulcers: p. 889)*

2. **(A)** Cefazolin is used as prophylaxis for the majority of clean surgical procedures especially those that involve the head and neck, gastroduodenal, biliary tract, gynecologic, and clean procedures. For cases in which there is an increased likelihood of encountering gram-negative organisms or anaerobic bacteria, a second-generation cephalosporin is recommended to provide broader coverage. Vancomycin is an alternative if the patient has an allergy to cephalosporins/penicillin or where high rates of methicillin-resistant organisms are known to occur. *(Lampris & Maddix, 2012, Ch. 51)*

3. **(D)** The clinical scenario reveals contamination of the abdomen at the time of injury with a potential source of gram-negative bacteria. Causes of septic shock may include traumatic injuries, infections, and systemic inflammatory response syndrome. Vasoactive mediators that are released cause a decrease in vascular tone, which leads to a relative hypovolemia resulting in hypotension and decreased cardiac output. Therapy will require empiric antibiotic use guided by knowledge of the source of infection and most likely pathogens. Although hypovolemic or hemorrhagic shock is the most commonly encountered clinical cause of shock in the surgical/trauma patient, the timelines and clinical presentation rule it out. Cardiogenic shock represents pump failure and is inconsistent with the clinical presentation. Neurogenic shock is usually found in association with spinal cord injuries at the cervical or high thoracic region. *(Chen et al., 2014, Chs. 5 and 12)*

4. **(D)** Cardiac tamponade is classically described by the triad of jugular venous distention (JVD), arterial hypotension, and muffled heart sounds. In the emergency department, suspicion of this clinical entity is usually confirmed by echocardiography. Echocardiography is the most sensitive and specific diagnostic test to be ordered when this entity is suspected. Pericardiocentesis, under ultrasound guidance, can be performed emergently to buy time until a definitive procedure can be performed. Clinical findings include tachycardia, hypotension, pulsus paradoxus, and Kussmaul's sign. *(Shabetai, 2010, Ch. 30, pp. 383–384)*

5. **(C)** A breast abscess is commonly seen in conjunction with lactation. When a breast abscess develops in the nonlactating breast inflammatory breast carcinoma must be considered in the differential. When a breast abscess develops the most common organism found is *Staphylococcus aureus*. Though incision and drainage, along with antibiotics, is typically sufficient, some patients may require removal of the involved ducts to prevent recurrence. *(Giuliano & Hurvitz, 2015, Ch. 17)*

6. **(D)** The case described is consistent with acute cholecystitis resulting from obstruction of the cystic duct. Typically symptoms include right upper quadrant (RUQ) pain, fever, and leukocytosis. Biliary colic is characterized by intermittent obstruction

without inflammation resulting in intermittent episodes of RUQ pain without fever or elevation in the white blood cell count. Choledocholithiasis is characterized by jaundice secondary to obstruction of the common bile duct; in ascending cholangitis, the common bile duct obstruction is complicated by infection resulting in RUQ pain, jaundice, and fever (Charcot's triad). In severe cases patients may also develop shock with mental status changes in addition to Charcot's triad, the latter is known as Reynold's pentad. *(Pham & Hunter, 2014, Ch. 32)*

7. **(D)** Pancreatic carcinoma involving the head of the pancreas presents with weight loss, jaundice, and midepigastric pain. Jaundice is less frequently encountered when the pancreatic tumor involves the body of the pancreas. A palpable, nontender gallbladder (Courvoisier sign) is more often associated with a pancreatic malignancy than cholelithiasis. *(Goldin et al., 2013, p. 358)*

8. **(B)** The abdominal ultrasound will show dilated intrahepatic and extrahepatic ducts secondary to obstruction of the common bile duct in choledocholithiasis. Ultrasound findings of a thickened gallbladder wall and pericholecystic fluid are seen with acute cholecystitis. Air in the lumen of the gallbladder is seen in acute emphysematous cholecystitis. *(Pham & Hunter, 2014, Ch. 32)*

9. **(D)** Ultrasonography is the first-line study in the evaluation of patients presenting with signs and symptoms of biliary disease. The sensitivity and specificity is 95%. It can detect stones, dilation of biliary ducts, thickening of the gallbladder, and pericolic collections of fluid and can also provide information pertaining to associated liver or pancreatic pathology. *(Elsey & Schmidt, 2014, p. 388)*

10. **(D)** The presenting symptoms associated with ascending cholangitis include fever, chills, right upper quadrant pain, and jaundice (Charcot's triad); the symptoms are secondary to an infected obstruction of the common bile duct. With spread of the infection, the patient may also develop hypotension and mental status changes; these additional symptoms in conjunction with Charcot's triad are known as Reynolds' pentad. Additional symptoms of common bile duct obstruction include light-colored stools and dark, tea-colored urine. *(Sharma, Whang, & Gold, 2014, pp. 396–397)*

11. **(B)** Acute pancreatitis typically presents with severe, steady midepigastric abdominal pain that radiates through the back; pain is associated with fever, nausea, and vomiting. The most common causes of acute pancreatitis are gallstones and alcohol. Laboratory studies will show elevated WBC and serum amylase levels. Amylase elevations are nonspecific and can be elevated with perforated ulcers and mesenteric ischemia. A perforated ulcer will show evidence of free air on plain film; mesenteric ischemia will not present with fever or an elevated WBC unless there is the presence of infarcted bowel at which point the patient would appear septic. Acute cholecystitis may be associated with elevations in amylase but they are typically only a modest increase. *(Valsangkar & Thayer, 2014, p. 431)*

12. **(C)** The bedside index for severity in acute pancreatitis score (BISAP) allows for prediction of mortality within the first 24 hours. It utilizes patient age, elevations in blood urea nitrogen (BUN), pleural effusions as detected on imaging, presence of the systemic inflammatory response (SIRS), and alteration in mental status. Scores >3 are associated with higher mortality, development of multiorgan dysfunction syndrome, and pancreatic necrosis. Ranson's criteria were developed to grade the severity of pancreatitis by utilizing laboratory and clinical findings. These are measured when the patient is admitted and within the next 48 hours. In addition to the original five criteria, an additional six variables are employed. Upon admission, the patient's age, WBC, glucose, LDH, and aspartate aminotransferase (AST) are evaluated. Within the next 48 hours, the HCT, BUN, calcium, PO_2 on room air, base deficit, and estimated fluid sequestration are measured. When less than two Ranson's signs are present, mortality is virtually zero; however, it increases to more than 50% when seven or more are present. While Ranson's criteria are the most commonly used predictive criteria for the severity of acute pancreatitis, final predictions cannot be assessed until 48 hours following admission. The acute physiology and chronic health evaluation II (APACHE II) is another classification of severity of disease, which can be assessed at any time. This system evaluates variables in temperature, mean

arterial pressure, heart rate, respiratory rate, oxygenation, arterial pH, serum sodium, serum potassium, serum creatinine, hematocrit, WBC, and Glasgow Coma Scale (neurologic evaluation). The Atlanta classification is used to establish an initial diagnosis of acute pancreatitis and employs amylase or lipase elevations, abdominal pain characteristic of acute pancreatitis, and computerized tomography or other imaging demonstrating findings compatible with acute pancreatitis. (*Valsangkar & Thayer, 2014, pp. 431–434*)

13. **(D)** Pancreatic pseudocysts are the most common complication associated with acute pancreatitis. A pseudocyst should be suspected for a patient who has continued abdominal pain, the development of an abdominal mass, and continued elevations of amylase or lipase levels following an episode of acute pancreatitis. An adynamic ileus would be associated with abdominal distention and changes in bowel sounds; an infected area of necrosis within the pancreatic gland would be associated with fever. Pancreatic cancer may be seen in conjunction with chronic pancreatitis. Laparoscopic drainage is a minimally invasive approach that is considered the standard of care. (*Ilbawi & Horvath, 2014, pp. 1414–1415*)

14. **(B)** Fibroadenomas are among the most common benign lesions found in young female patients. They occur usually from the late teens into the early 30s, although they have been found to a lesser degree in all age groups. This lesion is firm, ovoid, freely movable, and varies in size. In most instances when the lesion is less than 3 cm, and the patient is <21 years of age, imaging alone can be used to establish the diagnosis. Any fibroadenoma >4 cm requires core needle biopsy to establish a diagnosis and may be removed at the request of the patient. Those lesions >5 cm are usually excised, as the majority are symptomatic (pain/breast discomfort). (*Dixon & Macaskill, 2015, pp. 52–53*)

15. **(B)** Meckel diverticulum is prevalent in 2% of the population, has a 2:1 male:female predominance, and is usually located 2 ft from the ileocecal valve. The most common clinical presentations are bleeding, intestinal obstruction, and inflammation. Bright red or maroon bleeding is the most frequent complication in children younger than 2 years of age. (*Ferri, 2013, p. 662*)

16. **(A)** Most Crohn disease patients have the triad of abdominal pain, diarrhea, and weight loss. Intermittent or constant abdominal pain is the most common presenting symptom. Perianal involvement with fistulas is common with Crohn disease, but bleeding is uncommon. Bloody diarrhea is more commonly associated with ulcerative colitis. Rectal bleeding is commonly associated with colorectal carcinoma and hemorrhoidal disease. As Crohn disease can affect any part of the alimentary canal from the mouth to anus, surgical intervention is reserved for complications of the disease. (*Mellinger et al., 2013, pp. 277–278*)

17. **(D)** Obstipation and failure to pass flatus are actually symptoms of both paralytic ileus and small bowel obstruction (SBO). Patients with a paralytic ileus usually have minimal abdominal pain and hypoactive or absent bowel sounds due to hypomotility while those with an SBO will have crampy abdominal pain and increased high-pitched bowel sounds due to increased peristalsis. Plain abdominal radiographs in paralytic ileus will show gas throughout the small and large bowel as opposed to air confined to the small intestine only in SBO. (*Mellinger et al., 2013, pp. 277–278*)

18. **(A)** The first priority in proven or suspected small bowel obstruction is the correction of fluid and electrolyte abnormalities. Often, large volumes of fluid must be infused. The patient must be given sufficient fluid not only for maintenance requirements but also to correct losses from vomiting and nasogastric output and third-space loss. Urine output should be closely monitored for the adequacy of hydration. If the patient has a partial small bowel obstruction, no detectable hernia on examination and a history of operation, resolution may occur with fluid replacement and nasogastric tube placement, making an operation unnecessary. If the patient has no apparent etiology for obstruction, a cause should be determined by upper gastrointestinal and small bowel radiograph series. Laboratory data cannot confirm the diagnosis of bowel obstruction but are useful to rule out other diagnoses. A patient with a complete small bowel obstruction should undergo operation at the earliest opportunity, once the fluid and electrolyte repair is sufficient to establish adequate urine output. (*Mellinger et al., 2013, p. 282*)

19. (C) For a patient with diverticular disease, the preferred study to make the diagnosis and detect an associated abscess is a CT scan. A barium enema or endoscopic procedure is contraindicated due to increased risk of perforation during an acute exacerbation. *(Dayton et al., 2013, p. 307)*

20. (B) Most patients with diverticular disease respond to medical therapy with antibiotics. Patients who have required admission for two episodes of diverticulitis are recommended to undergo elective surgical resection to avoid complications. Patients with complications such as obstruction, perforation, or abscess require emergent surgery. Patients with bleeding require surgical intervention only if the bleeding does not stop spontaneously or with medical interventions. *(Dayton et al., 2013, p. 308)*

21. (D) Villous adenomas may contain cancer in 33% of cases, and when greater than 3 cm in size, this risk goes up to 50%. *(Dayton et al., 2013, p. 314)*

22. (D) A patient with a first-degree relative who is diagnosed with colorectal cancer or adenomatous polyps before the age of 60 years puts the patient at an increased risk for colorectal carcinoma. Accordingly, she should undergo a screening colonoscopy at age 40 or 10 years younger than the age her family member was first diagnosed with colorectal cancer. Colonoscopy should be repeated every 5 years for patients in the moderate-risk category. *(Colorectal Cancer Prevention & Early Detection, American Cancer Society, 2015)*

23. (B) Right-sided colon lesions can grow to large sizes due to the liquid characteristic of stool in this region. Large exophytic lesions can result in occult blood loss with the subsequent development of iron-deficiency anemia. The triad of weight loss, anemia, and a palpable mass in the right lower quadrant should raise suspicion for right colon carcinoma. *(Dayton et al., 2013, pp. 315–317)*

24. (D) Routine follow-up after surgical resection of a colon cancer includes annual colonoscopy not sigmoidoscopy, which only assesses the distal colon. Yearly colonoscopy aids in the early detection of metachronous cancers and premalignant polyps. The tumor marker for colon cancer is carcinoembryonic antigen (CEA) not carbohydrate antigen

19-9 (CA 19-9), which is used for pancreatic cancer. There is no role for annual chest films or fecal occult blood testing to monitor for a recurrence. *(Tejani & Cohen, 2013, p. 185)*

25. (C) Ulcerative colitis is characterized by confluent inflammation that is confined to the mucosal and submucosal layers of the colon. The rectum is almost always involved but rarely is associated with perianal fistulas. Crohn disease is characterized by transmural inflammation that can involve any part of the gastrointestinal tract from the mouth to the anus. Crohn disease is associated with segmental involvement with "skip" lesions. Strictures and perianal fistulas are also commonly seen with Crohn disease. Both diseases are characterized by exacerbations and remissions. *(Dayton et al., 2013, p. 312)*

26. (D) The current procedure of choice is a proctocolectomy with ileoanal pull through which will preserve anal sphincter function and avoid a permanent ileostomy. A local resection is inadequate due to continuous involvement of the colon with ulcerative colitis. *(Dayton et al., 2013, p. 311)*

27. (B) The diagnosis of large bowel obstruction (LBO) can be made on plain radiographs when there is a competent ileocecal valve that prevents decompression of the colon into the small bowel. When plain radiographs are suspicious for volvulus or ileocolic intussusception then a contrast enema should be performed. The contrast medium should preferably be water-soluble in case there is a perforation, and so that it does not interfere with future studies as they become warranted. *(Henning, 2016, p. 155)*

28. (D) Massive distention of the cecum, as detected on plain radiograph, is typically seen in "closed loop" obstructions of the colon where the ileocecal valve is competent. When distention approaches 12 cm, there is an increased risk of perforation and/or gangrene. Expedient surgical intervention is indicated. Although observation with intravenous fluids and nasogastric decompression are important adjuncts to management, surgical exploration is the only way to rapidly address this emergent situation and prevent ischemia and/or perforation. *(Dayton et al., 2013, pp. 314–315)*

29. **(B)** A volvulus is an obstruction of the colon due to a loop of bowel that has rotated more than 180 degrees on its axis with the mesentery. The most common site for a volvulus is the sigmoid colon (65%). A sigmoid volvulus is associated with abdominal pain and distention. Plain films of the abdomen would show a characteristic "bent inner tube" appearance though CT scan is required for definite location of the involved segment. Definitive treatment will require surgical fixation with resection of the redundant segment of colon. *(Gore et al., 2015, pp. 1107–1108)*

30. **(C)** Hemorrhoids are classified as external (distal to the dentate line and covered with anoderm) and internal (proximal to the dentate line and covered with insensate anorectal mucosa). Internal hemorrhoids are further classified on the basis of their extent of prolapse. First-degree hemorrhoids bulge into the anal canal and may prolapse in association with straining. Second-degree hemorrhoids prolapse through the anus but reduce spontaneously. Third-degree hemorrhoids prolapse through the anal canal and require manual manipulation for reduction. Fourth-degree hemorrhoids prolapse and cannot be reduced, as such they are at increased risk for strangulation. *(Beck & Beck, 2013, p. 301)*

31. **(A)** Anal fissures are linear tears in the lining of the anal canal. They are painful due to their location below the dentate line. Pain is worse with defection and associated with steaks of bright red blood on the stool or on the paper with wiping. Examination of the area is often difficult because of increased pain and sphincter spasm. Anal fissures are treated conservatively with mild analgesic medications, laxatives or stool softeners, and Sitz baths. Botulinum toxin has been used in the management of chronic fissures. For patients with refractory symptoms, a lateral internal sphincterotomy will release the sphincter spasm and allow the fissure to heal. There is a small risk of fecal incontinence following a sphincterotomy. *(Rintala & Pakarinen, 2012, p. 1317)*

32. **(A)** While adenocarcinoma, like other lung cancer types, is more likely to appear in smokers; it is the most common lung cancer seen in nonsmokers, particularly women. It generally originates in the periphery of the lung and can invade the chest wall and cause malignant pleural effusions. *(Dunn & Rothenberger, 2015, p. 1181)*

33. **(C)** Current recommendations, based upon literature review, recommend a laparoscopic myotomy (Heller myotomy) and partial fundoplication as the procedure of choice in the surgical management of achalasia. Partial fundoplication is added to the procedure in order to prevent the incidence of associated gastroesophageal reflux disease (GERD). Peroral endoscopic myotomy (POEM), as a procedure of choice, is still under investigation and its full usefulness as a definitive management strategy is under investigation. *(Jobe et al., 2015, pp. 997–1000)*

34. **(C)** Superficial thrombophlebitis is not uncommon. Appropriate initial management includes warm soaks and/or compresses, and anti-inflammatory medications. Anticoagulation is not indicated unless there is extension into the deep venous system as shown by duplex ultrasonography. Surgical excision of the affected segment may be performed when there is recurrent disease despite appropriate and timely anticoagulation. *(Hingorani & Ascher, 2015, p. 154)*

35. **(C)** A unilateral recurrent laryngeal nerve injury will result in paralysis of the vocal cord on that side causing hoarseness and difficulty with phonation. Bilateral recurrent laryngeal nerve injuries, though rare can result in abduction of both vocal cords, which can cause complete obstruction of the airway requiring an emergent intubation or tracheostomy. Acute postoperative cervical hematomas require emergent attention and the wound as well as the cervical fascia must be opened to relieve the extrinsic compression delayed complications. Hypocalcemia and wound seroma are also recognized complications of parathyroidectomy but do not cause respiratory distress. *(Carneiro & Irwin, 2014, pp. 233–236)*

36. **(A)** Diagnostic lobectomy, instead of observation, is recommended when a "cold" nodule is present and molecular testing is unavailable. Where pathology reveals the lesion is confined to the thyroid, without invasion of the capsule or vascular structures, no further treatment is required. If the lesion is follicular or papillary, then a completion thyroidectomy is suggested as definitive treatment. *(Lal & Clark, 2015, p. 1539)*

37. **(C)** Though papillary carcinoma is the most common type of thyroid malignancy, it is medullary carcinoma of the thyroid that is associated with MEN2. There are three subtypes of MEN2 that include MEN2A, MEN2B, and familial medullary thyroid cancer. An autosomal dominant mutation of the RET proto-oncogene on chromosome 10 is found as the genetic defect in all of these disorders. *(Lal & Clark, 2015, p. 1540)*

38. **(A)** α-Blockade is the first step in preparing a patient for resection of a pheochromocytoma. While β-blockers are also indicated to control the heart rate, they should only be started once the α-blockers have been initiated. Secondary to the effects of the pheochromocytoma, patients are severely vasoconstricted with an increased systemic vascular resistance (SVR). The heart rate and stroke volume are increased in order to compensate for the increased SVR. If β-blockers are initiated first, then cardiovascular collapse may occur because of the loss of the compensatory mechanisms. *(Wait & Lal, 2013, p. 422)*

39. **(B)** Hypokalemia is a common electrolyte disturbance in surgical patients. Symptoms of hypokalemia may include constipation, neuromuscular weakness, diminished tendon reflexes, paralysis, and postoperative arrhythmias. Concomitant deficiencies in magnesium can contribute significantly to the development of hypokalemia as well as hypocalcemia. In the surgical patient with persistent hypokalemia refractory to potassium administration, one should check magnesium levels and correct as appropriate. *(Antonenko et al., 2013, pp. 67–68)*

40. **(D)** Third-space fluid losses that occur with inflammatory conditions such as peritonitis result in an isotonic volume depletion; the recommended intravenous fluid used to replace those losses is lactated Ringer's solution or 0.9% normal saline. Glucose containing solutions should never be used for resuscitation. *(Antonenko et al., 2013, pp. 63–64)*

41. **(D)** Nonoperative management in hemodynamically stable patients with low-grade splenic injuries is preferred. This modality of therapy avoids a laparotomy and preserves splenic function. Postsplenectomy vaccination for encapsulated bacteria (*Streptococcus* and *Meningococcus*) should be administered to prevent overwhelming postsplenectomy infections. *(Dolich et al., 2013, p. 177)*

42. **(B)** Though only 30% of patients with esophageal varices will experience upper GI bleeding they are an important consideration in the differential diagnosis. Patients will require aggressive resuscitation with crystalloids and blood products. Every attempt should be made to identify the etiology of bleeding through endoscopy as it can be both diagnostic and therapeutic. Endoscopic approaches at controlling variceal bleeding are successful in 80% of cases. *(Chapman et al., 2013, pp. 380–381)*

43. **(D)** Due to the effectiveness of endoscopic and TIPS intervention in reducing portal pressures, and recurrent variceal bleeding, the use of shunts has become infrequent today. However, of the shunts listed if one needs to be performed the distal splenorenal shunts are associated with lower rates of encephalopathy. *(Chapman et al., 2013, pp. 383–384)*

44. **(D)** Although all of the conditions listed involve the spleen, by far the most common cause of surgical splenectomy is trauma. Traumatic injury to the spleen resulting in splenectomy is a common surgical condition. Blood dyscrasias make up the second most common etiology for splenectomy. It should be recognized though that the goal of treating patients with splenic injuries is preservation of the spleen when possible. *(Maung & Kaplan, 2013, UpToDate)*

45. **(B)** The most common site for an acute embolic occlusion is the femoral artery. The majority of arterial emboli originate in the heart and are associated with atrial fibrillation. They may also occur from mural thrombi in the left ventricle due to an akinetic or dyskinetic portion of the myocardium following a myocardial infarction. *(McKinsey et al., 2013, pp. 461–463)*

46. **(C)** Hematemesis warrants further investigation with upper gastrointestinal endoscopy to both determine the site of bleeding and provide potential therapy by endoscopic electrocautery or injection. *(Doherty, 2015c, pp. 529–530)*

47. **(D)** Obstruction of the lumen of the appendix is the underlying pathophysiology for the development of acute appendicitis; the most common cause of the luminal obstruction is lymphoid hyperplasia, which occurs in 60% of patients; the second most common cause is a fecalith. *(Mellinger et al., 2013, p. 294)*

48. **(B)** Umbilical hernias must be repaired when there is incarceration, strangulation, perforation, and evisceration as they are absolute indications for surgery. In cases where there is a large defect (>1.5 cm) it can be observed until age 5 and if not closed by then surgical repair should be undertaken. *(Cilley, 2012, p. 964)*

49. **(A)** Achalasia is characterized by progressive dysphagia, which is painless in contrast to esophageal cancer, which is characterized by odynophagia. While patients with achalasia have regurgitation of food, there is minimal loss of weight. Esophageal cancer is associated with anorexia and weight loss. Patients with achalasia typically drink large amounts of liquids to force their food down and have problems with aspiration pneumonia. Patients with reflux esophagitis will complain of epigastric or substernal pain that is worse when supine or leaning forward. *(Jobe et al., 2015 p. 942)*

50. **(B)** This vignette is consistent with an emergent resection in an unprepared patient. The most appropriate therapy for an acute perforation is a Hartmann procedure, which includes resection of the affected portion of the bowel, a temporary diverting colostomy, and oversewing of the distal rectal stump; the second stage of the procedure will involve taking down the colostomy with anastomosis to the rectal stump. *(Dayton et al., 2013, p. 308)*

51. **(C)** The patient has >2 systemic inflammatory response (SIRS) criteria in addition to shock and hypoperfusion of organs as demonstrated by his elevated lactic acid level. Though pancreatitis can be a precursor to the SIRS response in this case the constellation of findings points to septic shock. Aggressive resuscitation and implementation of the surviving sepsis parameters are indicated. *(Dellinger et al., 2013, p. 596)*

52. **(B)** Patients who have septic shock and are not responsive to fluid administration require pressors to maintain a mean arterial pressure ≥65 mm Hg. The pressor of choice to accomplish this is norepinephrine (Levophed). Epinephrine can be added to

or substituted for norepinephrine. In addition vasopressin can be added to norepinephrine in an attempt to reduce pressor requirements or to raise the MAP. Dopamine can also be utilized when tachyarrhythmias occur in cases of relative bradycardia. It should never be used in low doses to attempt to stimulate urine production as studies show this to be ineffective. *(Dellinger et al., 2013, p. 596)*

53. **(C)** Typically a chest radiograph is obtained in cases of suspected pneumothorax, in this case insertion of a tube thoracostomy is the best approach to management as the patient most likely has a tension pneumothorax. The patient is cyanotic and has labored respirations and physical examination clearly points to a right-sided tension pneumothorax. In addition to a chest radiograph bedside ultrasound of the lung may also be diagnostic but both are not utilized in tension pneumothorax as it is a clinical diagnosis. *(Dolich et al., 2013, pp. 186, 193)*

54. **(B)** Flail chest occurs when two or more ribs are segmentally fractured. On physical examination, they will have paradoxical respirations where the affected segment rises with expiration and falls with inspiration. When respiratory failure occurs it is usually in association with an underlying pulmonary contusion. Management typically includes tube thoracostomy for pneumothorax or hemothorax, pain management, pulmonary toileting, and mechanical respiration. Due to altered pulmonary parenchymal fluid dynamics at the point of pulmonary contusion fluid restriction is warranted when possible. *(Dolich et al., 2013, p. 193)*

55. **(B)** This patient is described as a transient responder as he initially responded to volume resuscitation but then had recurrent hypotension. Any patient with blunt abdominal trauma who is hypotensive or a transient responder must be assumed to have ongoing hemorrhage most often due to an injury of the spleen or liver. When suspected blunt abdominal trauma results in injury to solid abdominal viscera, and the patient is hemodynamically stable then evaluation with computerized tomography is indicated. Otherwise bedside imaging with ultrasound can be utilized to detect free intraperitoneal fluid prior to taking the patient to the operating room for definitive intervention. *(Dolich et al, 2013, pp. 195–197)*

56. **(A)** The most common cause of immediate pulmonary complications (can extend up to 48 hours postoperatively) is atelectasis. It has been found to occur in up to 90% of patients who have had general anesthesia. Features of consolidation on physical examination as well as the presence of a postoperative fever may be present. The best way to address the issue of postoperative atelectasis is by preoperative training in the use of incentive spirometry extending to its use during the postoperative period, appropriate pain management, early mobilization, and chest physiotherapy. *(Dolich, 2013, pp. 48–49)*

57. **(D)** In addition to myasthenia gravis, tumors of the thymus gland can produce varied paraneoplastic syndromes. Approximately 30% of patients with a thymoma will have myasthenia gravis and 15% of patients with myasthenia gravis will develop a thymoma. *(Theodore & Jablons, 2015)*

58. **(A)** Surgical patient populations, particularly those admitted for severe trauma, burns, crush injuries or in those who develop impaired renal function; must be closely monitored for the development of hyperkalemia. When hyperkalemia results in EKG changes the use of intravenous calcium will antagonize its tissue effects and not result in changes to overall serum concentration. *(Shires, 2015, pp. 77–78)*

59. **(D)** Pilonidal cysts occur most frequently at the intergluteal cleft and may be associated with active infection. Though they have a high rate of recurrence they should be treated initially with incision and drainage. Definitive care of a chronic cyst or infection will require unroofing of the sinus tract with curettage of the base. The wound is usually left open, kept clean, and allowed to close by secondary intention. *(Dunn & Rothenberger, 2015, p. 1233)*

60. **(D)** Obturator hernias may cause intestinal obstruction as they become trapped within the obturator foramen. The intestinal obstruction is at times described as intermittent and associated with paresthesias along the medial thigh (Howship–Romberg sign) due to compression of the obturator nerve. *(Deveney, 2015, p. 780)*

61. **(C)** Squamous cell carcinoma is the most frequent lung cancer in males and is highly associated to smoking history. Its location is typically central and

may present with bulky lymph nodes, laryngeal nerve involvement (hoarseness), cough, hemoptysis, and wheezing due to high-grade compressive airway obstruction. *(Nason et al., 2015, pp. 616, 623)*

62. **(A)** Lung cancer can present in many different ways with many different associated signs and symptoms. The most common symptoms associated with lung cancer are cough, dyspnea, wheezing, hemoptysis, pneumonia, and lung abscess. Other nonpulmonary symptoms may also be found that involve the heart, mediastinum, esophagus, superior vena cava, or chest wall. *(Nason et al., 2015, Ch. 19)*

63. **(B)** The most important factor in dealing with solitary pulmonary nodules (SPN) is whether or not there is a change in size over time. The review of old chest radiographic images is paramount to making this determination. With the availability of CT imaging of the chest it has become important in the further classification of solitary pulmonary nodules. Plain radiographs are insufficient as CT scan is required to categorize SPNs with regard to their size, location, and whether or not there are multiple lesions. *(Nason et al., 2015, Ch. 19)*

64. **(A)** The signs and symptoms described in this patient most likely represent a superior sulcus tumor of the lung. Tumors in this location can involve the stellate ganglion resulting in Horner's syndrome, atypical chest or shoulder pain from first rib and chest wall involvement, and radicular pain in the arm on the affected side due to invasion of T1 brachial plexus nerve roots. *(Nason et al., 2015, Ch. 19)*

65. **(D)** In the classic presentation of acute appendicitis patients will complain of poorly localized periumbilical pain that localizes to the right lower quadrant (RLQ). Anorexia and nausea are common symptoms with vomiting a less frequent occurrence. Physical examination typically finds pain at McBurney's point and may be associated with other findings such as Rovsing's sign or the iliopsoas sign. Diagnostic tests do not contribute much to the diagnostic process in typical presentations and are not cost effective unless utilized in patients in whom the diagnosis is not as clear. *(Mellinger et al., 2013, pp. 317–318)*

66. **(C)** Open repair of an abdominal aortic aneurysm (AAA) requires loss of the inferior mesenteric

artery. In cases where there is insufficient collateralization via the marginal artery via the superior mesenteric artery, colonic ischemia may develop. Colonic ischemia is characterized by early bowel movements postoperatively. When faced with a patient who has had an early bowel movement perioperatively sigmoidoscopy must be performed so as to detect ischemia early. The detection of infarcted colon will require emergent surgical intervention with resection. *(McKinsey et al., 2013, p. 480)*

67. **(C)** Indirect inguinal hernias are the most common hernias in both males and females. Femoral hernias occur most commonly in females but they do not occur more commonly than indirect inguinal hernias. *(Neumayer et al., 2013, pp. 229–231)*

68. **(D)** Meckel diverticulum is the most common congenital lesion of the small intestine. The "rule of two's," as it applies to Meckel diverticulum is that: it occurs in 2% of the population, is 2:1 male: female predominant, is located 2 ft from the ileocecal valve, is usually 2 cm in size, and may contain two tissue types (pancreatic and gastric). Though symptoms related to Meckel diverticulum are rare the most common symptoms include obstruction, hemorrhage, inflammation, and umbilical fistula. *(Mellinger et al., 2013, pp. 314–315)*

69. **(D)** Peptic ulcer disease includes ulcers of both the stomach and duodenum. In cases where the presentation of peptic ulcer disease is massive, upper gastrointestinal hemorrhage resuscitation with crystalloids and blood products is paramount. Once the patient has been adequately resuscitated upper endoscopy should be performed. Endoscopy can be both diagnostic and therapeutic. When gastric ulcers are identified they should be biopsied as 2% to 4% may contain underlying malignancies. *(Paige et al., 2013, pp. 271–272)*

70. **(D)** Physical examination by itself is unreliable in the diagnosis of deep vein thrombosis (DVT). Some clinical signs of DVT include leg redness, leg warmth, pain, tenderness, and swelling (unilateral or bilateral). When DVT is suspected on clinical grounds patients should undergo a real time duplex B-mode ultrasound evaluation of the lower extremities. *(Tisherman et al., 2013, pp. 149–150)*

71. **(C)** Patients with deep vein thrombosis complicated by pulmonary embolism (PE) require appropriate anticoagulation. In cases where there are contraindications to anticoagulation, continued thrombosis/PE despite adequate anticoagulation, or bleeding while on anticoagulation then patient should have inferior vena cava (IVC) filter placed. *(Tisherman et al., 2013, p. 150)*

72. **(A)** The most common cause of small bowel obstruction (SBO) is adhesions. At times intrinsic luminal etiologies prompted by the ingestion or formation of foreign bodies can also cause a SBO. These causes include phytobezoars and large gallstones. In the case of large gallstones an inflamed gallbladder forms a fistula to the small bowel and the stone passes into the intestine where it eventually becomes trapped at the ileocecal valve causing obstruction. *(Mellinger et al., 2013, pp. 300–302)*

73. **(A)** Moderate or severe symptoms of benign prostatic hyperplasia (BPH) can be managed conservatively by expectant observation. As part of their observation conservative management with α α-blockers may be included. Providers need to be careful with the addition of any antihypertensive medication as α-blockers in combination with some antihypertensives may cause profound hypotension. *(Meng et al., 2015, p. 952)*

74. **(A)** Surgical wounds that leak serous fluid in a spontaneous manner should raise suspicions for a surgical wound failure with disruption of the fascia. As in this case it is possible for the fascia to disrupt while the skin stays intact. This condition must be recognized as soon as possible and the patient returned to the operating room for closure. *(Eddy et al., 2013, p. 49)*

75. **(A)** Instrumentation of the esophagus and ingestion of foreign bodies are common causes of esophageal perforation. Penetrating trauma only accounts for 10% of esophageal perforations but when present may result in a pericardial crunching sound heard best to the left of the sternal border and at the cardiac apex. In addition patients may complain of retrosternal or chest pain that localizes to the side of the perforation. *(Nagji et al., 2010, p. 457)*

76. **(C)** This patient has a protein rich pleural effusion with a high red blood cell count (RBC) and low pH. This type of pleural fluid analysis is most compatible with an exudate. Exudates are most frequently caused by inflammatory conditions or malignancies. When there are a high number of RBCs in the fluid, not in association with trauma or a traumatic pleural tap, then those effusions are typically malignant in nature. *(Nason et al., 2015, Ch. 19)*

77. **(B)** The combination of dysphagia, night sweats, and constitutional symptoms like fatigue should raise suspicion for lymphoma, particularly when imaging reveals a lesion in the superior mediastinum. Superior mediastinal lesions can be remembered by the mnemonic of the 4 T's: thyroid tumors, teratomas, thymomas, and "terrible" lymphomas. *(Nason et al., 2015, Ch. 19)*

78. **(C)** Choledocholithiasis, a stone in the common bile duct, can result in the development of cholangitis, an ascending infection of the biliary tree. When stones of the common bile duct are detected via imaging then an endoscopic retrograde cholangiopancreatography (ERCP) should be performed. ERCP in combination with sphincterotomy can remove the stone without the need for open surgery. *(Hines et al., 2013, pp. 358–359)*

79. **(A)** Perforated colon lesions often lead to the development of intra-abdominal abscesses. These collections stimulate a prolonged systemic inflammatory response that can lead to widespread endothelial damage. When the lungs sustain endothelial damage they develop an inability to oxygenate properly despite increasing the oxygen provided to the patient. It is this refractory hypoxemia in a septic patient that characterizes the presence of acute respiratory distress syndrome. *(Burchard et al., 2013, pp. 124–125)*

80. **(B)** A child who presents with signs and symptoms of small bowel obstruction and a "sausage-shaped" mass has intussusception. Intussusception is a telescoping of small bowel that can be caused by Meckel diverticulum. In addition to a Meckel diverticulum serving as the lead point for an intussusception, it may cause obstruction due to the development of a volvulus around the diverticulum or around a mesodiverticular band. *(Mellinger et al., 2013, pp. 314–315)*

81. **(A)** The presence of obstructive symptoms and haustral markings identified on plain radiographs of the abdomen point to the presence of a large bowel obstruction. The most common causes of large bowel obstruction are colon cancer, diverticular disease, and volvulus. Partial obstruction of the large bowel, when there is an incompetent ileocecal valve, can be managed conservatively with nasogastric decompression and intravenous fluids. Closed-loop obstructions where there is a competent ileocecal valve must be managed surgically for fear of rupture of the cecum. Volvulus is also a surgical emergency and must be decompressed or risk ischemia and/or perforation. *(Dayton et al., 2013, pp. 334–336)*

82. **(C)** Critically ill patients will at times require insertion of central venous catheters due to lack of access, infusion of medications not indicated for peripheral venous use, and hemodynamic monitoring. Acute complications associated with central venous catheter insertion include pneumothorax, hemothorax (vascular injury), catheter malpositioning, air embolization, and arrhythmia. The most concerning long-term complication is a central line–associated bloodstream infection (CLABSI). This patient has all of the symptoms associated with a pneumothorax on the side of catheter insertion. It is imperative that the practitioner always associates acute changes in a patient's condition occurring shortly after a procedure, with the potential it being directly related to the procedure just performed. *(Tisherman et al., 2013, p. 145)*

83. **(A)** Penetrating trauma of the chest associated with hemodynamic instability requires aggressive resuscitation to restore perfusion to vital organs. Patients with severe hemorrhage and cardiac tamponade may find standard resuscitation inadequate to restore perfusion. In cases where patients lose vital signs just prior to arrival to the emergency department (ED) or shortly after arrival then immediate thoracostomy may be required. Immediate ED thoracostomy allows for cross clamping of the aorta, release of cardiac tamponade with pericardiotomy, open heart massage, intracardiac medications, direct control of source of hemorrhage, and relief of air embolism if present. The use of tube thoracostomy is insufficient in cardiac arrest secondary to trauma unless the arrest is due to tension pneumothorax. *(Dolich et al., 2013, p. 145)*

84. (A) Patients with known cardiac history, particularly previous myocardial infarction, present an increased operative mortality and morbidity in the face of elective surgery. Postoperative myocardial ischemia will occur between 5% and 10% of the time and has an associated mortality of 50%. Patients who have had a myocardial infarction within 3 months of elective surgery have a 30% risk of further acute events occurring including cardiac death. Allowing time after a myocardial infarction has occurred is the best strategy to decrease the cardiac mortality associated with it. Waiting at least 6 months reduces cardiac risk to 5% so elective surgical procedures should be performed after this time period has elapsed. *(Eddy et al., 2013, p. 31)*

85. (A) The development of a milky white pleural effusion after attempted or successful central line placement can be associated with injury to the thoracic duct. Most commonly thoracic duct injury is related to injury during a surgical procedure performed in the region, especially cardiothoracic and esophageal. It is treated with a tube thoracostomy, low-fat diet, and occasionally requires hyperalimentation. Copious chylous drainage or drainage for more than 7 days should prompt serious consideration of operative intervention. *(Nason et al., 2015, pp. 685–687)*

REFERENCES

American Cancer Society. Colorectal cancer prevention and early detection. Accessed April 5th, 2015. http://www.cancer.org/acs/groups/cid/documents/webcontent/003170-pdf.pdf

Antonenko D, Brandt MM, Reines HD, Santey H, Tillou A. Fluids, electrolytes, and acid-base balance. In: Lawrence PF, Bell RM, Dayton MT, Hebert J, eds. *Essentials of General Surgery*. 5th ed. Philadelphia, PA: Lippincott Williams & Wilkins; 2013:63–64.

Antonenko D, Brandt MM, Reines HD, Santey H, Tillou A. Fluids, electrolytes, and acid-base balance. In: Lawrence PF, Bell RM, Dayton MT, Hebert J, eds. *Essentials of General Surgery*. 5th ed. Philadelphia, PA: Lippincott Williams & Wilkins; 2013:67–68.

Beck D, Beck DE. *Handbook of Colorectal Surgery*. 3rd ed. London, England: JP Medical Ltd.; 2013:301.

Burchard KW, Brasel K, Capella J, Pritts TA. Shock: cell metabolic failure in critical illness. In: Lawrence PF, ed. *Essentials of General Surgery*. 5th ed. Philadelphia, PA: Lippincott Williams & Wilkins; 2013:124–125.

Carneiro P, Irwin GL. Complications of thyroidectomy and parathyroidectomy. In: Cohn SM, Dolich MO, eds. *Complications in Surgery and Trauma*. 2nd ed. Boca Raton, Fl: CRC Press; 2014.

Chapman WC, Alseidi AA, Hiatt JR, Nauta RJ, Stone MD. Liver. In: Lawrence PF, Bell RM, Dayton MT, Hebert J, eds. *Essentials of General Surgery*. 5th ed. Philadelphia, PA: Lippincott Williams & Wilkins; 2013:380–381.

Chapman WC, Alseidi AA, Hiatt JR, Nauta RJ, Stone MD. Liver. In: Lawrence PF, Bell RM, Dayton MT, Hebert J, eds. *Essentials of General Surgery*. 5th ed. Philadelphia, PA: Lippincott Williams & Wilkins; 2013:383–384.

Chen CL, Cooper MA, Shapiro ML, Angood PB, Makary MA. Patient safety. In: Brunicardi F, Andersen DK, Billiar TR, et al., eds. *Schwartz's Principles of Surgery*. 10th ed. New York, NY: McGraw-Hill; 2014.

Cilley RE. Disorders of the umbilicus. In: Coran AG, Adzick NS, Krummel TM, Laberge JM, Shamberger RC, Caldamone AA, eds. *Pediatric Surgery*. 7th ed. Philadelphia, PA: Elsevier-Saunders; 2012:964.

Dayton MT, Isenberg GA, Rakinic J, et al. Colon, rectum, and anus. In: Lawrence PF, ed. *Essentials of General Surgery*. 5th ed. Philadelphia, PA: Lippincott Williams & Wilkins; 2013:307.

Dayton MT, Isenberg GA, Rakinic J, et al. Colon, rectum, and anus. In: Lawrence PF, ed. *Essentials of General Surgery*. 5th ed. Philadelphia, PA: Lippincott Williams & Wilkins; 2013:308.

Dayton MT, Isenberg GA, Rakinic J, et al. Colon, rectum, and anus. In: Lawrence PF, ed. *Essentials of General Surgery*. 5th ed. Philadelphia, PA: Lippincott Williams & Wilkins; 2013:311.

Dayton MT, Isenberg GA, Rakinic J, et al. Colon, rectum, and anus. In: Lawrence PF, ed. *Essentials of General Surgery*. 5th ed. Philadelphia, PA: Lippincott Williams & Wilkins; 2013:312.

Dayton MT, Isenberg GA, Rakinic J, et al. Colon, rectum, and anus. In: Lawrence PF, ed. *Essentials of General Surgery*. 5th ed. Philadelphia, PA: Lippincott Williams & Wilkins; 2013:314.

Dayton MT, Isenberg GA, Rakinic J, et al. Colon, rectum, and anus. In: Lawrence PF, ed. *Essentials of General Surgery*. 5th ed. Philadelphia, PA: Lippincott Williams & Wilkins; 2013: 314–315.

Dayton MT, Isenberg GA, Rakinic J, et al. Colon, rectum, and anus. In: Lawrence PF, ed. *Essentials of General Surgery*. 5th ed. Philadelphia, PA: Lippincott Williams & Wilkins; 2013:315–317.

Dayton MT, Isenberg GA, Rakinic J, et al. Colon, rectum, and anus. In: Lawrence PF, ed. *Essentials of General Surgery.* 5th ed. Philadelphia, PA: Lippincott Williams & Wilkins; 2013:334–336.

Dellinger RR, Levy MM, Rhodes A, et al. Surviving sepsis campaign: international guidelines for management of severe sepsis and septic shock: 2012. *Critical Care Medicine.* 2013; 41(2):580–637, 596.

Dempsey DT. Stomach. In: Brunicardi FC, Andersen DK, Billiar TR, et al., eds. *Schwartz's Principles of Surgery.* 10th ed. New York, NY: McGraw-Hill; 2014.

Deveney KE. Chapter 32: Hernias & Other Lesions of the Abdominal Wall. In. Doherty GM ed. *Current Diagnosis & Treatment.* 14th ed. New York, NY: McGraw-Hill; 2015.

Dixon JM, Macaskill EJ. Management of benign breast disease. In: Riker AI, ed. *Breast Disease: Comprehensive Management.* 1st ed. New York, NY: Springer Science + Business Media; 2015:52–53.

Doherty GM. Fluid & electrolyte management. In: Doherty GM, ed. *Current Diagnosis and Treatment: Surgery.* 14th ed. New York, NY: The McGraw-Hill Companies; 2015a.

Doherty GM. Pancreas. In: Doherty GM, ed. *Current Diagnosis & Treatment: Surgery.* 14th ed. New York, NY: McGraw-Hill; 2015b.

Doherty GM. Chapter 23: Stomach & Duodenum. In. Doherty GM ed. *Current Diagnosis & Treatment.* 14th ed. New York, NY: McGraw-Hill; 2015c.

Dolich MO, Bjerke HS, Chipman JG, Luchette FA, Patterson LA. Trauma. In: Lawrence PF, Bell RM, Dayton MT, Hebert J, eds. *Essentials of General Surgery.* 5th ed. Philadelphia, PA: Lippincott Williams & Wilkins; 2013:145, 175, 177, 186, 193, 195–197.

Dunn KMB, Rothenberger DA. Chapter 29: Colon Rectum, and Anus. In: Brunicardi FC, Andersen DK, Billiar TR, et al., eds. *Schwartz's Principles of Surgery.* 10th ed. New York, NY: McGraw-Hill; 2015.

Eddy VA, Arnell TD, Harris KA, Hassan I, Morrison JE. Perioperative evaluation and management of surgical patients. In: Lawrence PF, ed. *Essentials of General Surgery.* 5th ed. Philadelphia, PA: Lippincott Williams & Wilkins; 2013:31.

Eddy VA, Arnell TD, Harris KA, Hassan I, Morrison JE. Perioperative evaluation and management of surgical patients. In: Lawrence PF, ed. *Essentials of General Surgery.* 5th ed. Philadelphia, PA: Lippincott Williams & Wilkins; 2013:49.

Elsey JK, Schmidt DR. Acute cholecystitis. In: Cameron JL, Cameron AM, eds. *Current Surgical Therapy.* 11th ed. Philadelphia, PA: Elsevier-Saunders; 2014:388.

Ferri FF. Ferri's clinical advisor: 5 books in 1. Meckel diverticulum. In: *Ferri's Clinical Advisor: 5 Books in 1.* 15th ed. Philadelphia, PA: Elsevier-Mosby; 2013:662.

Ferri FF. Ferri's clinical advisor: 5 books in 1. Pressure ulcers. In: *Ferri's Clinical Advisor: 5 Books in 1.* 15th ed. Philadelphia, PA: Elsevier-Mosby; 2013:889.

Giuliano AE, Hurvitz SA. Breast disorders. In: Doherty GM, ed. *CURRENT Diagnosis & Treatment: Surgery.* 14th ed. New York, NY: McGraw-Hill; 2015.

Goldin SB, et al. Pancreas: In: Lawrence PF, ed. *Essentials of General Surgery.* 5th ed. Philadelphia, PA: Lippincott Williams & Wilkins; 2013; p. 358.

Gore RM, Szucs RA, Wolf EL, Scholz FJ, Eisenberg RL, Rubesin SE. Miscellaneous abnormalities of the colon. In: Gore RM, Levine MS, eds. *Textbook of Gastrointestinal Radiology: Expert Consult.* 4th ed. Philadelphia, PA: Elsevier-Saunders; 2015:1003.

Gore RM, Szucs RA, Wolf EL, Scholz FJ, Eisenberg RL, Rubesin SE. Miscellaneous abnormalities of the colon. In: Gore RM, Levine MS, eds. *Textbook of Gastrointestinal Radiology: Expert Consult.* 4th ed. Philadelphia, PA: Elsevier-Saunders; 2015:1007–1108.

Henning W. Chapter 16: Recognizing Bowel Obstruction and Ileus; In: *Learning Radiology:* Recognizing the Basics. 3rd ed. Philadelphia, PA: Elsevier: Saunders; 2016.

Hines OJ, Bingener J, Cason FD, Edwards M, Hopkins MA. Biliary tract. In: Lawrence PF, ed. *Essentials of General Surgery.* 5th ed. Philadelphia, PA: Lippincott Williams & Wilkins; 2013:358–359.

Hingorani A, Ascher E. Superficial thrombophlebitis. In: Gahtan V, Costanza MJ, eds. *Essentials of Vascular Surgery for the General Surgeon* (eBook). New York, NY: Springer; 2014:154.

Ilbawi A, Horvath KD. Laparoscopic management of pancreatic pseudocyst. In: Cameron JL, Cameron AM, eds. *Current Surgical Therapy.* 11th ed. Philadelphia, PA: Elsevier-Saunders; 2014:1414–1415.

Jobe BA, Hunter JG, Watson DL. Esophagus and diaphragmatic hernia. In: Brunicardi FC, Andersen DK, Billiar TR, et al., eds. *Schwartz's Principles of Surgery.* 10th ed. New York, NY: McGraw-Hill; 2015.

Lal G, Clark OH. Chapter 38: Thyroid, Parathyroid, and Adrenal Gland. In: Brunicardi FC, Andersen DK, Billiar TR, et al., eds. *Schwartz's Principles of Surgery.* 10th ed. New York, NY: McGraw-Hill; 2015.

Lampiris HW, Maddix DS. Chapter 51: Clinical use of antimicrobial agents: Antimicrobial prophylaxis. In: Katzung BG, Masters SB, Trevor AJ, eds. *Basic & Clinical Pharmacology.* 12th ed. New York, NY: McGraw-Hill; 2012.

Li CM, McCoy JA, Hsu HK. Esophagus. In: Lawrence PF, ed. *Essentials of General Surgery.* 5th ed. Philadelphia, PA: Lippincott Williams & Wilkins; 2013:277–278.

Maung AA, Kaplan LJ. Surgical management of splenic injury in the adult trauma patient. In: Frankel HL, Collins KA, eds. UptoDate. New York, NY: Wolters Kluwer; 2013.

McKinsey JF, Alexander J, Byer A, et al. Diseases of the vascular system. In: Lawrence PF, Bell RM, Dayton MT, Hebert J, eds. *Essentials of General Surgery.* 5th ed. Philadelphia, PA: Lippincott Williams & Wilkins; 2013: 461–463.

McKinsey JF, Alexander J, Byer A, et al. Diseases of the vascular system. In: Lawrence PF, ed. *Essentials of General Surgery*. 5th ed. Philadelphia, PA: Lippincott Williams & Wilkins; 2013:480.

Mellinger JD, Dubé S, Friel C, et al. Small intestine and appendix. In: Lawrence PF, ed. *Essentials of General Surgery*. 5th ed. Philadelphia, PA: Lippincott Williams & Wilkins; 2013:277–278.

Mellinger JD, Dubé S, Friel C, et al. Small intestine and appendix. In: Lawrence PF, ed. *Essentials of General Surgery*. 5th ed. Philadelphia, PA: Lippincott Williams & Wilkins; 2013:282, 294, 300–302, 314–315, 317–318.

Meng MV, Walsh TJ, Chi TO. Urologic disorders. In: Papadakis MA, McPhee SJ, Rabow MW, eds. *Current Medical Diagnosis & Treatment*. 54th ed. New York, NY: McGraw-Hill; 2015:952.

Nagji AS, Lau CL, Kozower BD. Esophageal perforation. In: Rabinovici R, Frankel HL, Kirton O, eds. *Trauma Critical Care and Surgical Emergencies: A Case and Evidence-Based Textbook*. London, England: Informa UK; 2010:457.

Nason KS, Maddaus MA, Luketich JD. Chest Wall, Lung, Mediastinum, and Pleura, In: Brunicardi FC, Andersen DK, Billiar TR, et al., eds. *Schwartz's Principles of Surgery*. 10th ed. New York, NY: McGraw-Hill; 2015. Accessed online, December 1, 2015.

Neumayer L, Dangleben DA, Fraser S, Gefen J, Maa J, Mann BD. Abdominal wall, including hernia. In: Lawrence PF, ed. *Essentials of General Surgery*. 5th ed. Philadelphia, PA: Lippincott Williams & Wilkins; 2013:229–231.

Neumayer L, Dangleben DA, Fraser S, Gefen J, Maa J, Mann BD. Abdominal wall, including hernia. In: Lawrence PF, ed. *Essentials of General Surgery*. 5th ed. Philadelphia, PA: Lippincott Williams & Wilkins; 2013:238.

Paige JT, Farell TM, Jones DB, Shebrain S, Steele KE. Stomach and duodenum. In: Lawrence PF, ed. *Essentials of General Surgery*. 5th ed. Philadelphia, PA: Lippincott Williams & Wilkins; 2013:271–272.

Pham TH, Hunter JG. Gallbladder and the extrahepatic biliary system. In: Brunicardi F, Andersen DK, Billiar TR, et al., eds. *Schwartz's Principles of Surgery*. 10th ed. New York, NY: McGraw-Hill; 2014.

Rintala RJ, Pakarinen MP. Other disorders of the anus and rectum, anorectal function. In: Coran AG, Adzick NS, Krummel TM, Laberge JM, Shamberger RC, Caldamone AA, eds. *Pediatric Surgery*. 7th ed. Philadelphia, PA: Elsevier-Saunders; 2012.

Shabetai R. Pericardial disease. In: Jeremias A, Brown DL, eds. *Cardiac Intensive Care*. 2nd ed. Philadelphia, PA: Saunders-Elsevier; 2010:383–384.

Sharma G, Whang EE, Gold JS. Acute cholangitis. In: Cameron JL, Cameron AM, eds. *Current Surgical Therapy*. 11th ed. Philadelphia, PA: Elsevier-Saunders; 2014:396–397.

Shires GT. Chapter 3: Fluid and Electrolyte Management of the Surgical Patient. In: Brunicardi FC, Andersen DK, Billiar TR, et al., eds. *Schwartz's Principles of Surgery*. 10th ed. New York, NY: McGraw-Hill; 2015.

Tejani MA, Cohen SJ. Colon and rectum carcinoma surveillance counterpoint: USA. In: Johnson FE, Browman GP, Audisio RA, et al., eds. *Patient Surveillance After Cancer Treatment* (eBook). New York, NY: Springer Science + Business Media; 2013:185.

Theodore PR, Jablons D. Thoracic wall, pleura, mediastinum & lung. In: Doherty GM. *Current Diagnosis and Treatment: Surgery*. 14th ed. New York, NY: McGraw-Hill Education; 2015.

Tisherman SA, Brunsvold M, Daley BJ, Morrison JE, Schenarts PJ, Wohitmann C. Surgical critical care. In: Lawrence PF, ed. *Essentials of General Surgery*. 5th ed. Philadelphia, PA: Lippincott Williams & Wilkins; 2013:145.

Tisherman SA, Brunsvold M, Daley BJ, Morrison JE, Schenarts PJ, Wohitmann C. Surgical critical care. In: Lawrence PF, ed. *Essentials of General Surgery*. 5th ed. Philadelphia, PA: Lippincott Williams & Wilkins; 2013:149–150.

Tisherman SA, Brunsvold M, Daley BJ, Morrison JE, Schenarts PJ, Wohitmann C. Surgical critical care. In: Lawrence PF, ed. *Essentials of General Surgery*. 5th ed. Philadelphia, PA: Lippincott Williams & Wilkins; 2013:150.

Valsangkar N, Thayer SP. Acute pancreatitis. In: Cameron JL, Cameron AM, eds. *Current Surgical Therapy*. 11th ed. Philadelphia, PA: Elsevier-Saunders; 2014:431.

Valsangkar N, Thayer SP. Acute pancreatitis. In: Cameron JL, Cameron AM, eds. *Current Surgical Therapy*. 11th ed. Philadelphia, PA: Elsevier-Saunders; 2014:431–434.

Wait RB, Lal A. Surgical endocrinology: adrenal glands. In: Lawrence PF, ed. *Essentials of General Surgery*. 5th ed. Philadelphia, PA: Lippincott Williams & Wilkins; 2013: 422.

CHAPTER 17

Orthopedics and Rheumatology

Ian McLeod, MEd, MS, PA-C, ATC

DIRECTIONS: Each of the numbered questions or incomplete statements is followed by possible answers or completions of the statement. Select the ONE-lettered answer or completion that is BEST in each case.

1. A 20-year-old male presents with complaints of left lateral ankle pain following an injury that occurred when he was landing from a jump while playing basketball. On examination, there is tenderness over the anterior talofibular ligament. The calcaneofibular and posterior talofibular ligaments are nontender to palpation. Anterior drawer testing is positive for pain and loss of endpoint. Inversion subtalar tilt test does not cause any pain and there is a firm endpoint. Based upon this information, what was the most likely mechanism of injury?

   (A) Eversion
   (B) Inversion
   (C) Plantar flexion
   (D) Eversion and plantar flexion
   (E) Inversion and plantar flexion

2. A 33-year-old man complains of left anterior shoulder pain for 4 weeks. The pain is made worse with overhead activities. On examination, you note maximal pain in the shoulder with palpation between the greater and lesser tubercle. Pain in the shoulder is exacerbated when the arm is held at the side, elbow flexed to 90 degrees, and the patient is asked to supinate and flex the forearm against your resistance. Based on this presentation, what is the most likely diagnosis?

   (A) Rotator cuff tendonitis
   (B) Acromioclavicular sprain
   (C) Anterior shoulder dislocation
   (D) Rotator cuff tear
   (E) Bicipital tendonitis

3. A 62-year-old man presents complaining of progressively worse right shoulder pain for 5 weeks. The pain is located anterolaterally and is aggravated by overhead activities. The patient notes significant pain when trying to sleep with his arm in a forward-flexed position and his hand behind his head. The patient notes weakness of the right arm and states that he has noticed that he uses the arm less because of the pain. On physical examination, you elevate the patient's arms to 90 degrees, abduct to 30 degrees, and internally rotate the arms with the thumbs pointing downward. When you apply downward pressure to both arms you note weakness on the right side and the patient reports exacerbation of his shoulder pain. When the patient has his arms at his side and elbows flexed to 90 degrees you ask him to resist inward and outward pressure to the forearms; during this maneuver he has full strength and no complaints of pain. Based on this presentation, what is the most likely injured structure?

   (A) Infraspinatus tendon
   (B) Supraspinatus tendon
   (C) Teres minor tendon
   (D) Subscapularis tendon
   (E) Bicipital tendon

4. A 73-year-old woman presents to the emergency department following a fall in her home. She tripped over a throw rug, fell forward and landed with her arms extended and hands outstretched. She presents complaining of left wrist pain. Based upon the radiograph shown in Figure 17-1, what is the most likely diagnosis?

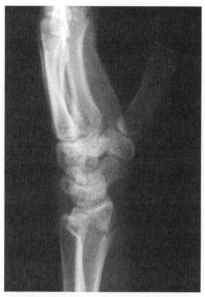

Figure 17-1. Reproduced with permission, from Chin HW, Visotsky J: Wrist fractures. *Emerg Med Clin N Amer*;11:(3)1993.

(A) Barton fracture

(B) Colles fracture

(C) Smith fracture

(D) Boxer fracture

(E) Monteggia fracture

5. Idiopathic osteonecrosis of the femoral head is the most likely diagnosis in which of the following patients?

(A) 5-year-old boy who complains of significant hip and knee pain

(B) 6-year-old boy who reports a limp and aching in the groin and proximal thigh

(C) 7-year-old obese girl who manifests a painless limp

(D) 12-year-old girl who complains of progressively worsening hip pain, fever, and chills

(E) 18-year-old boy who complains of bilateral hip pain that is worse in the morning and is relieved with activity

6. A 22-year-old female was playing basketball when she tripped and landed on the pavement with her hands outstretched. She presents complaining of abrasions on the right thenar eminence and "wrist pain." Physical examination reveals tenderness to palpation between the extensor pollicis longus and extensor pollicis brevis. Assessment of the median, ulnar, and radial nerves reveals no sensor or motor changes when compared with the left hand. Radial and ulnar pulses are 2+ bilaterally with capillary refill less than 2 seconds on all five digits of the right hand. Posterior–anterior view radiographs of the wrist and posterior–anterior wrist radiographs with the wrist in ulnar deviation reveal no fractures or dislocations. What is the appropriate management for this patient at this time?

(A) Immediate orthopedic referral

(B) Cock-up splint until symptoms resolve

(C) Physical therapy referral for assessment and treatment

(D) Thumb spica splint and repeat radiographs in 2 weeks

(E) No further treatment is necessary because the radiographs were negative and no vascular or neurological abnormalities were noted on examination

7. A 55-year-old male patient of northern European descent presents with painless limitation of movement in the ring finger of the right hand. The patient states that over the past 9 months his ring finger has been gradually pulled into a bent position. He has tried to straighten his finger but has been unable to do so. He can bend his finger and make a fist without difficulty. Examination of the palmar aspect of the right hand reveals a taut cord that begins in the palmar region and crosses the metacarpophalangeal joint of the ring finger. There is a palmar skin nodule at the base of the taut band. Palpation of the nodule and taut band does not elicit tenderness. You are able to passively flex the ring finger to its end range of motion but any attempt to extend the ring finger beyond its initial resting position is restricted due to a firm end feel. What is the most likely diagnosis?

(A) Jersey finger

(B) Trigger finger

(C) Dupuytren contracture

(D) Gamekeeper finger

(E) Ganglion cyst

8. A 37-year-old flight attendant presents complaining of worsening foot pain for 3 weeks. The pain is located on the plantar surface of her forefoot and is described as severe, "burning" pain. The pain also radiates into her third and fourth toes. The patient states that, at first, she thought she had a pebble in her shoe, but when she removed her shoe, she could not find any obvious offending agent in her shoe. On physical examination, you are able to reproduce the pain by grasping the medial and lateral aspect of the foot in your hand and squeezing the metatarsal heads together. There is no tenderness with palpation of the metatarsal shafts. What is the most likely diagnosis?

(A) Hammer toe

(B) Morton neuroma

(C) Metatarsalgia

(D) Metatarsal stress fracture

(E) Metatarsophalangeal synovitis

9. A 27-year-old woman with no significant medical history presents complaining of left elbow pain for 3 days. The patient states that over the last 3 days, her left elbow has become increasingly red, swollen, and painful. The patient is left-hand dominant. The patient is employed as a chiropractor, she is sexually active but denies a history of sexually transmitted infections. The patient is currently having her menses, denies any recent foreign travel, and acknowledges that while she regularly plays tennis, she does not recall any history of elbow trauma. On physical examination, you discover an elbow joint that is markedly erythematous, warm to touch, and tender to palpation. Range of motion is decreased secondary to edema and pain. Radiographs of the elbow reveal only soft tissue swelling but no fracture or dislocation. Joint aspiration is performed and a gram-negative diplococcus is identified on cytological examination. What is the most likely cause of this patient's septic arthritis?

(A) *Staphylococcus aureus*

(B) *Escherichia coli*

(C) *Neisseria gonorrhoeae*

(D) *Pseudomonas aeruginosa*

(E) Methicillin-resistant *Staphylococcus aureus*

10. A 53-year-old woman presents with pain in her right wrist. The pain is aggravated by movement of the thumb and when she makes a fist. She also notes that when she moves her thumb, there is an occasional locking sensation in the radial aspect of her wrist. Physical examination of the wrist reveals swelling and tenderness over the distal radius. Full flexion of the thumb into the palm combined with ulnar deviation of the wrist, produces pain. Radiographic evaluation of the wrist shows no bone abnormalities. Which of the following would be the treatment of choice in this patient presentation?

(A) Immobilization of the wrist with a thumb spica splint

(B) Tendon sheath corticosteroid injection

(C) Operative treatment to restore functionality

(D) Prompt neurological evaluation

(E) Proceed to bone scan to evaluate the area of pain

11. The following photo (Fig. 17-2) depicts what type of deformity involving the fourth finger?

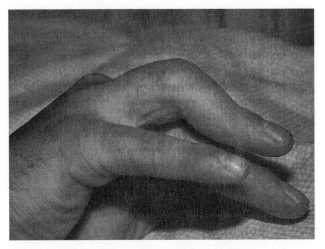

Figure 17-2. Reproduced, with permission, from Knoop KJ, Stack LB, Storrow AB, et al. The *Atlas of Emergency Medicine*. 3rd ed. New York, NY: McGraw-Hill Education, 2010. Figure 11-41. Photographer: E. Lee Edstrom, MD.

(A) Boutonniere

(B) Swan neck

(C) Mallet

(D) Heberden's

(E) Jersey

12. A 62-year-old man complains of low back pain that radiates from his back down into his buttock and into his right leg. On physical examination, you note sensory loss on the first dorsal web space between the first and second toes and decreased ability to dorsiflex (extend) the first toe on the right side. The straight-leg raise test elicits pain at 45 degrees of elevation. Based on the information contained in this scenario, between which pairing of vertebrae is the disc herniation most likely to have occurred?

   (A) L2–L3
   (B) L3–L4
   (C) L4–L5
   (D) L5–S1
   (E) S1–S2

13. You have been following a 52-year-old woman with a complaint of back pain over the past 7 weeks. During the first 5 weeks of her condition, the back pain was steadily declining and her neurological findings on physical examination were decreasing. Over the past 2 weeks, she has complained of worsening pain that is currently unrelenting, especially at night. On physical examination, she has increased lumbar pain with both the straight-leg raise and crossed straight-leg raise tests. Her muscle weakness has likewise accelerated over the past 2 weeks, and she is no longer able to heel walk using her left ankle. What is the most appropriate management strategy at this time?

   (A) Conservative therapy including application of ice and physical therapy referral for muscle stretching and strengthening
   (B) Plain radiographs of the lumbar spine
   (C) Computed tomography (CT) of the lumbar spine
   (D) Magnetic resonance imaging (MRI) of the lumbar spine
   (E) Lower extremity nerve conduction testing

14. A 62-year-old man presents with complaints of an acute onset of pain in his left first metatarsophalangeal joint. The joint is erythematous to inspection. Pain is elicited with active and passive range of motion assessment, and the patient is unable to bear weight on his foot secondary to the pain. Examination of the joint fluid by polarized light reveals needle-like and negatively birefringent crystals. What would be the most appropriate intervention at this time?

   (A) Parenteral vancomycin for 4 to 6 weeks
   (B) Indomethacin 50 mg every 8 hours as needed for pain for 10 days
   (C) Prednisone 50 mg once daily for 5 days
   (D) Moist heat application
   (E) Allopurinol 100 mg once daily until symptoms resolve

15. A 27-year-old man with a history of intermittent gout, mild obesity, and alcohol dependency complains of lumbar back pain for 2 days. On physical examination, you note a man who is in moderate distress. He is sitting still on the examination table. Vital signs reveal a temperature of 101.5°F orally, pulse of 99/min regular, respirations of 20/min unlabored, pulse oximetry of 99% on room air, body mass index (BMI) of 28.5. Lungs are clear to auscultation; heart demonstrates a regular rate and rhythm without murmurs. Abdominal examination reveals normoactive bowel sounds and no rigidity or guarding. There are areas of erythema and ecchymosis in the antecubital crease on his right arm with red streaking extending proximally from the antecubital crease. Examination of the back reveals no erythema or muscle spasm. You elicit pinpoint tenderness over the fourth lumbar vertebra to palpation. There is only mild discomfort to palpation in the paraspinous muscles in the lumbar region. The patient has full range of motion to flexion and extension at the waist. Straight-leg raise test elicits pain in the hamstring region at 80 degrees on the right leg but the cross straight-leg raise test is negative. There are no sensory changes noted in the lower extremities bilaterally and the deep tendon reflexes (DTRs) are 2+ in the patellar and Achilles bilaterally. Anal sphincter tone is within normal limits. What is the best treatment choice for this patient at this time?

   (A) Conservative management, including nonsteroidal anti-inflammatory drugs (NSAIDs) and a work excuse for 3 days
   (B) Narcotic pain medication plus physical therapy referral
   (C) Ciprofloxacin 750 mg once a day for 14 days

(D) Parenteral antibiotics for 4 to 6 weeks

(E) Parenteral antibiotics weekly for 6 months

16. A 10-year-old boy is brought to the emergency department after falling during the recess at school. The patient states he on the monkey bars when he lost his grip and fell to the ground. He landed with all of his weight on his right foot. He complains of pain in his right ankle and is unable to put any weight on his right lower extremity. Based upon the x-ray shown in Figure 17-3, how would you classify this patient's fracture?

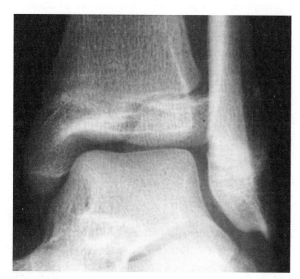

Figure 17-3. Reproduced with permission from Shah BR, Lucchesi M. *Atlas of Pediatric Emergency Medicine.* New York, NY: McGraw-Hill Education, 2006. Figure 133-5.

(A) Salter–Harris type I

(B) Salter–Harris type II

(C) Salter–Harris type III

(D) Salter–Harris type IV

(E) Salter–Harris type V

17. A 25-year-old man was involved in a motor vehicle collision and complains of right leg pain. The car was traveling approximately 50 miles per hour when the driver lost control of the vehicle, causing it to leave the road and run head-on into a tree. At the time of the accident, he was restrained by his seat belt and sitting in the front passenger seat. The force of the collision caused the dashboard to be driven violently back against the patient's knees. The patient localizes his pain to the right hip. On the basis of this mechanism of injury and location

of pain complaints, what would you expect to find when you inspect the right leg?

(A) Flexed, abducted, and externally rotated

(B) Shortened, abducted, and externally rotated

(C) Shortened, abducted, and internally rotated

(D) Shortened and externally rotated

(E) Shortened, adducted, and internally rotated

18. A 42-year-old automobile mechanic presents complaining of neck pain that radiates down the lateral aspect of his arm and into his left hand. The patient states that the pain has become progressively more constant over the past 3 weeks. He feels that he is "loosing strength" in his left arm and that parts of his left hand are feeling numb. He states that his symptoms seem to lessen when he places his hand on top of his head. Physical examination reveals vital signs that are within normal limits; no muscle atrophy or spasm is noted in the neck or upper extremities bilaterally. Sensory ability is diminished in the dorsolateral aspect of the thumb and index finger left hand. Biceps muscle strength is 5/5 on the right and 4/5 on the left. Wrist extension strength is 5/5 on the right and 4/5 on the left. Tricep strength is 5/5 bilaterally. Tricep reflexes are +2 bilaterally, right-sided biceps and brachioradialis reflexes are 2+, and left-sided biceps and brachioradialis reflexes are 1+. On the basis of this presentation, what spinal root is most likely involved?

(A) C5

(B) C6

(C) C7

(D) C8

(E) T1

19. Nonsteroidal anti-inflammatory agents are frequently utilized in treating the patient with osteoarthritis. In addition to the potential for bleeding and gastrointestinal effects, the primary concern, especially in the elderly patient, is irreversible damage to which of the following?

(A) Eyes

(B) Heart

(C) Kidneys

(D) Peripheral vascular system

(E) Central nervous system

20. A 7-year-old boy is brought to the emergency department after sustaining a fall onto his outstretched hand. He complains of pain involving the entire arm and refuses to move his arm, which is held in anatomical position with the elbow flexed at 90 degrees. On physical examination, there is notable tenderness over the elbow with associated swelling and pain on attempted rotation. There is no apparent tenderness to palpation involving the wrist or shoulder. The child refuses to participate with range of motion evaluation. Radiographic evaluation of the elbow shows the presence of a positive posterior fat pad sign. What is the most likely diagnosis with this patient's presentation?

    (A) Nursemaid elbow
    (B) Lateral epicondylitis
    (C) Medial epicondylitis
    (D) Radial head dislocation
    (E) Occult fracture of the radial head

21. A 35-year-old man presents with complaints of swelling and pain in left knee. The patient states that he sustained a twisting injury in a football game 3 days ago. The injury did not take him out of the game; he was able to continue participating with minimal difficulty. Over the last 2 days, the pain has progressed. He notes a catching sensation and pain that is more medially located. On physical examination, the patient is found to have tenderness over the medial joint line and limited range of motion. Forced flexion and circumduction of the joint cause a painful click. What is the most likely diagnosis in this patient presentation?

    (A) Anterior cruciate ligament tear
    (B) Medial meniscus tear
    (C) Pes anserine bursitis
    (D) Tibial plateau fracture
    (E) Medial collateral ligament tear

22. Which of the following motor, sensory, and reflex findings are most likely to be found in a patient with lumbar radiculopathy of the L4–L5 disc?

    (A) Weakness of the anterior tibialis, numbness of the shin, and an asymmetric knee reflex

    (B) Weakness of the great toe flexor and gastrocsoleus, inability to sustain tiptoe walking, and an asymmetrical ankle reflex
    (C) Weakness of the great toe extensor, numbness on the top of the foot and first web space, no reflex findings
    (D) Perianal numbness, urinary and bowel incontinence
    (E) Ankle clonus

23. Which of the following characteristics help to distinguish the "pseudoclaudication" of a patient with spinal stenosis from true claudication?

    (A) Insidious onset of symptoms
    (B) Worsening of pain by lumbar flexion
    (C) Radiation of pain to the upper back
    (D) Preservation of pedal pulses
    (E) Localizing maximum area of discomfort to the lower back

24. A 15-year-old boy was playing football and was hit during a play, causing an abduction injury of his left lower leg. He locates the pain along the medial aspect of the knee, and there is a minimal level of joint effusion. Which of the following tests would assess for stability of the medial collateral ligament?

    (A) Valgus stress test
    (B) Varus stress test
    (C) Apprehension sign
    (D) Lachman test
    (E) Anterior drawer sign

25. A 12-year-old obese boy presents with pain in the right thigh and medial knee. The pain has been over a 6-week period. The pain is described as aching in nature. Over the last month, the patient reports he has been walking with a limp. On physical examination, the right knee is found to be unremarkable. A slight limp noted with gait. Radiographs of the right knee are normal. Which of the following is the most appropriate step in the evaluation of this patient?

(A) Examine and x-ray the right hip

(B) X-ray the left knee for comparison

(C) Obtain a computed tomography (CT) scan of the right knee

(D) Obtain a magnetic resonance image of the right knee

(E) Reassure the parents and observe the patient for progression

26. Treatment of scoliosis is usually employed for patients with curvature greater than which of the following curve magnitudes?

(A) 20 degrees

(B) 30 degrees

(C) 40 degrees

(D) 50 degrees

(E) 60 degrees

27. A 24-year-old man presents with low back pain of 2 days' duration. The patient is a manual laborer and reports lifting a heavy box while at work the previous day. Initially, the patient had no complaints, but the following day, stiffness and pain began. The patient denies radiation of the pain, numbness, or difficulty with urination. He denies previous complaints of back pain or injury. On physical examination, there is noted paravertebral muscle spasm and slight decrease in range of motion of the spine. Deep tendon reflexes are equal bilaterally, and no sensory deficits are noted. Which of the following is the most appropriate intervention?

(A) Magnetic resonance imaging (MRI) of the lumbar spine

(B) Plain radiographs of the lumbar spine

(C) Return the patient to work with no limitations

(D) Refer the patient for trigger point injections

(E) Initiate a short period of rest, analgesia, and progressive functional program

28. Which of the following is most diagnostic of a septic joint?

(A) Synovial fluid analysis

(B) Plain radiograph

(C) Ultrasound of the joint

(D) Computed tomography (CT) scan of the joint

(E) Magnetic resonance imaging (MRI) of the joint

29. An 8-year-old boy presents with complaint of a painful right wrist of 2 days' duration. The mother of the child reports that the child jumped off a swing landing on his outstretched arms. He immediately complained of pain in the right wrist and now has some mild swelling on the radial aspect of the wrist. Radiographic evaluation of the wrist presents an area of impaction on the distal radius, with a slight bend in the opposing cortex. Which of the following best describes this type of fracture?

(A) Greenstick fracture

(B) Torus fracture

(C) Plastic deformation

(D) Radial neck fracture

(E) Monteggia fracture

30. A 39-year-old woman presents with complaints of pain in her left foot of 4 weeks' duration. The patient works as a cashier in a department store, which requires her to be on her feet for long periods. She notes that the pain is most severe on the bottom of her foot and is worse upon arising in the morning and then it subsides with ambulation. On examination, there is no pain with medial and lateral compression of the calcaneus. Active and passive foot and ankle range of motion are pain free and equal bilaterally. Resisted foot and ankle range of motion is 5/5 and pain free. The patient has a benign medical history and no other complaints. Which of the following is the most likely diagnosis of this patient?

(A) Heel spur

(B) Achilles tendonitis

(C) Tarsal tunnel syndrome

(D) Plantar fasciitis

(E) Calcaneal stress fracture

31. A 17-year-old boy presents with complaints of pain located in his fifth digit. He was involved in an altercation and states that his hand was injured from punching someone. On physical examination of the patient's hand, there is tenderness, swelling, and pain with palpation of the fifth metacarpal. Based upon the radiograph shown in Figure 17-4, what is the most appropriate initial intervention for stabilizing the injured structure?

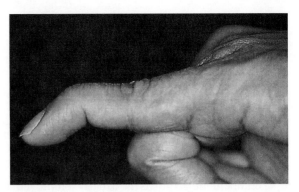

Figure 17-5. Reproduced, with permission, from Knoop KJ, Stack LB, Storrow AB, et al. *The Atlas of Emergency Medicine.* 3rd ed. New York, NY: McGraw-Hill Education, 2010. Figure 11–51. Photographer: Kevin J. Knoop, MD, MS.

(A)   Rupture or avulsion of the insertion of the extensor tendon at the base of the distal phalanx

(B)   Rupture or avulsion of the insertion of the flexor tendon at the base of the distal phalanx

(C)   Fracture of the middle phalanx

(D)   Dislocation of the distal interphalangeal joint

(E)   Fracture of the proximal phalanx

33. A 10-year-old boy presents to the emergency department status post a fall from his bicycle. The patient complains of pain located in his right knee with an associated 2- × 2-cm abrasion just inferior to the patella. There is no swelling noted of the knee. The child is not cooperative with examination of the extremity. Radiograph is taken of the right knee, and there is no finding of fracture or joint changes. Incidentally, a lesion is noted at the distal femur and is depicted on the Figure 17-6. Based upon the information provided and the radiographic presentation, what is the most likely diagnosis?

(A)   Osteoid osteoma

(B)   Chondrosarcoma

(C)   Osteosarcoma

(D)   Osteochondroma

(E)   Ewing sarcoma

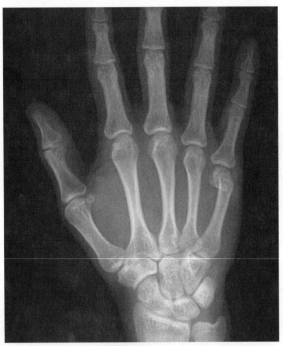

Figure 17-4. Reproduced, with permission, from Knoop KJ, Stack LB, Storrow AB, et al. The Atlas of Emergency Medicine. 3rd ed. New York: McGraw-Hill Education, 2010. Figure 11.32. Photographer: Cathleen M. Vossler, MD.

(A)   Thumb spica splint

(B)   Volar wrist splint

(C)   Ulnar gutter splint

(D)   Wrist and thumb spica cast

(E)   Buddy taping of fourth and fifth finger

32. A 33-year-old male presents with complaints of right index finger pain localized to the distal phalanx and an inability to actively extend the distal interphalangeal joint. Injury to the finger occurred when it was struck by a baseball. Based upon the information provided and Figure 17-5, what is the most likely anatomical structural cause of the deformity?

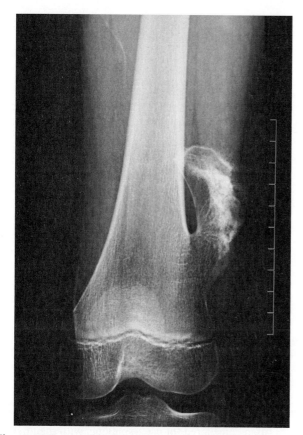

Figure 17-6. Reproduced, with permission, from Skinner HB, McMahon PJ. *Current Diagnosis & Treatment in Orthopedics.* 5th ed. New York, NY: McGraw-Hill Education, 2014. Figure 5-15.

34. A 39-year-old woman presents with complaints of left anterior knee pain of 4 weeks' duration. She has noted difficulty with going up and down the staircase. The patient also notes increased pain in the knee upon arising after being seated for a period. The pain may then improve with walking. The patient denies joint crepitus or locking sensation. On physical examination, there is no swelling or obvious joint distortion. The pain is reproduced with placing the knee in slight flexion and gentle pressure placed on the patella as the patient contracts the quadriceps. The knee appears stable, with no signs of crepitus, joint laxity, or internal derangement. Radiographs of the left knee are essentially benign. What course of treatment is best for this patient?

(A) Crutches for 6 weeks, keeping the joint nonweight bearing

(B) Cortisone injection

(C) Physical therapy to strengthen the quadriceps

(D) Physical therapy to strengthen the lower back

(E) Progress to orthopedic evaluation for consideration of internal derangement of the knee

35. A 17-year-old volleyball player complains of acute onset of right knee pain. During a game, she jumped to block a ball and when she landed, her knee gave out. The patient felt a shifting sensation and heard a "pop" at the time of the injury and immediately experienced pain inside her knee joint. Her knee swelled rapidly following the injury. Examination reveals a moderate knee joint effusion. Anterior drawer and Lachman testing are positive for lack of end feel. Posterior drawer, valgus and varus stress testing at 0 and 30 degrees do not cause pain and demonstrate a firm end feel. Lateral displacement of the patella while her knee is fully extended does not cause patient pain or apprehension. What structure is most likely to have been compromised?

(A) Medial patellar retinaculum

(B) Posterior cruciate ligament

(C) Anterior cruciate ligament

(D) Medial collateral ligament

(E) Arcuate complex

36. Which of the following clinical manifestations is most characteristic of polymyalgia rheumatica (PMR)?

(A) Subcutaneous inflammatory lesions

(B) Pain and stiffness of proximal muscle groups

(C) Insidious onset of symmetrical joint involvement

(D) Widespread musculoskeletal pain and tender points

(E) Symmetrical weakness initially in the legs that progresses caudally

37. A 53-year-old obese man presents with a third attack of gout within 1 year. Following the treatment of this acute attack, further laboratory testing is performed and the patient is found to have an elevated serum uric acid level and a 24-hour uric acid secretion of 950 mg (normal 250 to 750 mg per 24 hours). Which of the following medications would be most appropriate to initiate for prevention of further gouty attacks?

(A) Colchicine

(B) Probenecid

(C) Prednisone

(D) Allopurinol

(E) Indomethacin

38. A 32-year-old woman with history of anxiety presents with worsening fatigue and sleep disturbance associated with unbearable "pain all over the body" for the past several months. The physical examination is essentially unremarkable except for localized painful tenderness to palpation over the trapezius, upper back, and buttocks. Which of the following is the most likely diagnosis?

(A) Fibromyalgia

(B) Polymyositis

(C) Paget disease

(D) Polymyalgia rheumatica

(E) Systemic lupus erythematosus

39. A 28-year-old female presents with decreased appetite, weight loss, fever, and joint pain. Physical examination reveals thinning of her hair a facial rash depicted in Figure 17-7. Which of the following tests will be the most valuable in confirming your suspected diagnosis?

(A) Gliadin antibody

(B) Antibody to double-stranded DNA (anti-dsDNA)

(C) Antinuclear antibody (ANA)

(D) Anticentromere antibody

(E) Antiribosomal P antibody

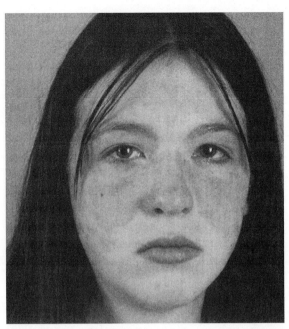

Figure 17-7. Reproduced, with permission from, Wolff K, Johnson RA, Suurmond D. *Fitzpatrick's Color Atlas & Synopsis of Clinical Dermatology.* 5th ed. New York, NY, McGraw-Hill Education, 2005; p. 385.

40. Tumor necrosis factor (TNF) inhibitors are most often considered for use in patients with rheumatoid arthritis (RA) that does not respond to initial therapy. Which of the following screenings should occur before a patient is placed on this class of medication?

(A) Chest x-ray

(B) Allergy testing

(C) Liver function tests

(D) Purified protein derivative (PPD) test

(E) Serum BUN (blood urea nitrogen) and creatinine test

41. A 44-year-old male presents with complaints of heartburn, joint aches, and finger stiffness. The heartburn has been present for approximately a year but has been progressively worsening heartburn over the past 3 to 4 months. Initially, he would experience intermittent heartburn but now it occurs after every meal. He reports a long-standing history of skin coloration changes involving his fingers when they are exposed to a cold environment that has never been formally diagnosed. He is concerned about his fingers due to recent bouts of swelling and difficulty making a fist because his fingers feel tight. Which of the following is the most likely diagnosis?

(A) Sarcoidosis

(B) Scleroderma

(C) Dermatomyositis

(D) Eosinophilic fasciitis

(E) Eosinophilia–myalgia syndrome

42. A 6-year-old girl is diagnosed with juvenile idiopathic arthritis (JIA). Which of the following referrals is indicated, especially if the patient also has a positive antinuclear antibody test?

(A) Ophthalmologist for a screening eye examination

(B) Otolaryngologist for a screening hearing examination

(C) Dermatologist for evaluation of skin expression of the disease

(D) Endocrinologist for evaluation of potential growth restriction

(E) Gastroenterologist for evaluation of potential peptic ulcer disease

43. You are evaluating a patient for a lateral ankle pain after they rolled their ankle inwards (Figure 17-8). The patient was unable to weight bear for four steps immediately after the injury and at the time of the evaluation. Tenderness in which area would indicate the need for radiographs?

(A) 1

(B) 2

(C) 3

(D) 4

(E) 5

44. A 65-year-old man presents with complaints of acute onset of pain and swelling of the right great toe. He denies recent alcohol ingestion or trauma to the area. On physical examination, the patient is afebrile, and the first metatarsophalangeal joint is erythematous, swollen, and warm to the touch. Laboratory evaluation reveals a WBC (white blood cells) count of 12,000/mL and a normal differential. Serum uric acid level is found to be 5 mg/dL. Synovial fluid analysis reveals the presence of rhomboid-shaped crystals. Which of the following is the most likely diagnosis?

(A) Acute gout

(B) Pseudogout

(C) Psoriatic arthritis

(D) Infectious arthritis

(E) Rheumatoid arthritis

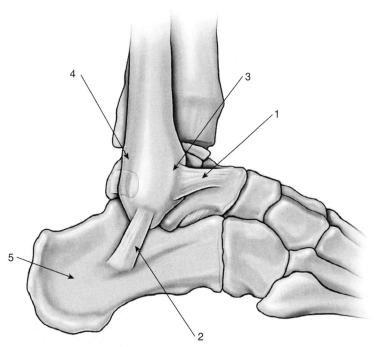

Figure 17-8. Reproduced, with permission, from Morton DA. *The Big Picture: Gross Anatomy.* New York, NY: McGraw-Hill Education, 2011. Figure 37–5B.

45. Which of the following treatment options for osteoporosis has the added benefit of reducing the risk of breast cancer?

    (A) Calcitonin
    (B) Raloxifene
    (C) Alendronate
    (D) Teriparatide
    (E) Conjugated estrogen

46. Which of the following patterns of stiffness is most characteristic of patients with rheumatoid arthritis?

    (A) Morning stiffness lasting at least 1 hour
    (B) Exacerbation of joint stiffness with walking
    (C) Frequent, brief episodes of stiffness after inactivity
    (D) Stiffness reflected by a major delay in muscle relaxation
    (E) Stiffness evidenced by increased resistance to passive movement

47. Related infections that have been identified as triggers of reactive arthritis include sexually transmitted infections and which of the following other types of infections?

    (A) Ear infections
    (B) Eye infections
    (C) Enteric infections
    (D) Musculoskeletal infections
    (E) Central nervous system infections

48. A 59-year-old woman with a known history of rheumatoid arthritis presents with relatively severe complaints of pain, notable bony deformity of the hands with extra-articular findings of cutaneous nodules, scleritis, and pleurisy. On physical examination, the patient is found to have splenomegaly. Which of the following is the most appropriate laboratory evaluation in order to further evaluate the suspected diagnosis?

    (A) Complete blood count (CBC)
    (B) Uric acid
    (C) C-reactive protein
    (D) Antinuclear antibodies
    (E) Erythrocyte sedimentation rate

49. A 45-year-old woman with recent diagnosis of rheumatoid arthritis has begun treatment with celecoxib. She has been on this medication for 3 months and notes that her pain continues. Early signs of joint involvement are present in the patient's hands. Which of the following medications is the most appropriate to add to her treatment?

    (A) Aspirin
    (B) Rituximab
    (C) Etanercept
    (D) Leflunomide
    (E) Methotrexate

50. A 12-year-old girl presents with complaints of intermittent pain and stiffness involving her hands. This pain has been progressively worsening over the past 3 years. She relates that for the past 2 months she has been feeling increasingly tired and has experienced swelling and stiffness of her hands, which appears worse in the morning and is relieved as the day progresses. The physical examination shows she has a low-grade fever. There are multiple symmetrical joint swelling of the proximal interphalangeal and metacarpophalangeal joints with associated warmth, tenderness, and effusion. Initial laboratory findings include a complete blood count (CBC) that reveals mild anemia, an elevated erythrocyte sedimentation rate, a positive rheumatoid factor, and a negative antinuclear antibody (ANA) test. X-rays of the hands and wrists show soft tissue swelling and periarticular osteopenia. Which of the following is the most likely diagnosis?

    (A) Reactive arthritis
    (B) Infectious arthritis
    (C) Systemic juvenile idiopathic arthritis
    (D) Polyarticular juvenile idiopathic arthritis
    (E) Pauciarticular juvenile idiopathic arthritis

51. A 48-year-old woman presents with a chief complaint of gradually progressing difficulty in climbing stairs over the past 3 months. The physical examination shows there is notable proximal muscle weakness of the upper and lower extremities. The remainder of the examination is unremarkable. The laboratory evaluation shows an elevated serum creatinine phosphokinase level, and a muscle biopsy reveals lymphoid inflammatory infiltrates. Which of the following is the appropriate initial treatment of choice in this patient?

(A) Prednisone

(B) Azathioprine

(C) Methotrexate

(D) Immunoglobulin

(E) Hydroxychloroquine

52. A 47-year-old obese male presents with complaints of left toe pain and swelling. Pain onset occurred 2 days ago. Patient denies any form of trauma. He reports that any form of contact to the first toe region is exquisitely painful. While obtaining additional historical information you identify that the day prior to the onset of the pain and swelling he had eaten a significant amount of shrimp. Based upon the information that has been provided and the photo shown in Figure 17-9, which of the following is the correct term to describe his condition?

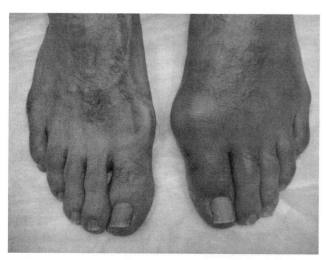

Figure 17-9. Reproduced, with permission, from *DeGowin's Diagnostic Examination*. 10th ed. Plate 30.

(A) Crepitus

(B) Podagra

(C) Xerostomia

(D) Paronychi

(E) Chondrocalcinosis

53. Which of the following is an established risk factor for osteoporosis and is also an indication for measuring bone density?

(A) Obesity

(B) Alcoholism

(C) Hypercalcemia

(D) History of scoliosis

(E) Short-term corticosteroid therapy

54. A 22-year-old man presents with an insidious onset of low back pain over the last 6 months. He describes the pain as dull and has difficulty localizing the pain. The pain often radiates to his thighs. The pain is worse in the morning and associated with stiffening that lessens during the day. The patient notes that there is no history of trauma. The initial laboratory evaluation shows an elevated erythrocyte sedimentation rate, positive HLA-B27, and a negative rheumatoid factor. Plain films of the lumbar spine reveal bilateral blurring of the sacroiliac joints. Which of the following is the most likely diagnosis?

(A) Systemic lupus

(B) Lumbar disc disease

(C) Rheumatoid arthritis

(D) Ankylosing spondylitis

(E) Polymyalgia rheumatica

55. A 65-year-old woman with long-standing rheumatoid arthritis presents for a preoperative evaluation appointment. She is scheduled for a total joint arthroplasty in 2 weeks. Which of the following is the most appropriate intervention to detect an associated condition that may lead to complications during anesthesia?

(A) HLA (human leukocyte antigen) typing

(B) Slit-lamp examination

(C) Thoracoscopic lung biopsy

(D) Repeat rheumatoid factor

(E) Flexion and extension x-rays of cervical spine

56. Which of the following clinical manifestations is associated with systemic disorders that are HLA-B27 related, including ankylosing spondylitis, reactive arthritis, psoriasis, and Behçet syndrome?

(A) Uveitis

(B) Dysentery

(C) Vasculitis

(D) Hyperuricemia

(E) Thoracic involvement

57. A 67-year-old man presents with pain and stiffness in his shoulders and hips lasting for several weeks with no history of trauma. He also has complaints of headache, throat pain, and jaw claudication. It is imperative to diagnose this patient promptly in order to prevent which of the following complications?

(A) Anemia
(B) Cerebral aneurysms
(C) Mononeuritis multiplex
(D) Ischemic optic neuropathy
(E) Respiratory tract complications

58. Which of the following is a cause of inflammatory polyarthritis?

(A) Gout
(B) Osteoarthritis
(C) Reactive arthritis
(D) Psoriatic arthritis
(E) Systemic lupus erythematosus

59. A 65-year-old woman presents with severe midback pain of 2 weeks duration. She has no history of trauma. Radiographic evaluation reveals compression fractures of T11 and T12. A complete blood count, erythrocyte sedimentation rate, serum protein, serum calcium, phosphate, and parathyroid hormone levels are all within normal ranges. In addition to ordering a dual-energy x-ray absorptiometry (DEXA) scan, which of the following laboratory evaluations is most helpful in evaluating this patient for secondary causes of this presentation?

(A) Bone biopsy
(B) Rheumatoid factor
(C) Serum magnesium
(D) 25-hydroxyvitamin D
(E) Antinuclear antibodies test

60. Which of the following HLA haplotypes is strongly associated with rheumatoid arthritis?

(A) HLA-B8
(B) HLA-B27
(C) HLA-B51
(D) HLA-DR4
(E) HLA-DRB3

61. Reactive arthritis most commonly presents with a tetrad of urethritis, conjunctivitis, mucocutaneous lesions, and oligoarthritis. Which of the following joints are most commonly involved with this condition?

(A) Sacroiliac joints
(B) Metatarsophalangeal joints
(C) Large weight-bearing joints
(D) Metacarpophalangeal joints
(E) Distal interphalangeal joints

62. A 58-year-old postmenopausal woman presents for a routine annual examination. She is concerned about osteoporosis and is currently taking no medications. While counseling the patient about calcium intake along with the appropriate amount of vitamin D, what amount of calcium per day should be recommended for this patient?

(A) 700 mg
(B) 1,000 mg
(C) 1,200 mg
(D) 1,500 mg
(E) 2,000 mg

63. Which of the following medications has been shown to have a definite association with the potential development of systemic lupus erythematosus?

(A) Isoniazid
(B) Penicillin
(C) Gold salts
(D) Allopurinol
(E) Griseofulvin

64. A 52-year-old man with hypertension associated with recent unexplained weight loss presents with fever, malaise, and gradual onset of pain and weakness of his leg muscles for the past month. Physical examination reveals a mottled reticular pattern overlying portions of both calves and an area of ulceration with surrounding induration on the left lateral malleolus. Initial laboratory results reveal mild normochromic anemia, leukocytosis, and elevation of C-reactive protein, BUN, and creatinine. Which of the following is the most appropriate diagnostic evaluation to confirm the suspected diagnosis?

(A) HLA-B27 typing
(B) Rheumatoid factor

(C) MRI of sacroiliac joints

(D) Antinuclear antibodies test

(E) Tissue biopsy of area of induration

65. Patients diagnosed with Sjögren syndrome should be counseled to avoid which of the following class of medications?

(A) Penicillins

(B) Decongestants

(C) Antihistamines

(D) Corticosteroids

(E) Fluoroquinolones

66. A 10-year-old boy presents with complaints of left posterior heel pain for 3 months. Pain onset was insidious. His parents describe him as a very active child and that currently he his participating in a youth soccer league and a youth basketball league. Pain is increased with weight-bearing activities, especially running and jumping. His parents report that he will limp at times, especially if he has both soccer and basketball practice the same day. Pain will decrease with rest and ice. Pain is the least severe when he first awakes in the morning. He denies night pain. Examination of the left foot and ankle region reveals no erythema, swelling, or obvious deformities. Pain is reproduced with calcaneal compression. Active and passive foot and ankle range of motion is pain free and equal bilaterally. What is the most likely diagnosis?

(A) Achilles tendonitis

(B) Calcaneal apophysitis

(C) Plantar fasciitis

(D) Calcaneal osteomyelitis

(E) Retrocalcaneal bursitis

67. Inflammation of a growth plate typically caused by repetitive activity is defined as:

(A) Apophysitis

(B) Epicondylitis

(C) Epicondylosis

(D) Osteomyelitis

(E) Osteochondritis

68. A 35-year-old male presents to the emergency department with complaint of pain and numbness in both legs after a traumatic fall. He also tells you that he is having problems controlling his bladder and has urinated in his clothes involuntarily. Upon physical examination, you note bilateral lower extremity sensory and motor deficits across multiple myotomes and dermatomes. There is poor sphincter tone with digital rectal examination. Which is the most appropriate initial treatment?

(A) Emergency surgery consult

(B) Nonsteroidal anti-inflammatory drugs (NSAIDs) and activity restriction for 5 to 7 days

(C) Epidural corticosteroid injections

(D) Physical therapy referral

(E) Parenteral antibiotics

69. A patient has been attempting to self-manage their lateral elbow pain which they believe is due to "tennis elbow." Part of the self-management has included the utilization of a "tennis elbow brace" that is depicted in Figure 17-10. The patient is concerned because they have developed numbness on the dorsal aspect of the hand between the first and second metacarpals. You suspect this numbness is iatrogenically induced through the use of their brace. What structure is most likely injured?

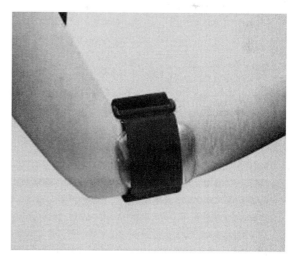

Figure 17-10. Reproduced, with permission, from Hoogenboom BJ, Voight ML, Prentice WE. *Musculoskeletal Interventions: Techniques for Therapeutic Exercise.* 3rd ed. New York, NY: McGraw-Hill Education, 2014. Figure 21–23.

(A) Radial nerve

(B) Ulnar nerve

(C) Musculocutaneous nerve

(D) Median nerve

(E) Axillary nerve

70. A 50-year-old female presents with complaints of left shoulder pain that has been present for 6 months. She denies history of traumatic injury. The pain has been progressively worsening. Shoulder pain and tightness restrict her from being able to reach out the side and perform overhead activities. Physical examination of the left shoulder reveals a significant limitation of both active and passive shoulder external rotation range of motion and a moderate limitation of both active and passive shoulder flexion. Resisted shoulder range of motion testing is pain free and demonstrates no strength loss. What is the most likely diagnosis?

    (A) Subacromial impingement syndrome
    (B) Bicipital tendonitis
    (C) Infraspinatus rotator cuff tear
    (D) Supraspinatus rotator cuff tear
    (E) Adhesive capsulitis

71. You diagnosis a patient as having adhesive capsulitis and based upon history and physical examination make the determination that the patient is in the inflammatory phase. What would be the most appropriate initial therapeutic intervention for the patient at this time?

    (A) Subacromial corticosteroid injection
    (B) Glenohumeral intra-articular corticosteroid injection
    (C) Orthopedic surgery referral for a manipulation under anesthesia
    (D) Sling immobilization for 4 to 6 weeks
    (E) Referral for chiropractic manipulation

72. A 48-year-old male presents for evaluation of injury to his Achilles tendon. The injury occurred yesterday while he was playing tennis. He was attempting to change direction when he felt a "pop" in Achilles tendon region and he felt like he was kicked in the back part of his leg. Since the injury he has been unable to put any weight on the involved extremity. He provides additional history that for the past 6 months his primary care provider has been treating him for Achilles tendonitis. Which of the following most likely contributed to his traumatic injury?

    (A) Corticosteroid injection into the Achilles tendon
    (B) Short course of nonsteroidal anti-inflammatory drugs (NSAIDs)

    (C) Physical therapy
    (D) Daily ice application
    (E) Heel lift support

73. Which of the following medication classes is associated with increased risk of tendinopathy and tendon ruptures?

    (A) Tetracyclines
    (B) Aminoglycosides
    (C) Fluoroquinolones
    (D) Macrolides
    (E) Clindamycin

74. A 56-year-old diabetic female presents for evaluation of a recurrent catching sensation involving the ring finger of her right hand. When she attempts to make a fist it feels like her ring finger "gets stuck" halfway through the motion, if she keeps trying to flex her ring finger she will feel a pop and will then be able to fully flex the ring finger and make a fist. On examination, there is no obvious erythema involving the ring finger. The skin is not warm to touch. You palpate a nontender nodule just distal to the palmar crease of the ring finger. Which of the following is the most likely diagnosis?

    (A) Stenosing flexor tenosynovitis
    (B) Flexor tendon rupture
    (C) Palmar fascia fibrosis
    (D) Metacarpophalangeal joint sprain
    (E) Flexor tendon sheath infection

75. A 32-year-old male presents with complaints of low back pain for 5 years. The pain has been progressively worsening. He does not remember a traumatic event associated with the initial pain onset. The back pain is worse in the morning. There is associated stiffness of the low back region that takes several hours to loosen up. He has found that working out at the gym in the morning the back pain and stiffness will improve. During your examination, you identify a loss of lumbar flexion range of motion. Due to the duration of his symptoms and motion limitation radiographs of the lumbar spine are obtained and the lateral view is depicted in Figure 17-11. Which of the following laboratory tests would support the diagnosis?

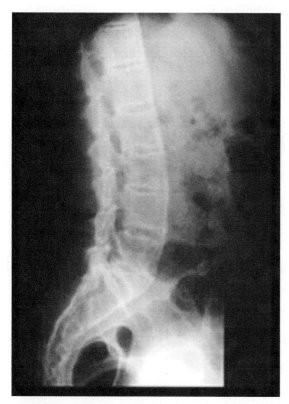

Figure 17-11. Current medical diagnosis & treatment 2015 > Rheumatologic & immunologic disorders > eFigure 20-23.

(A) Antinuclear antibody (ANA)

(B) Human leukocyte antigen B27 (HLA-B27)

(C) Rheumatoid factor (RF)

(D) Erythrocyte sedimentation rate (ESR)

(E) Antibodies to cyclic citrullinated peptides (anti-CCP)

76. You are in the process of evaluating a 19-year-old runner for leg pain that has been present for 4 weeks. Initially the pain was present only when running but now the pain is constant. There is no history of traumatic injury. Palpation of the tibia identifies a focal area of bony tenderness that correlates with the patients pain complaints. Radiographs of the tibia and fibula are negative for a cortical fracture line. Based upon the information provided which of the following would be the most appropriate diagnostic study to order next?

(A) Magnetic resonance imaging (MRI)

(B) Pre- and postexercise compartmental pressures

(C) Computed tomography (CT) scan

(D) Radionuclide bone scan

(E) Musculoskeletal ultrasound (US)

77. A 52-year-old woman presents to your primary care clinic with complaints of cervical pain. The cervical pain onset was gradual and she has been experiencing the pain for the past 6 months. The pain is present for a majority of the day and is exacerbated when she extends her neck to look upward. Utilization of a cervical pillow allows her to sleep pain free at night. Physical examination reveals limitation of cervical extension as well as right and left cervical rotation due to pain. Due to the range of motion limitations you order cervical radiographs and the lateral view is depicted in Figure 17-12. Based on the information provided which of the following is the most likely diagnosis?

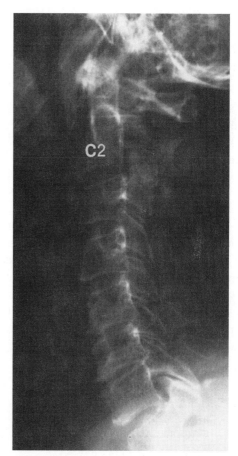

Figure 17-12. Reproduced, with permission, from Chen MYM, Pope TL, Ott DJ. *Basic Radiology.* 2nd ed. New York, NY: McGraw-Hill Education, 2011. Figure 13-11.

(A) Ankylosing spondylitis

(B) Cervical spondylolisthesis

(C) Cervical osteoarthritis

(D) Metastatic tumor

(E) Torticollis

78. You are evaluating a 13-year-old male for progressively worsening thoracic pain that has been present for the past 6 months. The patient characterizes the pain as a dull ache that is present all of the time. If he tries to lean backward and extend his upper back, the pain will become sharp. His parents have noticed that his upper back has been becoming progressively more rounded over the past several years. Radiographs (x-rays) of the thoracic spine reveal anterior wedging of four adjacent thoracic vertebrae, the degree of wedging ranges from 7 to 10 degrees. What is the most likely cause of his pain?

(A) Ankylosing spondylitis

(B) Postural kyphosis

(C) Thoracic scoliosis

(D) Scheuermann kyphosis

(E) Thoracolumbar scoliosis

79. An 18-year-old patient presents to the emergency department after sustaining a contusion to the anterolateral aspect of his lower leg (tib-fib region) 12 hours ago. The contusion occurred when a lacrosse ball hits him. Despite ice, over the counter NSAIDs and elevation of the involved extremity, his pain has been progressively worsening. Examination of the leg reveals a tense skin along the anterolateral aspect of the leg and pain with passive stretch of the ankle dorsiflexors. Radiographs are obtained and there is no evidence of fracture. During the course of your evaluation the patients pedal pulse on the involved extremity has diminished from 2+ to 1+. What would be most appropriate test to confirm your suspected diagnosis?

(A) Compartmental pressure testing

(B) Ankle-brachial index (ABI)

(C) Magnetic resonance imaging (MRI)

(D) Lower extremity vascular Doppler ultrasound (US)

(E) Serum creatine kinase (CK)

80. A 25-year-old male presents to the emergency department with complaints of left shoulder pain and limited function. He injured the shoulder 3 hours ago while wrestling. When the injury occurred he felt a shifting sensation inside his shoulder and since that point in time he has been unable to move his left upper extremity. On examination, you note fullness in the anterior aspect of the left shoulder

and that the shoulder is slightly abducted and externally rotated. You obtain radiograph of the shoulder which is depicted in Figure 17-13. What structure is most at risk based upon the injury he has sustained?

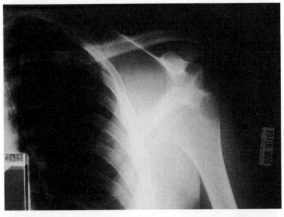

Figure 17-13. Reproduced, with permission, from Knoop KJ, Stack LB, Storrow AB, et al. The atlas of emergency medicine. 3rd ed. New York, NY: McGraw-Hill Education, 2010. Figure 11–5. Photographer: Kevin J. Knoop, MD, MS.

(A) Axillary nerve

(B) Ulnar nerve

(C) Median nerve

(D) Radial nerve

(E) Musculocutaneous

81. A father is concerned because his 5-year-old son is favoring his right elbow and is very reluctant to use his right arm. The child localizes his pain the lateral aspect of the elbow. The child denies a traumatic fall and denies direct trauma to the area. The father reports that the pain began after he lifted his son off the ground by grabbing on his wrists and pulling him upward. What is the most likely diagnosis?

(A) Radial head subluxation

(B) Lateral epicondylitis

(C) Radial head fracture

(D) Ulnar nerve injury

(E) Olecranon apophysitis

82. Corticosteroid use can predispose a patient to which of the following?

(A) Osteonecrosis

(B) Osteoarthritis

(C) Adhesive capsulitis

(D) Ankylosing spondylitis

(E) Rheumatoid arthritis

83. A 59-year-old male presents with complaints of pain and stiffness involving the fingers that is worse when he first awakens in the morning. A majority of the pain and stiffness is localized to the distal interphalangeal (DIP) joints. He has been self-managing the pain with oral nonsteroidal anti-inflammatory drugs (NSAIDs). On physical examination, you note enlargement of the DIP joints that is depicted on Figure 17-14. The DIP joints are tender with palpation but not warm to touch. What is the appropriate term for these enlargements?

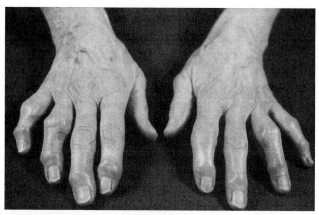

Figure 17-14. Reproduced, with permission, from Kasper D, Fauci A, Hauser S, et al. Harrison's Principles of Internal Medicine. 19th ed. New York: McGraw-Hill Education, 2015. Figure 394-2.

(A) Podagra

(B) Bouchard nodes

(C) Heberden nodes

(D) Schmorl nodes

(E) Gottron papules

84. A 65-year-old male presents with complaints of right knee pain. Pain onset was gradual and initially began several years ago. The pain has been progressively increasing and in the past 6 months has begun to limit his activity level. Examination of the right knee reveals a mild joint effusion. There is no erythema and the knee is not warm to touch. Active and passive knee flexion is limited approximately 5 degrees from end range due to knee tightness. Weight-bearing radiograph of the right knee is

obtained and demonstrated in Figure 17-15. What would be the most appropriate initial therapeutic intervention at this time?

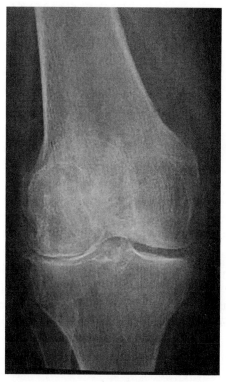

Figure 17-15. Reproduced, with permission, from Maitin IB. Current diagnosis & treatment: physical medicine & rehabilitation. New York, NY: McGraw-Hill Education, 2015. Figure 33-4.

(A) Intra-articular hyaluronate injections

(B) Oral opioids

(C) Oral nonsteroidal anti-inflammatory drugs (NSAIDs)

(D) Intra-articular corticosteroid injection

(E) Total knee replacement

85. A 67-year-old female is in for follow-up after sustaining a humeral shaft fracture 1 week ago. She is concerned because over the past several days she has developed an inability to extend her wrist. What nerve has she likely injured?

(A) Axillary

(B) Median

(C) Ulnar

(D) Radial

(E) Musculocutaneous

Answers and Explanations

1. **(E)** The most common mechanism of injury for an ankle sprain is combined inversion and plantar flexion. This mechanism injures the anterior talofibular ligament rather than the calcaneofibular ligament. Injury to the anterior talofibular ligament will result tenderness when the ligament is palpated. Pain and loss of a firm endpoint with anterior drawer testing is consistent with injury to the anterior talofibular ligament. Pure inversion mechanism of injury stresses the calcaneofibular ligament and pure eversion mechanism of injury stresses the middle portion of the deltoid ligament. Pure plantar flexion injuries are much more likely to cause injury to the midfoot (Lisfranc sprain) and rarely injure the ankle ligaments. The combined mechanism of the eversion and plantar flexion injures the anterior portion of the deltoid ligament. *(Luke & Ma, 2014, Ch. 41)*

2. **(E)** Bicipital tendonitis is an inflammation of the long head of the biceps tendon and tendon sheath, which causes anterior shoulder pain that, resembles and often accompanies coexisting rotator cuff tendonitis. Tenderness with bicipital tendonitis is reproduced with Yergason test. During Yergason test, the shoulder pain is exacerbated when the arm is held at the side, elbow flexed to 90 degrees, and the patient is asked to supinate and flex the forearm against your resistance. Rotator cuff injuries often accompany bicipital tendonitis, and bicipital tendonitis can occur secondary to compensation for rotator cuff disorders or labral tears. In this case, the pain is clearly reproduced in a pattern suggestive of bicipital tendonitis. Acromioclavicular sprains can result in pain with overhead activities but the area of palpable tenderness will be over the acromioclavicular joint, not the biceps tendon. The cross arm test is the provocative test that would reproduce the shoulder pain associated with an acromioclavicular joint sprain. There is no historical component that would suggest a recent shoulder dislocation and there is no mention of positive apprehension test, which would be indicative of anterior shoulder instability. *(Boyd, Martinez, & Feden, 2011, Ch. 37)*

3. **(B)** The maneuver described is commonly referred to as the supraspinatus strength test or the "empty the can" test. Weakness in this maneuver is suggestive of injury to supraspinatus tendon. The teres minor and infraspinatus tendons are external rotators and are often tested with the arm at 90 degrees of elbow flexion with the patient attempting to externally rotate against resistance. The subscapularis is also tested at 90 degrees of elbow flexion with resistance applied as the patient attempts to internally rotate against resistance. *(Bickley & Szilagyi, 2013, p. 625)*

4. **(B)** Distal radius fractures are commonly associated with falls, especially falls on an outstretched hand. Middle-aged and elderly patients, especially those with osteoporosis, are susceptible to these injuries. A Colles fracture is classically described as dorsally angulated and displaced distal radius metaphysical fracture. A Smith fracture, sometimes referred to as a reverse Colles fracture, is an extra-articular metaphysical fracture of the radius with volar angulation and displacement. Barton fracture is a displaced unstable articular fracture-subluxation of the distal radius with volar displacement. A boxer fracture classically involves the fifth metacarpal bone and is associated with a closed hand trauma. A Monteggia fracture involves a fracture of the ulna shaft and a dislocation of the radial head. *(Escarza et al., 2011, Ch. 266)*

5. **(B)** Legg–Calvé–Perthes disease is idiopathic osteonecrosis of the femoral head in children. The

condition typically affects children between the ages of 4 and 8 years, but the range of onset is 2 to 12 years of age. It is unilateral in 90% of patients and four times more common in male population. Typically, the patient presents with a limp that worsens with activity and is thus more noticeable at the end of the day. If the child reports pain, it is typically an aching in the groin or proximal thigh. *(Sarwark, 2010, Sect. 9, pp. 1122–1126)*

6. **(D)** The scaphoid bone is based on the proximal row of carpal bones but extends into the distal row, making it more vulnerable to injury when a patient falls on an outstretched hand. The scaphoid bone is the most frequently injured carpal bone, accounting for 60% to 70% of all carpal fractures. At the time of initial injury, 10% to 15% of scaphoid fractures may not be visible on plain radiographs. Patients with pain in the anatomical snuffbox to palpation or axial loading, even with normal radiographs, should be treated as though they have a scaphoid fracture and placed in a thumb spica splint. Repeat radiographs should be taken after 1 to 2 weeks. If radiographs are still normal but tenderness over the scaphoid bone persists, an MRI should be ordered. Fractures of the scaphoid have a high incidence of nonunion and osteonecrosis because the major blood supply enters in the distal segment of the bone and can be disrupted with injury/fracture and thus conservative management is warranted. *(Sarwark, 2010, Sect. 4, pp. 484–487)*

7. **(C)** Dupuytren contracture is a painless nodular thickening and contracture of the palmar fascia that leads to a gradually progressive loss of active and passive finger extension range of motion. Males of northern European descent are the patient population that is most commonly affected. Jersey finger and trigger finger involve tendon ruptures at the distal interphalangeal joint that result in loss of active motion but passive motion is maintained. Patients with trigger finger classically complain of pain and catching when they flex their finger. Gamekeeper injuries typically occur at the first metacarpophalangeal joint and involve injury to the ulnar collateral ligament. Ganglion cysts of flexor tendon sheath can present as a tender mass in the palm but rarely do they limit active or passive range of motion. *(Sarwark, 2010, Sect. 4, pp. 447–449)*

8. **(B)** The symptom profile points toward a diagnosis of Morton neuroma. Morton neuroma is a perineural fibrosis of the common digital nerve as it passes between the metatarsal heads. It commonly occurs between the third and fourth toes and is associated with dysesthesias into the affected toes. Many patients state that they feel as though they are "walking on a marble" or that they feel as if they have a pebble in their shoe. Symptoms are made worse by wearing high-heeled or tight, restrictive shoes. Hammer toe presents as a flexion deformity of the proximal interphalangeal joint. Tenderness over the plantar aspect of the metatarsal head(s) would be the expected physical examination finding with metatarsalgia. Focal bone tenderness, most commonly along the metatarsal shaft, would consistent with a metatarsal stress fracture. Metatarsophalangeal synovitis should be suspected when there is tenderness and swelling of the involved metatarsophalangeal joint. *(Sarwark, 2010, Sect. 7, pp. 827–829)*

9. **(C)** Gonococcal arthritis usually occurs in otherwise healthy individuals, is two to three times more common in women than in men, is especially common during menses and pregnancy, and is rare after age 40. There are two forms of gonococcal arthritis. Septic arthritis, the purulent monoarthritis form, occurs approximately 40% of the time; and the bacteremic form, characterized by a triad of migratory polyarthritis, tenosynovitis, and dermatitis, occurs approximately 60% of the time. Septic monoarthritis most frequently involves the knee, elbow, wrist, or ankle. Less than one-fourth of patients have any genitourinary symptoms. Patients with septic arthritis complain of pain, swelling, and redness beginning days to weeks after gonococcal infection. *Staphylococcus aureus* is a gram-positive organism that is the most common cause of nongonococcal septic arthritis. *Escherichia coli* and *Pseudomonas aeruginosa* are the most common nongonococcal gram-negative isolates in adults. Gram-negative septic arthritis occurs with more frequency in injection drug users and immunocompromised patients. *(Hellmann & Imboden, 2014, Ch. 20)*

10. **(A)** This patient presentation is most consistent with De Quervain tendinitis or tenosynovitis of the abductor pollicis longus and extensor pollicis brevis. The thickening of the tendon sheath and resultant tendon inflammation causes pain, swelling, and a

triggering phenomenon of locking or sticking. This disorder is more common in middle-aged women and in repetitive motion injuries. On physical examination, the finding of a positive Finkelstein test, which is pain with full flexion of the thumb into the palm, with ulnar deviation of the wrist, is diagnostic of De Quervain tendinitis. Initial treatment is aimed at immobilization of the wrist to allow for pain and inflammatory relief. A course of nonsteroidal anti-inflammatory drugs (NSAIDs) is helpful for pain relief as well. Corticosteroid injection is reserved for patients who fail with immobilization and NSAID use. Operative treatment should be considered only if injections are not helpful. Radiographic evaluation is not helpful in the evaluation or treatment of this condition. (*Sarwark, 2010, Sect. 4, pp. 443–446*)

11. **(B)** A Boutonniere deformity classically presents as persistent flexion of the proximal interphalangeal joint with hyperextension of the distal interphalangeal joint. A swan neck deformity classically manifests as hyperextension of the proximal interphalangeal joint with fixed flexion of the distal interphalangeal joint. Heberden nodes are found on the dorsolateral aspects of the distal interphalangeal joints and can lead to flexion or deviation deformities at the involved joint. Jersey finger involves a flexor tendon rupture most commonly at the distal phalanx with a resultant inability to flex at the distal interphalangeal joint but no deformity or loss of function at the proximal interphalangeal joint. Mallet finger is an extensor tendon injury that presents as flexion deformity at distal interphalangeal joint with the patient unable to extend at the involved joint, there is no deformity or loss of function at the proximal interphalangeal joint. (*Bickley & Szilagyi, 2013, p. 649*)

12. **(C)** Disc herniation at the L4–L5 level will affect the L5 nerve root. L5 nerve root irritation causes sensory changes in the first dorsal web space between the first and second toes and motor weakness with first toe dorsiflexion (extension). Disc herniation at the L2–L3 level will affect the L3 nerve root. L3 nerve root irritation causes sensory changes in the anterolateral thigh, motor weakness with knee extension, and diminished patellar tendon reflex. Disc herniation at the L3–L4 level will affect the L4 nerve root. L4 nerve root irritation causes sensory changes in the medial calf, motor weakness with dorsiflexion of the ankle, and diminished

patellar tendon reflex. Disc herniation at the L5–S1 level affects the S1 nerve, which causes sensory changes on the lateral aspect of the foot, motor weakness with plantar flexion of the ankle, and diminished Achilles reflex. Disc herniation at the S1–S2 level will affect the S2 nerve. S2 nerve root irritation causes sensory changes in the posterior thigh and motor weakness with knee flexion. (*Luke & Ma, 2014, Ch. 41*)

13. **(D)** The patient's symptoms and signs have worsened over the past 2 weeks. In particular, she has experienced the following "red flags": failure to improve after 4 to 6 weeks of conservative therapy, unrelenting night pain, and progressive motor or sensory deficit. Conservative therapy is not warranted in the face of these red flags. Plain radiographs are not highly sensitive or specific. They are reasonably useful to identify compression fractures and degenerative changes in the spine. CT is relatively good for revealing most bony spinal pathology. Lower extremity nerve conduction testing can be utilized to assess the physiologic function of the nerve root but will not provide insight regarding the pathologic anatomical changes at the lumbar spine. MRI provides the most detailed images of the soft tissues of the disc and nerve roots. Since the symptom profile points toward a nerve root irritation more than a bony abnormality, MRI would be the appropriate choice at this time. (*Luke & Ma, 2014, Ch. 41*)

14. **(B)** The presence of needle-like and negatively birefringent crystals visualized under polarized light combined with the patient's history and physical examination findings is consistent with an acute gout attack involving the first metatarsophalangeal joint. Although serial measurements of the serum uric acid detect hyperuricemia in 95% of patients, a single uric acid determination during an acute flare of gout is normal in up to 25% of cases. Initial management of an acute gout attack is an oral nonsteroidal anti-inflammatory drug such as indomethacin or oral low-dose colchicine. Oral glucocorticoids such as prednisone should be utilized only when a patient presents with contraindications to the use of both nonsteroidal anti-inflammatories and colchicine. Gout is an inflammatory arthropathy so heat application should be avoided because of the potential for increasing the inflammatory response. Allopurinol is a urate-lowering medication and is of

no benefit when initiated during an acute gout attack. *(Hellmann & Imboden, 2014, Ch. 20)*

15. **(D)** The patient demonstrates an elevated temperature with evidence of infection and proximal lymphangitis from wounds in the antecubital crease. Intravenous drug use should be suspected with this presentation. Osteomyelitis is a serious infection of the bone. Osteomyelitis resulting from bacteremia is a disease associated with injection drug users that commonly develops in the spine. Patients with osteomyelitis often present with sudden onset of fever, chills, and pain and tenderness over the involved bone. Traditionally, antibiotics have been administered parenterally for at least 4 to 6 weeks. Parenteral weekly antibiotics or oral antibiotics will not be sufficient to effectively treat the infection. Straight-leg raise test is positive for lumbar radiculopathy if pain in the sciatic distribution is reproduced between 30 and 70 degrees passive flexion of the straight leg. The patients' complaints of hamstring pain with the straight-leg raise are most likely due to stretching of the hamstring musculature. *(Hellmann & Imboden, 2014, Ch. 20)*

16. **(C)** In a Salter–Harris type III fracture the fracture line extends intra-articularly from the epiphysis, through the physis, with the cleavage plane continuing along the physis to the periphery. Salter–Harris type I fractures occur when the epiphysis separates from the metaphysis. Salter–Harris type II fractures occur when the fracture line extends a variable distance along the physis and then out through a piece of metaphyseal bone. In Salter–Harris type IV injuries the fracture line originates at the articular surface and extends through the epiphysis, the entire thickness of the physis, and continues through the metaphysis. In Salter–Harris type V injuries there is a compression of the physis with minimal displacement of the epiphysis. *(Hopkins-Mann et al., 2011, Ch. 133)*

17. **(E)** The mechanism of injury suggests a posterior hip dislocation. In a posterior hip dislocation, the femur is dislocated posterior to the acetabulum when the thigh is flexed, as may occur in a head-on MVA when the patient's knee is violently impacted by the dashboard. The significant clinical findings of a posterior hip dislocation are an extremity that is shortened, adducted, and internally rotated. An anterior hip dislocation classically presents as a flexed, abducted, and externally rotated leg. A fractured femoral neck is classically externally rotated and shortened. *(Vanderhave, 2015, Ch. 40)*

18. **(C)** Cervical radiculopathy is referred neurogenic pain in the distribution of a cervical nerve root with or without associated numbness, weakness, or loss of reflexes. The usual cause in young adults is herniation of a cervical disk that entraps the root as it enters the foramen. C6 root irritation manifests pain in the neck, shoulder, lateral aspect of the arm, and radial aspect of the forearm. Sensory changes are seen in the dorsolateral aspect of the thumb and index finger. Biceps and wrist extensors/pollicis longus are noted to have muscle weakness or atrophy. Biceps and brachioradialis DTRs manifest changes with C6 root irritation. C7 nerve root irritation often presents with pain in the neck, shoulder, medial border of the scapula, lateral aspect of the arm, and dorsum of the hand. Sensory changes are in the longer finger and dorsum of the hand. Muscle weakness is noted with triceps and finger extensors, and DTR changes are noted in the triceps. C5 radiculopathy presents with pain in the neck, shoulder, and anterolateral aspect of the arm. Sensory changes are seen in the deltoid region; muscle atrophy is seen in the deltoid and biceps. DTR changes with a C5 root irritation are manifested in the biceps reflex. *(Sarwark, 2010, Sect. 8, pp. 922–924)*

19. **(C)** Nonsteroidal anti-inflammatory drugs (NSAIDs) are metabolized in the liver and excreted via the kidneys. Elderly patients are more at risk of developing irreversible damage to the renal system. Renal function physiologically decreases with the advancing age. With decreased clearance of the medication, renal damage ensues and leads to accumulation of the drug and further renal damage. Renal function should be monitored in the elderly patient receiving high doses of any NSAIDs. Hepatic failure is also a concern with the use of NSAID, especially where there is potential for overdose. There is no documented evidence of damage to the eyes, heart, peripheral vascular system, or central nervous system. *(Hellmann & Imboden, 2014, Ch. 20)*

20. **(E)** The most likely diagnosis in this patient presentation is an occult fracture of the radial head. This is supported by the mechanism of injury, physical examination, and radiographic findings. On physical

examination, tenderness over the radial head with local swelling and pain with rotation and flexion of the forearm is usually present. Fractures of the radial head may be subtle on initial radiographs. The finding of an anterior fat pad may be a normal finding, but the finding of a posterior fat is pathological and usually indicates an occult fracture of the radial head. Nursemaid elbow is more commonly seen in children 1 to 3 years of age and is associated with injury that is pulling in nature on the hand with the elbow in full extension. Lateral and medial epicondylitis are typically overuse injuries that occur in patients 35 to 50 years of age. Radial head dislocation may be associated with fracture of the radial head; the supporting evidence in this case does not support dislocation. Radial head dislocation is typically posteriorly and evident on radiographs. (*Black et al., 2015, Ch. 39*)

21. **(B)** This patient presentation is most consistent with a medial meniscus tear. Medial meniscus tears are more likely to present with a twisting injury of the knee. Patients usually are ambulatory after the injury, with pain and swelling progressing 2 to 3 days after the injury. The pain is usually located in the medial or lateral side of the knee and is associated with a catching or locking sensation caused by swelling or mechanical blockage from torn meniscus. On physical examination, there is tenderness over the medial or lateral joint line. The McMurray test is positive when forced flexion and circumduction of the joint causes a painful click. Anterior cruciate ligament can result from a twisting injury as well but would be more likely associated with hemarthrosis and a positive Lachman test or anterior drawer sign. Pes anserine bursitis more commonly presents with tenderness distal to the medial joint line and is more likely associated with overuse. Tibial plateau fracture would present with bony tenderness and a result of high-energy fracture. Medial collateral ligament tear would present with pain and instability with valgus stress on the joint. (*Sarwark, 2010, Sect. 6, pp. 684–688*)

22. **(C)** The radiculopathy found with L4–L5 disc herniation presents with weakness of the great toe extensor, numbness on the top of the foot and first web space, and no reflex findings. Radiculopathy of the L3–L4 disc presents with weakness of the anterior tibialis, numbness of the shin, and an asymmetric knee reflex. Radiculopathy of the

L5–S1 disc presents with weakness of the great toe flexor and gastrocsoleus, inability to sustain tiptoe walking, and an asymmetrical ankle reflex. Cauda equina syndrome is associated with perianal numbness and urinary and bowel incontinence. Ankle clonus is more likely to be associated with demyelinating conditions. (*Sarwark, 2010, p. 719*)

23. **(D)** The pain of spinal stenosis presents in the lower back, radiating to the buttocks and thighs, and is aggravated with walking and alleviated with rest or lumbar flexion. Distinguishing "pseudoclaudication" of a patient with spinal stenosis from true vascular insufficiency is best supported by the preservation of pedal pulses and the location of pain in the thighs. (*Sarwark, 2010, Sect. 6, pp. 661–662*)

24. **(A)** Evaluating the medial collateral ligament is best completed by applying valgus stress to the knee extended and then flexed at 30 degrees and then evaluating the stability. If the knee shows exaggerated laxity, there is more likelihood that the medial collateral ligament is torn. Varus stress evaluates the integrity of the lateral collateral ligament. The apprehension sign evaluates for patellar instability. The Lachman test and anterior drawer sign are to evaluate for anterior cruciate ligament tears. (*Sarwark, 2010, Sect. 6, pp. 663–666*)

25. **(A)** This patient presentation is most suggestive of slipped capital femoral epiphysis of the right hip. This condition is commonly seen during adolescence (11–13 years), and obesity is also a contributing factor. The patient more commonly presents with referred pain to the medial knee and thigh with an associated limp. The combination of a thickened growth plate from the influence of growth hormone causing a weaker bone, lack of sexual maturity to stabilize the physis, obesity adding mechanical stress, and the mechanics of the joint adds to the increased likelihood of slippage of the epiphysis. Examination of the hip along with radiographic studies is imperative to further evaluate this patient. Hip examination would reveal loss of abduction and internal rotation of the hip. Radiographically, a frog-legged lateral view is best for detecting slippage. Establishing the degree of slippage is imperative to determining the treatment. In this patient presentation, a radiograph of the left knee is not necessary. Further radiographic evaluation of the

knee with CT scan or MRI is not necessary. Reassuring the parents and observing this patient is not advisable, as prompt evaluation and treatment is imperative due to the progressiveness of this disease. *(Sarwark, 2010, Sect. 9, pp. 1180–1183)*

26. **(A)** The treatment of scoliosis depends on the magnitude of the curvature of the spine and risk of progression. Curvatures less than 20 degrees usually do not require intervention. Curvature at 20 to 40 degrees in a skeletally immature patient may respond to bracing. Curvatures greater than 60 degrees may require surgical intervention. *(Erickson & Caprio, 2013, Ch. 26)*

27. **(E)** The initial treatment of a patient with low back pain without neurological deficit consists of conservative management despite the causation. Muscle strain, ligament sprain, or early disc disease is all treated with rest, analgesia, and progressive functional activities. Diagnostic evaluation to include radiographs, and MRI of the lumbar spine is reserved for the patient who does not respond to conservative management. Returning the patient to work, especially manual labor, would be counterproductive for the pain. Trigger point injections are not proven to show benefit in the treatment of acute low back pain. *(Sarwark, 2010, Sect. 8, pp. 940–943)*

28. **(A)** The evaluation of septic arthritis is best accomplished with synovial fluid analysis and culture. Radiological imaging can be normal when infection present. Ultrasound, CT scan, and MRI can all confirm the presence of joint effusion but none of these tests have the ability to determine if the effusion is due to joint sepsis. *(Hellmann & Imboden, 2014, Ch. 20)*

29. **(B)** This patient's scenario is consistent with a torus fracture of the radius. Torus fractures commonly present as a "buckle" of the cortex and are due to force or compression of the bone. This type of fracture is more common to occur in a pediatric patient because of the "softer" nature of the bone. Torus fractures usually do not create alignment issues and heal within 3 weeks with simple immobilization. A greenstick fracture involves disruption of one side of the cortex with angulation of the bone; this type of fracture does not separate the ends of the bone. Plastic deformation is the change in the natural shape of the bone with a detectable suture line;

there is no "buckle" with this type of fracture. Radial neck fracture would present with angulation of the radial head and is proximally located. Monteggia fracture refers to an ulnar fracture with associated radial head dislocation from the capitulum. *(Erickson & Caprio, 2013, Ch. 26)*

30. **(D)** This patient presentation is typical of the pain associated with plantar fasciitis, where the pain is located on the bottom of the foot and more commonly is severe on initially getting up in the morning and lessens with ambulation. In most cases of plantar fasciitis, there is maximal pain along the plantar medial aspect of the heel, corresponding to the origin of the plantar fascia at the medial calcaneal tuberosity. Heel spurs are more likely to be associated with continued pain. Achilles tendonitis is more likely to occur over the bony prominence of the calcaneus and have pain with passive stretch of the Achilles as well as pain with resisted plantar flexion. Tarsal tunnel syndrome is associated with compression of the posterior tibial nerve and with diffuse pain, paresthesias, and burning of the medial ankle and is worse after walking and occurs at night. A calcaneal stress fracture will have pain with calcaneal compression and the pain will increase with ambulation. *(Sarwark, 2010, Sect. 7, pp. 839–843)*

31. **(C)** The radiograph demonstrates a fifth metacarpal neck fracture. Ulnar gutter splints are utilized to immobilize fractures involving the fifth metacarpal. Thumb spica splints are utilized for fractures of the first metacarpal. Fractures involving the second, third, and fourth metacarpals can be immobilized with a volar splint. Casts should not be applied during the first 48 to 72 hours to reduce the risk of compartment syndrome. Buddy taping the fourth and fifth fingers will not provide enough stability to allow fracture healing. *(Coleman & Reiland, 2011, Ch. 28)*

32. **(A)** Mallet finger is caused by rupture or avulsion of the insertion of the extensor tendon. It is also known as baseball finger due to the cause of injury commonly associated with a ball striking the finger, causing sudden passive flexion of the actively extended distal interphalangeal joint. The presentation is a distal interphalangeal joint that is unable to extend at the joint. Treatment of this extensor tendon injury is best accomplished with continuous splinting of the DIP joint in extension for 8 weeks. Jersey

finger is caused by rupture or avulsion of the flexor tendon at the base of the distal phalanx. It occurs when an individual is holding onto a piece of clothing or an object and the distal interphalangeal joint is forcibly extended. The presentation with a jersey finger is inability to actively flex the distal interphalangeal joint. Jersey finger injuries should be referred for orthopedic consultation and surgical repair. *(Sarwark, 2010, Sect. 4, pp. 461–464 and 501–503)*

33. **(D)** This patient presentation is more consistent with osteochondroma, which is the most common bone tumor in children and is typically associated with a pain-free mass. The tumor appears as a pedunculated or sessile lesion that resembles a cartilaginous cap on a bony stalk. This tumor has a very rare malignant tendency and is excised only if it interferes with function. Osteoid osteoma is a benign bone lesion and typically produces pain that is more pronounced at night. Osteoid osteoma lesions are commonly identified in the tibial diaphysis, proximal femur, and spine. Radiographs demonstrate a radiolucent nidus with a sclerotic, reactive rim. Chondrosarcoma is a malignant bone tumor with a peak incidence in the fifth and sixth decades of life. Common locations include the knee, shoulder, pelvis, and spine. On x-ray they will demonstrate cortical thickening and stippling consistent with cartilage deposition. Osteosarcoma typically occurs about the knee and is the most common primary malignant bone tumor. On x-ray the tumor appears as a destructive lesion demonstrating some bone formation. Ewing sarcoma typically presents with pain, fever, and leukocytosis which in some instances results in them being mistaken as an osteomyelitis. Common locations for Ewing sarcoma are the pelvis, knee, proximal humerus and femur diaphysis. Radiographs reveal a destructive lesion that frequents the diametaphyseal region. *(Srinivasan et al., 2010, Ch. 40)*

34. **(C)** This patient presentation is most likely patellofemoral syndrome. The typical presentation includes anterior knee pain of vague location; the pain is increased by flexion load such as stair climbing and the patient has a positive "theatre sign." Theatre sign consists of pain after being seated for prolonged period. Treatment of patellofemoral syndrome is initially conservative and aimed at strengthening the quadriceps. Referral to physical

therapy is helpful with regaining strength and implementing therapeutics. Injection of the joint with corticosteroid would be less likely associated with the initial approach and weight-bearing exercises should be avoided in the acute phase. Immobilizing the joint is counterproductive. *(Sarwark, 2010, Sect. 6, pp. 704–707)*

35. **(C)** Anterior cruciate ligament injuries can occur due to contact and noncontact mechanisms. It is common for individuals to describe a shifting sensation and pop at the time of injury. Laxity with anterior drawer and Lachman testing is consistent with a tear of the anterior cruciate ligament. Firm end feel with posterior drawer, valgus and varus testing rules out injury to the posterior cruciate ligament, medial collateral ligament, and lateral collateral ligament. The lack of pain and apprehension with patellar apprehension testing rules out a patellar subluxation/dislocation injury. *(Sarwark, 2010, Sect. 6, pp. 640–643)*

36. **(B)** An abrupt onset of proximal muscle pain and stiffness in the shoulder and pelvic girdle areas, usually associated with fever, malaise, and weight loss, is characteristic of polymyalgia rheumatica. Subcutaneous inflammatory lesions denote erythema nodosum. These lesions are associated with pregnancy and several systemic disorders, such as sarcoidosis, tuberculosis (TB), and streptococcal infections. Insidious onset of symmetrical joint involvement is most commonly associated with rheumatoid arthritis. Widespread musculoskeletal pain and tender points, referred to as "trigger points," are seen with fibromyalgia syndrome. Trigger points may be found anywhere on the body but are most common in the neck, shoulders, hands, low back, and knees. Symmetrical weakness initially in the legs that progresses caudally is characteristic of Guillain–Barré syndrome. *(Hellmann & Imboden, 2014 , Ch. 20)*

37. **(D)** Medications used to prevent gout exacerbations include allopurinol and uricosuric drugs, such as probenecid. Allopurinol inhibits the production of uric acid and is indicated for patients who overproduce uric acid, and uricosuric drugs are used in patients who undersecrete uric acid. Criterion to classify a patient as an overproducer of uric acid is a 24-hour uric acid excretion test. The result showing uric acid excretion of 800 mg or greater indicates that the patient is an overproducer. In this

patient scenario, there is an overproduction of uric acid, making the case for the use of allopurinol. If this patient's 24-hour uric acid excretion was less than 800 mg, the use of a uricosuric drug would then be appropriate. Prednisone, colchicine, and indomethacin are alternative treatments for acute attacks of gout and are not used for preventive measures. *(Hellmann & Imboden, 2014, Ch. 20)*

38. **(A)** Fibromyalgia is the most likely diagnosis in this patient. It is most frequently seen in woman between the ages of 20 and 50. Patients complain of chronic musculoskeletal pain commonly associated with fatigue and sleep disturbances as well as headaches and numbness. Physical examination is normal except for the presence of multiple "trigger points." Polymyositis most commonly presents with weakness rather than pain, and although it may present at any age, it is most common in the fifth and sixth decades of life. Paget disease is most commonly diagnosed after the age of 40 and is usually asymptomatic and mild, but if symptomatic, presents with bone pain. Polymyalgia rheumatica is commonly seen in patients older than 50 years and presents with shoulder and pelvic pain. Systemic lupus erythematosus does affect mainly young female patients but involves multiple organ systems that include skin lesions, joint symptoms, ocular manifestations as well as lung, heart, and neurological symptoms. *(Hellmann & Imboden, 2014, Ch. 20)*

39. **(B)** Autoantibody production is the primary immunological abnormality seen in patients with systemic lupus erythematosus (SLE); the antinuclear antibody (ANA) is the most characteristic of SLE and seen in 95% of patients with SLE but is not specific for the diagnosis of SLE. A positive ANA can also be found in patients with lupoid hepatitis, scleroderma, rheumatoid arthritis, Sjögren disease, dermatomyositis, and polyarteritis. ANA testing should be employed as the initial screening test in a patient suspected of having SLE. A negative total ANA test is strong evidence against the diagnosis of SLE, whereas a positive test is not confirmatory of the diagnosis. The most specific antibody tests for SLE are antibodies to double-stranded DNA (anti-dsDNAs) and anti-Smith (anti-SM). Although these tests are more specific for SLE, they are less sensitive than the ANA test. Anti-dsDNA is positive in 60% of patients with SLE and anti-SM is positive in 30% of patients.

Anti-dsDNA is more likely to reflect disease activity. Gliadin antibody assay is utilized to assess patients with suspected celiac disease. Anticentromere antibody is associated with CREST (calcinosis, Raynaud phenomenon, esophageal dysmotility, sclerodactyly, and telangiectasia) syndrome in scleroderma. Antibodies to ribonucleoprotein are present in patients with a mixture of overlapping rheumatological symptoms known as "mixed connective tissue disease." *(Hellmann & Imboden, 2014, Ch. 20)*

40. **(D)** Patients being treated for rheumatoid arthritis with tumor necrosis factor (TNF) inhibitors are at increased risk for developing an opportunistic infection, such as tuberculosis (TB). It is recommended that screening for the presence of latent TB occur before TNF inhibitors are started. There is no specific indication to order a chest x-ray, allergy testing, liver function tests, or serum BUN and creatinine prior to initiation of TNF inhibitors. *(Hellmann & Imboden, 2014, Ch. 20)*

41. **(B)** Scleroderma is characterized by diffuse thickening of the skin and is associated with areas of telangiectasia and changes in skin pigmentation. Most patients with scleroderma also have associated Raynaud phenomenon and gastrointestinal involvement. Sarcoidosis more commonly presents with pulmonary symptoms and erythema nodosum. Dermatomyositis presents with scaly patches over the dorsum of the hands (Gottron sign) and lilac discoloration of the eyelids (heliotrope rash). Eosinophilic fasciitis is a rare disorder associated with skin changes similar to those seen in scleroderma; however, there is no association with Raynaud phenomenon. Eosinophilia–myalgia syndrome is associated with chronic ingestion of tryptophan, which is an amino acid previously found in over-the-counter preparations for insomnia and premenstrual syndrome, now banned by the Food and Drug Administration. Cutaneous findings in eosinophilia–myalgia syndrome present with a range of expression from hives to swelling of the extremities. *(Hellmann & Imboden, 2014, Ch. 20)*

42. **(A)** The most common type of juvenile idiopathic arthritis (JIA) is the pauciarticular form that is oligoarticular, involving four or less joints. A risk with this form of JIA is the development of insidious, asymptomatic uveitis, which may lead to

blindness if not detected and treated. Routine ophthalmologic screening with slit-lamp examination is recommended every 3 months if the patient has a positive antinuclear antibody (ANA) and every 6 months if the patient has a negative ANA. Patients with JRA are not at increased risk of hearing impairment; thus a referral to the otolaryngologist is unnecessary. Patients with JIA who have a systemic presentation do have a characteristic rash, but a dermatology consultation is usually not warranted. Growth restriction may occur with any form of JIA, more commonly found in systemic onset and polyarticular onset JIA. There is no current method to predict which patients will have growth restriction, and a routine referral is not often indicated. Even though the use of nonsteroidal anti-inflammatory drugs (NSAIDs) is the first line of treatment in JIA, they are usually well tolerated in children as long as the medication is taken with food. Referral to a gastroenterologist is not indicated. *(Soep, 2013, Ch. 29)*

43. **(D)** The Ottawa ankle rules are a set of clinical prediction rules that guide the need for radiographs in patients presenting with traumatic ankle injuries. If the patient is unable to weight bear for four steps immediately after the injury or at the time of evaluation and there is: (1) bony tenderness along the posterior edge of the lateral or medial malleolus or if there is (2) bony tenderness over the navicular then ankle radiographs should be obtained. *(Luke & Ma, 2014, Ch. 41)*

44. **(B)** Pseudogout presents similarly to acute gout and is best diagnosed by the finding of the rhomboid-shaped crystals of calcium pyrophosphate in joint aspirates. Joints commonly involved in pseudogout are the knees and wrists and other joints such as the metacarpophalangeals, hips, shoulders, ankles, and elbows. The diagnosis of pseudogout is further supported by the finding of a normal serum uric acid level. Acute gout would more likely be associated with an elevated serum uric acid level. Psoriatic arthritis commonly presents with asymmetrical oligoarticular involvement of two to four joints, and in a higher percentage of patients, there is known presence of the dermatological expression of psoriasis. Infectious arthritis is ruled out with the findings of an afebrile patient and WBC count of 12,000/mL. In acute infectious arthritis, the WBCs would be expected to be elevated in the range of 50,000 to 200,000/mL. Rheumatoid arthritis usually presents with symmetrical polyarticular involvement of three or more joints. *(Hellmann & Imboden, 2014, Ch. 20)*

45. **(B)** Raloxifene, a selective estrogen receptor modulator, has the added benefit of reducing the risk of breast cancer while increasing bone density and reducing the risk of vertebral fractures in patients with osteoporosis. Calcitonin, bisphosphonates (alendronate), and teriparatide, although utilized in the treatment of osteoporosis, do not have an added benefit of reducing the risk of breast cancer. Conjugated estrogens, such as Premarin (Wyeth pharmaceuticals, Philadelphia, PA), may actually increase the risk of breast cancer in patients. *(Chrousos, 2012, Ch. 40)*

46. **(A)** Morning stiffness lasting at least 1 hour is characteristic of rheumatoid arthritis (RA). Exacerbation of joint stiffness with weight-bearing (such as walking) and frequent, brief episodes of stiffness (lasting >30 minutes) after inactivity are both more characteristic of degenerative joint disease, not RA. Stiffness reflected by a major delay in relaxation after muscle contraction is seen in myotonic dystrophy. Stiffness evidenced by increased resistance to passive movement describes the "rigidity" associated with parkinsonism. *(Hellmann & Imboden, 2014, Ch. 20)*

47. **(C)** Reactive arthritis, previously known as Reiter syndrome, typically presents with the clinical triad of urethritis, conjunctivitis, and arthritis. Most cases of reactive arthritis are associated with either a sexually transmitted infection (STI) or an enteric infection. Common STI etiological triggers are *Chlamydia trachomatis* or *Ureaplasma urealyticum*. Enterically *Shigella, Salmonella, Yersinia,* or *Campylobacter* is an organism associated with reactive arthritis. Common ear, eye, musculoskeletal, and central nervous system infections are usually not associated with reactive arthritis. *(Hellmann & Imboden, 2014, Ch. 20)*

48. **(A)** This patient presentation of known rheumatoid arthritis with severe deformities, extra-articular findings, and splenomegaly is most likely Felty syndrome. Felty syndrome is characterized by the triad of deforming rheumatoid arthritis, splenomegaly, and neutropenia. The appropriate laboratory test to order would be a CBC to evaluate for neutropenia. Uric acid

testing is helpful in evaluating gout but is not relevant to this patient presentation. Ordering an erythrocyte sedimentation rate or C-reactive protein is not necessarily helpful in diagnosing Felty syndrome; in an acute inflammatory flare, both would most likely be elevated. Antinuclear antibodies could be present in 20% to 40% of patients but are not diagnostic of Felty syndrome. *(Hellmann & Imboden, 2014, Ch. 20)*

49. **(E)** The treatment of rheumatoid arthritis (RA) is aimed at reduction of pain, preservation of function, and prevention of deformity. Although nonsteroidal anti-inflammatory drugs (NSAIDs) provide symptomatic relief, they do not alter progression or prevent erosion of the joint. Consequently, in addition to NSAID therapy, disease-modifying antirheumatological drugs (DMARDs) should also be initiated as soon as the diagnosis is confirmed. The most common initial DMARD used as treatment of choice in RA is methotrexate. Aspirin should not be added because of the increased risk of gastrointestinal side effects as well as having no effect on altering RA disease progression. Rituximab is a biological DMARD and is indicated to be added in patients with RA refractory to treatment with combination therapy of methotrexate and a tumor necrosis factor inhibitor (TNF). Etanercept is a TNF inhibitor. This class of medication is often added in patients with RA who are not responding to methotrexate therapy alone. Leflunomide is a pyrimidine synthesis inhibitor that is approved for the treatment of RA; however, it is contraindicated for use in premenopausal women secondary to its carcinogenic and teratogenic potential. *(Hellmann & Imboden, 2014, Ch. 20)*

50. **(D)** The most likely diagnosis in this patient is polyarticular juvenile idiopathic arthritis (JIA). This form of JIA is seen in approximately 25% of patients with JIA. It is characterized by symmetrical involvement of five or more joints. Two subsets of the disease exist that are distinguished by the presence or absence of rheumatoid factor. A positive rheumatoid factor is most commonly seen in girls with later disease onset (at least 8 years old). An antinuclear antibody (ANA) test may be positive but is more likely to be positive with the pauciarticular form. In the early stage of the disease, the x-ray may be normal or show soft tissue swelling and periarticular osteopenia. In addition to the positive ANA of pauciarticular JIA patients, the arthritis must be present in four or fewer joints. Early onset disease is commonly seen in girls aged 1 to 5 years and has a positive ANA; up to 30% of patients will also have eye involvement. Late-onset disease is more common in male patients, with involvement of the large joints. Systemic JIA, also known as "Still disease," is seen in about 10% to 15% of children with JIA. It is characterized by daily intermittent fever spikes and a transient, nonpruritic, pale pink, blanching macular, or maculopapular rash found on the trunk. A positive rheumatoid factor is rare in this form of JIA. Reactive arthritis is usually associated with a recent viral or bacterial infection. Infectious arthritis more commonly presents as monoarticular and is usually acute in onset. *(Soep, 2013, Ch. 29)*

51. **(A)** The most likely diagnosis in this patient is polymyositis. This is supported by the finding of a gradual progressive proximal muscle weakness and elevation of creatinine phosphokinase level. The finding of lymphoid inflammatory infiltrates on muscle biopsy confirms the diagnosis. Initial treatment of choice in this condition is the use of a corticosteroid (prednisone). Patients who do not respond to prednisone may then benefit from the use of methotrexate or azathioprine. Both intravenous immune globulin and hydroxychloroquine are effective for the treatment of patients with dermatomyositis that is resistant to prednisone therapy. *(Hellmann & Imboden, 2014, Ch. 20)*

52. **(B)** Podagra is the term utilized to denote the involvement of the great toe in cases of gout. *Crepitus* refers to a sound or feeling associated with the movement of joints due to joint irregularities. *Xerostomia* is the term applied to symptoms of dryness of the mouth, which may be seen in Sjögren syndrome. *Paronychia* is the term used to identify an area of soft tissue infection along the nail margin and most commonly due to a hangnail or ingrown nail. *Chondrocalcinosis* refers to the presence of calcium-containing salts in articular cartilage associated with metabolic diseases, such as pseudogout. *(Hellmann & Imboden, 2014, Ch. 20)*

53. **(B)** Risk factors for osteoporosis and indications for measuring bone density include alcoholism. Low body mass index (BMI >19 kg/m^2), not obesity; hypocalcemia, not hypercalcemia; loss of height or

thoracic kyphosis, not scoliosis; and long-term corticosteroid therapy (more than 6 mg of prednisone for more than 1 month), not short-term corticosteroid therapy are also indications for measuring bone density. *(Fitzgerald, 2014, Ch. 26)*

54. **(D)** Ankylosing spondylosis is the most likely diagnosis in this patient. This condition is a chronic inflammatory disorder of the joints of the axial skeleton and commonly presents in the late teens or twenties. Male patients have a higher incidence than do female patients. A common presentation is pain in the lower back with radiation to the thighs and associated limitation of movement that may lessen during the day. Laboratory findings include an elevated erythrocyte sedimentation rate and positive HLA-B27. The HLA-B27 is not a specific test for ankylosing spondylitis; a small percentage of the normal population has a positive finding of this antigen. The earliest radiographic findings occur in the sacroiliac joints, with the detection of erosion and blurring of the joint space. Systemic lupus commonly affects women of childbearing years and presents with exacerbations and remissions of arthritis, rash, fatigue, and the potential for organ system involvement. Lumbar disc disease is usually seen in the age group of 35 to 45 years and is more likely to be associated with trauma. Rheumatoid arthritis does have the potential to affect this age group, but it would more likely be associated with smaller joints of the hands, along with a positive rheumatoid factor. Polymyalgia rheumatica more commonly affects patients older than 50 years and is associated with fatigue, malaise, chronic pain, and stiffness of the proximal muscles, shoulders, neck, and pelvic girdle. *(Hellmann & Imboden, 2014, Ch. 20)*

55. **(E)** Cervical spine disease in long-standing rheumatoid arthritis (RA) may lead to C1–C2 subluxation and spinal cord compression. Flexion and extension x-rays of the cervical spine will detect the possibility of subluxation to avoid potential complications with neck movement during anesthesia. Although HLA-DR4 is associated with RA, it has no prognostic value in detecting potential complications with anesthesia. Slit-lamp examination will diagnose scleritis or episcleritis, which is a nonarticular manifestation of RA, but the presence of either of these conditions is also not associated with increased risk

from anesthesia. Although lung disease may develop in patients with RA, thoracoscopic lung biopsy is not indicated prior to anesthesia. Patients with RA who are seropositive are more likely to have severe erosive disease, rheumatoid nodules, and extra-articular manifestations but are not at increased risk, per se, during anesthesia. *(Hellmann & Imboden, 2014, Ch. 20)*

56. **(A)** Uveitis is an associated finding in patients with ankylosing spondylitis, reactive arthritis, psoriasis, and Behçet disease. These disorders can cause a nongranulomatous anterior uveitis that usually presents unilaterally with pain, redness, photophobia, and visual loss. Uveitis associated with Behçet disease can be aggressive and result in blindness. Dysentery is more likely to be associated with reactive arthritis. Vasculitis is seen with Behçet disease. Hyperuricemia may be found with psoriasis. Thoracic involvement is often found in ankylosing spondylitis. *(Hellmann & Imboden, 2014, Ch. 20)*

57. **(D)** The most urgent need for diagnosis of a patient with symptoms of polymyalgia rheumatica (PMR) and giant cell arteritis is to prevent blindness caused by ischemic optic neuropathy as a result of occlusive arteritis of the ophthalmic artery. Early diagnosis is imperative as the neurological damage to the optic nerve is not reversible. Most patients with this diagnosis will have a normochromic-normocytic anemia, but this does not create urgency in treatment. Cerebral aneurysms are not common findings with PMR; large vessels such as the subclavian and aorta may be involved in giant cell arthritis in 15% of patients. Mononeuritis multiplex commonly presents with painful paralysis of a shoulder, and respiratory tract complications are more nonclassic findings with the presentation of PMR. *(Hellmann & Imboden, 2014, Ch. 20)*

58. **(E)** Inflammatory causes of polyarthritis include systemic lupus erythematosus and rheumatoid arthritis. Gout, although inflammatory, is most commonly monoarticular. Osteoarthritis is a noninflammatory process that is also usually monoarticular. Both reactive arthritis and psoriatic arthritis involve two to four joints and are therefore classified as oligoarticular. *(Hellmann & Imboden, 2014, Ch. 20)*

59. **(D)** This patient has typical findings associated with osteoporosis. Most patients with osteoporosis are

asymptomatic until fractures present. Fractures occur spontaneously and are associated with back pain of varied degrees. Serum calcium, phosphate, and parathyroid hormone levels are often normal. Since vitamin D deficiency state is common in osteoporosis, a 25-hydroxyvitamin D should be ordered. Bone biopsy is not indicated with this patient; this would be reserved for evaluating for osteomalacia. Rheumatoid factor and antinuclear antibodies would not be of importance with this patient presentation. Serum magnesium is associated more with evaluating for parathyroid or thyroid disorder and has no value with osteoporosis. *(Fitzgerald, 2014, Ch. 26)*

60. **(D)** Rheumatoid arthritis (RA) is associated with HLA-DR4. Patients with a positive DR4 will most likely have more serious and seropositive RA disease. HLA-B8 is associated with Graves hyperthyroidism and myasthenia gravis. HLA-B27 is associated with multiple diseases that are classified as spondyloarthropathies, including ankylosing spondylitis, reactive arthritis (Reiter syndrome), and psoriatic spondylitis. HLA-B51 is associated with Behçet disease, and HLA-DRB3 is associated with type 1 diabetes mellitus. *(Hellmann & Imboden, 2014, Ch. 20)*

61. **(C)** The most common joints involved in reactive arthritis are the large weight-bearing joints of the knees and ankles. The sacroiliac joints are involved in only 20% of patients with reactive arthritis. The small joints of the feet, such as metatarsophalangeal joints, are not likely joints involved in reactive arthritis. Metacarpophalangeal joints are primarily involved in rheumatoid arthritis or systemic lupus erythematosus. Distal interphalangeal joints are commonly involved in osteoarthritis and psoriatic arthritis. *(Hellmann & Imboden, 2014, Ch. 20)*

62. **(D)** The recommended calcium intake for postmenopausal women not on estrogen replacement therapy is 1,500 mg. For premenopausal women and postmenopausal women on estrogen replacement therapy, the recommended adult dose is 1,000 mg. The average adult has a daily dietary intake of 700 mg of calcium, which falls below the standard recommendation. Calcium is found in dairy products, green leafy vegetables, and fish with bones. There is no current recommendation for 2,000 mg of calcium intake. *(Baron, 2014, Ch. 29)*

63. **(A)** Drugs that have a definite association with systemic lupus erythematosus include isoniazid. Penicillin, gold salts, allopurinol, and griseofulvin are all classified as having an unlikely association. *(Hellmann & Imboden, 2014, Ch. 20)*

64. **(E)** This patient most likely has polyarteritis nodosa (PN). A major obstacle in making the diagnosis is the absence of a disease-specific serological test. The diagnosis requires confirmation with either a tissue biopsy or angiogram. HLA-B27 antigens are not associated with the suspected diagnosis. While classic PN will have low titers of rheumatoid factor and antinuclear antibodies, both are nonspecific findings and will not confirm the diagnosis. An MRI of the sacroiliac joints is indicated in evaluation of the early stages of suspected ankylosing spondylitis and plays no role in the evaluation of PN. *(Hellmann & Imboden, 2008, pp. 738–739)*

65. **(B)** Sjögren syndrome is an autoimmune disorder that commonly presents with dryness of the eyes, mouth, and other areas of the body covered by mucous membrane. Because of the chronic dysfunction of the exocrine glands and chronicity of dryness of the eyes and the mouth, patients should be counseled to avoid decongestants and atropinic drugs. The use of these medications can further exacerbate their symptoms. Penicillins, antihistamines, corticosteroids, and fluoroquinolones are not directly associated with encouraging exocrine dysfunction. *(Hellmann & Imboden, 2014, Ch. 20)*

66. **(B)** Calcaneal apophysitis commonly affects young active children. Pain is localized to the posterior aspect of the calcaneus. Pain is increased with activity. Calcaneal apophysitis is uncommon in girls 9 years of age and older and in boys 11 years of age and older because the calcaneal apophysis has closed. Achilles tendonitis will present with focal tenderness over the Achilles tendon combined with pain and possible range of motion loss with passive range of motion assessment. Retrocalcaneal bursitis will have a similar presentation to Achilles tendonitis with the pain being reproduced with palpation in the retrocalcaneal region and not over the Achilles tendon. The pain associated with plantar fasciitis is on the plantar aspect of the heel and classically the pain is the most severe upon first awakening in the

morning. Pain associated with osteomyelitis is constant and activity limiting. *(Sarwark, 2010)*

67. **(A)** Apophysitis denotes inflammation of a growth plate, most commonly due to repetitive activity. Epicondylitis is an acute inflammatory process involving the attachment site of a tendon on an epicondyle. Epicondylosis is a chronic inflammatory process involving the attachment site of a tendon on an epicondyle. Osteomyelitis is an infection of involving bone. Osteochondritis occurs at the articular surface of a bone and involves varying degrees of articular cartilage inflammation. *(Coel et al., 2013, Ch. 27)*

68. **(A)** This patient likely has cauda equina syndrome which is caused by a sudden decrease in the volume of the lumbar spinal canal resulting in compression of multiple nerve roots. Involvement of the sacral roots (S2–S4) that control bladder and anal sphincter function make it a surgical emergency. Failure to surgically decompress the spinal canal can lead to permanent bladder and bowel dysfunction. Physical therapy and/or NSAIDs and activity restriction are appropriate recommendations for mechanical low back pain and discogenic back pain that do not involve the sacral nerve roots. Epidural corticosteroid injections would not be appropriate due to the emergent nature of cauda equina syndrome. Parenteral antibiotics are indicated for the treatment of osteomyelitis of the lumbar spine. *(Cowan & Thompson, 2010, Ch. 36)*

69. **(A)** The sensory distribution of the radial nerve in the hand is the dorsal aspect between the first and second digits. Sensory distribution of the ulnar nerve in the hand is the fifth digit and medial half of the fourth digit. The sensory distribution for the axillary nerve is the lateral shoulder. The sensory distribution of the median nerve is the palmar aspect of the hand between the first, second, and third digits. The sensory distribution for the musculocutaneous nerve is the radial side of the forearm. *(Waxman, 2013, Appendix C)*

70. **(E)** Adhesive capsulitis, also known as a frozen shoulder, presents as a loss of both active and passive glenohumeral range of motion. Typical age of onset is between 40 and 60 years of age. The most common motion that is limited is external rotation which can be attributed to contracture of the coracohumeral ligament. Patients may report pain with resisted range of motion assessment but rarely will they present with a strength deficit. With subacromial impingement syndrome and bicipital tendonitis there will be no significant active or passive range of motion deficits. Tears involving either the infraspinatus or the supraspinatus will present with a strength deficit and preservation of passive range of motion. *(Sarwark, 2010, Sect. 2, pp. 291–293)*

71. **(B)** Intra-articular glucocorticoid injections are shown to be beneficial in the treatment of adhesive capsulitis. Therapeutic benefits of intra-articular injections include reduced pain and improved range of motion. Subacromial corticosteroid injections have not shown to be beneficial because the pathological process of adhesive capsulitis involves the glenohumeral joint and the glenohumeral capsule neither of which structure are targeted with a subacromial injection. Surgical manipulation under anesthesia has proven to be beneficial but due to the risk of humeral fractures it should not be the first-line treatment. Chiropractic manipulation is not recommended in the treatment of adhesive capsulitis because the restricted range of motion is due to contracture of the joint capsule and not a misalignment of anatomical structures. Sling immobilization would likely reduce a patients pain complaints but it will likely lead to further range of motion loss which will be detrimental to the long-term recovery process. *(Prestgaard, 2015)*

72. **(A)** Corticosteroids are known to cause tendon degeneration especially when they are injected directly into a tendon. There is no risk of tendon degeneration with NSAID use. Physical therapy and daily ice application are appropriate for the management of Achilles tendonitis and do not increase the risk of tendon rupture. Heel lift supports are beneficial in the treatment of Achilles tendonitis because they reduce the tension on the tendon. There is no risk of tendon rupture associated with utilization of a heel lift. *(Ham & Maughan, 2015)*

73. **(B)** The FDA requires manufacturers to include a boxed warning indicating the increased risk of tendinopathy and tendon rupture associated with

fluoroquinolones. None of the other medications increase the risk of tendinopathy or tendon rupture. *(Hooper, 2015)*

74. **(A)** The history provided by the patient is the classic complaint associated with a trigger finger which is medically termed stenosing flexor tenosynovitis. A flexor tendon rupture would present as a complete inability to flex the involved finger. Palmar fascia fibrosis is commonly referred to as Dupuytren's contracture and will present as a flexor contracture of the involved finger with a palpable cord within the palmar fascia. A metacarpophalangeal (MCP) joint sprain should be suspected when there is a history of a traumatic injury and there is tenderness of the MCP joint. Severe pain and tenderness with palpation of the flexor tendon sheath associated with recent history of a puncture of bite wound would raise concern for an infection of the flexor tendon sheath. *(Blazar & Aggarwal, 2015)*

75. **(B)** This patient's presentation is suggestive of ankylosing spondylitis (AK) and up to 90% of patients with ankylosing spondylitis are positive for HLA-B27. While patients with AK may demonstrate an elevated erythrocyte sedimentation rate (ESR) it is nonspecific finding. Ankylosing spondylitis is a seronegative spondyloarthropathy, therefore rheumatoid factor (RF), antinuclear antibody (ANA), and antibodies to cyclic citrullinated peptides (anti-CCP) will be negative and would only be beneficial in ruling out other differential diagnoses. *(Qubti & Flynn, 2013, Ch. 17)*

76. **(A)** This patient likely has a tibial stress injury, dependent upon the severity of the injury there may or may not be a cortical fracture line. Radiographs should be obtained as the initial diagnostic study but they have a low sensitivity, especially during the earlier stages of injury when a cortical fracture line has yet to develop. Magnetic resonance imaging (MRI) has supplanted radionuclide bone scans as the imaging study of choice because MRIs have equal sensitivity and a higher level of specificity. Computed tomography (CT) scans should be utilized if there is concern for extensive bony injury because of the greater anatomic detail that is available with CT scans. Musculoskeletal ultrasound is gaining in popularity but there is not an established body of research at this time regarding the sensitivity and specificity of US as it relates to the diagnosis of stress injuries to bone. *(deWeber, 2015)*

77. **(C)** The radiographs demonstrate degenerative disc space narrowing and osteophytes at the C5–C6 and C6–C7 disk space levels which are characteristic of cervical osteoarthritis. In addition, the insidious onset of her pain and range of motion limitations are consistent with cervical osteoarthritis. Radiographic changes associated with ankylosing spondylitis include calcification of the anterior spinal ligaments and fusion of the cervical spine. Cervical spondylolisthesis will be visualized as slippage of one vertebra in relation to the other. There is no evidence of destructive or lytic lesions on the radiographs that would indicate the presence of a metastatic tumor. Metastatic tumors will also cause night pain that interferes with the ability to sleep. Torticollis involves spasm or contracture of the sternocleidomastoid muscle with patients demonstrating a head tilt toward the affected side and head rotation to the unaffected side. *(Sarwark, 2010, Sect. 8, pp. 925–928)*

78. **(D)** Scheuermann kyphosis is most common in boys and is diagnosed radiographically a kyphotic curve with anterior wedging of more than 5 degrees in a minimum of three successive vertebrae. Postural kyphosis is more common in girls and the patient is able to correct the curvature voluntarily. Ankylosing spondylitis results in straightening and fusion of the involved spinal segment. Scoliosis is the term used to describe a lateral curvature of the spine. *(Sarwark, 2010, Sect. 9, pp. 1118–1121)*

79. **(A)** The clinical presentation is consistent with an acute anterior compartment syndrome. Compartmental pressure testing will allow confirmation of the suspected diagnosis and will also assist in determining if emergent fasciotomy is warranted. Ankle brachial index (ABI), magnetic resonance imaging (MRI), and lower extremity vascular Doppler ultrasound (US) can all provide valuable information however none of those modalities are capable of measuring compartmental pressure. If muscle damage has occurred serum creatine kinase (CK) levels will be elevated but this is a nonspecific finding. *(Stracciolini & Hammerberg, 2014)*

80. **(A)** Nerve injuries occur in 10% to 25% of acute anterior shoulder dislocations. The axillary nerve is the most commonly injured nerve due to it being placed under traction when the humeral head dislocates anteriorly. Weakness with abduction and/or decreased sensation along the lateral aspect of the shoulder should raise suspicion for injury to the axillary nerve. *(Rudzinski et al., 2011, Ch. 268)*

81. **(A)** Radial head subluxation, also known as "nursemaids elbow," is the most common elbow injury in children 5 years and younger. Children in this age range are prone to the injury because of increased ligamentous laxity. The mechanism that leads to radial head subluxation is traction of the forearm when the elbow is extended and the forearm is pronated. Children that have sustained a radial head subluxation are reluctant to use the involved upper extremity until the radial head is reduced and returned to its normal anatomical position. Lateral epicondylitis is caused by repetitive microtrauma to the common extensor tendon due to overuse. Radial head fractures occur when an individual falls on an outstretched hand. The ulnar nerve is located on the medial aspect of the elbow and injury to the nerve will typically manifest as tingling, numbness and/or pain in the fourth and fifth fingers (ulnar nerve distribution), and weakness of the intrinsic hand muscles. Olecranon apophysitis develops due to repetitive traction stress placed on the olecranon, for example throwing, and occurs due to overuse. In addition, pain associated with an olecranon avulsion would be localized to the posterior aspect of the elbow. *(Sarwark, 2010, Sect. 9, pp. 1001–1005)*

82. **(A)** Osteonecrosis is a complication of corticosteroid use. All of the other conditions listed carry an indication for either oral or intra-articular corticosteroid therapy. *(Hellmann & Imboden, 2014, Ch. 20)*

83. **(B)** Heberden nodes are a bony enlargement of the distal interphalangeal (DIP) joints associated with osteoarthritis. Bouchard nodes are a bony enlargement of the proximal interphalangeal (PIP) joints associated with osteoarthritis. Schmorl nodes are a protrusion of the intervertebral disc cartilage into the adjacent vertebral body endplate that can be found in a number of vertebral disorders. Podagra describes the inflammation and erythema associated with an acute gout flare involving the first metatarsophalangeal (MTP) joint. Gottron papules are characterized by multiple erythematous to violaceous papules on the dorsum of the interphalangeal joints and metacarpophalangeal joints associated with dermatomyositis. *(Hellmann & Imboden, 2014, Ch. 20)*

84. **(C)** Of the clinical interventions listed above, oral nonsteroidal anti-inflammatory drugs (NSAIDs) are most appropriate treatment intervention at this time. Ideally, the lowest dose necessary to provide symptom relief should be utilized. Older patient and those with underlying comorbidities (e.g., hypertension, type II diabetes) should be closely monitored for possible adverse effects. Intra-articular corticosteroids are indicated for patients that cannot take oral NSAIDs or in patients that have not achieved satisfactory symptomatic relief with oral NSAIDs. Intra-articular hyaluronate injections are utilized for patients that have failed on initial pharmacological intervention (oral NSAIDs and intra-articular corticosteroid injections). Oral opioids should be utilized as a last resort for patients that have failed all other pharmacological interventions. Total knee replacements are reserved for patients with severe osteoarthritis that have failed oral and intra-articular medications. *(Kalunian, 2015)*

85. **(D)** The radial nerve lies in close proximity to the midhumeral shaft as it passes through the spiral groove and therefore it is the most common nerve injury associated with humeral shaft fractures. Injury to the radial nerve manifests as a wrist drop. Injuries to the ulnar nerve can occur with humeral shaft fractures but they are less common than radial nerve injuries and would manifest as grip weakness. Injuries to the median nerve can occur with humeral shaft fractures but they are less common than radial nerve injuries and would manifest as thumb opposition weakness. The axillary nerve is in close proximity to the humeral head and is the most common nerve injury associated proximal humeral fractures. Injury to the axillary nerve manifests as weakness with shoulder abduction. Injuries to the musculocutaneous nerves due to humeral shaft fractures are very rare. If the musculocutaneous nerve is injured it would manifest as weakness with elbow flexion and forearm supination. *(Rudzinski et al., 2011, Ch. 268)*

REFERENCES

Baron RB. Chapter 29: Nutritional disorders. In: Papadakis MA, McPhee SJ, Rabow MW, eds. *Current Medical Diagnosis & Treatment 2015*. New York, NY: McGraw-Hill; 2014.

Bickley LS, Szilagyi PG. *Bates' Guide to Physical Examination and History Taking*. 11th ed. Philadelphia, PA: Lippincott Williams & Wilkins; 2013.

Black W, Hosey RG, Johnson JR, Evans-Rankin K, Rankin WM. Chapter 39: Common upper & lower extremity fractures. In: South-Paul JE, Matheny SC, Lewis EL, eds. *Current Diagnosis & Treatment: Family Medicine*. 4th ed. New York, NY: McGraw-Hill; 2015.

Blazar PE & Aggarwal R. Trigger finger (stenosing flexor tenosynovitis). In: UpToDate, 2015.

Boyd AS, Martinez RA, Feden JP. Chapter 37: Acute musculoskeletal complaints. In: South-Paul JE, Matheny SC, Lewis EL, eds. *Current Diagnosis & Treatment In Family Medicine*. 3rd ed. New York, NY: McGraw-Hill; 2011.

Chrousos GP. Chapter 40: The gonadal hormones & inhibitors. In: Katzung BG, Masters SB, Trevor AJ, eds. *Basic & Clinical Pharmacology*. 12th ed. New York, NY: McGraw-Hill; 2012.

Coel RA, Hoang QB, Vidal A. Chapter 27: Sports medicine. In: Hay WW Jr, Levin MJ, Deterding RR, Abzug MJ, eds. *Current Diagnosis & Treatment: Pediatrics*. 22nd ed. New York, NY: McGraw-Hill; 2013.

Coleman R, Reiland A. Chapter 28: Orthopedic emergencies. In: Stone C, Humphries RL, eds. *Current Diagnosis & Treatment Emergency Medicine*. 7th ed. New York, NY: McGraw-Hill; 2011.

Cowan JA Jr, Thompson B. Chapter 36: Neurosurgery. In: Doherty GM, ed. *Current Diagnosis & Treatment: Surgery*. 13th ed. New York, NY: McGraw-Hill; 2010.

deWeber K. Overview of stress fracture. In: UpToDate, 2015.

Erickson MA, Caprio B. Chapter 26: Orthopedics. In: Hay WW Jr, Levin MJ, Deterding RR, Abzug MJ, eds. *Current Diagnosis & Treatment: Pediatrics*. 22nd ed. New York, NY: McGraw-Hill; 2013.

Escarza R, Loeffel MF III, Uehara DT. Chapter 266: Wrist injuries. In: Tintinalli JE, Stapczynski J, Ma O, Cline DM, Cydulka RK, Meckler GD, eds. *Tintinalli's Emergency Medicine: A Comprehensive Study Guide*. 7th ed. New York, NY: McGraw-Hill; 2011.

Fitzgerald PA. Chapter 26: Endocrine disorders. In: Papadakis MA, McPhee SJ, Rabow MW, eds. *Current Medical Diagnosis & Treatment 2015*. New York, NY: McGraw-Hill; 2014.

Ham P & Maughan KL. Achilles tendinopathy and tendon rupture. In: UpToDate, 2015.

Hellmann DB, Imboden JB Jr. Chapter 20: Rheumatologic & immunologic disorders. In: Papadakis MA, McPhee SJ, Rabow MW, eds. *Current Medical Diagnosis & Treatment 2015*. New York, NY: McGraw-Hill; 2014.

Hopkins-Mann C, Ogunnaike-Joseph D, Moro-Sutherland D. Chapter 133: Musculoskeletal disorders in children. In: Tintinalli JE, Stapczynski J, Ma O, Cline DM, Cydulka RK, Meckler GD, eds. *Tintinalli's Emergency Medicine: A Comprehensive Study Guide*. 7th ed. New York, NY: McGraw-Hill; 2011.

Hooper, DC. Fluorquinolones. In: UpToDate, 2015.

Kalunian KC. Initial pharmacologic therapy of osteoarthritis. In: UpToDate, 2015.

Luke A, Ma C. Chapter 41: Sports medicine & outpatient orthopedics. In: Papadakis MA, McPhee SJ, Rabow MW, eds. *Current Medical Diagnosis & Treatment 2015*. New York, NY: McGraw-Hill; 2014.

Prestgaard TA. Frozen shoulder (adhesive capsulitis). In: UpToDate, 2015.

Qubti M, Flynn JA. Chapter 17: Ankylosing spondylitis & the arthritis of inflammatory bowel disease. In: Imboden JB, Hellmann DB, Stone JH, eds. *Current Rheumatology Diagnosis & Treatment*. 3rd ed. New York, NY: McGraw-Hill; 2013.

Rudzinski JP, Pittman LM, Uehara DT. Chapter 268: Shoulder and humerus injuries. In: Tintinalli JE, Stapczynski J, Ma O, Cline DM, Cydulka RK, Meckler GD, eds. *Tintinalli's Emergency Medicine: A Comprehensive Study Guide*. 7th ed. New York, NY: McGraw-Hill; 2011.

Sarwark JF. In: Rosemont IL, ed. *Essentials of Musculoskeletal Care*. 4th ed. Rosemont IL: American Academy of Orthopaedic Surgeons; 2010.

Soep JB. Chapter 29: Rheumatic diseases. In: Hay WW Jr, Levin MJ, Deterding RR, Abzug MJ, eds. *Current Diagnosis & Treatment: Pediatrics*. 22nd ed. New York, NY: McGraw-Hill; 2013.

Sarwark JF. In: Rosemont IL, ed. *Essentials of Musculoskeletal Care*. 4th ed. American Academy of Orthopaedic Surgeons; 2010.

Srinivasan RC, Tolhurst S, Vanderhave KL. Chapter 40: Orthopedic surgery. In: Doherty GM, ed. *Current Diagnosis & Treatment: Surgery*. 13th ed. New York, NY: McGraw-Hill; 2010.

Stracciolini A & Hammerberg EM. Acute compartment syndrome of the extremities. In: UpToDate, 2014.

Vanderhave K. Chapter 40: Orthopedic surgery. In: Doherty GM, ed. *Current Diagnosis & Treatment: Surgery*. 14th ed. New York, NY: McGraw-Hill; 2015.

Waxman SG. Appendix C: Spinal nerves and plexuses. In: Waxman SG, ed. *Clinical Neuroanatomy*. 27th ed. New York, NY: McGraw-Hill; 2013.

CHAPTER 18

Ophthalmology/Otolaryngology

Linda S. MacConnell, PA-C, MPAS, MAEd

DIRECTIONS: Each of the numbered questions or incomplete statements is followed by possible answers or completions of the statement. Select the ONE-lettered answer or completion that is BEST in each case.

1. A 39-year-old male states that he was holding his baby daughter and she put her fingers in his right eye. He now presents to the ED with acute eye pain and photophobia. His right eye appears grossly normal except for increased tearing. Which of the following is the diagnostic study of choice in this patient?

    (A) Schiotz or applanation tonometry
    (B) Fundoscopic examination and refraction
    (C) Fluorescein staining
    (D) Schirmer test
    (E) Visual acuity testing

2. A patient develops acute eye pain and photophobia after mild trauma to the eye. Examination of the eye is grossly normal except for photophobia and tearing. This patient is most likely suffering from which of the following conditions?

    (A) Subconjunctival hemorrhage
    (B) Hyphema or blood in the anterior chamber
    (C) Conjunctival abrasion
    (D) Corneal abrasion
    (E) Ophthalmoplegia

3. A patient is seen in the emergency department following mild to moderate trauma to the eye. The patient states that his pain is 8/10. Examination is essentially normal except for epiphora and significant photophobia. What is the most appropriate treatment for this patient?

    (A) Antibiotic ointments or drops
    (B) Emergent consultation with an ophthalmologist
    (C) Complete bed rest and avoidance of ASA and other NSAIDs
    (D) Medications to cause miosis such as pilocarpine
    (E) Oral or topical NSAIDs for pain relief

4. When seeing a 64-year-old gentleman for a routine follow-up of hypertension and hyperlipidemia, examination of the retina shows white lesions with irregular borders. They are moderate in size. What are these lesions are called?

    (A) Hard exudates
    (B) Cotton-wool patches
    (C) Drusen
    (D) Intraluminal plaques
    (E) Retinal infiltrates

5. A 5-year-old child presents to your pediatric practice with her parents complaining of a 2-day history of fever (101°F), sore throat, and tearing and mild erythema of both eyes. Since it is summer, she has been taking swimming lessons in a public pool. There is no cough, nasal congestion, pain, or photophobia. Your examination shows a small amount of exudate in the eyes bilaterally along with a large amount of clear discharge. There are conjunctival follicles present in both eyes and follicles of the pharyngeal mucosa. There is nontender adenopathy in the preauricular area. What is the most likely diagnosis for this patient?

    (A) Viral conjunctivitis
    (B) Bacterial conjunctivitis
    (C) Allergic conjunctivitis
    (D) Bacterial pharyngitis
    (E) Blepharitis

6. A 5-year-old patient in your pediatric practice is seen with her parents who states there is a 2-day history of fever (101°F), sore throat, and tearing and mild erythema of both eyes. She has been swimming in a public pool. There is scant exudate present bilaterally and a large amount of watery discharge. There are conjunctival and pharyngeal mucosa follicles present. Nontender preauricular adenopathy is present. What is the most appropriate treatment for this patient?

(A) Oral antibiotics

(B) Topical or systemic antiviral medications

(C) Symptomatic treatment only

(D) Ocular antihistamines for treatment of allergies

7. A 40-year-old female presents with a foreign-body sensation in the right eye. Over the last 3 weeks, she has had gradually increasing painless swelling around the right lower eyelid. Your examination shows a nontender discrete nodule on the right lower eyelid. There is no evidence of injection or discharge and her visual acuity is normal. The most likely diagnosis is:

(A) Blepharitis

(B) Pterygium

(C) Chalazion

(D) Dacryocystitis

(E) Hordeolum

8. After a recent bout of gastroenteritis characterized by vomiting and diarrhea, a 60-year-old male patient presents with bright red blood visible on the lateral right sclera. Blood pressure is normal as is his visual acuity. What is your treatment plan?

(A) Emergency consultation with an ophthalmologist

(B) Computed tomography (CT) scan to rule out intracranial hemorrhage

(C) Provide reassurance to the patient; no treatment is needed

(D) Complete intraocular examination with dilation

(E) Complete blood cell count and bleeding studies

9. A 16-year-old presents with her mother and complains of pain, irritation, and decreased hearing in the right ear since waking this morning. Upon examining the patient with an otoscope, a moth is noted in the right external auditory canal. You are not able to completely visualize the tympanic membrane. What is the most appropriate treatment?

(A) Insert a wick and topical antibiotics

(B) Debrox insertion and remove with suction

(C) Insert 2% lidocaine solution and use suction or forceps for removal

(D) Irrigate with tepid saline

10. A 45-year-old female relates a history of recurring bouts of uveitis, primarily posterior. Chemistry panel shows elevated serum calcium and uric acid levels. As part of the workup, a chest x-ray is obtained and reveals bilateral hilar adenopathy. Her uveitis is most likely secondary to what diagnosis?

(A) Sarcoidosis

(B) Alpha-1 antitrypsin deficiency

(C) Silicosis

(D) Tuberculosis

(E) Histoplasmosis

11. Which of the following is the most common cause of permanent blindness in people greater than 65 years of age in the United States?

(A) Glaucoma

(B) Cataracts

(C) Diabetic retinopathy

(D) Age-related macular degeneration

(E) Retinal detachment

12. A 22-year-old mixed martial arts practitioner presents after an injury during a match which has resulted in a fluctuant, mildly tender edematous lesion of the anterior-superior outer portion of the right pinna. Which of the following is the most appropriate treatment?

(A) Refer to otolaryngology for definitive treatment with I & D and pressure dressing

(B) Perform I & D only if the pinna becomes erythematous and extremely tender

(C) Prescribe a 10-day course of amoxicillin/ clavulanate (augmentin) and schedule a follow-up appointment in 2 weeks

(D) Apply a soft bulky dressing to the pinna and recommend no further treatment, but have the patient follow-up only if he develops a temperature greater than 101 degrees

13. While working in the ER you are triaging a patient who experienced facial trauma. You note blood in the anterior chamber of the patient's left eye. What is a possible complication for this patient?

(A) Retinal detachment

(B) Cataract formation

(C) Glaucoma

(D) Chronic conjunctivitis

(E) Complications are extremely rare and most patients return to normal vision

14. A 7-year-old boy presents with his mother for evaluation of severe left ear pain for 2 days. There is no fever and there are no upper respiratory infection type symptoms. You are not able to visualize the tympanic membrane well, but upon examination there is tenderness with movement of the tragus and several palpable preauricular nodes. What is the most likely diagnosis?

(A) Ramsay-Hunt syndrome

(B) Acute otitis media

(C) Perforated tympanic membrane

(D) Acute otitis externa

(E) Eustachian tube dysfunction

15. A 48-year-old male patient is diagnosed with shingles involving cranial nerve V. During the examination you note that the tip of his nose is involved. At this point, it is crucial to rule out involvement of:

(A) The opposite pinna

(B) Nasal septum

(C) Ipsilateral epitrochlear node

(D) Tympanic membrane

(E) Cornea

16. While working in a university health clinic, you are evaluating a 19-year-old female student with complainant of sore throat, fatigue for 14 days. She has a low-grade fever of 100°F. Examination shows exudative pharyngitis along with tender anterior and posterior lymphadenopathy. A rapid strep antigen test is negative. What is the next step in treating this patient?

(A) Review history for recurring tonsillitis

(B) Perform a monospot test (heterophile antibody)

(C) Advise the patient that it is viral and treat presumptively

(D) Treat with penicillin

(E) Await confirmation of culture before definitive treatment

17. You are evaluating a patient for recurring bouts of vertigo. The attacks generally last less than half an hour and are associated with decreased low-frequency hearing in the left ear along with nonpulsatile tinnitus in the ipsilateral ear. You obtain an audiogram which shows a low-frequency hearing loss in the left ear only. Which of the following is the most likely diagnosis based on the patient history?

(A) Benign paroxysmal positional vertigo

(B) Ménière syndrome

(C) Vestibular neuronitis

(D) Labyrinthitis

(E) Acoustic neuroma

18. A 19-year-old female presents with pain, redness, and swelling of the upper eyelid for the last 3 days. There are no visual changes or photophobia. Examination reveals a tender, erythematous, and outward-pointing edema of the right eyelid. The most likely diagnosis is which of the following?

(A) Hordeolum

(B) Chalazion

(C) Subconjunctival hemorrhage

(D) Entropion

(E) Blepharitis

19. What pathogen is most likely associated with acute onset pain, redness, and outward-pointing edema of the eyelids?

(A) *Aspergillus* species

(B) *Staphylococcus aureus*

(C) *Haemophilus influenzae*

(D) *Candida albicans*

(E) *Streptococcus aureus*

20. After being involved in an altercation the night before a 24-year-old male presents to the ER with persistent double vision. His left periorbital area displays significant ecchymosis and edema. Based on the history, what other findings do you expect on physical examination and what diagnostic test will confirm the diagnosis?

    (A) Hyphema; Schiotz tonometer

    (B) Hyphema; plain radiograph

    (C) Restricted ocular movement; CT scan

    (D) Restricted ocular movement; plain radiography

    (E) Ruptured globe; retinal angiography

21. A 45-year-old woman suddenly experiences severe pain in the right eye along with blurred vision, nausea, and vomiting. Intraocular pressure is 58 mm Hg and there is a moderately dilated right pupil, decreased visual acuity, shallow anterior chamber, and steamy cornea noted during physical examination. Based on this information, what is the most likely diagnosis?

    (A) Retinal detachment

    (B) Retinal artery occlusion

    (C) Uveitis

    (D) Primary open angle glaucoma

    (E) Primary acute angle closure glaucoma

22. A 75-year-old man presents with sudden unilateral vision loss. His history includes some prior episodes of visual loss that completely resolved spontaneously. In the past, to evaluate these episodes, he underwent a carotid ultrasound which confirmed a suspected diagnosis of bilateral carotid stenosis. Considering the patient's current painless sudden visual loss, which of the following findings would you expect to find with fundoscopic examination?

    (A) Retinal lines that have the appearance of a "ripple on a pond" or a "billowing sail"

    (B) A pale or milky retina with a cherry-red fovea

    (C) Enlarged physiologic cup, occupying more than half of the disc's diameter

    (D) A swollen disc with blurred margins; no visible physiologic cup

    (E) Yellowish-orange to creamy-pink disc with sharp margins and a centrally located physiologic cup

23. Your patient is a 70-year-old female. She states that her children and grandchildren have asked her to seek medical attention as she seems to be losing her hearing. She is in generally good health and her only medications are a multiple vitamin along with calcium and vitamin D. You examine her ears and find the external auditory canals to be free of cerumen and the tympanic membranes to be normal in appearance. What other complaint is the patient most likely to experience?

    (A) Otalgia

    (B) Tinnitus

    (C) Vertigo

    (D) Pressure sensation in the ears

    (E) Tympanic membrane perforation

24. You determine that a patient with bilateral hearing loss should undergo an audiogram for a more complete evaluation of her hearing loss. As part of the examination, you perform Weber and Rinne tests and find that Weber is equal in both ears and air conduction is greater than bone conduction is greater in both ears. Therefore, you suspect that her hearing loss, if any, is most likely:

    (A) Conductive

    (B) Sensorineural

    (C) There is no hearing loss; Weber and Rinne tests are both normal

    (D) Mixed hearing loss (sensorineural and conductive)

    (E) Idiopathic

25. A 35-year-old woman presents with a history of a self-limited upper respiratory illness 3 weeks prior to this visit. She now complains of persistent weakness, difficulty chewing and malaise which worsen at the end of the day. She complains that she has difficulty keeping her right eye open toward the latter part of the day. Taking a nap usually helps to alleviate the patient's symptoms. Upon examination, you notice that the right eyelid covers the top part of her pupil. Pupillary reactions are normal. A complete neurological evaluation is otherwise negative.

Which evaluation is most likely to confirm your suspected diagnosis?

(A) CT scan of the brain

(B) Lumbar puncture

(C) Fundoscopic examination

(D) Tensilon test

(E) Psychiatric evaluation

26. A 28-year-old man presents with bilateral conjunctivitis, dysuria, pain in his lower back and right Achilles tendonitis. What is the most likely diagnosis?

(A) Ankylosing spondylitis

(B) Reiter syndrome

(C) Behçet disease

(D) Polyarteritis nodosa

(E) Gonococcal disease

27. A 2-year-old child is brought to your office by her parents. You notice mild but obvious strabismus. Unless she undergoes ophthalmologic treatment, what is the likely outcome?

(A) Amblyopia

(B) Esotropia

(C) Exotropia

(D) Hypophoria

(E) Crossed eyes

28. A previously healthy 14-month-old little boy is brought into your pediatric clinic with his mother who states that he has nasal blockage and "stinky green" nasal drainage from the left nostril only for 2 days. Apart from the unilateral purulent nasal drainage, the remainder of the examination is normal. What is the most likely diagnosis?

(A) Nasal polyps

(B) Frontal sinusitis

(C) Nasal foreign-body impaction

(D) Deviated nasal septum

(E) Choanal atresia

29. A woman in her third trimester of pregnancy believes that she may have been exposed to cytomegalovirus at some point in her pregnancy.

Exposure to cytomegalovirus increases the risk of which of the following disorders?

(A) Limb deformity

(B) Sensorineural hearing loss

(C) Neonatal sepsis

(D) Intraventricular hemorrhage

(E) Cleft palate

30. A 36-year-old female presents to the occupational health clinic with a history of a fleck of metal in the right eye obtained while working in a fabrication plant. You note a large area of subconjunctival hemorrhage and a central abrasion of the sclera. How would you rule out perforation of the globe?

(A) Apply gentle pressure to the globe to see if there is an extrusion

(B) Perform a magnetic resonance imaging test

(C) Perform a Schiotz tonometry test

(D) Perform a test using fluorescein dye

(E) Do nothing until cleared by an ophthalmologist

31. A 12-year-old girl was seen a week ago with an upper respiratory infection, which has failed to improve. She now presents with an elevated temperature (101.4°F), bilateral facial pain, congestion, and purulent nasal drainage. At this point what is the most appropriate therapy?

(A) 10 days of amoxicillin

(B) Sinus CT

(C) 10 days of ciprofloxacin

(D) Warm facial compresses and sinus washes

(E) 10 days of cefaclor

32. A child with notching of the maxillary incisors (Hutchinson's teeth or incisors) most likely has:

(A) A history of congenital syphilis

(B) A history of intraoral infection with Mycoplasma pneumonia

(C) A history of in utero exposure to tetracycline

(D) Been given a sulfa product before the age of 2 months

(E) Continued using a pacifier past the age of 2 years

33. A 70-year-old woman with a history of glaucoma and diabetic retinopathy presents to the ED stating that she fell down and bumped her head earlier in the evening. She is now experiencing a sensation of flashing lights and floaters in her right eye. She has decreased visual acuity and feels there is a curtain over her visual field. Fundoscopic examination is difficult and therefore nondiagnostic. What is the next step that you should take?

- (A) Emergency ophthalmology referral
- (B) Fasting blood glucose
- (C) CT scan of the head
- (D) Neurological examination
- (E) Admission to the hospital for head injury observation

34. The next patient is a 72-year-old gentleman with poorly controlled type 2 diabetes on oral medications. He has been treated for the past 3 weeks with ear drops for external otitis, but the infection continues to worsen. Your examination today reveals profuse foul-smelling purulent drainage along with granulation tissue in the auditory canal. What is the next step in managing this patient?

- (A) Debride the canal and start on an oral antipseudomonal antibiotic such as ofloxacin.
- (B) Perform a gram stain and culture of the discharge.
- (C) Request an emergent CT of the head.
- (D) Prescribe oral, antibiotics, topical otic antibiotics and provide pain management.
- (E) Improve management of the patient's diabetes and your conservative therapy will become more efficacious.

35. For which of the following conditions is a lateral cervical x-ray with a soft tissue technique a useful part of the workup?

- (A) Allergic rhinitis
- (B) Epiglottitis
- (C) Asthma
- (D) Quinsy
- (E) Croup

36. A 60-year-old female with a history of well-controlled diabetes presents with acute episode of left

facial paralysis. She is still able to wrinkle and elevate her forehead bilaterally. She has been in good health recently and has not experienced otalgia. The ears are normal both grossly and to otoscopic examination. Tuning forks yield negative Weber and Rinne. Eye examination is also completely normal to include visual acuity, extraocular movements, and pupillary responses. Based on physical examination findings, what is the most likely diagnosis?

- (A) Bell's palsy
- (B) Ramsay-Hunt syndrome
- (C) Cerebrovascular accident
- (D) Peripheral facial nerve palsy
- (E) Diabetic neuropathy

37. A 17-year-old female presents with sneezing, clear rhinorrhea, itchy watery nose, and eyes. You examine the young woman and find clear nasal drainage and pale, boggy, edematous turbinates. What is the most likely diagnosis?

- (A) Viral upper respiratory infection
- (B) Nasal foreign body
- (C) Asthma
- (D) Allergic rhinitis
- (E) Rhinitis medicamentosa

38. A 35-year-old female presents complaining that she experiences several minutes of vertigo-associated turning over in bed for the last 3 days. She denies hearing loss, otalgia, and tinnitus. The Dix–Hallpike maneuver shows rotary nystagmus diminishing with repeated testing. What is the most likely diagnosis?

- (A) Central nervous system (CNS) lesion.
- (B) Benign positional vertigo
- (C) Labyrinthitis
- (D) Ménière syndrome
- (E) Vestibular neuronitis

39. A 44-year-old male presents with unilateral hearing loss, tinnitus, unsteadiness, and imbalance which has been slowly developing over the last few months. You appropriately order an audiogram and find a unilateral sensorineural hearing loss with poor speech discrimination. What is the most likely cause of the patient's hearing loss?

(A) Megaloblastoma

(B) Impacted cerumen

(C) Otosclerosis

(D) Labyrinthitis

(E) Acoustic neuroma

40. A 43-year-old male presents with "lifelong" history of chronic ear infections and episodic purulent drainage from his right ear canal. The patient currently is without symptoms. Examination of the ear shows a clear external canal, but the tympanic membrane is retracted and there is a pocket of white material and an opacity of the pars flaccida. The Weber test lateralizes to the right and Rinne shows AC > BC on the left and BC > AC on the right. What is this finding called?

(A) Tympanosclerosis

(B) Otosclerosis

(C) Cholesteatoma

(D) Keratosis obturans

(E) Malignant otitis externa

41. A patient presents in your clinic with a rash 2 days after having a sore throat and a fever examination reveals Pastia's lines, a "strawberry tongue," and circumoral pallor. Labs show a positive ASO titer. The patient is on no medications to have caused the rash or prevented it. What is your diagnosis?

(A) Scarlet fever

(B) Erythema infectiosum

(C) Infectious mononucleosis

(D) Rubella

(E) Rubeola

42. You are evaluating a patient with eye pain and after taking a history, measuring visual acuity, extraocular movement and grossly examining the eye, you apply fluorescein stain and examine with a Wood's lamp. You see what looks like a "tree branch" pattern. What is the most likely diagnosis?

(A) Glaucoma

(B) Hypopyon

(C) Hyphema

(D) Herpetic keratitis

(E) Iritis

43. You are seeing a 19-year-old male for follow-up from urgent care where he was seen 2 days earlier with a sore throat. The patient is febrile (102°F), has a muffled (hot potato) voice, and extreme difficulty opening his mouth (trismus). He opens it just far enough for you to note uvular deviation. What is your diagnosis?

(A) Torus palatinus

(B) Gingival hyperplasia

(C) Koplik spots

(D) Ranula

(E) Peritonsillar abscess

44. A 35-year-old man presents with a sudden marked decrease in hearing in his left ear. There is no history of trauma, otorrhea, or vertigo. The physical examination appears to be normal except for the tuning fork tests. The Weber test lateralizes to the better ear and the Rinne test shows that air conduction is better than bone conduction bilaterally. After confirming findings with an audiometric evaluation, what is the most appropriate therapy?

(A) Broad-spectrum antibiotic

(B) Nasal steroids

(C) Decongestant

(D) Oral steroids

(E) Antihistamines

45. Gingival hyperplasia may be a complication of chronic administration of which of the following medications?

(A) Phenytoin (Dilantin)

(B) Valproic acid (Depakote)

(C) Phenobarbital

(D) Clonazepam (Klonopin)

(E) Carbamazepine (Tegretol)

46. A 4-year-old girl presents with fever, rash, bilateral occipital, and posterior cervical adenopathy along with conjunctivitis. What is the pathognomonic physical examination finding for measles (rubeola)?

(A) Gray pharyngeal membrane

(B) Exudative pharyngitis

(C) Koplik spots

(D) Steeple sign

(E) Thumbprint sign

47. A 65-year-old gentleman presents with an acute onset of right facial nerve paralysis. Physical examination shows vesicular lesions on the ipsilateral pinna. What is the most likely diagnosis?

(A) Bell's palsy

(B) Ramsay-Hunt syndrome

(C) Moebius syndrome

(D) Millard–Gubler syndrome

(E) Melkersson–Rosenthal syndrome

48. What is the treatment of choice for a patient presenting with acute facial nerve paralysis, and painful vesicular lesions of the ipsilateral pinna?

(A) Antibiotics

(B) Antifungals

(C) Beta blockers

(D) Oral corticosteroids

(E) Ear drops

49. A 50-year-old woman presents with a progressive sense of decreased hearing in her right ear over the course of the last 20 years. Her father had hearing problems at a young age as well, but never underwent any type of workup. She denies any history of ear problems or infection as a child, ear trauma, or excessive noise exposure. The entire physical examination of the ear is normal and the tympanogram testing is within normal limits. The Weber test lateralizes to the ear with the decreased hearing (the right). Air conduction is greater than bone conduction in the left ear, but the right ear shows bone conduction better than air conduction. What is the most likely diagnosis?

(A) Serous otitis media

(B) Otosclerosis

(C) Presbycusis

(D) Myringosclerosis

(E) Idiopathic hearing loss

50. Your patient is a 35-year-old male who recently underwent restoration of teeth #28, 29, and 30. He has a 24-hour history of fever, dysphagia, odynophagia, and drooling secondary to inability to swallow his own secretions. Examination of the patient shows a toxic-appearing male with trismus, edema of the neck, and submandibular area along with poor dentition, foul smelling breath, and gingivitis. The tongue, which is painful for the patient to move is displaced posteriorly, and a temperature of 103°F is noted. What is the most likely diagnosis?

(A) Sialadenitis

(B) Peritonsillar abscess

(C) Retropharyngeal abscess

(D) Epiglottitis

(E) Ludwig's angina

51. A 49-year-old female complains of 2-week history of severe left ear pain. She states that chewing exacerbates her ear pain. Her hearing is unchanged. Examination shows tenderness to palpation anteriorly of an otherwise normal appearing external canal meatus. The examination of the tympanic membrane is normal. The patient's diagnosis is most likely:

(A) Otitis externa

(B) Otitis media

(C) Temporomandibular joint disorder

(D) Furuncle of the canal

(E) Chondritis

52. Your patient who is 30 weeks pregnant complains of recent onset of severe nasal congestion. She denies rhinorrhea, facial pain, and fever. She has not had previous nasal symptoms until about a month ago. It has been becoming progressively worse. Her ENT examination is essentially normal. What is your diagnosis?

(A) Allergic rhinitis

(B) Perennial rhinitis

(C) Vasomotor rhinitis

(D) Rhinitis of pregnancy

(E) Chronic rhinitis

53. While examining a 6-year-old female, you note an alarming finding suggestive of cystic fibrosis. Which of the following nasal conditions is suggestive of this disease?

(A) Chronic rhinitis

(B) Nasal polyps

(C) Choanal atresia

(D) Perennial allergic rhinitis

(E) Acute sinusitis

54. A 14-year-old is seen for several severe nosebleeds in the past few weeks. There is a large reddish-brown mass within the left posterior nasal cavity. What is the most likely diagnosis for this mass?

(A) Blood clot

(B) Inverting papilloma

(C) Hemorrhagic polyp

(D) Septal hematoma

(E) Juvenile angiofibroma

55. What is the most common site for epistaxis in adults?

(A) Woodruff's plexus

(B) Anterior ethmoid

(C) Hasselbach's plexus

(D) Sphenopalatine artery

(E) Kiesselbach's plexus

56. You are examining a 64-year-old male patient with a 45 pack-year history of tobacco (both cigarette and smokeless tobacco) use. The patient complains of a 2-month history of a 2- × 0.5-cm white lesion on the right lateral ventral area of the tongue. Upon lifting the tongue with gauze, you note that the lesion is adherent to the tongue and cannot be rubbed off. What is the most likely diagnosis?

(A) Squamous cell carcinoma

(B) Hairy tongue

(C) Leukoplakia

(D) Oral candidiasis

(E) Geographic tongue

57. You are examining a 64-year-old male patient with a 45 pack-year history of tobacco (both cigarette and smokeless tobacco) use. The patient complains of a 2-month history of a 2- × 0.5-cm white lesion on the right lateral ventral area of the tongue. Upon lifting the tongue with gauze, you note that the lesion is adherent to the tongue and cannot be rubbed off. After a careful history and physical

examination, what is the most appropriate intervention?

(A) Place the patient on an antifungal medication

(B) Obtain a facial and neck CT with enhancement

(C) Advise the patient to decrease trauma to the tongue and prescribe a mouthwash containing oral corticosteroids and an antibiotic

(D) Incisional or excisional biopsy

(E) Reassure the patient that it will resolve without treatment

58. A 23-year-old male patient states that he was injured during an altercation about 5 to 6 days ago. He was hit in the face during the disagreement. He states that the nasal swelling that he had experienced has decreased, but he has had increasingly more difficulty breathing through his nose. Upon examination, you note soft fluctuant swelling of the septum bilaterally. There is no tenderness to palpation. What is the most appropriate intervention?

(A) Intranasal steroids for 2 to 3 weeks to reduce nasal inflammation

(B) Broad-spectrum antibiotic to prevent abscess formation

(C) Emergent referral to otolaryngology (ENT) provider

(D) CT scan to rule out complex nasal fracture

(E) Needle aspiration of the fluctuant area with cultures

59. An 18-month-old little girl, described by her mother as an active explorer, presents with foul smelling unilateral nasal drainage and decreased activity. What is the most likely cause of the patient's symptoms?

(A) Ethmoid sinusitis

(B) Nasal polyp

(C) Impacted foreign body

(D) Maxillary sinusitis

(E) Acute viral rhinitis

60. Your next patient is a 26-year-old otherwise healthy male who suffered a nondisplaced nasal fracture 3 weeks ago. He now presents with clear right-sided rhinorrhea. He states that his nose has healed completely and feels fine at this time. He states that he is experiencing short gushes of salty tasting liquid from his right nostril several times a day. Sometimes he can produce the liquid by leaning forward. What test should be run on this patient?

    (A) "Bull's eye" test
    (B) Specific gravity
    (C) Gram stain
    (D) Culture and sensitivity
    (E) Glucose dipstick

61. Which of the following is the most common cause of chronic cough in adults?

    (A) Common cold
    (B) Sinusitis
    (C) Asthma
    (D) Postnasal drip syndrome
    (E) Gastroesophageal reflux disease

62. Which of the following patients should undergo audiologic evaluation?

    (A) A 35-year-old female with a history of tympanostomy tubes as a child
    (B) A 6-year-old little girl with otitis media
    (C) A 69-year-old healthy female
    (D) A 40-year-old male whose father developed hearing loss in his mid-60s
    (E) A 58-year-old male with chronic cerumen impaction

63. A 66-year-old male with poorly controlled diabetes mellitus presents to the emergency department with a sudden onset and rapid progression of sore throat with severe pain with swallowing saliva. Upon examining the throat, you note mild erythema. Which of the following is true?

    (A) Treatment is supportive and based on symptom relief
    (B) Inpatient treatment is needed
    (C) Patient should be given IM ceftriaxone and prednisone and follow-up in 48 hours

    (D) Laryngoscopy is absolutely contraindicated
    (E) Needle biopsy should be performed

64. A 17-year-old Asian male presents to the clinic complaining of increasingly painful left ear for the prior 3 days which has now become severely painful. He is a swimmer on the school swim team. The pain is now so severe that the ear is painful to touch. The left ear displays tenderness on motion of the tragus and there is significant edema along with a small amount of purulent drainage. Culture of the ear would most likely grow:

    (A) *Pseudomonas aeruginosa*
    (B) *Staphylococcus aureus*
    (C) *Haemophilus influenzae*
    (D) *Moraxella catarrhalis*
    (E) *Streptococcus pneumoniae*

65. A 14-year-old boy presents to follow-up on unilateral tonsillitis from a previous visit. He was previously treated with a 10-day course of amoxicillin. Over the last 6 weeks, since finishing his antibiotics, his right tonsil has continued to enlarge. Other than the enlarged right tonsil, the pharynx is normal without exudate or inflammation. Careful palpation of the oropharynx reveals a nontender right tonsil 50% larger than the left tonsil. There is nontender right cervical adenopathy. Complete blood cell count and differential is within normal limits. What is the most appropriate management for this patient?

    (A) Reassure the patient and his mother that this is normal after tonsillitis and the tonsil will return to normal size as the patient gets older.
    (B) Order a monospot.
    (C) Order a soft tissue lateral radiograph to rule out a retropharyngeal abscess.
    (D) Prescribe an alternative antibiotic and schedule routine follow-up.
    (E) Obtain an urgent surgical consult for tonsillectomy.

66. A 42-year-old male presents complaining of chronic nasal blockage. History reveals that he has been using 12-hour nasal spray every 6 hours for several months. He initially used the spray as directed, but with continued usage, he finds that he has to use it

more frequently, as he cannot breathe without it. He has no clear or purulent drainage and denies epistaxis. What is your diagnosis?

(A) Deviated septum

(B) Allergic rhinitis

(C) Nasal polyps

(D) Rhinitis medicamentosa

(E) Chronic sinusitis

67. Oral carcinomas in general, _____ _____.

(A) Are treated primarily with radiation if they are small

(B) Are related to tobacco use and excessive alcohol consumption

(C) Are more likely to result from leukoplakia than erythroplakia

(D) Are rapidly growing tumors with early metastatic potential

(E) Range from well to poorly differentiated adenocarcinomas

68. A 54-year-old morbidly obese gentleman presents complaining of persistent fatigue all day long despite a full night sleep obtained with short-acting sleeping pills which worsen his symptoms. His medical history is significant for poorly controlled hypertension. Every morning he awakens with a sore throat and a headache. Which of the following is the most likely condition this patient is suffering from?

(A) Endogenous depression

(B) Diabetes mellitus

(C) Hypothyroid

(D) Obstructive sleep apnea

(E) Cushing's syndrome

69. Your patient is a 39-year-old second grade teacher who states that she developed acute hoarseness 3 days ago. Prior to that, she had a cold, the symptoms of

which are improving. There is no history of smoking or other tobacco use. What is the most important intervention for the patient at this time?

(A) Discuss that due to her occupation, she is at increased risk of leukoplakia of the vocal cords

(B) She should be placed on an antibiotic as she most likely has a bacterial infection

(C) Discuss her increased risk of vocal cord paralysis

(D) Recommend the patient be placed on a course of oral steroids with a taper

(E) Advise the patient to avoid singing or shouting until her normal voice returns

70. Your patient is a 35-year-old male who is HIV positive. He states that he has a loss of appetite and odynophagia. You examine the mouth and find white plaques on the tongue and buccal mucosa. Gentle scraping with a tongue blade removes the white plaques revealing erythematous raw areas underneath. What is the most likely diagnosis?

(A) Candidiasis

(B) Squamous cell carcinoma

(C) Basal cell carcinoma

(D) Hairy leukoplakia

(E) Diphtheria

71. Your patient, who is a 39-year-old truck driver presents stating that he has had a growth for at least 8 years on his eyes. Your examination shows a fleshy triangular area of conjunctivae encroaching onto the nasal aspect of the cornea bilaterally. It has begun affecting his vision. What is the best intervention at this time?

(A) Artificial tears

(B) Excision

(C) Iridotomy

(D) Topical NSAIDs

(E) Reassurance, this is a benign condition

Answers and Explanations

1. **(C)** Fluorescein staining is the diagnostic evaluation of choice to diagnose corneal abrasions which, based on the history, is the patient's most likely diagnosis. While ophthalmic evaluation and refraction should be performed in all patients with eye complaints they do not definitively diagnose a suspected corneal abrasion. Tonometry is used to measure intraocular pressure in patients and is an evaluation for glaucoma. Schirmer test is used when a person experiences very dry eyes or excessive watering of the eyes and measures the function of the lacrimal glands. *(Hua & Doll, 2010, pp. 81–83)*

2. **(C)** Corneal abrasion can result from relatively insignificant trauma and causes ACUTE pain and photophobia. Subconjunctival hemorrhages are not painful and do not cause photophobia. Hyphema will also produce pain and photophobia, but blood will be visible in the pupil and/or iris, it causes decreased and blurry vision and usually results from more significant trauma or systemic disease. The conjunctiva is far less innervated than the cornea and lacerations are less painful than corneal abrasions. *(Hua & Doll, 2010, pp. 81–83)*

3. **(C)** Corneal abrasions are treated with antibiotic drops and occasionally patching. Ophthalmology referral is generally not necessary. Complete bed rest and avoidance of anticoagulating medications are appropriate treatment of hyphema or blood in the anterior chamber. Agents which cause mydriasis, not miosis, are appropriate adjuncts to treatment for corneal abrasion. *(Hua & Doll, 2010, pp. 81–83)*

4. **(B)** Hypertension sometimes produces fluffy grayish or white lesions of the retina called cotton-wool spots. Hard exudates are usually small and round and are sharply outlined bright yellow retinal lesions. Drusen are little round yellow spots, maybe hard or softly outlined and are associated with age-related macular degeneration. Preretinal hemorrhages appear as a horizontal line of demarcation and obscure the underlying retinal vessels. *(http://www.kellogg.umich.edu/theeyeshaveit/optic-fundus/yellow-white.html)*

5. **(A)** Fever, pharyngitis, conjunctivitis, and findings of preauricular lymph nodes point to viral conjunctivitis. Common in children, it is sometimes associated with contaminated swimming pools. Bacterial conjunctivitis is characterized by erythematous conjunctiva, along with significant purulent discharge and is usually unilateral. Allergic conjunctivitis is associated with pruritus along with clear watery drainage. Bacterial pharyngitis is most commonly associated with pharyngeal erythema and exudate, along with tender anterior cervical adenopathy. *(Kaufman, 2011, pp. 290–293)*

6. **(C)** Viral conjunctivitis is usually self-limited and treated symptomatically with antipyretics as needed. Topical antibiotics, while indicated for bacterial conjunctivitis are not indicated for viral conjunctivitis. Topical acyclovir is sometimes indicated in the treatment of herpes viral conjunctivitis, characterized by unilateral pain, injection, mild photophobia, and mucoid discharge and photophobia. The patient in question did not exhibit these symptoms. If the patient notes itchy eyes, consideration might have been given to ocular antihistamines. *(Kaufman, 2011, pp. 290–293)*

7. **(C)** A chalazion is a granulomatous sterile inflammation of a merino main gland. Chalazions develop gradually producing hard, painless discreet swelling of the upper or lower eyelid. Pterygia do not affect

the eyelids, they are conjunctival lesions. Dacryocystitis is a localized infectious process of the lacrimal sac. They are warm and tender. Hordeolum is acutely developing inflammatory lesion. Blepharitis usually occurs bilaterally and involves the entire upper or lower eyelid. Pterygiums are conjunctival lesions not involving the eyelids. Dacryocystitis produces a warm, tender localized infection of the lacrimal sac. Hordeola are acutely developing inflammatory lesions. *(Jackson, 2011, pp. 427–432)*

8. **(C)** A subconjunctival hemorrhage is associated with acute onset of symptoms, the patient is usually alarmed. The hemorrhage was brought on by vomiting associated with the acute bout of gastroenteritis, but may sometimes appear spontaneously, or after a cough or a sneeze. The patient has a subconjunctival hemorrhage and no emergent consultation is needed. CT is unnecessary. Extensive examination is not required. With hemorrhage limited to the conjunctiva, no further evaluation of coagulation is needed. *(Walker & Adhikari, 2011)*

9. **(C)** Two percent lidocaine will paralyze the insect, which may then be removed with suction or forceps. Topical antibiotics are only indicated in otitis externa of bacterial etiology. Wicks are indicated with significant edema to the canal, but not in the case of a foreign body. Debrox is not used with foreign bodies, but is helpful dissolving impacted cerumen. Saline irrigation should not be performed with any organic foreign bodies like beans or insects as the water may cause them to expand. *(Ifran, 2012, p. 332)*

10. **(A)** The etiology of uveitis is generally immunologic. Posterior uveitis is generally associated with sarcoidosis, toxoplasmosis, tuberculosis and syphilis. Of these, sarcoid presents with hilar lymphadenopathy, elevated ACE, calcium and uric acid levels. Alpha-1 antitrypsin deficiency is not associated with uveitis, but rather COPD. Silicosis is a pulmonary disease caused by inhalation of silicon dioxide dust. Elevated serum calcium and uric acid is not seen. Radiographs typically show bilateral alveolar filling and a ground-glass appearance. Tuberculosis may present with hilar lymphadenopathy, but elevated ACE, calcium, and uric acid levels are not characteristic of tuberculosis. Histoplasmosis

may rarely involve asymptomatic ocular involvement. CBC may show anemia and elevated lactate dehydrogenase and alkaline phosphatase. *(Ishaq et al., 2012, pp. 92–97)*

11. **(D)** In developed countries, age-related macular degeneration (ARMD) is the leading cause of blindness in patients over the age of 65. ARMD causes loss of fine/central vision and the lateral/peripheral vision is retained. There is no cure for ARMD. Early diagnosis and treatment of glaucoma is effective in protecting vision. Cataracts are the leading cause of blindness in the world, but not in the United States. Cataract surgery improves vision in 95% of people with cataracts in the developed world. Diabetic retinopathy is very common and is the leading cause of blindness in adults aged 20 to 65. The vast majority (90%) retinal detachments are effectively repaired with surgery. *(Riordan-Eva, 2014, p. 177)*

12. **(A)** The most appropriate course of action for this patient is to refer immediately for I & D by an ENT specialist for the best results. The cartilage of the pinna requires vascular supply from the perichondrium. If deprived of blood, the devascularized tissue can become permanently damaged resulting in the so-called "cauliflower ear." This is frequently caused by blunt trauma such as that experienced by wrestlers, boxers, and martial artists. Although antibiotics are frequently given in addition to I & D, they will not prevent tissue necrosis. A pressure dressing is applied after I & D. *(Kubota et al., 2010, pp. 863–866)*

13. **(C)** Acute angle closure glaucoma may be brought on by hemorrhage causing excessive red blood cells in the anterior chamber damaging the trabecular meshwork. Globe rupture and intraocular foreign body may occur during injury, not retinal detachment. Cataracts are not a complication of hyphema. Hyphema does not involve the conjunctiva so chronic conjunctivitis is not a concern. The patient requires complete rest and daily ophthalmologic assessment until there is total resolution. *(Riordan-Eva, 2014, p. 188)*

14. **(D)** Tenderness of the tragus and preauricular adenopathy, are present with otitis externa (OE), but not acute otitis media. Eustachian tube dysfunction

causes middle ear pressure. Ramsay-Hunt syndrome is a herpes zoster infection of the ear canal and the lesions would be visible. Ramsay-Hunt syndrome is characterized by visible vesicular lesions of the ear canal, auricle, and/or mucous membrane of the oropharynx. It is extremely rare in children, particularly with the advent of varicella immunization. Otitis media does not usually present with canal edema or drainage blocking visualization of the tympanic membrane and does not typically cause tenderness of the tragus. Often only mildly tender, a perforated TM would cause pain in the middle ear and there would generally be no pain with manipulation of the tragus. The tympanic membrane is often minimally tender once the perforation occurs. Typically there is a history of pain relieved by the perforation. Generally there is no pain with manipulation of the tragus. Eustachian tube dysfunction causes middle ear pressure, generally without pain. (*Rosenfeld et al., 2014, pp. S1–S24*)

15. **(E)** Involvement of the tip of the nose with herpes virus is known as Hutchinson's sign. It is suggestive of involvement of the cornea with herpes and urgent referral to an ophthalmologist is recommended. The patient has shingles (herpes zoster) which follows dermatomes and is generally unilateral. Ruling out involvement of the nasal septum is not crucial. Involvement of the tip of the nose or lid margins should lead one to suspect corneal involvement. Tympanic membrane involvement is not crucial to rule out and is not related to herpes zoster ophthalmicus. (*Riordan-Eva, 2014, p. 170*)

16. **(B)** Mononucleosis is a frequent cause of exudative pharyngitis in the absence of strep pharyngitis. It is often associated with anterior and posterior cervical adenopathy along with generalized lymphadenopathy and an enlarged spleen. Obtaining a monospot can provide the definitive diagnosis. While reviewing the history is certainly an aspect of every patient encounter, reviewing the history for similar episodes is unlikely to lead to a diagnosis for this patient. Although the patient does likely have a viral infection, it is appropriate to evaluate for mononucleosis. A rapid strep test was negative and the course of this patient's illness has run longer than strep pharyngitis usually runs. A monospot test is rapid and easy to obtain. There is no benefit to withholding the test at this time. (*Ferri, 2014, p. 728*)

17. **(B)** Ménière syndrome is characterized by bouts of vertigo along with unilateral low-frequency sensorineural hearing loss with tinnitus in the affected ear. Eustachian tube dysfunction usually results in a conductive hearing loss. Benign paroxysmal vertigo (BPPV) is not associated with unilateral hearing loss. The vertigo of BPPV is associated with positional change. Vestibular neuronitis and labyrinthitis present with acute severe vertigo and often nausea and vomiting and neither is associated with unilateral hearing loss. An acoustic neuroma is usually associated with a hearing loss across all frequencies which is generally insidious in onset. (*Herraiz et al., 2010, pp. 162–167*)

18. **(A)** The lesion described is a hordeolum. A chalazion is a granulomatous lesion and is nontender. It is associated with redness and swelling of the conjunctiva. Blepharitis presents bilaterally and is a chronic condition. Subconjunctival hemorrhage affects the conjunctiva only. Entropion is inward turning of the lower eyelid which presents in older people. (*Lindsley et al., 2010*)

19. **(B)** The lesion, a hordeolum is most likely caused by a staphylococcal infection, typically *Staphylococcus aureus*. (*Lindsley et al., 2010*)

20. **(C)** A history of facial/orbital trauma that results in diplopia is suggestive of an orbital blowout fracture with entrapment. One would expect restricted extraocular movements. Plain films could help identify injury to the bones, the CT is the best assessment of orbital trauma. (*Greenberg & Daniel, 2011*)

21. **(E)** Based on the patient's symptoms, abnormal findings on eye examination and the significantly elevated intraocular pressure of 70 mm Hg (normal being 10–21 mm Hg), the diagnosis is acute angle closure glaucoma. This is an ophthalmic emergency. Retinal artery occlusion and detachment are painless and the fundoscopic findings are different. (*Riordan-Eva, 2014, pp. 171–172*)

22. **(A)** The central retinal artery occlusion occurs when small emboli become lodged in retinal arterioles. Recurrent small emboli frequently cause amaurosis fugax or transient visual loss. Fundoscopic examination will show a pale retina with a cherry-red spot at the fovea. (*Riordan-Eva, 2014, p. 176*)

23. **(B)** The patient most likely has age-related sensorineural hearing loss or presbycusis. This is often associated with tinnitus. There is usually no pain or pressure sensation associated with presbycusis. Isolated age-related hearing loss is not associated with vertigo. The examination findings indicated that the tympanic membranes were normal. *(Manes, www.clinicalkey.com/#!/topic/presbycusis)*

24. **(B)** This woman's hearing loss is most likely age-related sensorineural hearing loss, or presbycusis. In a conductive hearing loss, the Weber is transmitted to the ear with decreased hearing and the bone conduction is greater than the air conduction (even with bilateral conductive losses). The patient's history states that there is a hearing loss. *(Isaacson, 2010)*

25. **(D)** Myasthenia gravis (MG) is a relatively common disorder, occurring in about 2–7 in 10,000 people. It affects patients in all age groups and both sexes, but is more common in women in their 20s and 30s and in men in their 50s and 60s. The male to female ratio is about 3:2. Patients present with ptosis, diplopia, difficulty swallowing and chewing, weakness and fatigability of muscles. The weakness increases during repeated use (fatigue) or late in the day and may improve following rest or sleep. The diagnostic modality of choice is Tensilon or edrophonium testing. *(Drachman & Amato, 2015, Ch. 461)*

26. **(B)** Reiter syndrome is a disorder that consists of a triad of the following symptoms: arthritis, conjunctivitis, and urinary tract symptoms. It is sometimes referred to as a reactive arthritis, responding to an infection elsewhere in the body particularly in the GI or genitourinary tract. The diagnosis is based on history and physical examination findings. *(Hellman & Imboden, 2010, p. 776)*

27. **(A)** Amblyopia is the permanent decrease in visual acuity in a child caused by abnormal visual exposure during the maturation process. During this time it is important for the retina and central nervous system to integrate. Strabismus, which can cause blurred retinal image in one or both eyes can lead to this permanent visual disorder. *(Coats & Paysse, 2014)*

28. **(C)** Nasal drainage which is purulent and unilateral in a child or someone with cognitive compromise should be considered to be a foreign-body impaction until proven otherwise. Nasal polyps do not typically cause purulent drainage. However, if a child presents with nasal polyposis, consideration should be given a workup for cystic fibrosis, possibly including a sweat chloride test. *(Weinberger & Terris, 2010, Ch. 15)*

29. **(B)** Congenital CMV infections are generally not apparent at birth. Five percent to 25% of asymptomatic infants with CMV infections develop significant hearing, visual, or dental abnormalities over the next several years. Hepatic pathology is also common in exposed infected infants, but of the options given, sensorineural hearing loss is the most likely complication of CMV infection. *(Picone O et al., 2013)*

30. **(D)** Perform a special fluorescein dye examination of the eye. This test is called a Seidel test. It consists of applying a fluorescein dye strip gently to the area of injury and then viewing it under a slit lamp with a cobalt blue light. If a perforation or leak is present, the fluorescein dye will be diluted by aqueous fluid from the injured site. If a globe rupture is suspected, an eye shield should be immediately placed over the affected eye and further examination deferred to avoid putting pressure on the eyes. An MRI is not indicated if there is a metallic object in the eye. *(Fraghihi et al., 2012)*

31. **(A)** The patient has developed acute sinusitis secondary to her previous upper respiratory infection and amoxicillin is the first-line antibiotic recommended. Based on the history and PE findings, CT is not needed at this time. Oral ciprofloxacin is not indicated in pediatric patients for sinusitis; the only indication for which a fluoroquinolone (i.e., ciprofloxacin) is licensed by the U.S. Food and Drug Administration for use in patients younger than 18 years are complicated urinary tract infections, pyelonephritis, and postexposure treatment for inhalation anthrax. Cefaclor is not indicated for sinusitis. Although warm facial compresses and sinus washes are helpful adjunct treatments, an antibiotic is indicated in this patient. *(Friedman et al., 2013)*

32. **(A)** Notching of the incisors is sometimes but not always caused by congenital syphilis. None of the other listed options cause Hutchinson's incisors.

(http://www.fpnotebook.com/Dental/Teeth/ HtchnsnsTth.htm)

33. **(A)** Patients with retinal detachment frequently complain of unilateral photopsia or a sensation of flashing light, an increased number of floaters (posterior vitreous detachment), decreased visual acuity and metamorphopsia, or wavy distortion of an object. Emergency referral to an ophthalmologist is warranted if a retinal detachment is suspected. *(Arroyo, 2013)*

34. **(C)** A CT scan is imperative at this time to confirm the diagnosis of malignant external otitis. Granulation tissue in the canal is suggestive of this condition as are cranial nerve palsies. In addition, the diagnosis is suggested by the patient's history of poorly controlled diabetes. Persistent external otitis can evolve into osteomyelitis of the skull base. *(Hollis & Evans, 2011, pp. 1212–1217)*

35. **(B)** Epiglottitis will show a "thumb sign" on the lateral C-spine x-ray. The thumbprint sign or "thumb sign" describes a swollen, enlarged epiglottis; usually with dilated hypopharynx and normal subglottic structures. *(Verbruggen et al., 2012, pp. 143–148)*

36. **(C)** Sparing of the forehead in facial paralysis as in this patient is indicative of a lesion superior to the nucleus of the VII cranial nerve such as a brain tumor or a stroke. Ramsay-Hunt is accompanied by painful vesicular lesions. *(Jauch et al., 2010)*

37. **(D)** Allergic rhinitis is associated with pale edematous, boggy nasal mucosa, along with clear rhinorrhea. Viral rhinitis is associated with erythematous turbinates, asthma produces expiratory wheezing and coughing, and a nasal foreign body causes foul smelling unilateral nasal drainage. *(Rachelefsky & Farrar, 2013)*

38. **(B)** The description is consistent with positional vertigo which is assumed to be caused by tiny canaliths in the inner ear. It is a benign, self-limited condition, and can be treated with an 80% success with canalith repositioning procedure. The Dix–Hallpike maneuver is a positional testing that is used to confirm the diagnosis. The vertigo must be positional in nature. Ménière syndrome is associated with unilateral tinnitus and hearing loss in addition to vertigo, which is not positional. Vertigo associated with labyrinthitis and vestibular neuronitis is not positional. Central lesions do not typically have an association of the vertigo and nystagmus. Vestibular nystagmus should differentiate positional vertigo from a central lesion. *(Johnson & Lalwani, 2012, Ch. 56)*

39. **(E)** Vestibular schwannoma or acoustic neuroma causes asymmetric (unilateral) sensorineural hearing loss, tinnitus, and disequilibrium. The audiometric findings of sensorineural hearing loss with poor speech discrimination along with tinnitus and unsteadiness should cause one to obtain an MRI with gadolinium enhancement as soon as possible to rule out acoustic neuroma or schwannoma of the vestibular nerve. There is no condition known as megaloblastoma. Impacted cerumen may cause mild dizziness and possibly conductive hearing loss. Otosclerosis has a hereditary disposition and conductive hearing loss. Labyrinthitis is not associated with hearing loss. *(Johnson & Lalwani, 2012, Ch. 61)*

40. **(C)** A cholesteatoma is a squamous epithelial–lined sac that gradually increases in size and can eventually erode through bones, for example, the ossicular chain or nerves (i.e., facial nerve). It may become infected and drain intermittently. It is sometimes a complication of chronic otitis media or may result from perforation of the tympanic membrane involving the margin or pars flaccida. Myringosclerosis (scarring of the tympanic membrane) presents as white one-dimensional translucent patches on the TM. Tympanosclerosis and otosclerosis involve pathology of the middle ear. Keratosis obturans is accumulation of scaly sloughed-off keratin in the external auditory canal. *(Chang, 2012, Ch. 50)*

41. **(A)** Strawberry tongue: erythematous and sometimes edematous tongue with prominent papillae (Strawberry tongue), pink or red linear lesions seen in the body folds, especially the antecubital and axillary folds (Pastia's lines), and a positive antistreptolysin test, indicating previous streptococcal infection, clinch the diagnosis of Scarlet fever. *(Usatine et al., 2013, Ch. 34)*

42. **(C)** The "tree branch" is the classical presentation of herpetic infection of the cornea. This patient

should be evaluated by an ophthalmologist as soon as possible. Glaucoma may give a shallow anterior angle. Hyphema is blood, hypopyon is pus in the anterior chamber, behind the cornea. Iritis gives perilimbal injection. *(Riordan-Eva, 2014, Ch. 7)*

43. **(E)** Trismus and muffled or "hot potato" voice developing in a patient with a sore throat are the clues to the diagnosis. Along with the uvular deviation, this trio provides a classic description of a peritonsillar abscess. Palatal tori are completely benign midline palatal masses that are asymptomatic. Koplik spots are pathognomonic for measles. Gingival hyperplasia is seen on the gingiva and an oral ranula produces swelling of the floor of the mouth that is usually nonpainful. Speaking, chewing, breathing, and swallowing may be affected because of the upward and medial displacement of the tongue. *(Lustig & Schindler, 2010, p. 205)*

44. **(D)** Weber testing lateralizing to the good ear suggests a sensorineural hearing loss. The cause is unknown, but generally thought to be viral or vascular. The only therapy shown to be efficacious for sudden onset sensorineural hearing loss is oral corticosteroids given as soon as possible. None of the other listed treatments is efficacious for sensorineural hearing loss and only serve to delay appropriate treatment. *(Lustig & Schlinder, 2014c, Ch. 8)*

45. **(A)** Gingival hyperplasia is a known possible complication of dilantin. The prevalence of phenytoin-induced gingival hyperplasia is estimated at 15% to 50% in patients taking the medication. *(Mejia, 2014)*

46. **(C)** Koplik spots are pathognomonic of measles and consist of bluish-white dots ~1 mm in diameter surrounded by erythema. The lesions appear first on the buccal mucosa opposite the lower molars but rapidly increase in number to involve the entire buccal mucosa. They fade with the onset of rash. They may even be used to isolate children to prevent epidemics as they appear prior to maximum infectivity. Gray pharyngeal pseudomembrane is pathognomonic of diphtheria. Exudative pharyngitis is seen with mononucleosis and streptococcal pharyngitis. Steeple sign is seen in croup, and a thumbprint sign is seen with epiglottitis. *(Moss, 2012, Ch. 192)*

47. **(B)** Herpes zoster oticus (Ramsay-Hunt syndrome) consists of acute facial palsy combined with otalgia and varicella- or vesicular-type lesions. There is intense ear pain, pathognomonic lesions on the pinna, and facial paralysis. The cause is the herpes varicella virus. *(Jauch et al., 2010, Ch. 5)*

48. **(D)** The patient has Ramsay-Hunt syndrome which is most appropriately treated with oral corticosteroids, antiviral medications, and pain medications. *(Jauch et al., 2010, Ch. 5)*

49. **(B)** Otosclerosis is a progressive, familiar condition in which the bones of the middle ear (the ossicles) soften and then harden (or sclerose) at the joints. This results in increased impedance to the passage of sound through the ossicles causing conductive hearing loss. Diagnosis may be made based on the family history of hearing loss which proves via tuning forks or audiometry to be conductive. The physical examination would show normal tympanic membranes. Presbycusis and "idiopathic hearing loss" or sudden onset sensorineural hearing loss cause sensorineural loss and myringosclerosis does not generally produce any hearing loss. Serous otitis media would be apparent on pneumatoscopy. *(Driscoll & Carlson, 2012, Ch. 51)*

50. **(E)** Ludwig's angina, most likely secondary to dental infection is a cellulitis of the floor of the mouth which if left untreated could completely obstruct the airway. The submental, sublingual, and submandibular spaces are infected bilaterally. Patients usually present with poor dental hygiene, dysphagia, odynophagia, trismus, and edema of the upper midline neck and the floor of mouth. Clinical examination reveals edema of the entire upper neck and floor of mouth. Infection progresses rapidly and can posteriorly displace the tongue, causing airway compromise. The appropriate plan includes CT of the neck, IV antibiotics, and preparation for intubation. *(Lustig & Schindler, 2014b, pp. 223–224)*

51. **(C)** TMD is a common cause of pain referred to the ear. It may be an inflammatory response to dental procedures or caused by bruxism. The tipoffs to this diagnosis are the pain increased by eating and normal ear examination apart from tenderness over the TMJ within the ear canal. In a retrospective study of 4,528 patients with TMD, the most

common presenting signs and symptoms were: pain (96.1%), ear discomfort or dysfunction (82.4%), headache (79.3%), TMJ discomfort or dysfunction (75.0%). *(Tsai et al., 2015)*

52. **(D)** Rhinitis of pregnancy is common and can peak in the third trimester of pregnancy. Rising levels of estrogen cause an increase in hyaluronic acid in the nasal tissue thus increasing nasal edema and congestion. The obstetrician may recommend treatment with decongestants or nasal steroids, however, treatment is generally optional as the condition resolves postpartum. *(Shah & Emanuel, 2012)*

53. **(B)** Finding nasal polyposis in a child is a "red flag" condition and should make the clinician suspicious of possible cystic fibrosis. Usually this disease is diagnosed in early childhood generally with lung involvement and often failure to thrive. The children may also experience chronic sinusitis and recurring ear infections. Polyps generally appear between the ages of 5 and 14. Alert clinicians should order a sweat chloride test. *(Lustig & Schindler, 2014a, p. 216)*

54. **(E)** A nasal mass in a postpubescent male (13–21 years) is typical of juvenile angiofibromas, which are benign vascular tumors. They tend to present in adolescent males. The patient usually presents complaining of severe unilateral epistaxis and obstruction. Any biopsy done should be in the OR based on the possibility of severe hemorrhage. *(Tewfik & Garni, 2014)*

55. **(E)** The most common site of epistaxis is in the anterior septum where a confluence of veins creates a superficial venous plexus known as the Kiesselbach plexus. *(Manes, 2010, pp. 203–212)*

56. **(C)** The lesion described, an adherent white lesion represents leukoplakia. It should be considered as a premalignant lesion as 1% to 20% of the lesions progress to carcinoma in 10 years. *(Goldstein & Goldstein, 2014)*

57. **(D)** Based on this lesion's description as an adherent white lesion, one cannot rule out leukoplakia without pathologic evaluation. It should be considered as a premalignant lesion as 1% to 20% of the lesions progress to carcinoma in 10 years. An incisional or excisional biopsy must be performed as there is a possibility for progression to oral carcinoma. *(Goldstein & Goldstein, 2014)*

58. **(C)** Emergency referral for surgical drainage of the nasal septal hematoma is required. Drains and packing must be placed to prevent reaccumulation of the hematoma. Additionally, the integrity of the nasal septal cartilage must be evaluated. Failure to drain the subperichondrial hematoma would cause necrosis of the nasal cartilage and result in saddle nose deformity. *(Ngo & Schraga, 2014)*

59. **(C)** Foreign bodies in the nose create foul smelling purulent and sometimes bloody unilateral nasal drainage. Unilateral purulent nasal drainage should be considered a foreign body until proven otherwise and clinicians must always rule out nasal foreign bodies with a complaint of unilateral purulent nasal drainage, particularly in a child or a patient with decreased cognitive abilities. *(Cohen & Agrawal, 2011, Ch. 116)*

60. **(E)** Injuries to the nasal bone and nasal process of the frontal bone may lead to a fracture through the cribriform or ethmoid bones. Cerebrospinal fluid (CSF) is typically unilateral and comes in short rapid gushes, or as a steady flow. CSF contains glucose which can be easily measured with a urine glucose dipstick. *(Welch, 2014)*

61. **(D)** Postnasal drainage is the most common cause of a chronic cough in an adult. Asthma is the second most common cause and gastroesophageal reflux is the third cause. *(Sarko & Stapczynski, 2011, Ch. 65)*

62. **(C)** Routine audiology screening is recommended in all adults who have reached the age of 65. None of the other patients requires an audiogram based on their presentations. *(Jerger, 2010, pp. 424–425)*

63. **(B)** Epiglottitis should be suspected when there is rapid onset of severe sore throat, or when the pain and odynophagia is disproportional to the physical examination findings. It is more common in patients who have diabetes. Contrary to children, indirect laryngoscopy is generally safe in adults. The patient should be hospitalized for airway maintenance, and IV treatment. Fewer than 10% of adults require intubation. *(Verbruggen et al., 2012, pp. 143–148)*

64. **(A)** External otitis is usually caused by gram-negative rods like Pseudomonas or Proteus. *(Kaushik, 2010)*

65. **(E)** Lymphoma may present as unilateral tonsillar enlargement. The rapidly enlarging tonsil and lack of other infectious symptoms suggests a malignant process. Performing a tonsillectomy will provide a biopsy specimen. *(Suurna, 2012, Ch. 21)*

66. **(D)** Chronic use of nasal decongestant sprays for more than 5 to 7 days will usually result in rebound nasal congestion if they are not continued. This is called rhinitis medicamentosa. Treatment is based on stopping the use of the nasal inhaler. *(Weinberger & Terris, 2015)*

67. **(B)** Squamous cell carcinoma accounts for 90% of oral cancer. Alcohol and tobacco use are the major risk factors. Leukoplakia represents early invasive squamous cell carcinoma or dysplasia in 2% to 6% of cases. Erythroplakia is more aggressive and undergoes malignant transformation more frequently. Local resection is the treatment of choice for smaller lesions, and radiation is not generally used as first-line treatment for small lesions. *(Amagasa et al., 2011)*

68. **(D)** Obstructive sleep apnea (OSA) is caused by loss of pharyngeal muscle tone which causes it to collapse during inspiration. This causes narrowing of the airway. OSA is particularly common in overweight middle-aged males. It is frequently associated with poorly controlled hypertension. There is usually daytime hypersomnolence. Alcohol and hypnotic/sedatives may increase the symptoms. *(Chesnutt & Prendergast, 2014)*

69. **(E)** Acute laryngitis is a common cause of hoarseness and often persists for a week or more after resolution of other symptoms of an upper respiratory infection. The patient should be warned to avoid vigorous use of the voice such as singing, shouting, or excessive talking until their voice returns to normal, since persistent use may lead to the formation of traumatic vocal fold hemorrhage, polyps, and cysts. Leukoplakia is related to tobacco and alcohol use, along with dental irritation. Most cases of laryngitis are viral in etiology and this patient's symptoms were resolving, therefore antibiotic treatment is not indicated. Laryngitis is not a risk factor for vocal cord paralysis. There are many causes of vocal cord paralysis, but laryngitis, even if protracted is not one of them. *(Reveiz & Cardona, 2013)*

70. **(A)** Candidiasis produces a thick white coating on the tongue that is easily scraped off, revealing a raw erythematous area underneath. Candida is common is immunocompromised patients. Oral cancers, most commonly squamous cell carcinomas are more common in abusers of tobacco and alcohol over the age of 50. *Corynebacterium diphtheriae* produces a red throat and gray exudate or the uvula, pharynx, and tongue. Although this patient is HIV positive and therefore at risk for hairy leukoplakia, the feathery white lesions of hairy leukoplakia cannot be scraped off. *(Giannini & Shetty, 2011, pp. 231–240)*

71. **(B)** The patient stated that the lesion was affecting his vision. Therefore, and especially as the patient is a truck driver, he requires excision of this lesion. Artificial tears along with topical NSAIDs or corticosteroids may help symptoms of an irritated pterygium, but do not provide definitive treatment. An iridotomy is the recommended treatment for acute angle closure glaucoma. *(Riordan-Eva, 2014, Ch. 7)*

REFERENCES

Amagasa T, Yamashiro M, Uzawa N. Oral premalignant lesions: from a clinical perspective. *Int J Clin Oncol.* 2011;16(1):5–14.

Arroyo JG. Retinal detachment. In: Trobe J, Park L, eds. *UpToDate.* Waltham, MA: UpToDate; 2014.

Chang C. Chapter 50: Cholesteatoma. In: Lalwani AK, ed. *CURRENT Diagnosis & Treatment in Otolaryngology—Head & Neck Surgery.* 3rd ed. New York, NY: McGraw-Hill; 2012. http://accessmedicine.mhmedical.com/content.aspx?bookid=386&Sectionid=39944092. Accessed April 23, 2015.

Chesnutt MS, Prendergast TJ. Pulmonary disorders. In: Papadakis MA, McPhee SJ, Rabow MW, eds. *Current Medical Diagnosis & Treatment 2015.* New York, NY: McGraw-Hill; 2014. http://accessmedicine.mhmedical.com/content.aspx?bookid=1019&Sectionid=57668601. Accessed April 27, 2015.

Coats DK, Paysse EA. Evaluation and management of strabismus in children. In: Saunders RA, Torchia MM, eds. *UpToDate.* Waltham, MA: UpToDate; 2014.

Cohen JS, Agrawal D. Chapter 116: The nose and sinuses. In: Tintinalli JE, Stapczynski JS, Ma OJ, Cline DC, Cydulka R, Meckler GD, eds. *Tintinalli's Emergency Medicine: A Comprehensive Study Guide.* 3rd ed. New York, NY: McGraw-Hill; 2011. http://accessmedicine.mhmedical.com/content.aspx?bookid=348&Sectionid=40381588. Accessed April 27, 2015.

Drachman DB, Amato AA. Chapter 461: Myasthenia gravis and other diseases of the neuromuscular junction. In: Kasper D, Fauci A, Hauser S, Longo D, Jameson J, Loscalzo J, eds. *Harrison's Principles of Internal Medicine.* 19th ed. New York, NY: McGraw-Hill; 2015. http://accessmedicine.mhmedical.com/content.aspx?bookid=1130&Sectionid=79756727. Accessed April 23, 2015.

Driscoll CW, Carlson ML. Chapter 51: Otosclerosis. In: Lalwani AK, ed. *CURRENT Diagnosis & Treatment in Otolaryngology—Head & Neck Surgery.* 3rd ed. New York, NY: McGraw-Hill; 2012. http://accessmedicine.mhmedical.com/content.aspx?bookid=386&Sectionid=39944093. Accessed April 23, 2015.

Ferri FF. *Ferri's Clinical Advisor.* Philadelphia, PA: Elsevier-Mosby; 2014.

Fraghihi H, Hajizadeh F, Esfahani MR, et al. Posttraumatic endophthalmitis: report No 2. *Retina.* 2012;32(1):146–151.

Friedman NR, Scholes MA, Yoon PJ. Ear, nose, & throat. In: Hay WW Jr, Levin MJ, Deterding RR, Abzug MJ, eds. *CURRENT Diagnosis & Treatment: Pediatrics.* 22nd ed. New York, NY: McGraw-Hill; 2013. http://accessmedicine.mhmedical.com/content.aspx?bookid=1016&Sectionid=61597764. Accessed April 23, 2015.

Giannini PJ, Shetty KV. Diagnosis and management of oral candidiasis. *Otolaryngol Clin North Am.* 2011;44(1):231–240.

Goldstein BG, Goldstein AO. Oral lesions. UpToDate, In: Dellavalle RP, Deschler DG, Corona R, eds. *UpToDate.* Waltham, MA; 2014: Accessed October 7, 2014.

Greenberg RD, Daniel KJ. Chapter 31: *Eye Emergencies in CURRENT Diagnosis & Treatment Emergency Medicine.* 7th ed. 2011. http://accessmedicine.mhmedical.com/book.aspx?bookid=385. Accessed April 22, 2015.

Hellman DB, Imboden JB. Musculoskeletal & immunologic disorders. In: McPhee SJ, Papadakis MA, eds. *Current Medical Diagnosis and Treatment.* 49th ed. New York, NY: McGraw-Hill; 2010.

Herraiz C, Plaza G, Aparicio JM, Gallego I, Marcos S, Ruiz C. Transtympanic steroids for Meniere's disease. *Oto Neurotol.* 2010;31(1):162–167.

Hollis S, Evans K. Management of malignant (necrotizing) otitis externa. *J Laryngol Otol.* 2011;125(12):1212–1217.

Hua L, Doll T. A series of 3 cases of corneal abrasion with multiple etiologies. *Optometry.* 2010;81(2):83–85.

Irfan M. Ear foreign body: tackling the uncommons. *Med J Malaysia.* 2012;67(3):332.

Isaacson B. Hearing loss. *Med Clin North Am.* 2010;94(5):973–988.

Ishaq M, Muhammad JS, Mahmood K. Uveitis is not just an ophthalmologist's concern. *J Pak Med Assoc.* 2012;62(2):92–97.

Jackson J. Chapter 65: *Pfenninger and Fowler's Procedures for Primary Care.* Philadelphia, PA: Mosby; 2011:427–432. downloaded from www.clinicalkey.com/#!/content/book/3-s2.0-B9780323052672000650?scrollTo=%23top April 21, 2015.

Jauch EC, Barbabella SP, Fernandez FJ, Knoop KJ. Chapter 5: Ear, nose, and throat conditions. In: Knoop KJ, Stack LB, Storrow AB, Thurman R, eds. *The Atlas of Emergency Medicine.* 3rd ed. New York, NY: McGraw-Hill; 2010. http://accessmedicine.mhmedical.com/content.aspx?bookid=351&Sectionid=39619704. Accessed April 23, 2015.

Jerger J. New horizons in speech audiometry? *J Am Acad Audiol.* 2010;21(7):424–425.

Johnson J, Lalwani AK. Chapter 56: Vestibular disorders. In: Lalwani AK, ed. *CURRENT Diagnosis & Treatment in Otolaryngology—Head & Neck Surgery.* 3rd ed. New York, NY: McGraw-Hill; 2012. http://accessmedicine.mhmedical.com/content.aspx?bookid=386&Sectionid=39944099. Accessed October 27, 2014.

Johnson J, Lalwani AK. Chapter 61: Vestibular schwannoma (acoustic neuroma). In: Lalwani AK, ed. *CURRENT Diagnosis & Treatment in Otolaryngology—Head & Neck Surgery.* 3rd ed. New York, NY: McGraw-Hill; 2012. http://accessmedicine.mhmedical.com/content.aspx?bookid=386&Sectionid=39944105. Accessed October 27, 2014.

Kaufman H. Adenovirus advances: new diagnostic and therapeutic options. *Current Opin Ophthalmol.* 2011;22(4):290–293.

Kaushik V, Malik T, Saeed SR. Interventions for acute otitis externa. *CochraneDatabase Syst Rev.* 2010;(1):CD004740.

Kubota T, Ohta N, Fukase S, Kon Y, Aoyagi M. Treatment of auricular hematoma by OK-432. *Otolaryngol Head Neck Surg.* 2010;142(6):863–866.

Lindsley K, Nichols JJ, Dickersin K. Interventions for acute internal hordeolum. *Cochrane Database Syst Rev.* 2010;(9):CD007742.

Lustig LR, Schindler JS. Ear, nose, & throat disorders. In: McPhee SJ, Papadakis MA, eds. *Current Medical Diagnosis and Treatment.* 49th ed. New York, NY: McGraw-Hill; 2010.

Lustig LR, Schindler JS. Ear, nose, & throat disorders. In: Papadakis MA, McPhee SJ, Rabow MW, eds. *Current Medical Diagnosis & Treatment 2014.* New York, NY: McGraw-Hill; 2014a:216.

Lustig LR, Schindler JS. Ear, nose, & throat disorders. In: Papadakis MA, McPhee SJ, Rabow MW, eds. *Current Medical Diagnosis & Treatment 2014.* New York, NY: McGraw-Hill; 2014b:223–224.

Lustig LR, Schindler JS. Ear, nose, & throat disorders. In: Papadakis MA, McPhee SJ, Rabow MW, eds. *Current Medical Diagnosis & Treatment 2015.* New York, NY: McGraw-Hill; 2014c. http://accessmedicine.mhmedical.com/content.aspx? bookid=1019&Sectionid=57668600. Accessed April 23, 2015.

Manes RP. Evaluating and managing the patient with nose-bleeds. *Med Clin North Am.* 2010;94(5):903–912.

Manes RP. www.clinicalkey.com/#!/topic/presbycusis. Accessed April 23, 2015.

Mejia L. *Drug-Induced Gingival Hyperplasia.* http://emedicine. medscape.com/article/1076264. Accessed October 27, 2014.

Moss WJ. Chapter 192: Measles (rubeola). In: Longo DL, Fauci AS, Kasper DL, Hauser SL, Jameson J, Loscalzo J, eds. *Harrison's Principles of Internal Medicine.*18th ed. New York, NY: McGraw-Hill; 2012. http://accessmedicine. mhmedical.com/content.aspx?bookid=331&Sectionid =40726951. Accessed October 27, 2014.

Ngo J, Schraga E. 2014. http://emedicine.medscape.com/ article/149280-overview. Accessed April 27, 2015.

Picone O, Vauloup-Fellous C, Cordier AG, et al. A series of 238 cytomegalovirus primary infections during pregnancy: description and outcome. *Prenat Diagn.* 2013;33(8):751–758.

Rachelefsky G, Farrar JR. A control model to evaluate pharma-cotherapy for allergic rhinitis in children. *JAMA Pediatr.* 2013;167(4):380–386.

Reveiz L, Cardona AF. Antibiotics for acute laryngitis in adults. *Cochrane Database Syst Rev.* 2013;3:CD004783.

Riordan-Eva P. Chapter 7: Disorders of the eyes & lids. In: Papadakis MA, McPhee SJ, Rabow MW, eds. *CURRENT Medical Diagnosis & Treatment 2014.* New York, NY: McGraw-Hill; 2014. http://accessmedicine.mhmedical.com/ content.aspx?bookid=330&Sectionid=44291009. Accessed August 18, 2014.

Rosenfeld RM, Schwartz SR, Cannon CR, et al. Clinical practice guideline: acute otitis externa. *Otolaryngol Head Neck Surg.* 2014;150(1 Suppl):S1–S24.

Sarko J, Stapczynski J. Chapter 65: Respiratory distress. In: Tintinalli JE, Stapczynski JS, Ma OJ, Cline DC, Cydulka R, Meckler GD, eds. *Tintinalli's Emergency Medicine: A Comprehensive Study Guide.* 7th ed. New York, NY: McGraw-Hill; 2011. http://accessmedicine.mhmedical.com/content.

aspx?bookid=348&Sectionid=40381531. Accessed April 27, 2015.

Shah SB, Emanuel IA. Chapter 14: Nonallergic & allergic rhi-nitis. In: Lalwani AK, ed. *CURRENT Diagnosis & Treatment in Otolaryngology—Head & Neck Surgery.* 3rd ed. New York, NY: McGraw-Hill; 2012. http://accessmedicine.mhmedical. com/content.aspx?bookid=386&Sectionid=39944047. Accessed April 23, 2015.

Suurna MV. Chapter 21: Management of adenotonsillar disease. In: Lalwani AK, ed. *CURRENT Diagnosis & Treatment in Otolaryngology—Head & Neck Surgery.* 3rd ed. New York, NY: McGraw-Hill; 2012. http://accessmedicine.mhmedical. com/content.aspx?bookid=386&Sectionid=39944057. Accessed April 27, 2015.

Tewfik TL, Garni MA. 2014. http://emedicine.medscape.com/ article/872580-overview#a0112. Accessed April 27, 2015.

Tsai V, Sinert R, Heffer S. Temporomandibular joint syndrome clinical presentation. 2015. http://emedicine.medscape.com/ article/809598-clinical. Accessed April 23, 2015.

Usatine RP, Smith MA, Chumley HS, Mayeaux EJ Jr. Chapter 34: Scarlet fever and strawberry tongue. In: Usatine RP, Smith MA, Chumley HS, Mayeaux EJ Jr, eds. *The Color Atlas of Family Medicine.* 2nd ed. New York, NY: McGraw-Hill; 2013. http://accessmedicine.mhmedical.com/content.aspx?bookid =685&Sectionid=45361073. Accessed October 27, 2014.

Verbruggen K, Halewyck S, Deron P, Foulon I, Gordts F. Epiglottitis and related complications in adults. Case reports and review of the literature. *B-ENT.* 2012;8(2):143–148.

Walker RA, Adhikari S. Eye emergencies. *Chapter 36: Tintinalli's Emergency Medicine: A Comprehensive Study Guide.* 7th ed. 2011. http://accessmedicine.mhmedical.com/content.aspx? sectionid=40381722&bookid=348&jumpsection-ID=40404823&Resultclick=2. Accessed April 21, 2015.

Weinberger PM, Terris DJ. Chapter 15: Otolaryngology—head & neck surgery. In: Doherty GM, ed. *CURRENT Diagnosis & Treatment: Surgery.* 13th ed. New York, NY: McGraw-Hill; 2010. http://accessmedicine.mhmedical.com/content.aspx? bookid=343&Sectionid=39702802. Accessed April 23, 2015.

Weinberger PM, Terris DJ. Otolaryngology: head & neck sur-gery. In: Doherty GM, ed. *CURRENT Diagnosis & Treatment: Surgery.* 14th ed. New York, NY: McGraw-Hill; 2015. http:// accessmedicine.mhmedical.com/content.aspx?bookid =1202&Sectionid=71517698. Accessed April 27, 2015.

Welch KC. 2014. http://emedicine.medscape.com/ article/861126-workup Accessed April 27, 2015.

CHAPTER 19

Urology

Anne E. Schempp, MPAS, PA-C

DIRECTIONS: Each of the numbered questions or incomplete statements is followed by possible answers or completions of the statement. Select the ONE-lettered answer or completion that is BEST in each case.

1. What is the most common composition of renal calculi?

    (A) Calcium
    (B) Cystine
    (C) Protein
    (D) Struvite
    (E) Uric acid

2. A 32-year-old female presents with fever, chills, and flank pain for 24 hours. She developed dysuria and urinary frequency 3 days prior and states that both have worsened. Which of the following findings most specifically confirms the likely diagnosis?

    (A) 3+ red blood cells
    (B) 3+ white blood cells
    (C) Epithelial cells
    (D) Hyaline casts
    (E) White blood cell casts

3. What is the most common pathogen associated with acute cystitis in female patients?

    (A) *Chlamydia trachomatis*
    (B) *Escherichia coli*
    (C) Proteus species
    (D) Pseudomonas species
    (E) *Staphylococcus epidermidis*

4. Which of the following is the most likely presenting symptom of bladder cancer?

    (A) Dysuria
    (B) Foul-smelling urine
    (C) Hematuria
    (D) Oliguria
    (E) Urinary frequency

5. A 26-year-old male presents with complaints of burning with urination, joint pain, and red eye for the past week. Based on the combination of these presenting symptoms, which of the following is the most likely diagnosis?

    (A) Balanitis
    (B) Gonorrhea
    (C) Reactive arthritis
    (D) Rheumatoid disease
    (E) Tertiary syphilis

6. Which of the following sexually transmitted disorders manifests as a painless genital ulcer?

    (A) Chancroid
    (B) Genital herpes
    (C) Genital warts
    (D) Molluscum contagiosum
    (E) Syphilis

7. Which of the following conditions is defined as the inability to reduce the foreskin of the penis once it has been retracted?

    (A) Balanitis
    (B) Hypospadias
    (C) Paraphimosis
    (D) Phimosis
    (E) Urethral meatal stricture

8. Which of the following findings would be of most concern if found while examining a 26-year-old healthy male patient?

   (A) A left testis sitting higher than the right
   (B) A nontender mass on a testis
   (C) A tender epididymis
   (D) An enlarged, fluid-filled scrotum
   (E) Dilated veins within the spermatic cord

9. Which anatomical portion of the prostate becomes hyperplastic in the process of benign prostatic hyperplasia?

   (A) Anterior fibromuscular area
   (B) Central zone
   (C) Peripheral zone
   (D) Prostatic capsule
   (E) Transition zone

10. A 38-year-old man presents with an abrupt onset of myalgia, low-back pain, and perineal pain. The patient also reports urinary symptoms of frequency, urgency, and dysuria. A urinalysis reveals 3+ white blood cells and urine culture confirms the presence of gram-negative bacteria. What is the initial therapeutic approach for this patient?

    (A) Fluoroquinolone for 4 weeks
    (B) Fluoroquinolone and α-blocker for 8 weeks
    (C) Hospitalization with intravenous cephalosporin
    (D) Nonsteroidal anti-inflammatory drugs and hot sitz baths for 48 hours
    (E) Penicillin intramuscular injection immediately

11. A 20-year-old college football player presents with a chief complaint of a dull ache in his scrotum after prolonged standing on the sideline. It seems to get worse with vigorous activity and is relieved by lying down. Dilated veins in the left scrotum are observed on inspection, and both testicles are palpable and without masses. What is the most likely diagnosis?

    (A) Hydrocele
    (B) Prostadynia
    (C) Spermatocele
    (D) Testicular mass
    (E) Varicocele

12. A 72-year-old man presents to the office with a chief complaint of a 3-month history of nocturia. He states that he is upset by the dribbling he experiences after voiding, has been getting up three times a night to urinate, and sometimes he finds himself straining to void. What is the most reasonable initial therapeutic approach for this patient?

    (A) Finasteride (Proscar)
    (B) Fluid restriction before sleeping
    (C) Tamsulosin (Flomax)
    (D) Transurethral resection of the prostate
    (E) Watchful waiting

13. A 6-month-old boy is brought to the office by his mother for a follow-up check for a right undescended testicle that has been absent since birth. This examination is consistent with previous examinations, revealing an empty right hemiscrotum. Even with surgical treatment, which of the following conditions is the patient at a higher risk of developing in later years?

    (A) Epididymitis
    (B) Hypospadias
    (C) Orchitis
    (D) Retrograde ejaculation
    (E) Testicular torsion

14. A 65-year-old woman presents with a complaint of blood in her urine intermittently for the last month. She denies fever, chills, flank pain, dysuria, or frequency. Social history is positive for a 45 pack-year history but she reports stopping smoking tobacco last year. What is the most likely cause of her hematuria?

    (A) Acute cystitis
    (B) Acute pyelonephritis
    (C) Bladder cancer
    (D) Renal calculus
    (E) Urethral prolapse

15. A 32-year-old man presents with a complaint of urinary frequency and suprapubic pain. He states that he has been feeling poorly for the past 4 days with intermittent fever, chills, and persistent malaise. He denies feeling this way before. Physical examination is significant for a temperature of 101°F. Genital examination is normal except for finding of

a tender, enlarged prostate on digital rectal examination. What is the most likely diagnosis?

(A) Acute bacterial prostatitis

(B) Benign prostatic hypertrophy

(C) Chronic bacterial prostatitis

(D) Gonorrhea

(E) Prostatic abscess

16. A 34-year-old female at 32 weeks' gestation presents for an obstetric check. She denies urinary symptoms other than frequency, which she has had for the past 6 months and attributes to her pregnancy. Her urine dipstick, today and at her last visit were positive for leukocyte esterase. Urine culture proved bacteria count at $>10^5$ CFU/mL. She was treated with an appropriate antibiotic for 7 days. Which of the following is best for the management of the patient at this point in her care?

(A) Extend antibiotic for 14 days total treatment

(B) Perform cystoscopy

(C) Perform intravenous pyelogram (IVP)

(D) Repeat urine culture after treatment

(E) Refer to urology

17. A 16-year-old girl presents to the emergency department with a 1-day history of severe right flank pain with associated vomiting. She denies any fever, urgency, or dysuria. Her past medical history is unremarkable. Physical examination reveals guarding and rebound on the right lower abdomen, along with severe right costovertebral angle tenderness. Which of the following radiographic studies is indicated for this patient?

(A) Flat plate abdominal series

(B) Intravenous pyelogram (IVP)

(C) KUB (kidneys, ureter, bladder) radiograph

(D) Noncontrast spiral computed tomography (CT) pelvis

(E) Urine cytology

18. A 75-year-old woman, G_4P_4, presents to establish care. Appearing healthy, denies any additional problems. However, when specifically asked, she admits to having urinary incontinence for "a couple of years" and now describes symptoms that have recently worsened. The patient experiences the need to void almost hourly and she now uses four to five adult incontinence pads per day to manage the urine

she leaks. She denies leaking urine with coughing or sneezing. What is the most likely diagnosis?

(A) Acute cystitis

(B) Interstitial cystitis

(C) Rectal prolapse

(D) Stress incontinence

(E) Urge incontinence

19. A patient has a history of multiple episodes of renal calculi secondary to hypercalcemia. On laboratory analysis, levels of parathyroid hormone (PTH) are found to be consistently low. Which of the following is the most likely explanation for these laboratory findings?

(A) Dietary calcium excess

(B) Hyperthyroidism

(C) Malignancy

(D) Primary hyperparathyroidism

(E) Vitamin D intoxication

20. A 54-year-old woman presents with gross hematuria and right-sided flank pain. Physical examination is positive for a right upper quadrant palpable mass and negative for costovertebral angle tenderness. Gross blood is observed in the urine specimen. What is the most likely diagnosis?

(A) Angiomyolipoma

(B) Hepatic carcinoma

(C) Renal abscess

(D) Renal cell carcinoma

(E) Renal cyst

21. A 32-year-old man presents to the urgent care with a concern of scrotal tenderness that began 3 days ago that has now worsened. Physical examination reveals a temperature of 100.7°F, positive tenderness in the posterolateral aspect of the right testis, and swelling. There is no spermatic cord tenderness with palpation and no transillumination present. What is the most likely diagnosis?

(A) Epididymitis

(B) Epididymo-orchitis

(C) Hydrocele

(D) Orchitis

(E) Testicular torsion

22. A 21-year-old sexually active female presents with recurrent pain with urination. Initially treated with trimethoprim–sulfamethoxazole (Bactrim) for 3 days, her symptoms did not resolve. Urine culture sent at her return visit was negative for growth. Pelvic examination was negative for pain and no hyphae or clue cells are seen on microscopic examination of vaginal fluid. What organism should be considered as the most likely cause of her continued symptoms?

   (A) Candida species
   (B) *Chlamydia trachomatis*
   (C) *Escherichia coli*
   (D) *Gardnerella vaginalis*
   (E) Proteus species

23. A 43-year-old female patient presents with back pain and hematuria. The patient reports her mother was on dialysis before she died, but she herself denies history of urinary tract infections. The patient is afebrile and her physical examination is positive for diffuse back tenderness and bilateral flank masses with palpation. Urine dipstick is positive for 3+ blood and is negative for leukocytes and nitrites. What is this patient's most likely diagnosis?

   (A) Adult polycystic kidney disease
   (B) Horseshoe kidney
   (C) Nephrolithiasis
   (D) Renal cell carcinoma
   (E) Renal cyst

24. A 37-year-old woman returns for reevaluation after being treated for a urinary tract infection 5 days prior with oral antibiotics. She reports her symptoms have not gotten better and have even gotten worse with a new onset of fever and flank pain. Which of the following tests is an appropriate next step in her evaluation?

   (A) Renal ultrasound
   (B) Serum creatinine
   (C) Straight catheter sample for dipstick urinalysis
   (D) Urine culture and sensitivity
   (E) Urine cytology

25. When treating a patient for benign prostatic hyperplasia, which of the following classes of medications addresses the prostate and has the quickest onset of action?

   (A) Anticholinergics
   (B) α-Adrenergic antagonists
   (C) 5α-Reductase inhibitors
   (D) Herbal supplements
   (E) Phosphodiesterase inhibitors

26. A bone scan of a male patient with cancer is shown in Figure 19-1. Based on this finding on bone scan, which of the following is the most likely source of the primary cancer?

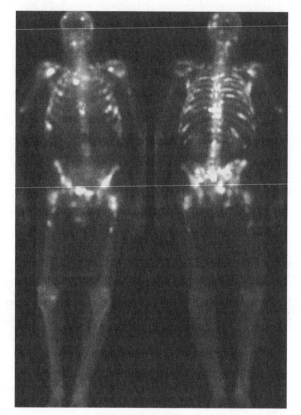

Figure 19-1.

   (A) Bladder
   (B) Prostate
   (C) Renal cell
   (D) Testis
   (E) Penile

27. A 32-year-old female presents with claims of "another UTI." The patient's complaint is narrowed to dysuria and increased frequency for the last 2 days. The patient denies fever and none is assessed by the nurse. The chart review reveals that this is the patient's fourth visit to the clinic in

the last 9 months. After treating her infection, which of the following is the best next step in her management?

(A) Admit the patient for inpatient care

(B) Obtain pelvic computed tomography

(C) Perform urodynamics

(D) Refer the patient to urology for evaluation

(E) Send urine for lab-confirmed microscopy

28. What is the most common cause of recurrent urinary tract infections in a 4-year-old girl?

(A) Bladder diverticulum

(B) Congenitally shortened urethra

(C) Renal calculus

(D) Resistant organism

(E) Vesicoureteral reflux

29. A 27-year-old woman with recurrent urinary tract infections presents with concerns about another infection. In previous infections, the patient has always been treated with the correct antibiotic according to culture and sensitivity results. Also, a recent work-up for genitourinary anatomic abnormalities was negative. Which of the following disorders could contribute to her recurrent infections?

(A) Antiphospholipid antibody syndrome

(B) Partner associated urinary infections

(C) Renal abscess

(D) Systemic lupus erythematosus

(E) Type 2 diabetes mellitus

30. What is the lowest number of colony forming units seen on urine culture that indicate a positive result?

(A) 10^2/mL

(B) 10^3/mL

(C) 10^4/mL

(D) 10^5/mL

(E) 10^8/mL

31. A 42-year-old woman, with a history of a struvite renal calculus, presents for evaluation of possible urinary tract infection. She reports intermittent, mild right flank pain for 4 days. Her urine dipstick is positive for microscopic hematuria, and the urine pH is 7.5. The kidney, ureter, bladder film (KUB) is positive for two visible stones in the right kidney. Considering this information, a culture of her urine would most likely be positive for which of the following organisms?

(A) *Chlamydia trachomatis*

(B) *Escherichia coli*

(C) *Gardnerella vaginalis*

(D) Proteus species

(E) *Streptococcus pneumoniae*

32. A 57-year-old female presents with complaints of increasing urinary urgency and pelvic pain. These symptoms have gradually worsened over the past 6 months to the point the patient gets up at night to void several times a night. The pain always improves after voiding. The patient is postmenopausal and denies any history of other urinary tract infections or leaking urine. On examination, there is no suprapubic pain with palpation and urinalysis is negative. For which of the following disorders is this patient most at risk?

(A) Bladder cancer

(B) Endometriosis

(C) Interstitial cystitis

(D) Overflow incontinence

(E) Urinary tract infection

33. Which of the following urinary findings will be observed in a patient with noninflammatory nonbacterial prostatitis?

(A) Negative urine culture with positive culture of expressed secretions

(B) Negative urine culture with negative culture of expressed secretions

(C) Negative urine culture with elevated erythrocytes on microscopic

(D) Positive urine culture with positive culture of expressed secretions

(E) Positive urine culture with negative culture of expressed secretions

34. Which of the following radiographic studies is indicated for the initial evaluation of a questionable palpable mass in the area of the kidney, with no other complaints by the patient?

    (A) Abdominal computed tomography
    (B) Abdominal magnetic resonance imaging
    (C) Intravenous pyelogram
    (D) Renal biopsy
    (E) Renal ultrasound

35. Which of the following history findings is seen in patients with erectile dysfunction and is linked to its mechanism of endothelial dysfunction?

    (A) Difficulty maintaining erection
    (B) Dyspareunia
    (C) Loss of libido
    (D) Pain with erection
    (E) Previous pelvic surgery

36. Which of the following history findings would trigger a workup for vesicoureteral reflux in a young female patient?

    (A) Dark-colored urine
    (B) Epigastric abdominal pain
    (C) Nocturnal enuresis
    (D) Painless hematuria
    (E) Recurrent cystitis

37. Upon genital examination of a newborn male, the urethral meatus is found located proximal to the tip of the glans on the ventral aspect of the penis. This finding is defined as which of the following conditions?

    (A) Epispadias
    (B) Hypospadias
    (C) Phimosis
    (D) Urethral stricture
    (E) Urethrorectal fistula

38. Which of the following physical examination findings is found with hydrocele?

    (A) Cystic scrotal mass
    (B) Fever
    (C) Enlargement with valsalva
    (D) Painful testis
    (E) Solid mass on upper pole of testis

39. Which of the following findings on digital rectal examination is most concerning for cancer of the prostate?

    (A) Bright red blood
    (B) Decreased sphincter tone
    (C) Enlargement
    (D) Nodularity
    (E) Pain

40. Which of the following is an obstructive voiding symptom associated with benign prostatic hyperplasia?

    (A) Frequency
    (B) Incontinence
    (C) Nocturia
    (D) Postvoid dripping
    (E) Urgency

41. What is the single most important sign on genital examination indicating a potential urethral injury in a male patient?

    (A) Blood at the urethral meatus
    (B) Pain on digital rectal examination
    (C) Penile pain
    (D) Suprapubic distention
    (E) Scrotal tenderness

42. A 14-year-old male presents complaining of sudden onset of pain and swelling in the left testis accompanied by nausea for approximately 30 minutes. He denies trauma, dysuria, or urinary frequency. On examination, the left testis appears to be riding higher than the right and is tender to palpation. The scrotal skin appears normal. Which of the following diagnostic tests should be performed next on the scrotum to confirm the most likely diagnosis?

    (A) Angiography
    (B) Color Doppler sonogram
    (C) Computed tomography
    (D) Magnetic resonance imaging
    (E) Radionuclide testing

43. A 28-year-old man presents with swelling in the left testis. He does admit to a small amount of discomfort in the left testis over the past few months. The patient states that he also noticed a sense of fullness for the past 3 months but denies acute pain, dysuria, or penile discharge. He states the swelling does not change based on activity or positioning. Based on this history, which of the following is the most likely diagnosis?

    (A) Epididymitis
    (B) Orchitis
    (C) Testicular torsion
    (D) Testicular tumor
    (E) Varicocele

44. A 56-year-old male presents to the emergency department with complaints of a painful erection for the past 3 hours in the absence of sexual activity. His past medical history is significant for sickle cell anemia. Based on this history, which of the following is the most likely diagnosis?

    (A) Balanitis
    (B) Paraphimosis
    (C) Penile fracture
    (D) Peyronie disease
    (E) Priapism

45. A 52-year-old male presents with concerns about problems with erections. After a full workup, he is diagnosed with organic erectile dysfunction. Which of the following modifications will decrease risk of progressive disease?

    (A) Begin low carbohydrate diet
    (B) Begin selective serotonin reuptake inhibitor
    (C) Increase alcohol consumption
    (D) Stop smoking
    (E) Use lower extremities compression stockings

46. Which of the following increases risk of squamous cell carcinoma of the penis?

    (A) Adolescent age
    (B) Coinfection with human immunodeficiency virus
    (C) Obesity
    (D) Paget disease of penis
    (E) Uncircumcised

47. Which of the following is the strongest risk factor for developing renal cell carcinoma?

    (A) Cigarette smoking
    (B) Diabetic nephropathy
    (C) Obesity
    (D) Polycystic kidney disease
    (E) Recurrent renal infections

48. Which of the following management options should be encouraged in all patients with urinary stone disease, regardless of stone composition?

    (A) Allopurinol
    (B) Fluid intake of 2 L daily
    (C) Increase physical exercise
    (D) Low calcium diet
    (E) Thiazide diuretics

49. Which of the following is an indication for circumcision?

    (A) Balanoposthitis
    (B) Cancer prevention
    (C) Hypospadias
    (D) Paraphimosis
    (E) Peyronie disease

50. When should a couple seek evaluation for male factors contributing to an inability to conceive?

    (A) After the female partner is evaluated with no suspected cause
    (B) After male is 35 years of age
    (C) After one month of frequent intercourse
    (D) After 1 year of regular unprotected intercourse
    (E) Before attempting to conceive

51. A 65-year-old female presents with complaint of urine leakage for the past 12 months. She states that she only notices leaking after sneezing or coughing, not with feelings of urgency. Urinalysis is normal. Which of the following treatments is appropriate at the initial stage of her treatment?

    (A) Anticholinergic agent
    (B) Intravesicular botulinum toxin A (Botox)
    (C) Pelvic floor muscle training
    (D) Surgical repair
    (E) Vaginal pessary

52. Which of the following conditions would be best evaluated using urodynamic testing?

(A) Bladder tumor

(B) Interstitial cystitis

(C) Neurogenic bladder

(D) Recurrent cystitis

(E) Urethral stricture

53. Which of the following laboratory findings is expected in a patient with prostatic enlargement causing obstruction?

(A) Decreased prostate-specific antigen

(B) Elevated serum creatinine

(C) Hematuria

(D) Leukocytosis

(E) Pyuria

54. A 14-year-old male presents with complaints of acute onset left-sided testicular pain and vomiting for the past 30 minutes. Ultrasound with Doppler reveals decreased blood flow to the affected testis without mass. A surgical repair must be performed within what window of time to have the best chance to salvage the testis?

(A) 15 minutes

(B) 1 hour

(C) 6 hours

(D) 24 hours

(E) 48 hours

55. On a pelvic computed tomography, a patient is found to have incidental bilateral hydronephrosis. Which of the following urinary symptoms would point to a urethral stricture as the cause of his findings?

(A) Dysuria

(B) Frequency

(C) Hesitancy

(D) Nocturia

(E) Urgency

56. Which type of incontinence would a male patient most likely experience secondary to uncontrolled benign prostatic hypertrophy?

(A) Neuropathic incontinence

(B) Nocturnal incontinence

(C) Overflow incontinence

(D) Stress incontinence

(E) Urge incontinence

57. What is the initial treatment of choice for an adult patient diagnosed with phimosis?

(A) Broad-spectrum antibiotics

(B) Circumcision

(C) Dorsal slit

(D) Immediate retraction of the foreskin

(E) Oral antifungal agents

58. A 28-year-old female presents with her fourth episode of culture confirmed cystitis in the past 6 months. Each episode clears completely with antibiotic treatment. She is currently trying to conceive with her partner and has a sulfa allergy. Which of the following regimens would be most appropriate for this patient as prophylaxis?

(A) 8 ounces cranberry juice daily

(B) Amoxicillin 100 mg daily

(C) Levofloxacin (Levaquin) 500 mg daily

(D) Nitrofurantoin (Macrobid) 50 mg daily

(E) Trimethoprim 100 mg daily

59. Which of the following antibiotics is best for urinary tract infection due to *Pseudomonas* species?

(A) Amoxicillin (Amoxil)

(B) Ciprofloxacin (Cipro)

(C) Metronidazole (Flagyl)

(D) Nitrofurantoin (Macrobid)

(E) Trimethoprim–sulfamethoxazole (Bactrim)

60. Most children achieve continence of the bladder by what age?

(A) 1 year

(B) 2 years

(C) 4 years

(D) 6 years

(E) 8 years

61. A 68-year-old male presents for concerns with inability to maintain erection. He uses nitroglycerin as needed for unstable angina prescribed by his cardiologist in addition to his antihypertensive medications. His serum testosterone level is within normal limits. Which of the following initial treatments for erectile dysfunction is appropriate for this patient?

(A) Intraurethral alprostadil (Muse)

(B) Penile prosthesis

(C) Tadalafil (Cialis)

(D) Testosterone gel (Androgel)

(E) Yohimbine (Yohimbe)

62. A 69-year-old presents for his annual physical. When reviewing his urinary review of systems, he only complains of diminished force of the urinary stream and denies frequency, nocturia, or dysuria. He states that this symptom does not bother him. His prostate-specific antigen (PSA) is 1.6 ng/mL. He scores a 6 on the American Urological Association symptom score. Which of the following treatment options is appropriate for this patient?

(A) Finasteride (Proscar)

(B) Oxybutin (Ditropan)

(C) Tamsulosin (Flomax)

(D) Transurethral resection of prostate (TURP)

(E) Watchful waiting

63. Which of the following medications used for benign prostatic hyperplasia will decrease the prostate-specific antigen by about 50% with regular use?

(A) Dutasteride (Avodart)

(B) Leuprolide (Lupron)

(C) Silodosin (Rapaflo)

(D) Terazosin (Hytrin)

(E) Trospium (Sanctura)

64. A 78-year-old female is diagnosed with overactive bladder and given a trial of oxybutin (Ditropan). She is suffering from mild dementia and, in addition to her complaints of dry mouth, the oxybutin seemed to worsen her confusion. What is the next appropriate medication of choice for her condition?

(A) Darifenacin (Enablex)

(B) Fesoterodine (Toviaz)

(C) Mirabegron (Myrbetriq)

(D) Oxybutin extended release (Ditropan XL)

(E) Tolterodine (Detrol)

65. A 72-year-old female presents with complaints of urine leakage for the past 4 months. She states that she leaks urine when she feels the urge to urinate and cannot stop it from occurring. Urinalysis is normal. In addition to bladder training, which of the following medications is first-line treatment for her symptoms?

(A) Darifenacin (Enablex)

(B) Finasteride (Proscar)

(C) Intravesicular botulinum toxin A (Botox)

(D) Oxybutin (Ditropan)

(E) Tamsulosin (Flomax)

Answers and Explanations

1. **(A)** Seventy-five percent to 85% of all kidney stones are composed of either calcium phosphate or calcium oxalate. Another 5% to 10% of kidney stones consist of uric acid. Calcium and uric acid stones are more common in the male population. About 1% of kidney stones consist mainly of cysteine and about 5% are made of struvite, which is a combination of magnesium, ammonium, and phosphate. Struvite stones frequently present as staghorn calculi, are associated with urinary tract infections, and are more common in women. Stones containing calcium are radiopaque; others are radiolucent. *(Asplin et al., 2012, Ch. 287)*

2. **(E)** White blood cell casts, in the presence of the acute symptoms (fever, chills, flank pain, and dysuria), provide strong evidence of acute pyelonephritis. Hyaline casts are nonspecific findings and can be found in patients without urologic pathology or in patients with glomerulonephritis. Although observed in many patients, the finding of pyuria is nonspecific and a patient with pyuria may or may not have infection. Red blood cells are rarely seen in acute pyelonephritis and the presence of hematuria usually suggests the presence of calculi or tumor. Epithelial cells are not associated with pyelonephritis. *(Lee & Vincenti, 2013, Ch. 33)*

3. **(B)** Women experience urinary tract infections at a much higher rate than their male counterparts. Cystitis most commonly is due to ascending colonization of the lower urinary tract. In women, the urethra is shorter and easily contaminated with fecal flora. Other factors that increase the risk of cystitis include extremes of age, sexual intercourse, diaphragm use, and pregnancy. *E. coli* is the most common pathogen in uncomplicated cystitis and accounts for 85% to 95% of uncomplicated urinary tract infections in women. Pseudomonas is more likely in patients with recurrent urinary tract infections and in hospitalized patients. *S. epidermidis* may indicate a contaminated specimen. *C. trachomatis* is more likely found in other conditions such as sexually transmitted urethritis rather than cystitis. Urinary tract infections due to *Proteus* species are rare and usually occur as a result of chronic catheterization. *(Russo & Johnson, 2012, Ch. 149)*

4. **(C)** The most common presenting symptom of bladder cancer is painless hematuria, which occurs in 85% to 90% of patients. Additional symptoms of bladder irritability, urinary frequency, urgency, and dysuria are possible presentations but are usually associated with invasive bladder cancer. Foul smelling urine and oliguria are not presenting symptoms of bladder cancer. *(Cornett & Dea, 2014, Ch. 39)*

5. **(C)** Both chlamydia and gonorrhea infections can result in urethritis. Gonococci can disseminate to the joints and cause septic arthritis. Chlamydia is typically asymptomatic in male patients but can cause chronic conjunctivitis in adolescents and young adults. Reactive arthritis, also known as Reiter syndrome, is a result of an untreated chlamydia infection, and is typically characterized in texts by the triad of urethritis, arthritis, and conjunctivitis. All of the symptoms may not be present or not identified at the time of presentation. Tertiary syphilis is characterized by neurologic and cardiovascular disease, gummas, auditory and ophthalmic involvement, and cutaneous lesions. Balanitis is an infection of the glans and foreskin in an uncircumcised male and can cause dysuria but not arthralgia or conjunctivitis. *(Gaydos & Quinn, 2012, Ch. 176)*

6. **(E)** Syphilis presents initially as a painless genital ulcer called a chancre. It occurs approximately 3 weeks after exposure to *Treponema pallidum.* It often goes unnoticed and resolves without treatment in 3 to 6 weeks. Chancroid is the painful lesion of *Haemophilus ducreyi.* It is a large sloughing ulcer with secondary infection and inflammation of the inguinal lymph nodes. Genital warts, caused by human papillomavirus (HPV), may be painless and manifest on the genitals without ulceration. Genital herpes manifests as painful vesicles upon outbreaks often with prodromal tingling in the area of the lesion. Molluscum contagiosum is painless, but manifests as umbilicated papules. *(Krieger, 2013, Ch. 16; Wang, 2012, Ch. 183)*

7. **(C)** Paraphimosis is the condition in which the foreskin (prepuce) cannot be reduced back over the glans once it has been retracted. Chronic inflammation is commonly the cause. Balanitis is commonly seen with phimosis but specifically refers to the inflammation of the glans penis. Phimosis is the inability to retract the foreskin from its original position. Urethral meatal stricture occurs following inflammation of the urethra from chronic infection or trauma. Hypospadias is a congenital condition associated with a ventral location of the urethral meatus proximal to the glans. *(McAninch, 2013, Ch. 41)*

8. **(B)** Although all of these findings might elicit some concern, the nontender testicular mass would be of most concern because it should be considered testicular cancer until proven otherwise. Testicular cancer affects predominantly young men in the age group ranging from 20 to 35 years. These tumors can metastasize early in their development and almost all will require chemotherapy to treat. A tender epididymis might indicate epididymitis. A fluid-filled scrotum is likely due to a hydrocele and can be surgically repaired. The dilated veins are an indication of a varicocele, a condition that usually does not require treatment unless considered a causative factor for infertility. The left testicle frequently rides higher than the right and is not pathologic. *(Walsh & Smith, 2013, Ch. 44)*

9. **(E)** Benign prostatic hyperplasia develops in the transition zone and involves, to varying degrees, both stromal and epithelial tissue. The hyperplastic process results in increased cell numbers. As enlargement progresses, mechanical obstruction results from intrusion of the transition zone into the urethral lumen. The peripheral zone is the primary site for prostate carcinoma—approximately 60% to 70% occur there. The remainder typically is found in the central zone. The prostatic capsule encompasses the entire gland and does not enlarge on its own. *(Cooperberg et al., 2013, Ch. 23)*

10. **(A)** Fluoroquinolones and sulfa drugs have high drug penetration into prostatic tissue and are recommended for 4 to 6 weeks for patients with acute bacterial prostatitis. Penicillins are not indicated in the treatment of acute bacterial prostatitis. Patients presenting as acutely ill and febrile and exhibiting symptoms of acute urinary retention would benefit from hospitalization with parenteral antibiotics. Patients with chronic bacterial prostatitis may benefit from a longer course of antibiotics combined with an α-blocker to reduce urinary symptoms. Nonsteroidal medications and sitz baths may relieve the symptoms associated with chronic prostatitis. *(Coyle & Prince, 2014, Ch. 94)*

11. **(E)** A varicocele is recognized by the presence of scrotal enlargement caused by dilation of the pampiniform venous plexus. Varicoceles present as a "bag of worms" in the spermatic cord, are more prominent when the patient stands, can cause a dull ache in the scrotum. More than 80% of the time, varicoceles occur on the left side. Hydrocele and spermatocele are caused by fluid collection and are usually asymptomatic. Testicular masses must always be included in the differential diagnosis of scrotal masses, as they generally present painless. Prostadynia is a noninflammatory condition that is seen in younger men but is caused by pelvic floor and voiding dysfunction. It is treated by α-blockers or biofeedback. *(Meng et al., 2014, Ch. 23)*

12. **(C)** A trial of tamsulosin, a selective α-blocker, is most reasonable, as it will provide the patient with the quickest improvement in symptoms without the systemic side effects (i.e., orthostatic hypotension) of a nonselective α-blocker. Finasteride, a 5α-reductase inhibitor, requires 6 months of therapy before seeing symptomatic improvement. Watchful waiting in this case is unlikely to resolve the patient's moderate symptoms and fluid restriction may decrease the nocturia but will likely not moderate the patient's other symptoms. Transurethral resection of the prostate is an optional treatment for benign prostatic hypertrophy but because of higher rates of morbidity, mortality, and risks of retrograde ejaculation, impotence, and incontinence, it is used after failure of medical therapy. *(Lee, 2014, Ch. 67)*

13. **(E)** Even with surgical treatment aimed at bringing the testis into the scrotum for easy examination, there are several consequences associated with cryptorchidism including infertility, malignancy, hernia, and torsion of the previously undescended testis because genetic abnormality is common in this disorder. An undescended testis can be brought down into the scrotum with surgical orchiopexy, which is usually performed on babies between the age of 9 and 15 months. Orchiopexy does not change the risk of developing cancer of the testis but does allow for better examination. A history of cryptorchidism does not increase the likelihood of epididymitis, orchitis, hypospadias, or retrograde ejaculation. *(Meng & Tanagho, 2013, Ch. 4)*

14. **(C)** Hematuria in the absence of other symptoms in women older than 60 years is consistent with a bladder malignancy. Bladder cancer causes episodic, gross hematuria that is usually painless. Cigarette smoking is a risk factor that also increases the incidence of bladder cancer. Painful hematuria associated with suprapubic discomfort or dysuria (or both) is more indicative of cystitis or urinary tract calculi. Pyelonephritis is associated with chills, fever, and flank pain. Urethral prolapse occurs more commonly in children. *(Deng & Tanagho, 2013, Ch. 42; Meng et al., 2014, Ch. 23)*

15. **(A)** Acute bacterial prostatitis is the most common urologic diagnosis in men younger than 50 years old. Patient presentation includes the sudden onset of constitutional and urinary symptoms along with prostate tenderness on examination. Chronic bacterial prostatitis presents without fever, and the digital rectal examination is often normal. Prostatic abscesses result from inappropriate treatment of a prior episode of acute bacterial prostatitis. Benign prostatic hyperplasia is age related, with symptoms presenting in the fifth decade of life and does not manifest with constitutional symptoms. Gonorrhea

can be a cause of urethritis, but rarely infects the prostate acutely. *(Meng et al., 2014, Ch. 23; Nguyen, 2013, Ch. 14)*

16. **(D)** Even though this patient was asymptomatic, she required antibiotic treatment due to the repeat positive dipstick findings and confirmed bacteria count on culture. After treating with the proper antibiotic, urine culture should be repeated to confirm clearing of infection. Pregnant women already carry a higher risk of pyelonephritis due to pregnancy-related changes to the urinary tract. A longer course of antibiotics is not indicated for pregnant patients. Imaging studies and referral are not indicated in this patient. *(Nguyen, 2013, Ch. 14)*

17. **(D)** The preferred study for an adolescent with suspected renal colic is the spiral CT. This study is performed quickly, delineates the number and location of calculi, and demonstrates the presence of hydronephrosis in the involved kidney. It can also identify stones too small to be picked up on other diagnostic studies. In the past, an intravenous pyelogram was generally performed. A KUB (kidneys, ureter, bladder) film may not pick up radiolucent stones. A "flat plate" is an older term for a KUB. Urine for cytology is used to examine the urine for cancerous cells shed from the urinary tract and is not a concern in this presentation. *(Gerst & Hricak, 2013, Ch. 6)*

18. **(E)** Urinary incontinence is defined as involuntary urine loss. Urge incontinence is the result of uninhibited urge sensations that are so strong that the patient experiences an involuntary urine loss. Women particularly experience this problem with the changes associated with aging in response to weakened pelvic muscles secondary to childbirth as well as estrogen depletion causing weakening of the detrusor muscle. The problem may be worsened by the use of diuretics to treat hypertension. Stress incontinence is associated with increases in intra-abdominal pressure with activities such as laughing, sneezing, and coughing, etc. Acute cystitis would present with an acute clinical presentation. Interstitial cystitis is a chronic condition that is characterized more with dysuria and discomfort rather than incontinence. Rectal prolapse can cause incontinence to stool, but not to urine. *(Lue & Tanagho, 2013, Ch. 30)*

19. **(C)** Malignancy and primary hyperparathyroidism account for more than two-thirds of the cases of hypercalcemia, however primary hyperparathyroidism is associated with an elevated PTH. Malignancy, vitamin D intoxication, and hyperthyroidism are associated with suppressed levels of PTH but malignancy is the most common disorder of the three. *(Fitzgerald, 2014, Ch. 26)*

20. **(D)** The triad of gross hematuria, flank pain, and palpable mass are the common findings associated with renal cell carcinoma although they are rarely seen all together. Of the three, a palpable mass is the least likely to be found, but when present is significant for advanced disease. Most renal masses are simple cysts but are not palpable and require no additional workup. Angiomyolipoma contains large amounts of fat as shown on CT. A renal abscess is associated with a patient presentation that includes fever and flank pain. Hepatic carcinoma may present with right upper quadrant mass, but will produce gross hematuria. *(Cornett & Dea, 2014, Ch. 39; Konety et al., 2013, Ch. 22)*

21. **(A)** Pain and swelling are prominent features of epididymitis; fever and abdominal pain may also be present. Epididymitis is caused by an ascending infection. Without treatment, it may continue to the testicles causing a significant swelling that could make it difficult for the clinician to distinguish anatomically between the epididymis and the testicles. At this point, the diagnosis is epididymo-orchitis. Orchitis alone is most commonly a viral etiology (mumps) and is observed in prepubertal boys. In men younger than 30 years, epididymitis can be confused with torsion. Hydrocele will transilluminate and testicular torsion will present with acute severe pain usually in younger male patients. *(Nguyen, 2013, Ch. 14)*

22. **(B)** *C. trachomatis* should be considered in recurrent episodes of dysuria when urine cultures and pelvic examination are found to be negative. Although the pelvic examination was negative for pain, chlamydial infection can sometimes be asymptomatic in women and does not always lead to pelvic inflammatory disease. Chlamydial cultures should be performed on this patient to confirm the suspicion especially in those at high risk and with symptoms of urethritis. *(Deng & Tanagho, 2013, Ch. 42)*

23. **(A)** Adult polycystic kidney disease is a hereditary condition that almost always has a bilateral presentation (95% of the cases). It does not appear until after the age of 40, and dialysis or kidney transplantation is necessary for survival. Although they can present with hematuria, renal cysts, renal cell carcinoma, and nephrolithiasis generally present unilaterally; all conditions listed other than nephrolithiasis are usually painless. A horseshoe kidney (fusion of the renal tissue) may be palpated bilaterally but otherwise presents asymptomatically. *(McAninch, 2013, Ch. 32)*

24. **(D)** Because this patient presents for urinary symptoms that did not improve with initial treatment, she will need to undergo repeat urinalysis with culture and sensitivity to identify the causative pathogen and treat accordingly. She will be treated empirically based on her previous treatments and patient-specific factors. Straight catheter sample for the urinalysis is unnecessary. Evaluation of the kidneys via imaging or laboratory analysis at this point is not indicated, as it is likely that the initial infection was not sufficiently treated with the first round of antibiotics. Urine cytology is used in evaluation for malignant cells and is not indicated in this patient. *(Gupta & Trautner, 2012, Ch. 288; Meng et al., 2014, Ch. 23)*

25. **(B)** When treating BPH, there are several options that improve symptom control but do not actually work on the prostate tissue itself. Only α-adrenergic antagonists and 5α-reductase inhibitors affect the actual prostate and α-adrenergic antagonists work faster and are more effective, and for that reason, are usually used as first-line treatment. *(Lee, 2014, Ch. 67)*

26. **(B)** Prostate cancer is the most common primary source for metastatic bone disease in men. Although rare, men may present with lumbar pain as their presenting symptom for prostate cancer and should be considered in the clinician's differential diagnosis. Renal cell carcinoma commonly metastasizes to the lungs. Germ cell tumors (testes) metastasize to the lymph nodes located along the renal hilum. Bladder tumors commonly metastasize to lung. Penile cancer is rare. *(Cornett & Dea, 2014, Ch. 39; Gottschalk et al., 2013, Ch. 26)*

27. **(D)** This patient should receive a referral, as this is her fourth recurrence for the same problem within the period of a year. A recurrence rate of more than three infections per year should be evaluated by a urologist to rule out any anatomic abnormality. Imaging studies performed next should be under the direction of urology. Confirmed microscopy is not indicated in this scenario and is not cost effective. *(Stoller, 2013, Ch. 17)*

28. **(E)** Vesicoureteral reflux (VUR) is the retrograde passage of urine from the bladder to the kidneys via the ureter because of an incompetent vesicoureteral sphincter. It occurs in children 25% to 40% of the time. Although it occurs in both boys and girls, it is more common in girls, with the ratio of female/male occurrence being approximately 4:1 after 1 year of age. Most damage to the kidney occurs before the age of 5 years, as scarring leads to progressive renal deterioration. Any child with recurrent urinary tract infections should undergo referral and evaluation for VUR. *(Tanagho & Nguyen, 2013, Ch. 13; Watnick & Dirkx, 2014, Ch. 22)*

29. **(E)** Urinary tract infections (UTIs) are more common in patients with diabetes mellitus, resulting in a two- to fivefold increased frequency of UTIs when compared with nondiabetic patients. It is believed that two separate defects are responsible for this difference. First, there is a change in urinary cytokine secretions; and second, there is an increased adherence of microorganisms to the uroepithelial cells found throughout the urinary tract. The remainder of the disorders above do not cause recurrent UTI. *(Gonzales & Nadler, 2014, Ch. 2; Gupta & Trautner, 2012, Ch. 288; Nguyen, 2013, Ch. 14)*

30. **(D)** A urine culture is positive for an offending organism when the colony forming counts exceed 10^5/mL, although this criterion is not essential in making the diagnosis. A clinical diagnosis may be made on the basis of patient's symptoms and physical examination and therefore a culture may be considered positive at a lower number, such as 10^2/mL, if the patient is symptomatic. *(Gupta & Trautner, 2012, Ch. 288; Porten & Greene, 2013, Ch. 5)*

31. **(D)** This patient has struvite stones, a more rare cause of urinary stone formation. They are frequently associated with recurrent urinary tract infections, visible stones, and high urine pH. These stones are formed by urease-producing organisms including *Proteus* and *Pseudomonas*, while being caused less commonly by *Klebsiella*, *Providencia*, *Staphylococci*, and *Mycoplasma*. Struvite stones are not typically caused by *E. coli* and *C. trachomatis*. *(Asplin et al., 2012, Ch. 287; Stoller, 2013, Ch. 17)*

32. **(C)** This patient is at risk for having interstitial cystitis (IC) or painful bladder syndrome (PBS). Pelvic pain increases the differential to include all of the responses, but pelvic/suprapubic pain that decreases with voiding is associated with IC/PBS. The physical examination is usually normal, and a urine specimen for this patient will most likely be negative. Endometriosis will present with cyclic pelvic pain and will most likely also have adnexal tenderness. A UTI will have increased frequency and urgency and a positive urine specimen. The patient lacks incontinence which rules out overflow type as the cause. Patients with bladder cancer may have urinary symptoms of frequency, urgency, and suprapubic pain and may also have a urine specimen with hematuria. Interstitial cystitis is a diagnosis of exclusion and suspected patients should be referred to urology for full evaluation. *(Meng et al., 2014, Ch. 23; Warren, 2012, Ch. e35)*

33. **(A)** Prostatitis includes a continuum of prostate characteristics ranging from acute episodes to prostadynia, a noninflammatory disorder. Patients with acute bacterial prostatitis will have an exquisitely tender prostate gland, and prostatic massage is contraindicated in these patients. Nonbacterial prostatitis has no evidence of an acute infection but will have a positive culture of expressed prostatic secretions. *(Meng et al., 2014, Ch. 23)*

34. **(E)** Renal masses are initially identified by ultrasound. Ultrasound will be able to distinguish between a solid mass and a cyst. It is not uncommon to find some texts state that an intravenous pyelogram is noted as the initial test. Intravenous pyelogram has limited value, especially in differentiating small tumors. Whether a mass or a cyst, these findings are usually referred to a urologist who will follow-up with their own IVP and CT. *(Gerst & Hricak, 2013, Ch. 6; Watnick & Dirkx, 2014, Ch. 22)*

35. (A) One common etiology of erectile dysfunction (ED) is endothelial damage that leads to poor vascular function. Obtaining an erection with difficulty maintaining is one of the first signs of this etiology elicited on history. Loss of libido would be associated with a hormonal cause of ED. Neither painful erections nor dyspareunia are associated with ED. Previous pelvic surgery could lead to vascular dysfunction, but not due to dysfunction in the endothelium. *(Meng et al., 2014, Ch. 23)*

36. (E) Particularly in young female patients, any history that points to recurrent infection, especially cystitis or pyelonephritis, should trigger an evaluation for vesicoureteral reflux (VUR). Dark-colored urine and painless hematuria are concerning history findings, but point more toward a renal cause of disease. Although incontinence can be a sign of cystitis, enuresis limited to night would likely not be present in the presence of infection. Epigastric abdominal pain is not seen in patients with VUR and any pain associated with VUR, if present, would most likely be located in the renal or suprapubic areas. *(Tanagho & Nguyen, 2013, Ch. 13)*

37. (B) Hypospadias is a congenital anomaly defined by the location of the urethral meatus on the ventral surface of the penis located proximal to the glans. Epispadias is when the meatus is located on the dorsal surface of the penis. Phimosis is defined by the inability to retract the foreskin. Urethral stricture is uncommon in newborns and refers to the narrowing of any part of the urethra. Urethrorectal fistula can be congenital and results in communication between the urethra and the rectum, usually due to the failure of the development of the urorectal septum. Air and fecal matter passing through the urethra are the findings associated with this condition and it does not result in an abnormality of the location of the meatus on the penis itself. *(McAninch, 2013, Ch. 41; Meng et al., 2014, Ch. 23)*

38. (E) Hydrocele is a cystic mass that often surrounds the entire testis. It is not associated with fever as does epididymitis nor does it increase with valsalva, as does varicocele. The testis is usually nontender. *(Meng et al., 2014, Ch. 23; Meng & Tanagho, 2013, Ch. 4)*

39. (D) Nodularity and/or induration, if found on digital rectal examination must be evaluated further for cancer of the prostate. Bright red blood and decrease sphincter tone are not red flags for prostate cancer, but may be indicative of other serious rectal pathology. Enlargement of the prostate, especially when also found to be smooth and firm, is an indication of benign prostatic hyperplasia. Pain on palpation of the prostate is an indication of an inflammatory process such as infection or chronic inflammation. *(Cooperberg et al., 2013, Ch. 23)*

40. (D) Benign prostatic hyperplasia (BPH) is a condition that causes obstructive urinary symptoms due to prostatic enlargement. These include hesitancy, decrease force of stream, feeling of incomplete emptying, straining to void, and postvoid leakage. Irritative voiding symptoms such as urgency, frequency, and nocturia can be found in BPH but are due to a bladder response that is secondary to an increase in outlet resistance. Incontinence can be found in BPH but is not considered an obstructive symptom. *(Cooperberg et al., 2013, Ch. 23; Meng et al., 2014, Ch. 23; Scher, 2012, Ch. 95)*

41. (A) All pelvis trauma or saddle injuries have the potential to cause injury to the meatus in a male patient. Blood at the meatus, however is a sign that there could be injury to one of many parts of the urethra that could complicate catheterization and must be identified before proceeding. Pain on rectal examination, penile pain, and scrotal tenderness may indicate further injury, but are not findings specific to the urethra. Suprapubic distension could indicate bladder or abdominal injury and pathology, but alone are not specific to urethral trauma. *(McAninch, 2013, Ch. 18)*

42. (B) This patient is most likely experiencing torsion of the left testis. In order to assess blood flow, the color Doppler sonogram must be performed to confirm this urgent diagnosis. If blood flow is decreased or absent, the condition must be surgically repaired within 6 hours. Radionuclide testing can be performed on a testicular finding after Doppler confirms flow for an evaluation of the epididymis. Neither angiography, CT, nor MRI are appropriate tests for this patient. *(Cornett & Dea, 2014, Ch. 39; McAninch, 2013, Ch. 3; Meng et al., 2014, Ch. 23)*

43. (D) The patient in this scenario most likely has a testicular tumor based on the presentation. Without acute pain, epididymitis, torsion, and orchitis are highly unlikely. Because he has a several month history of painless enlargement and fullness, a tumor that could be cancerous should be suspected. Varicocele can cause a sensation of fullness, but does decrease or resolve upon lying supine. *(Cornett & Dea, 2014, Ch. 39; Motzer & Bosl, 2012, Ch. 96)*

44. **(E)** Priapism is a condition that results in a painful, prolonged erection usually in the absence of sexual activity. It is commonly idiopathic or due to a side effect of intracavernosal injections but can occur due to thrombosis in conditions such as sickle cell anemia. Although paraphimosis and penile fracture can cause pain, they are not related to erection. Balanitis, an acute or chronic inflammation of the glans can be uncomfortable but also does not relate to erection. Peyronie disease is a chronic condition that causes a curvature of the penis with erection and is associated with fibrous plaques of the septum or the sheath of the corpus cavernosum. *(McAninch, 2013, Ch. 41; McVary, 2012, Ch. 48; Meng et al., 2014, Ch. 23)*

45. **(D)** Smoking cessation is one of the few risk factors for organic ED that can be modified. Increased physical activity, and decreased alcohol consumptions are two others. A low carbohydrate diet has not been shown to affect ED and SSRIs worsen the disorder. Lower extremity–compression stockings are effective for increased venous return due to venous insufficiency, but will not contribute to better arterial flow seen in some causes of organic ED. *(Lue, 2013, Ch. 39; McVary, 2012, Ch. 48)*

46. **(E)** Squamous cell carcinoma is by far the most common type of penile cancer (98%) and occurs almost exclusively in patients who are not circumcised. It occurs most frequent in the fifth decade of life and is associated with poor hygiene and possibly viral causes. Obesity alone is not a risk factor. Both Paget disease and Kaposi sarcoma can involve the penis and lead to cancerous lesions, but these are not squamous cell in origin. *(Presti, 2013, Ch. 24)*

47. **(A)** Although cystic kidney disease and environmental exposure have likely been found to contribute to renal cell carcinoma, cigarette smoking is the only risk that is consistently linked to the disease and increases risk two-fold. Nephropathy, obesity,

and recurrent infection are not implicated as causes of RCC. *(Cornett & Dea, 2014, Ch. 39; Konety et al., 2013, Ch. 22; Scher & Motzer, 2012, Ch. 94)*

48. **(B)** All patients with urinary stone disease, regardless of stone composition, should drink about 2 L of fluid daily, especially after meals when fluid levels are lowest. For patients with calcium stone disease, a low sodium and low protein diet is recommended rather than a low-calcium diet due to the secondary effects of low calcium diet on bone mineral density. Thiazide diuretics are indicated for calcium stone disease only as they lower urinary levels of calcium but can increase risk of recurrence with other types of stones. Increasing physical exercise does not affect stone development. Allopurinol is indicated in addition to dietary modifications for patient with hyperuricosuria but not for all stone formers. *(Asplin et al., 2012, Ch. 287; Stoller, 2013, Ch. 17)*

49. **(D)** In some countries, circumcisions are routinely performed usually for religious or cultural reasons. Paraphimosis, phimosis, and infection are the only true indications. Balanoposthitis can lead to phimosis when chronic but because it can be treated easily with medications and proper hygiene, is not itself an indication for circumcision. Hypospadias itself does not require removal of the foreskin for treatment. Although penile carcinoma occurs in those who have not been circumcised, it is due to poor hygiene and chronic infection. Peyronie disease affects the shaft of the penis and does not involve the foreskin in any way that would indicate a need for removal. *(Berger, 2014, Ch. 6; McAninch, 2013, Ch. 41)*

50. **(D)** The workup for male related factors contributing to infertility should begin after failing to conceive after 1 year of regular intercourse. Of the 15% of couples who experience infertility, 20% of those can be due strictly to a male factor and 30% may have a contributing male factor. Evaluation involves hormonal testing and semen analysis. *(Walsh & Smith, 2013, Ch. 44)*

51. **(C)** This patient is suffering from stress incontinence and should be treated nonmedically with pelvic floor exercises, weight loss, and caffeine reduction. If this does not manage her symptoms, surgical repair may be the next step. A vaginal pessary is used as a nonsurgical treatment option for pelvic organ prolapse,

not stress incontinence alone. In the absence of mixed urinary incontinence (a combination of both stress and urge), medication therapy for stress incontinence is not indicated. *(Harper et al., 2014, Ch. 4; Lue & Tanagho, 2013, Ch. 30)*

52. **(C)** Urodynamics testing is performed by urology to evaluate the activity of the bladder, the urethra sphincter, and the pelvic musculature. Urodynamics can be used in the evaluation of medication refractory incontinence as well. An evaluation for recurrent cystitis, bladder tumor, interstitial cystitis, and in some cases urethral stricture could undergo urethrocystoscopy. *(Lue & Tanagho, 2013, Ch. 28)*

53. **(B)** In a patient with prostatic enlargement, significant enough to cause obstruction, there is the potential for acute kidney injury causing a rise in the serum creatinine and BUN. This occurs in about 10% of all BPH patients. In fact, elevations of these two chemistries in male patients should prompt evaluation for BPH. The presence of red blood cells and leukocytes is not an indication of obstruction. PSA levels, in this case, would be elevated due to the presence of a large gland, not obstruction itself. *(Cooperberg et al., 2013, Ch. 23)*

54. **(C)** This patient has torsion of the left testis with compromised blood flow and should be treated with surgical intervention within 6 hours. After 6 hours, the rate at which the testis can be saved decreases dramatically and is virtually zero after 48 hours. *(Chamie et al., 2014, Ch. 40)*

55. **(C)** Hydronephrosis is an indication of an obstructive process that is causing changes in the renal pelvis or calyces. Urethral stricture, a cause of lower urinary tract obstruction, shares symptoms such as hesitancy with other obstructive processes like benign prostatic enlargement or tumor of the bladder or urethra. Urinary urgency, dysuria, and frequency are irritative voiding symptoms. Nocturia can be caused by several processes and is not specific to obstructive disease. *(Stoller, 2013, Ch. 12)*

56. **(C)** A patient with uncontrolled BPH would most likely suffer from overflow incontinence due to the overdistention of the bladder from urinary retention or outflow obstruction. Urge incontinence is due to detrusor muscle overactivity and stress incontinence is due to pelvic floor instability, neither of which is directly related to BPH. Neuropathic incontinence refers to incontinence that is due to disease or injury to the brain, spinal cord, or peripheral nerves and is not a feature of BPH. Nocturnal incontinence is not a category of incontinence. *(Lue & Tanagho, 2013, Ch. 30)*

57. **(A)** Phimosis is a condition in which, usually due to poor hygiene and bacterial causes, the foreskin cannot be retracted over the glands. Broad-spectrum antibiotics are first-line treatment and the dorsal slit is only performed if drainage of the penis is needed on an urgent basis. Circumcision may be performed but only after infection is cleared. Because the foreskin cannot be retracted, it cannot be reduced. *(McAninch, 2013, Ch. 41)*

58. **(D)** Recurrent cystitis, once confirmed and investigated for other causes, can be treated with low-dose daily antibiotics. Levofloxacin, nitrofurantoin, and trimethoprim are indicated for this treatment, while amoxicillin and cranberry are not recommended as monotherapy. Trimethoprim alone can be used in patients with a sulfa allergy but like levofloxacin, is pregnancy category C. Nitrofurantoin is pregnancy category B. *(Coyle & Prince, 2014, Ch. 94; Nguyen, 2013, Ch. 14)*

59. **(B)** Urinary infections due to *Pseudomonas* spp. should be treated by ciprofloxacin, carbenicillin, tetracycline, or gentamycin plus piperacillin to ensure proper coverage. Amoxicillin can be used in combination with clavulanate when treating urinary infections to decrease resistance. Trimethoprim–sulfamethoxazole has poor coverage for *Pseudomonas*. Nitrofurantoin is best used for prophylaxis. Metronidazole is not indicated for UTI unless needed to cover a confirmed atypical organism. *(Coyle & Prince, 2014, Ch. 94; Nguyen, 2013, Ch. 14)*

60. **(D)** Enuresis (bedwetting) is a common problem seen in children and is diagnosed in children older than 5 years who have been experiencing episodes at least twice a week for 3 months without other known causes. Treatment consists of bedwetting alarms, scheduled voiding, and medications when appropriate. *(Goldson & Reynolds, 2013, Ch. 3; McAninch, 2013, Ch. 3)*

61. **(A)** Intraurethral alprostadil, a prostaglandin E1, enhances blood flow of the corpora of the penis and is an appropriate treatment for this patient. Because this patient has unstable angina that could require the use of nitroglycerin, the use of phosphodiesterase inhibitors (sildenafil, tadalafil, vardenafil, avanafil) are contraindicated due to serious hypotension. A penile prosthesis is not an initial treatment option and should be reserved for patients refractory to medical therapy or vacuum erection device. Testosterone gel should only be used in the presence of androgen deficiency. The herbal supplement yohimbine has not been shown to be more effective than placebo in clinical trials and can cause adverse effects like anxiety, tachycardia, and hypertension that, for this patient, would be potentially dangerous. *(Lee, 2014, Ch. 66)*

62. **(E)** Because this patient only has one urinary symptom that does not affect his quality of life and has a "mild" score on the AUA Symptom Score, watchful waiting is an appropriate treatment for this patient. Medical therapy (finasteride and tamsulosin) is not indicated until the symptoms become more severe or alter the patient's quality of life. Oxybutin can be used in patients with BPH to control irritative voiding symptoms if present. Surgical intervention is appropriate after medical therapy fails to control symptoms. *(Lee, 2014, Ch. 67)*

63. **(A)** The class of 5α-reductase inhibitors (dutasteride, finasteride) works for BPH by reducing the size of the prostate by about 25%, which reduces the level of PSA. They are a good choice in patients with a significantly enlarged gland; usually over 40 g but take longer to see the maximum effects. α-Adrenergic antagonists (prazosin, terazosin, doxazosin, alfuzosin,

tamsulosin, silodosin) work by relaxing the smooth muscle of the prostate and the bladder neck to increase flow and work faster and are more effective than the 5α-reductase inhibitors. Anticholinergics (darifenacin, fesoterodine, oxybutin, solifenacin, tolterodine, trospium) can be added to treatment in patients with irritative voiding symptoms but are not used as monotherapy. *(Lee, 2014, Ch. 67)*

64. **(C)** Although the side effect of dry mouth could decrease with extended release formulation of oxybutin or by switching to tolterodine that is better tolerated by the elderly patients, the effects of the antimuscarinic agents (oxybutin, tolterodine, trospium, solifenacin, darifenacin, fesoterodine) on this patient's dementia are a concern. Therefore, the use mirabegron, a β₃-adrenergic agonist, is indicated. This class of medications works by increasing bladder capacity by smooth-muscle relaxation allowing the bladder to store more urine. *(Lee, 2014, Ch. 67)*

65. **(D)** This patient is experiencing symptoms of urge incontinence that is most frequently caused by detrusor muscle overactivity. Oxybutin is an anticholinergic medication that works by relaxing the smooth muscle in the bladder to counter the detrusor activity. Botox can be used in the treatment of urge incontinence but is considered third-line treatment and is used in those refractory to other first and second-line treatments. Darifenacin is a second-generation antimuscarinic and is used as a second-line option when patients cannot tolerate other agents. Finasteride and tamsulosin are agents that are used in men for benign prostatic hypertrophy. *(Lue & Tanagho, 2013, Ch. 30; Rovner et al., 2014, Ch. 68)*

REFERENCES

Asplin JR, Coe FL, Favus MJ. Chapter 287: Nephrolithiasis. In: Longo DL, Fauci AS, Kasper DL, Hauser SL, Jameson J, Loscalzo J, eds. *Harrison's Principles of Internal Medicine.* 18th ed. New York, NY: McGraw-Hill; 2012. http://access medicine.com. Accessed January 5, 2015.

Berger TG. Chapter 6: Dermatologic disorders. In: Papadakis MA, McPhee SJ, Rabow MW, eds. *Current Medical Diagnosis*

& Treatment 2015. New York, NY: McGraw-Hill; 2014. http://accessmedicine.com. Accessed January 6, 2015.

Chamie K, Rochelle J, Shuch B, Belldegrun AS. Chapter 40: Urology. In: Brunicardi F, Andersen DK, Billiar TR, et al., eds. *Schwartz's Principles of Surgery.* 10th ed. New York, NY: McGraw-Hill; 2014. http://accessmedicine.com. Accessed January 9, 2015.

Cooperberg MR, Presti JC, Jr, Shinohara K, Carroll PR. Chapter 23: Neoplasms of the prostate gland. In: McAninch JW, Lue TF, eds. *Smith and Tanagho's General Urology*. 18th ed. New York, NY: McGraw-Hill; 2013. http://accessmedicine.com. Accessed January 6, 2015.

Cornett PA, Dea TO. Chapter 39: Cancer. In: Papadakis MA, McPhee SJ, Rabow MW, eds. *Current Medical Diagnosis & Treatment 2015*. New York, NY: McGraw-Hill; 2014. http://accessmed icine.com. Accessed January 6, 2015.

Coyle EA, Prince RA. Chapter 94: Urinary tract infections and prostatitis. In: DiPiro JT, Talbert RL, Yee GC, Matzke GR, Wells BG, Posey L, eds. *Pharmacotherapy: A Pathophysiologic Approach*. 9th ed. New York, NY: McGraw-Hill; 2014. http://accesspharmacy.com. Accessed January 6, 2015.

Deng DY, Tanagho EA. Chapter 42: Disorders of the female urethra. In: McAninch JW, Lue TF, eds. *Smith and Tanagho's General Urology*. 18th ed. New York, NY: McGraw-Hill; 2013. http://accessmedicine.com. Accessed January 6, 2015.

Fitzgerald PA. Chapter 26: Endocrine Disorders. In: Papadakis MA, McPhee SJ, Rabow MW, eds. *Current Medical Diagnosis & Treatment 2015*. New York, NY: McGraw-Hill; 2014. http://accessmedicine.com. Accessed January 6, 2015.

Gaydos CA, Quinn TC. Chapter 176: Chlamydial infections. In: Longo DL, Fauci AS, Kasper DL, Hauser SL, Jameson J, Loscalzo J, eds. *Harrison's Principles of Internal Medicine*. 18th ed. New York, NY: McGraw-Hill; 2012. http://access medicine.com. Accessed January 5, 2015.

Gerst S, Hricak H. Chapter 6: Radiology of the urinary tract. In: McAninch JW, Lue TF, eds. *Smith and Tanagho's General Urology*. 18th ed. New York, NY: McGraw-Hill; 2013. http://accessmedicine.com. Accessed January 6, 2015.

Goldson E, Reynolds A. Chapter 3: Child development and behavior. In: Hay WW, Jr., Levin MJ, Deterding RR, Abzug MJ, eds. *CURRENT Diagnosis & Treatment: Pediatrics*. 22nd ed. New York, NY: McGraw-Hill; 2013. http://accessmedicine.com. Accessed January 6, 2015.

Gonzales R, Nadler PL. Chapter 2: Common symptoms. In: Papadakis MA, McPhee SJ, Rabow MW, eds. *Current Medical Diagnosis & Treatment 2015*. New York, NY: McGraw-Hill; 2014. http://accessmedicine.com. Accessed January 6, 2015.

Gottschalk AR, Speight JL, Roach M, III. Chapter 26: Radiotherapy of urologic tumors. In: McAninch JW, Lue TF, eds. *Smith and Tanagho's General Urology*. 18th ed. New York, NY: McGraw-Hill; 2013. http://accessmedicine.com. Accessed January 9, 2015.

Gupta K, Trautner BW. Chapter 288: Urinary tract infections, pyelonephritis, and prostatitis. In: Longo DL, Fauci AS, Kasper DL, Hauser SL, Jameson J, Loscalzo J, eds. *Harrison's Principles of Internal Medicine*, 18th ed. New York, NY: McGraw-Hill; 2012. http://accessmedicine.com. Accessed January 6, 2015.

Harper G, Johnston C, Landefeld C. Chapter 4: Geriatric disorders. In: Papadakis MA, McPhee SJ, Rabow MW, eds. *Current Medical Diagnosis & Treatment 2015*. New York,

NY: McGraw-Hill; 2014. http://accessmedicine.com. Accessed January 6, 2015.

Konety BR, Vaena DA, Williams RD. Chapter 22: Renal parenchymal neoplasms. In: McAninch JW, Lue TF, eds. *Smith and Tanagho's General Urology*. 18th ed. New York, NY: McGraw-Hill; 2013. http://accessmedicine.com. Accessed January 6, 2015.

Krieger JN. Chapter 16: Sexually transmitted diseases. In: McAninch JW, Lue TF, eds. *Smith and Tanagho's General Urology*. 18th ed. New York, NY: McGraw-Hill; 2013. http://accessmedicine.com. Accessed January 6, 2015.

Lee BK, Vincenti FG. Chapter 33: Diagnosis of medical renal diseases. In: McAninch JW, Lue TF, eds. *Smith and Tanagho's General Urology*. 18th ed. New York, NY: McGraw-Hill; 2013. http://accessmedicine.com. Accessed January 6, 2015.

Lee M. Chapter 66: Erectile dysfunction. In: DiPiro JT, Talbert RL, Yee GC, Matzke GR, Wells BG, Posey L, eds. *Pharmacotherapy: A Pathophysiologic Approach*. 9th ed. New York, NY: McGraw-Hill; 2014. http://accesspharmacy.com. Accessed January 6, 2015.

Lee M. Chapter 67: Benign prostatic hyperplasia. In: DiPiro JT, Talbert RL, Yee GC, Matzke GR, Wells BG, Posey L, eds. *Pharmacotherapy: A Pathophysiologic Approach*. 9th ed. New York, NY: McGraw-Hill; 2014. http://accesspharmacy.com. Accessed January 6, 2015.

Lue TF, Tanagho EA. Chapter 28: Neuropathic bladder disorders. In: McAninch JW, Lue TF, eds. *Smith and Tanagho's General Urology*. 18th ed. New York, NY: McGraw-Hill; 2013. http://accessmedicine.com. Accessed January 6, 2015.

Lue TF, Tanagho EA. Chapter 30: Urinary incontinence. In: McAninch JW, Lue TF, eds. *Smith and Tanagho's General Urology*. 18th ed. New York, NY: McGraw-Hill; 2013. http://accessmedicine.com. Accessed January 6, 2015.

Lue TF. Chapter 39: Male sexual dysfunction. In: McAninch JW, Lue TF, eds. *Smith and Tanagho's General Urology*. 18th ed. New York, NY: McGraw-Hill; 2013. http://accessmedicine.com. Accessed January 6, 2015.

McAninch JW. Chapter 3: Symptoms of disorders of the genitourinary tract. In: McAninch JW, Lue TF, eds. *Smith and Tanagho's General Urology*. 18th ed. New York, NY: McGraw-Hill; 2013. http://accessmedicine.com. Accessed January 6, 2015.

McAninch JW. Chapter 18: Injuries to the genitourinary tract. In: McAninch JW, Lue TF, eds. *Smith and Tanagho's General Urology*. 18th ed. New York, NY: McGraw-Hill; 2013. http://accessmedicine.com. Accessed January 6, 2015.

McAninch JW. Chapter 32: Disorders of the kidneys. In: McAninch JW, Lue TF. eds. *Smith and Tanagho's General Urology*. 18th ed. New York, NY: McGraw-Hill; 2013. http://accessmedicine.com. Accessed January 6, 2015.

McAninch JW. Chapter 41: Disorders of the penis and male urethra. In: McAninch JW, Lue TF, eds. *Smith and Tanagho's General Urology*. 18th ed. New York, NY: McGraw-Hill; 2013. http://accessmedicine.com. Accessed January 6, 2015.

McVary KT. Chapter 48: Sexual dysfunction. In: Longo DL, Fauci AS, Kasper DL, Hauser SL, Jameson J, Loscalzo J, eds. *Harrison's Principles of Internal Medicine*. 18th ed. New York, NY: McGraw-Hill; 2012. http://accessmedicine.com. Accessed January 6, 2015.

Meng MV, Tanagho EA. Chapter 4: Physical examination of the genitourinary tract. In: McAninch JW, Lue TF, eds. *Smith and Tanagho's General Urology*. 18th ed. New York, NY: McGraw-Hill; 2013. http://accessmedicine.com. Accessed January 6, 2015.

Meng MV, Walsh TJ, Chi TD. Chapter 23: Urologic Disorders. In: Papadakis MA, McPhee SJ, Rabow MW, eds. *Current Medical Diagnosis & Treatment 2015*. New York, NY: McGraw-Hill; 2014. http://accessmedicine.com. Accessed January 6, 2015.

Motzer RJ, Bosl GJ. Chapter 96: Testicular cancer. In: Longo DL, Fauci AS, Kasper DL, Hauser SL, Jameson J, Loscalzo J, eds. *Harrison's Principles of Internal Medicine*. 18th ed. New York, NY: McGraw-Hill; 2012. http://accessmedicine.com. Accessed January 6, 2015.

Nguyen HT. Chapter 14: Bacterial infections of the genitourinary tract. In: McAninch JW, Lue TF, eds. *Smith and Tanagho's General Urology*. 18th ed. New York, NY: McGraw-Hill; 2013. http://accessmedicine.com. Accessed January 6, 2015.

Porten SP, Greene KL. Chapter 5: Urologic laboratory examination. In: McAninch JW, Lue TF, eds. *Smith and Tanagho's General Urology*. 18th ed. New York, NY: McGraw-Hill; 2013. http://accessmedicine.com. Accessed January 6, 2015.

Presti JC. Chapter 24: Genital tumors. In: McAninch JW, Lue TF, eds. *Smith and Tanagho's General Urology*. 18th ed. New York, NY: McGraw-Hill; 2013. http://accessmedicine.com. Accessed January 6, 2015.

Rovner ES, Wyman J, Lam S. Chapter 68: Urinary incontinence. In: DiPiro JT, Talbert RL, Yee GC, Matzke GR, Wells BG, Posey L, eds. *Pharmacotherapy: A Pathophysiologic Approach*. 9th ed. New York, NY: McGraw-Hill; 2014. http://accesspharmacy.com. Accessed January 6, 2015.

Russo TA, Johnson JR. Chapter 149: Diseases caused by gram-negative enteric bacilli. In: Longo DL, Fauci AS, Kasper DL, Hauser SL, Jameson J, Loscalzo J, eds. *Harrison's Principles of Internal Medicine*. 18th ed. New York, NY: McGraw-Hill; 2012. http://accessmedicine.com. Accessed January 6, 2015.

Scher HI. Chapter 95: Benign and malignant diseases of the prostate. In: Longo DL, Fauci AS, Kasper DL, Hauser SL, Jameson J, Loscalzo J, eds. *Harrison's Principles of Internal Medicine*. 18th ed. New York, NY: McGraw-Hill; 2012. http://accessmedicine.com. Accessed January 6, 2015.

Scher HI, Motzer RJ. Chapter 94: Bladder and renal cell carcinomas. In: Longo DL, Fauci AS, Kasper DL, Hauser SL, Jameson J, Loscalzo J, eds. *Harrison's Principles of Internal Medicine*. 18th ed. New York, NY: McGraw-Hill; 2012. http://accessmedicine.com. Accessed January 6, 2015.

Stoller ML. Chapter 12: Urinary obstruction and stasis. In: McAninch JW, Lue TF, eds. *Smith and Tanagho's General Urology*. 18th ed. New York, NY: McGraw-Hill; 2013. http://accessmedicine.com. Accessed January 6, 2015.

Stoller ML. Chapter 17: Urinary stone disease. In: McAninch JW, Lue TF, eds. *Smith and Tanagho's General Urology*. 18th ed. New York, NY: McGraw-Hill; 2013. http://accessmedicine.com. Accessed January 6, 2015.

Tanagho EA, Nguyen HT. Chapter 13: Vesicoureteral reflux. In: McAninch JW, Lue TF, eds. *Smith and Tanagho's General Urology*. 18th ed. New York, NY: McGraw-Hill; 2013. http://accessmedicine.com. Accessed January 6, 2015.

Walsh TJ, Smith JF. Chapter 44: Male infertility. In: McAninch JW, Lue TF, eds. *Smith and Tanagho's General Urology*. 18th ed. New York, NY: McGraw-Hill; 2013. http://accessmedicine.com. Accessed January 6, 2015.

Wang F. Chapter 183: Molluscum contagiosum, monkeypox, and other poxvirus infections. In: Longo DL, Fauci AS, Kasper DL, Hauser SL, Jameson J, Loscalzo J, eds. *Harrison's Principles of Internal Medicine*. 18th ed. New York, NY: McGraw-Hill; 2012. http://accessmedicine.com. Accessed January 6, 2015.

Warren JW. Chapter e35: Interstitial cystitis/painful bladder syndrome. In: Longo DL, Fauci AS, Kasper DL, Hauser SL, Jameson J, Loscalzo J, eds. *Harrison's Principles of Internal Medicine*. 18th ed. New York, NY: McGraw-Hill; 2012. http://accessmedicine.com. Accessed January 6, 2015.

Watnick S, Dirkx T. Chapter 22: Kidney disease. In: Papadakis MA, McPhee SJ, Rabow MW, eds. *Current Medical Diagnosis & Treatment 2015*. New York, NY: McGraw-Hill; 2014. http://accessmed icine.com. Accessed January 6, 2015.

CHAPTER 20

Preventive Medicine

James F. Cawley, MPH, PA-C, DHL(hon)

DIRECTIONS: Each of the numbered questions or incomplete statements is followed by possible answers or completions of the statement. Select the ONE-lettered answer or completion that is BEST in each case.

1. The most powerful and consistent risk factor for the development of substance use disorders (SUD) is:

   (A) Poverty
   (B) Age
   (C) Depression
   (D) Family history

2. Which of the following statements related to the identification of intimate partner violence (IPV) is TRUE?

   (A) Women are at less risk for violence during pregnancy
   (B) Most cases of domestic violence are sporadic and isolated
   (C) Victims of intimate partner violence are more likely to delay seeking care
   (D) Patients with family history of IPV are less at risk

3. If death rates per 1,000 licensed drivers are plotted by age, the distribution of the curve is:

   (A) Bell shaped
   (B) J shaped
   (C) U shaped
   (D) Unimodal

4. A group of physicians conducted interviews of their patients regarding symptoms of gastritis following use of two different types of NSAIDs for a research study. They found no difference in amount or frequency of symptoms between the two agents. An external reviewer concluded that the study was flawed because of assessment bias. What would have prevented this flaw?

   (A) Random assignment of the patients
   (B) Better training of the interviewers
   (C) Masking interviewers to the treatment
   (D) Using a case-control method

5. The proportion of nondiseased individuals who are correctly identified as negative by a test describes the test's:

   (A) Validity
   (B) Specificity
   (C) Reliability
   (D) Sensitivity

6. One of your patients is a 30-year-old man who tells you he is planning to travel to the Dominican Republic for a 3-week hiking trip. The most appropriate medication to use for malarial prophylaxis is:

   (A) Atovaquone
   (B) Chloroquine
   (C) Mefloquine
   (D) Doxycycline

7. Researchers wish to study the association between consumption of saturated fat and myocardial infarction. They administer a food frequency questionnaire to all patients ($n = 15,000$) who come to a large Health Maintenance Organization (HMO) practice for annual checkups in 1980. The researchers use the food frequency data to calculate the usual amount of saturated fat consumed by each participant per week. Then, they follow these patients for 15 years and determine the number of myocardial infarctions that occur in this group. What type of study is the study described above?

(A) Case-control study

(B) Cohort study

(C) Randomized controlled trial

(D) Cross-sectional study

8. Which tick-borne public health threat, especially prevalent in the upper Midwest, New England, and some of the mid-Atlantic States, is a cause of an infection of neutrophils?

(A) Human granulocytic anaplasmosis

(B) Rocky Mountain spotted fever

(C) Psittacosis

(D) Cryptococcosis

9. The medical evaluation of a 32-year-old HIV-infected male patient reveals a tuberculin skin test reaction at 5 mm and indurated. His chest x-ray is normal. He is currently taking antiretroviral therapy that includes protease inhibitors. He has not previously received antituberculous therapy nor had any known contact with people with tuberculosis (TB). Which is the most appropriate intervention at this time?

(A) Isoniazid (INH) for 9 months

(B) No preventive therapy for TB needed

(C) Rifampin for 9 months

(D) Streptomycin for 6 months

Questions 10 and 11

On a Friday afternoon, a 30-year-old registered nurse is brought to your office in employee health for evaluation following a needle stick injury that occurred in the HIV clinic. The source patient involved is known to be infected with HIV and has advanced AIDS.

10. Which of the following factors carries the greatest risk for the transmission of HIV to the nurse?

(A) Depth of injury

(B) Presence of visible blood on the needle

(C) Prior immune status of the nurse

(D) Stage of illness of the source patient

11. What is the most appropriate course of action for this health worker?

(A) Reassure her of the low risk of infection

(B) Offer two-drug antiretroviral therapy (lamivudine [combivir])

(C) Draw HIV antibody test and refer to an infectious disease specialist on Monday

(D) Offer triple drug therapy to prevent seroconversion

12. The prevention of shingles is best accomplished by:

(A) Administration of herpes zoster (HZ) vaccine (zoster vaccine live [zostavax]) in patients older than 50 years

(B) Prophylactic use of acyclovir (zovirax) in patients older than 50 years who present with a painful rash

(C) Use of vitamins to boost immunity in adults

(D) Administration of measles–mumps–rubella–varicella (MMRV) (proQuad) vaccine in children ages 1 through 10 years

13. What is the most prevalent sexually transmitted infection (STI) in the United States and also accounts for many observed complications such as pelvic inflammatory disease (PID), infertility, ectopic pregnancy, and chronic pelvic pain?

(A) Syphilis

(B) Chlamydia

(C) Herpes simplex

(D) Gonorrhea

14. In the course of investigating a 24-year-old HIV-infected male, it was observed that the HBsAg was positive. The patient is asymptomatic, his physical examination reveals normal result, and has CD4 count of 800. Which test is the most helpful in

determining if he is in the acute phase of viral hepatitis?

(A) HBeAg
(B) HBsAg
(C) IgG anti-HBcAg
(D) IgM anti-HBcAg

15. The most important risk factor for heat-related illness is:

(A) Age older than 65 years
(B) Age younger than 1 year
(C) History of previous heat stroke
(D) Obesity

Questions 16 and 17

A new screening program was instituted in Virginia. The program used a screening test that is effective in detecting cancer C at an early stage. Assume that there is no effective treatment for this type of cancer and, therefore, that the program results in no change in the usual course of the disease. Assume also that the rates noted are calculated from all known cases of cancer C and that there were no changes in the quality of the death certification of this disease.

16. What would happen to the apparent incidence rate of cancer C in Virginia during the first year of the program?

(A) Increase
(B) Decrease
(C) Remain constant
(D) Insufficient information to answer the question

17. What will happen to the apparent prevalence rate of cancer C in Maryland during the first year of the program?

(A) Increase
(B) Decrease
(C) Remain constant
(D) Insufficient information to answer the question

18. What is the protozoal infection, the source of which is usually animal-urine–contaminated water and

which causes an acute severe febrile icteric hepatitis?

(A) Relapsing fever
(B) Typhoid fever
(C) *Vibrio vulnificus*
(D) Leptospirosis

19. The leading cause of childhood (*ages 5 through 14*) death in the United States is:

(A) Poisoning
(B) Malignant neoplasms
(C) Unintentional injury
(D) Birth defects

20. Which disease/health threat is the leading cause of disability-adjusted life years (DALYs) in the United States?

(A) Lung cancer
(B) Ischemic heart disease
(C) Unipolar depression
(D) Road traffic injuries
(E) HIV/AIDS

21. Which of the following is the best example of primary prevention?

(A) Immunization against measles
(B) Mammography to detect breast cancer
(C) Testing to detect C-reactive protein (CRP) for the identification of coronary heart disease
(D) Performing carotid endarterectomy for the prevention of stroke

22. Which is the pathogenic pathway in the development of colorectal cancer accounting for 15% of sporadic cases and nearly all cases of hereditary nonpolyposis colorectal cancer (HNPCC)?

(A) Chromosomal instability
(B) Familial adenomatous polyposis (FAP) mutation
(C) Microsatellite instability
(D) Telomere cutoff

23. Of the following major sexually transmitted illnesses, which has a safe and effective vaccine?

    (A) Syphilis
    (B) Chlamydia
    (C) Hepatitis B
    (D) Herpes simplex II

24. What is the type of rate that is defined as the number of new cases of a disease occurring in a population per unit time?

    (A) Epidemic
    (B) Prevalence
    (C) Incidence
    (D) Virulence

25. Which factor is most closely associated with the spread of tuberculosis?

    (A) Poverty
    (B) Alcoholism
    (C) Poor hygiene
    (D) Crowding

26. Which of the following risk factors for coronary heart disease has the highest attributable risk (risk of disease due to a specific factor)?

    (A) Smoking
    (B) Elevated cholesterol
    (C) Lack of physical exercise
    (D) High blood pressure

27. For which patient is pneumococcal vaccine (PPV 23) *not* beneficial?

    (A) A 15-month-old HIV-infected child
    (B) A 20-year-old patient about to undergo a splenectomy for thrombotic thrombocytopenic purpura (TTP)
    (C) A 5-year-old patient with sickle cell disease
    (D) A 10-year-old child with nephrotic syndrome

Questions 28 through 30

A drug company sponsors and executes a randomized controlled clinical trial to assess the efficacy of a new topical cream medication aimed at inducing new hair growth in men with male pattern baldness. The researchers determine that new hair growth must increase by at least 20% in the treatment group (as compared to placebo) to be considered marketable. They determine a sample size that will ensure 80% power for the purposes of statistical testing and carry this out at the 5% level of statistical significance.

28. The probability that this statistical test will fail to detect a clinically important difference in hair growth between the two groups, given that such a difference actually exists between populations from which the samples were drawn:

    (A) Increases as the specific effect size decreases
    (B) Increases as the sample size increases
    (C) Increases as alpha, the level of significance, increases
    (D) Increases as the power of the test increases

29. The probability that this statistical test will detect the specific difference in new hair growth, given that such a difference does actually exist between the populations represented in the study samples, is:

    (A) 0.95
    (B) 0.05
    (C) 0.20
    (D) 0.80

30. Which of the following statements best describes alpha, the level of significance?

    (A) The chance of detecting a statistically significant difference between the two study groups is 95%
    (B) If new hair growth does not differ between the study and placebo groups, the chance of detecting a statistically significant difference between the two samples is 5% or less
    (C) If new hair growth differs between the two groups, the chance that the statistical test will detect a true difference between the samples is at least 95%
    (D) A statistically significant result will be obtained 5% of the time that a true difference exists between the study populations

31. The incidence rate of lung cancer is 120/100,000 person-years for smokers and 10/100,000 person-years for nonsmokers. What is the risk of developing lung cancer for persons who smoke?

    (A) 5
    (B) 12
    (C) 50
    (D) 100

32. The most prevalent arboviral disease in the United States is:

    (A) West Nile virus encephalitis
    (B) Anaplasmosis
    (C) Lyme disease
    (D) Eastern equine encephalitis

33. Eating undercooked chicken or food that has been contaminated by the drippings of raw chicken is most commonly associated with infection with:

    (A) *Salmonella*
    (B) *Giardia lamblia*
    (C) *Campylobacter*
    (D) *Escherichia coli 0157:H7*

34. The leading cause of blindness among adults (person ages 20–74 years) is:

    (A) Senile macular degeneration
    (B) Diabetes mellitus
    (C) Retinal artery thrombosis
    (D) Glaucoma

35. A 60-year-old white man presents with a palpable prostate mass and a prostate specific antigen (PSA) level of 6.2 ng/mL. There are no indicators of high risk (i.e., marked PSA elevation, other suspicious symptoms, positive family history, African-American race).

    The recommended next step is:

    (A) Observation
    (B) Measuring the free-to-total PSA ratio
    (C) Rechecking the PSA in 6 months
    (D) Prostate biopsy

36. Which statement best defines a meta-analysis?

    (A) A collection of research evidence that combines quantitative and qualitative methods
    (B) A long-term examination of a cohort studied longitudinally without a comparison group
    (C) An examination of research data already collected
    (D) An investigation that pools data gathered from multiple studies

37. An investigation is begun to identify the cause of lung cancer among ship workers. Workers with the disease were matched with controls by age, place of residence, and type of occupational category. The frequency of smoking and exposure to asbestos was then compared in the two groups. This is what type of study?

    (A) Retrospective cohort
    (B) Case-control
    (C) Controlled clinical trial
    (D) Observational

38. U.S. Preventive Services Task Force recommendation for screening for colon cancer in adults calls for:

    (A) Fecal-occult blood or sigmoidoscopy after age 40
    (B) Sigmoidoscopy or colonoscopy after age 60 through 75
    (C) Colonoscopy after age 50 and biannually after that
    (D) Fecal-occult blood testing, sigmoidoscopy, or colonoscopy after age 50 through 75

39. Which of the following is classified as a zoonotic disease?

    (A) Clostridium difficile
    (B) Typhoid fever
    (C) Plague
    (D) Listeriosis

40. Level of resistance of a community/group of people to a particular infectious disease beyond that afforded by protection of an immunized individual defines:

    (A) Community protective effect
    (B) Innate immunity
    (C) Herd immunity
    (D) Natural resistance

Answers and Explanations

1. **(D)** While there are a wide array of factors including biologic factors, gender, age, employment status, education, and psychiatric history, the strongest association identified for substance use is a positive family history of either drug or alcohol abuse. *(Brown & Fleming, 2008, p. 266)*

2. **(C)** Domestic (or intimate partner violence) violence is prevalent among women; with up to 50% lifetime prevalence being reported. It is often misdiagnosed. Many studies have demonstrated that women are at a higher risk during pregnancy. Patients with a positive family history of violence are at an increased risk for violence even if not currently in an abusive relationship. *(Feldman, 2008, pp. 380–385)*

3. **(C)** Fatalities per 1,000 licensed drivers in the United States are highest among the youngest and oldest drivers, the graph plotting fatalities by age shows a U-shaped distribution. *(Messinger-Rapport & Baker, 2004, p. 267)*

4. **(C)** This study is flawed because the investigators making the assessments were aware of the treatments the patients were receiving. This is called assessment bias and can be minimized by masking (blinding) the assessment team to the treatment. Training the interviewers will help improve interrater reliability. *(Riegelman, 2005, pp. 25–29)*

5. **(B)** Specificity describes the test's ability to identify the absence of disease in nondiseased individuals. It is typically expressed as a percentage. Sensitivity is defined as the ability of the test to detect the presence of disease in those who have it. Reliability is the ability of a test to reproduce similar results in similar situations over time. Validity is a broad concept that describes the ability of a test to distinguish between those who have a disease and those who do not. Sensitivity and specificity are components of validity. *(Gordis, 2009, pp. 85–103)*

6. **(B)** Chloroquine is a standard prophylaxis for the prevention of malaria. The Dominican Republic is a country with a high risk for malaria; it is also a chloroquine-susceptible region as are most parts of Central America and Mexico. It is safe, efficacious, and has few major side effects. It is ideal for short visits to endemic regions. Mefloquine and doxycycline are medications generally used in chloroquine-resistant regions. *(White & Breman, 2008, pp. 192–193; http://www.cdc.gov/malaria/ diagnosis_treatment/treatment.html)*

7. **(B)** Cohort studies typically observe study subjects and follow them forward in time. Case-control studies compare the experiences of cases of a disease and controls and measure exposures using past records. Cross-sectional studies observe or measure population characteristics at one point in time. *(Gordis, 2009, pp. 167–170)*

8. **(A)** Human granulocytic anaplasmosis (formerly known as "ehrlichiosis") is caused by a rickettsial bacterium and transmitted by the bite of various tick species that often overlap with those that transmit other diseases such as Lyme disease and babesiosis. Rocky Mountain spotted fever is also a tick-borne infection and is also rickettsial in origin and causes a systemic febrile syndrome and a rash. Psittacosis is associated with exposure to parrots and other birds and is primarily pneumonia illness; cryptococcal disease typically causes fungal meningitis in immunosuppressed persons. *(Walker et al., 2008, pp. 1059–1061)*

9. **(A)** A positive tuberculin skin test of 5-mm induration or more is considered positive in a person who has HIV infection, has had contact with a person with TB, or who has a positive chest x-ray. HIV-infected persons are at an increased risk of TB and should be screened on a regular basis. Prophylaxis is warranted in this patient, and it is recommended that INH be used for 9 months. Rifampin is not recommended for use in patients taking protease inhibitors, as this reduces effective levels of the antiretroviral drug. *(Raviglione & O'Brian, 2008, pp. 1006–1009)*

10. **(A)** and **11. (D)** The risk of HIV transmission following a needle stick with the blood of an HIV-infected patient is about 1:300. Risks are higher with deep punctures, large inocula, and source patients with high viral loads. While treatment with zidovudine decreases seroconversion by 79%, some clinicians recommend triple combination therapy in high-risk situations as described in the case. *(Zolopa & Katz, 2010, pp. 1220–1221)*

12. **(A)** The use of the HZ vaccine is a useful option for the prevention of herpes zoster infection in older adults. The HZ vaccine was licensed in 2006 and has 14 times the antigenicity of the varicella-zoster virus (VZV) vaccine used in children. The MMRV vaccine or the VZV vaccine used in children would be inappropriate for use in an adult. Treating an older adult suspected on developing zoster with acyclovir may moderate the length and severity of the illness but would not prevent it. *(Wolfe, 2008, p. 410)*

13. **(B)** Chlamydia is by far the most prevalent STI in the United States, with over 900,000 cases reported to the Centers for Disease Control and Prevention (CDC) in 2004. By comparison, in the same year, there were 330,000 cases of gonorrhea reported. Approximately 70% of chlamydia and 50% of gonorrheal infections are asymptomatic. If not adequately treated, 20% to 40% of women with chlamydia and 10% to 40% of women with gonorrhea will develop PID. Syphilis is much less common and is not associated with the cited complications. *(Kodner, 2008, p. 297)*

14. **(D)** Antibodies to the hepatitis B core antigen appear early in the infection with the IgM fraction being the most prominent. The presence of the surface antigen and/or the e antigen does not provide sufficient information regarding the timing of the acquisition of the infection. *(Dienstag, 2008, pp. 1932–1935)*

15. **(A)** Older adults are the most susceptible to heat-related illness because of decreased response of the cardiovascular system during hot weather. *(Lang & Hensrud, 2004, p. 257)*

16. **(A)** and **17. (A)** In this example, given the stated assumptions, it is likely that the incidence (the number of newly diagnosed cases) would increase due to heightened awareness of the cancer brought about by the screening program. This sometimes is called overdiagnosis, and the rise in incidence represents an artifactual, not real, increase in the occurrence of the disease. If the duration of the disease was relatively long, for instance, more than a year, it is also likely that the prevalence of the disease would also rise (incidence = prevalence × duration). *(Riegelman, 2005, pp. 175–183)*

18. **(D)** Human leptospirosis typically presents as an acute illness with high fever, jaundice, abdominal pain, and myalgia and is caused by one of three spirochetal serovars. Leptospires are typically transmitted by the ingestion of food or drink contaminated by the urine of various animals including cattle, dogs, swine, and rats. The most severe form is anicteric hepatitis (Weil syndrome), which carries a 5% to 40% mortality rate. Typhoid fever is caused by *Salmonella* and presents with acute then chronic severe diarrhea. Relapsing fever is caused by a tick-borne spirochete of the *Borrelia* species and causes a systemic febrile illness. *Vibrio vulnificus* is caused by a cholera-related bacterial species that causes a necrotizing cutaneous infection. *(Speelman & Hartskeerl, 2008, pp. 1048–1049)*

19. **(C)** Unintentional injuries comprise the leading cause of mortality in the childhood age group followed in rank order by malignant neoplasms, congenital malformations, homicide, and suicide. *(Woolf, 2008, p. 12)*

20. **(B)** Burden of disease studies has been implemented in many countries using the disability-adjusted life year (DALY) to assess major health problems and estimate the leading causes of morbidity. The leading

cause of morbidity in the United States for both males and females by a wide margin is ischemic heart disease. *(McKenna et al., 2005, pp. 415–423)*

21. **(A)** Primary prevention is the concept of preventing disease before it occurs. Immunization prevents infectious diseases such as smallpox. Because of immunization strategies, smallpox has been eradicated from the globe. Mammography and testing for CRP are forms of secondary prevention, as disease already exists in the patient, and the goal is identification of disease at the earliest stage; surgery for carotid artery stenosis is essentially a therapeutic procedure consistent with tertiary prevention. *(Aschengrau & Seage, 2003, pp. 405–406)*

22. **(C)** Microsatellite instability due to mismatch repair gene inactivation is present in approximately 15% of sporadic CRCs and is the major cause of hereditary nonpolyposis colorectal cancer (HNPCC). Other distinct pathways involving genetic alterations in the development of colon cancer include chromosomal instability which arises from an accumulation of allelic losses or mutation and accounts for a small number of cases of sporadically occurring colon cancer. Hypermethylation of promoter regions of genes contributes to some sporadic cases. *(Ahren & Axell, 2015)*

23. **(C)** Hepatitis B is commonly sexually transmitted, accounting for roughly 55% of all cases. Hepatitis B is more efficiently transmitted through sexual contact than HIV. The likelihood of sexual transmission of hepatitis B is reduced with condom use. The hepatitis B immunization is a safe and effective vaccination and has been shown to decrease rates of transmission. No vaccines are available for syphilis or chlamydial infections. An effective vaccine for herpes simplex II, a viral infection, is still under development. *(Chentoufi, et al., 2012)*

24. **(C)** Incidence rates reflect the occurrence of new cases of a disease in the population and are often used to assess the risk of a disease to the public's health. Virulence refers to the pathological properties of infecting microorganisms. Epidemic refers to outbreaks of disease above normal levels. Prevalence is the number of existing cases of a disease in a population per unit time. *(Gordis, 2009, pp. 38–52)*

25. **(D)** While poverty, alcoholism, and poor hygiene are all known risk factors for contracting tuberculosis, it is crowding that has the highest correlation with the transmission of the tubercle bacillus. Making crowding the primary factor stems from evidence that shows that it is coughing from individuals with active tuberculosis that aerosolizes tubercle bacilli that are then inhaled by a susceptible person. Thus, close contact among individuals substantially enhances the likelihood of this occurrence. *(Raviglione & O'Brian, 2008, pp. 1006–1009)*

26. **(A)** When assessing the impact of a risk factor on a group of individuals, the use of the concept of attributable risk is useful. Attributable risk is the percentage of the risk, among those with the risk factor, associated with exposure to the risk factor. If a cause-and-effect relationship exists, then attributable risk is the percentage of disease that can be potentially eliminated if the risk factor is completely removed. *(Riegelman, 2005, pp. 60–65)*

27. **(A)** Pneumococcal vaccine is not recommended for children younger than 2 years or less. This would include the 15-month-old child with HIV infection. The other three patients should receive the immunization. The spleen is important in the immune defense of infections with polysaccharide antigens. Protection with pneumococcal vaccination is important in persons with various conditions conferring higher risk of pneumococcal infection such as those who are asplenic, have sickle cell disease, or who have chronic diseases such as renal failure (or the nephritic syndrome). *(Woolf et al., 2008, p. 392)*

28. **(A), 29. (D),** and **30. (B)** The probability that the statistical test will fail to detect a clinically important difference, given that this difference actually exists is the beta, shows the chance of a type II error. As the sample size or level of significance—the alpha—increases, the chance of a beta error decreases. Because it is the complement of power, beta decreases as power increases. The probability that the statistical test will detect a true difference is the power of the test, and in this question, is equal to 0.80. A statistical test carried out on these two samples will erroneously detect a difference between the two groups 5% of the time. The highly significant result of the statistical test indicates that the observed effect of the new medications unlikely

to have occurred by chance (less than 0.05% of the time). *(Riegelman, 2005, pp. 18, 68–73)*

31. **(B)** The formula for the calculation of relative risk is I_e/I_{non-e}, where I represents the incidence of disease and e represents exposure. In this case, $120/100,000 \div 10/100,000 = 12$. This indicates that the risk of developing lung cancer among those exposed is 12 times that of the rate of those not exposed. *(Gordis, 2009, pp. 203–205)*

32. **(A)** West Nile virus has become the most common mosquito-borne (arthropod-borne or arboviral) infectious disease in the United States since the 2002 epidemic and is far more prevalent than eastern equine encephalitis. Between 2001 and 2004, it spreads progressively annually across the United States and is now endemic in most parts of the United States. Anaplasmosis is a bacterial infection transmitted by ticks and infects white blood cells producing a systemic febrile illness. Lyme disease is caused by tick bites, usually produces a vivid rash, and is endemic particularly in states on the Eastern seaboard. *(Barlem, 2009a, p. 595)*

33. **(C)** *Campylobacter* is a bacterial pathogen that causes fever, diarrhea, and abdominal cramps and is the most commonly identified bacterial cause of diarrheal illness in the world. They live in the intestines of healthy birds, and most raw poultry meat has *Campylobacter* on it. Eating undercooked chicken, or other food that has been contaminated with juices dripping from raw chicken, is the most frequent source of this infection; this accounts for 70% of cases. Salmonellosis typically includes fever, diarrhea, and abdominal cramps. *Escherichia coli* O157:H7 has a reservoir in cattle and other similar animals. Illness typically follows consumption of food or water that has been contaminated with microscopic amounts of cow feces and consists of a severe and bloody diarrhea and painful abdominal cramps. *Giardia* is associated with contaminated water supplies and causes a chronic diarrheal disease. *(Barlem, 2009b, pp. 456–458; Centers for Disease Control and Prevention, 2013)*

34. **(B)** Diabetes mellitus is a prevalent disease and is by far the leading responsible factor for blindness in adults aged 20 through 65 years. It is classified as either proliferative or nonproliferative. The latter form is characterized by dilation of veins, microaneurysms, retinal hemorrhages, retinal edema, and hard exudates. It is the most common cause of legal blindness in maturity-onset diabetes. *(Powers, 2008, pp. 2287–2288)*

35. **(B)** If the patient is considered at low risk, that is does not have the aforementioned risk factors, it seems most appropriate to measure the free-to-total PSA level. If it is normal, then recheck the PSA level within 3 to 6 months. A less-aggressive approach is supported by evidence that men with prostate cancer who defer treatment demonstrate no increase in mortality from prostate cancer for 8 to 15 years. This may also be appropriate management in patients with apprehension about unnecessary diagnostic or therapeutic procedures. *(Molella, 2008, p. 479)*

36. **(D)** A meta-analysis is a study that combines data obtained from multiple studies. By combining data from two or more studies, the power of the inquiry is increased, thus allowing for a more accurate estimate of the strength of an association. A collection of research evidence that combines quantitative and qualitative methods refers to a systematic review. A long-term examination of a cohort studied longitudinally without a comparison group describes a prospective cohort study. A study that is an examination of research data already collected is usually referred to as a secondary data analysis. *(Riegelman, 2005, pp. 99–102)*

37. **(B)** This is an example of a case-control study. Case-control studies begin by identifying those who have developed or failed to develop the disease being investigated. After identifying those with and without the disease, they look back in time to determine the characteristics of individuals (such as smoking or exposure to asbestos) before the onset of disease. Controls are individuals who are matched with cases in all respects except that they are free of disease. A retrospective cohort study, also called a historic cohort study, is one where the medical records of groups of individuals who are alike in many ways but differ by a certain characteristic (such as smoking) are compared for a particular outcome (such as lung cancer). The key distinction from a case-control study is the time of collection of outcomes and exposure data.

Observational studies are those in which the investigator does not have the capability to manipulate the studies' subject but instead simply observes the outcomes of various effects. *(Gordis, 2009, pp. 177–198; Riegelman, 2005, pp. 11–13)*

38. **(D)** The current recommendation of the U.S. Preventive Services Task Force in terms of screening adults for colon cancer indicates that either fecal-occult blood testing, sigmoidoscopy, or colonoscopy be used after age 50 through 75. *(U.S. Preventive Services Task Force, 2014)*

39. **(C)** Zoonotic diseases are infectious diseases that can be transmitted or shared by animals and humans. Plague is a classic zoonosis caused by a bacterium transmitted by fleas that are carried by rats. The others are primarily infections of the gastrointestinal tract secondary to either antibiotic overgrowth or food-borne contamination. *(Dennis & Campbell, 2008, pp. 980–981)*

40. **(C)** Herd immunity is defined as the resistance of a group of individuals to a disease when there is a large proportion of the group being immune. This concept is important because it is nearly impossible to achieve 100% immunization rates. Therefore, when random mixing occurs, it is possible to halt the spread of a particular communicable disease because the infected person is likely to encounter fewer individuals who are susceptible. *(Gordis, 2009, pp. 24–25)*

REFERENCES

Ahren DJ, Axell L. Lynch Syndrome (hereditary nonpolyposis colorectal cancer): Clinical Manifestations and Diagnosis. Accessed at: http://www.uptodate.com/contents/lynch-syndrome-hereditary-nonpolyposis-colorectal-cancer-clinical-manifestations-and-diagnosis?source=search_result&search=lynch+syndrome&selectedTitle=1%7E78

Aschengrau A, Seage GR. *Essentials of Epidemiology for Public Health*. Sudbury, MA: Jones and Bartlett; 2003.

Barlem TF. Insect-and-animal-borne viral infections. In: Fauci AS, Braunwald E, Kasper DL, et al., eds. *Harrison's Manual of Medicine*. 17th ed. New York, NY: McGraw-Hill; 2009a.

Barlem TF. Inflammatory diarrhea. In: Fauci AS, Braunwald E, Kasper DL, et al., eds. *Harrison's Manual of Medicine*. 17th ed. New York, NY: McGraw-Hill; 2009b.

Brown RT, Fleming MF. Substance abuse. In: Woolf SH, Jonas S, Kaplan-Liss E, eds. *Health Promotion and Disease Prevention*. 2nd ed. Philadelphia, PA: Lippincott Williams & Wilkins; 2008.

Chentoufi AA, Kritzer E, Yo D, Newborn AB, BenMohamed L. Towards a Rational Design of an Asymptomatic Clinical Herpes Vaccine: The Old, the New, and the Unknown. *Clin Dev Immunol*. 2012; 2012: 187585. Published online 2012 Mar 26. doi: 10.1155/2012/187585.

Centers for Disease Control and Prevention (CDC). Incidence and trends of infection with pathogens transmitted commonly through food - foodborne diseases active surveillance network, 10 U.S. sites, 1996-2012. *MMWR Morb Mortal Wkly Rep*. 2013; 62:283.

Dennis D, Campbell G. Plague and other yersinia infections. In: Fauci A, Braunwald E, Kasper DL, et al., eds. *Harrison's Principles of Internal Medicine*. 17th ed. New York, NY: McGraw-Hill; 2008.

Dienstag J. Acute viral hepatitis. In: Fauci A, Braunwald E, Kasper DL, et al., eds. *Harrison's Principles of Internal Medicine*. 17th ed. New York, NY: McGraw-Hill; 2008.

Feldman MD. Intimate partner violence. In: Feldman MD, Christensen JF, eds. *Behavioral Medicine: A Guide for Clinical Practice*. 3rd ed. New York, NY: McGraw-Hill; 2008.

Gordis L. *Epidemiology*. 4th ed. Philadelphia, PA: Saunders Elsevier; 2009.

Kodner CM. Sexually transmitted infections. In: Woolf SH, Jonas S, Kaplan-Liss E, eds. *Health Promotion and Disease Prevention*. 2nd ed. Philadelphia, PA: Lippincott Williams & Wilkins; 2008.

Lang RS, Hensrud DD. *Clinical Preventive Medicine*. 2nd ed. Chicago, IL: AMA Press; 2004.

McKenna MT, Michaud CM, Murray CJ, et al. Assessing the burden of disease in the United States using disability-adjusted life years. *Am J Prev Med*. 2005;28:415–423.

Messinger-Rapport BJ, Baker PT. Safety in the home and automobile. In: Lang RS, Hensrud DD, eds. *Clinical Preventive Medicine*. 2nd ed. Chicago, IL: AMA Press; 2004.

Molella RG. Health and genetic risk assessment instruments. In: Woolf SH, Jonas S, Kaplan-Liss E, eds. *Health Promotion and Disease Prevention in Clinical Practice*. 2nd ed. Philadelphia, PA: Lippincott Williams & Wilkins; 2008.

Powers AC. Diabetes mellitus. In: Fauci A, Braunwald E, Kasper DL, et al., eds. *Harrison's Principles of Internal Medicine.* 17th ed. New York, NY: McGraw-Hill; 2008.

Raviglione MC, O'Brian R. Tuberculosis. In: Fauci A, Braunwald E, Kasper DL, et al., eds. *Harrison's Principles of Internal Medicine.* 17th ed. New York, NY: McGraw-Hill; 2008.

Riegelman RK. *Studying a Study and Testing a Test.* 5th ed. Philadelphia, PA: Lippincott Williams & Wilkins; 2005.

Speelman P, Hartskeerl K. Leptospirosis. In: Fauci A, Braunwald E, Kasper DL, et al., eds. *Harrison's Principles of Internal Medicine.* 17th ed. New York, NY: McGraw-Hill; 2008.

U.S. Preventive Services Task Force. *Screening for Colorectal Cancer: U.S. Preventive Services Task Force Recommendation Statement. AHRQ Publication 08–05124-EF-3.* Rockville, MD: Agency for Healthcare Research and Quality; 2014, p. 24.

Walker DH, Dumler SJ, Marris T. Rickettsial disease. In: Fauci A, Braunwald E, Kasper DL, et al., eds. *Harrison's Principles of Internal Medicine.* 17th ed. New York, NY: McGraw-Hill; 2008.

White NJ, Breman JG. 2008, pp. 192–193; http://www.cdc.gov/malaria/ diagnosis_treatment/treatment.html

White NJ, Breman JG. Malaria. In: Fauci A, Braunwald E, Kasper DL, et al., eds. *Harrison's Principles of Internal Medicine.* 17th ed. New York, NY: McGraw-Hill; 2008.

Wolfe R. Immunizations. In: Woolf SH, Jonas S, Kaplan-Liss E, eds. *Health Promotion and Disease Prevention.* 2nd ed. Philadelphia, PA: Lippincott Williams & Wilkins; 2008.

Woolf SH. Principles of risk assessment. In: Woolf SH, Jonas S, Kaplan-Liss E, eds. *Health Promotion and Disease Prevention.* 2nd ed. Philadelphia, PA: Lippincott Williams & Wilkins; 2008.

Woolf SH, Jonas S, Kaplan-Liss E. *Health Promotion and Disease Prevention.* 2nd ed. Philadelphia, PA: Lippincott Williams & Wilkins; 2008.

Zolopa AR, Katz MH. HIV infection and AIDS. In: McPhee SJ, Papadakis MA, eds. *Current Medical Diagnosis and Treatment.* 49th ed. New York, NY: McGraw-Hill; 2010.

CHAPTER 21

Basic Science

Raymond J. Pavlick Jr., PhD

DIRECTIONS: Each of the numbered questions or incomplete statements is followed by possible answers or completions of the statement. Select the ONE-lettered answer or completion that is BEST in each case.

1. A 42-year-old female with a past medical history of schizophrenia begins to experience signs and symptoms of primary polydipsia. Which of the following changes in the patient's plasma osmolality, plasma antidiuretic hormone (ADH), and urine osmolality have most likely occurred?

	Plasma Osmolality	Plasma ADH	Urine Osmolality
(A)	↓	↑	↑
(B)	↓	↓	↑
(C)	↓	↓	↓
(D)	↑	↑	↓
(E)	↑	↓	↓

↑, increased; ↓, decreased (compared to normal).

2. A 56-year-old female presents to the clinic with complaints of persistent headaches, blurred vision, progressive loss of peripheral vision, and excessive sweating. On physical examination, the patient is noted to have enlarged hands and feet, macrognathia, macroglossia, and a prominent forehead. Which of the following metabolic abnormalities is most likely present in this patient?

(A) Decreased hepatic gluconeogenesis
(B) Decreased lipolysis in adipose tissue
(C) Increased blood glucose concentration
(D) Increased glucose uptake by skeletal muscle
(E) Increased insulin sensitivity

3. A 56-year-old male with a 23-year history of type 2 diabetes mellitus presents with bilateral swelling of his lower extremities. Laboratory analysis determines the presence of nephrotic syndrome. Which of the following changes in Starling's forces is most likely contributing to the patient's edema?

(A) Decreased capillary hydrostatic pressure
(B) Decreased capillary oncotic pressure
(C) Decreased interstitial hydrostatic pressure
(D) Increased capillary hydrostatic pressure
(E) Increased capillary oncotic pressure

4. A 64-year-old male with a 15-year history of aortic insufficiency develops worsening symptoms of his condition. Which of the following changes in end-diastolic volume (EDV) and preload is the patient most likely experiencing?

	End-diastolic Volume (EDV)	Preload
(A)	↓	↑
(B)	↓	↓
(C)	↑	↓
(D)	↑	↑
(E)	↑	↔

↑, increased; ↓, decreased; ↔, no change (compared to normal).

5. A 24-year-old male is struck by a hockey puck directly on the bridge of his nose resulting in anosmia. In which of the following structures would the synaptic connections between first- and second-order neurons be interrupted?

(A) Hypothalamus
(B) Olfactory bulbs
(C) Olfactory tracts
(D) Primary olfactory cortex
(E) Thalamus

6. Which of the following normally occurs during the quiet (normal) expiratory phase of a respiratory cycle in a healthy adult patient?

   (A) External intercostal muscles contract
   (B) Internal intercostal muscles contract
   (C) Intrapleural pressure increases
   (D) Lungs expel their functional residual capacity (FRC)
   (E) Passive recoil of the lungs lowers alveolar pressure

7. According to the Frank–Starling law of the heart:

   (A) The majority of ventricular filling occurs passively
   (B) The ventricles completely empty with every beat
   (C) The ventricles eject more blood with increases in end-diastolic volume
   (D) The ventricles eject more blood with sympathetic stimulation
   (E) Venous return decreases with an elevated central venous pressure

8. A 47-year-old female with a 20-year history of Crohn's disease develops localized small bowel adenocarcinoma, prompting surgical resection of the ileum. Which of the following conditions is most likely to occur in this patient if not treated appropriately following the surgery and throughout her lifetime?

   (A) Anemia
   (B) Hemochromatosis
   (C) Hyperbilirubinemia
   (D) Nyctalopia
   (E) Osteomalacia

9. Which of the following is the major determinant of resistance to blood flow in the arterial circulation?

   (A) Blood volume
   (B) Length of blood vessels
   (C) Plasma protein concentration
   (D) Radius of blood vessels
   (E) Viscosity of the blood

10. An 11-year-old male recently had soft tissue surgery performed in the upper and anterior part of his neck. Three weeks after the operation, deviation of the tongue to the left side was noted upon sticking it out. The left side of the tongue was also observed to have marked atrophy. Which of the following was most likely injured during the operation?

    (A) Left glossopharyngeal nerve
    (B) Left hypoglossal nerve
    (C) Right accessory nerve
    (D) Right glossopharyngeal nerve
    (E) Right hypoglossal nerve

11. Which of the following set of plasma levels is most consistent in a 47-year-old female diagnosed with primary hyperparathyroidism due to a solitary parathyroid adenoma?

	1,25-(OH)$_2$D$_3$ (Vitamin D$_3$)	Calcium (Ca^{+2})	Phosphate (PO$_4$$^{-3}$)
(A)	↓	↓	↑
(B)	↓	↓	↓
(C)	↓	↑	↓
(D)	↑	↑	↓
(E)	↑	↑	↑

    ↓, decreased; ↑, increased (compared to normal).

12. A 59-year-old, right-handed African-American male with a 20-year history of type 2 diabetes mellitus is found on the floor by his wife. She asks him what's wrong and his only complaint is a headache. Examination reveals an alert, awake patient with anosognosia, left hemineglect, and right gaze preferences. There are also signs of left hemiparesis (upper extremity substantially weaker than lower extremity) and left hemisensory deficits in the upper extremity and face. Which of the following arterial vessels was most likely affected?

    (A) Left anterior cerebral
    (B) Left middle cerebral
    (C) Right anterior cerebral
    (D) Right anterior inferior cerebellar
    (E) Right middle cerebral

13. A 34-year-old male comes to the emergency department complaining of stabbing right-sided flank pain that started early in the morning and awoke him from his sleep. He does not report any fever of

chills. On ultrasound, he is found to have a ureteral stone. Which of the following changes in hydrostatic pressure in Bowman's space (capsule), glomerular filtration rate (GFR), and filtration fraction are most likely to occur in this patient?

	Hydrostatic Pressure in Bowman's Space	Glomerular Filtration Rate (GFR)	Filtration Fraction
(A)	↓	↑	↑
(B)	↓	↑	↓
(C)	↑	↓	↑
(D)	↑	↑	↓
(E)	↑	↓	↓

↓, decreased; ↑, increased (compared to normal).

14. A 24-year-old female presents to the emergency department with severe diarrhea that has been occurring over the last 2 to 3 days. When she is supine, her blood pressure is 90/60 mm Hg and her heart rate is 102 beats/min. When she moves to a standing position, her heart rate further increases to 128 beats/min. Which of the following triggered the further increase in heart rate upon standing?

(A) Decrease in contractility (inotropy)

(B) Decrease in venous return

(C) Increase in afterload

(D) Increase in arterial tone (vasoconstriction)

(E) Increase in contractility (inotropy)

15. An arterial blood gas obtained from a 25-year-old female patient yields the following values:

pH = 7.52 (normal: 7.35–7.45)
$PaCO_2$ = 20 mm Hg (normal: 33–45 mm Hg)
$[HCO_3^-]$ = 16 mEq/L (normal: 22–28 mEq/L)

Based on these data, which of the following is most likely occurring in this patient?

(A) Compensation by buffers acting like bases

(B) Development of an alkaline urine

(C) Development of severe hypoventilation

(D) Overproduction of fixed acid

(E) Respiratory compensation of a metabolic alkalosis

16. A 31-year-old male presents with a 3-day history of left leg pain and swelling after playing video games continuously for almost 10 hours a day for

4 consecutive days. On each day, he would sit on the bed with his legs outstretched. Doppler ultrasound of the left leg confirmed extensive deep venous thrombosis requiring thrombolysis and anticoagulation. Which of the following changes in Starling's forces is the most likely cause of edema in this patient?

(A) Decreased capillary hydrostatic pressure

(B) Decreased capillary oncotic pressure

(C) Increased capillary hydrostatic pressure

(D) Increased capillary oncotic pressure

(E) Increased interstitial hydrostatic pressure

17. A 56-year-old male presents to the emergency department with right upper quadrant pain, nausea, and mild jaundice. Which of the following is most likely to be elevated in the blood?

(A) Bilirubin

(B) Creatinine

(C) Glucose

(D) Ketones

(E) Uric acid

18. A 52-year-old female presents with vaginal discharge that is white curd-like in appearance but is not malodorous. She has a 19-year history of obesity and poorly controlled type 2 diabetes mellitus. Microscopic examination of the discharge with 10% potassium hydroxide demonstrates filaments and spores. Which of the following is the most likely etiologic agent?

(A) *Candida*

(B) *Gardnerella*

(C) *Lactobacillus*

(D) *Staphylococcus epidermidis*

(E) *Trichomonas vaginalis*

19. A premature infant is born by a diabetic mother with the inability to produce adequate amounts of pulmonary surfactant. Which of the following will most likely occur as a result of this condition?

(A) Collapse of small lung alveoli

(B) Decreased solubility of carbon dioxide in the alveoli

(C) Decreased solubility of oxygen in the alveoli

(D) Increased lung compliance

(E) Reduction of alveolar surface tension

20. A 19-year-old female starts her normal menstruation this month. Which of the following is the normal, physiological trigger for this event?

(A) Degeneration of the corpus luteum

(B) Elevation of progesterone in the blood

(C) Secretion of human chorionic gonadotropin (hCG)

(D) Secretion of oxytocin

(E) Surge in luteinizing hormone (LH) secretion

21. A 58-year-old male with a past medical history of gouty arthritis presents with a red, swollen joint at the base of the great toe. His diet for the past 7 to 10 days consisted of large quantities of seafood and beer. The increased metabolism of which of the following most likely contributed to the patient's symptoms?

(A) Amino acids

(B) Polysaccharides

(C) Purines

(D) Pyrimidines

(E) Triglycerides

22. A 52-year-old female diagnosed with ductal adenocarcinoma in the head of the pancreas develops jaundice and steatorrhea. Which of the following is most likely to be diminished in the blood?

(A) Calcium

(B) Iron

(C) Vitamin B_{12}

(D) Vitamin C

(E) Vitamin K

23. A 35-year-old female presents to the clinic with irritability, palpitations, and a 15-pound weight loss over the past 6 weeks. History reveals heat intolerance and irregular menstrual cycles. Physical examination demonstrates protrusion of the eyes, moist skin, a diffusely enlarged thyroid gland, and a fine tremor of the hands. Her resting heart rate is 125 beats/minute. Initial laboratory testing shows a low serum thyroid stimulating hormone (TSH) and an elevated serum free thyroxine (T_4). Radioactive iodine uptake (RAIU) at 24 hours was 54% (normal: 10–30%). Which of the following is the most likely mechanism responsible for this patient's condition?

(A) Ectopic thyroid gland

(B) Factitious administration of levothyroxine

(C) Pituitary adenoma

(D) Production of thyroid stimulating hormone receptor antibodies

(E) Synthesis of antithyroglobulin antibodies

24. A 23-year-old male was found to be apneic and unresponsive in the surgical recovery room following reconstructive knee surgery. The patient was cyanotic with small pinpoint pupils, but he still had a pulse. About 20 minutes earlier, he received intravenous (IV) morphine for pain relief. While he is being assessed and resuscitated, an arterial blood gas sample was obtained, yielding the following:

> pH = 7.23 (normal: 7.35–7.45)
> $PaCO_2$ = 62 mm Hg (normal: 33–45 mm Hg)
> [HCO_3^-] = 26 mEq/L (normal: 22–28 mEq/L)

The patient is most likely suffering from an acute form of which of the following?

(A) Metabolic acidosis

(B) Metabolic alkalosis

(C) Mixed metabolic acidosis and respiratory alkalosis

(D) Respiratory acidosis

(E) Respiratory alkalosis

25. Which of the following is most likely to occur following the administration of a drug that inhibits acetylcholinesterase at peripheral target tissues?

(A) Bronchodilation

(B) Dry mouth

(C) Gastrointestinal tract hypermotility

(D) Pupil dilation

(E) Urine retention

26. During a spirometry test, a patient is asked to forcibly expel as much air from the lungs as possible. Which of the following represents the amount of air that remains in the patient's lungs following this maximal forced expiration?

(A) Expiratory reserve volume

(B) Functional residual capacity

(C) Residual volume

(D) Tidal volume

(E) Vital capacity

27. The sinoatrial (SA) node is the heart's normal pace-maker and controls the heart rate because it:

(A) Develops the fastest rate of depolarization

(B) Is located in the right atrium of the heart

(C) Is the only cardiac pacemaker that causes atrial depolarization

(D) Is unaffected by hormonal regulation

(E) Receives both sympathetic and parasympathetic innervation

28. A 54-year-old male presents in the emergency department with a junctional escape rhythm. Which of the following events of the cardiac cycle is most likely to be hindered by the patient's dysrhythmia?

(A) Closure of the semilunar valves

(B) Development of the dicrotic notch

(C) Isovolumetric ventricular relaxation

(D) Opening of the atrioventricular valves

(E) Ventricular filling

29. Which of the following is the major method by which carbon dioxide is transported in the venous blood?

(A) As bicarbonate ions

(B) Bound to albumin

(C) Bound to carbonic anhydrase

(D) Bound to hemoglobin

(E) Dissolved in the plasma

30. Which of the following most accurately describes the function of high-density lipoprotein (HDL)?

(A) Decreases lipoprotein lipase activity in adipocytes

(B) Inhibits chylomicron synthesis in the small intestine

(C) Inhibits endogenous cholesterol production by the body

(D) Prevents cholesterol absorption from the intestines

(E) Transports cholesterol to the liver for biliary excretion

Answers and Explanations

1. **(C)** Primary polydipsia (also known as psychogenic polydipsia) is characterized by a primary increase in water intake. This disorder is most often seen in middle-aged females and in patients with psychiatric illnesses. Ingesting large volumes of water typically causes a decrease in plasma osmolality, as solutes such as sodium and chloride become diluted in the blood. An increase in plasma osmolality (>295 mOsm/L) is a primary stimulus for antidiuretic hormone (ADH) secretion from the posterior pituitary; hence, a decrease in plasma osmolality leads to reduced ADH secretion. In addition, volume expansion also reduces ADH secretion to allow for more water excretion via the urine. This patient would be expected to produce large volumes of dilute urine in an attempt to maintain water homeostasis due to the excessive intake of water. As a result, the urine osmolality will be decreased. *(Bichet, 2013; Costanzo, 2014, Ch. 9)*

2. **(C)** The signs and symptoms noted in this patient are classic manifestations of growth hormone excess after puberty (acromegaly), most likely due to a pituitary adenoma. Growth hormone has diabetogenic effects that result in an increase in blood glucose concentration, including increased hepatic gluconeogenesis, inhibition of glucose uptake by skeletal muscle, increased lipolysis in adipose tissue, and decreased insulin sensitivity by a number of tissues. *(Costanzo, 2014, Ch. 9; Melmed, 2013)*

3. **(B)** Nephrotic syndrome refers to a distinct constellation of clinical and laboratory features of renal disease. It is specifically defined by the presence of heavy proteinuria (protein excretion greater than 3.5 g/24 hours), hypoalbuminemia (less than 3 g/dL), and peripheral edema. Capillary oncotic pressure (also known as plasma colloid osmotic pressure) is determined largely by the concentration of plasma proteins and causes fluid to move from interstitial spaces into capillaries. As the concentration of plasma protein decreases (hypoalbuminemia) in this patient due to proteinuria, there is less absorption of fluid into the capillaries and more net filtration of fluid out of the capillaries. This excess volume of interstitial fluid exceeds the ability of the lymphatic system to return it to the circulation, resulting in the patient's edema. *(Costanzo, 2014, Ch. 4; Kelepouris & Rovin, 2014)*

4. **(D)** Aortic insufficiency is defined by incompetence of the aortic valve. This results in a portion of the stroke volume leaking back (regurgitating) to the left ventricle during diastole, thereby increasing the end-diastolic volume (EDV) each time the left ventricle fills during a cardiac cycle. This, in turn, results in volume overloading of the left ventricle and an increase in left ventricular wall stress (preload), which typically leads to left ventricular dilation and hypertrophy. *(Gaasch, 2014)*

5. **(B)** The injury most likely led to fractures of the nasal and ethmoid bones, resulting in severing of the axons of several olfactory receptor cells. These olfactory receptors cells (first-order neurons) have axons that pass through the cribriform plate of the ethmoid bone. Their axon terminals synapse with second-order neurons right above the ethmoid bone within the glomeruli of the olfactory bulbs, which lie on the inferior surface of the frontal lobes. The axons of these second-order neurons continue to pass through the olfactory tracts, on their way to the primary olfactory cortex. *(Mann & Lafraniere, 2014)*

6. **(C)** During quiet expiration there is no muscle activity required to expel air. Passive (elastic) recoil of the lungs and chest wall causes alveolar volume to decrease, thereby creating the pressure gradient (alveolar pressure > atmospheric pressure) to induce airflow out of the lungs. The amount of air expelled is the tidal volume; the FRC is what remains in the lungs following a quiet expiration. The intrapleural pressure increases (i.e., becomes less negative) during quiet expiration due to the passive recoil of the lungs and chest wall. *(Costanzo, 2014, Ch. 5)*

7. **(C)** The Frank–Starling law of the heart explains the relationship between end-diastolic volume and stroke volume. According to the relationship, the more the ventricles fill with blood during diastole (within physiological limits), the more forceful they will contract during systole. This is an intrinsic mechanism the heart uses to match cardiac output with venous return without any neural or hormonal influences. *(Costanzo, 2014, Ch. 4)*

8. **(A)** The ileum is the site where the majority of vitamin B_{12} absorption occurs (in conjunction with intrinsic factor) within the small intestine. Vitamin B_{12} is one of many essential substances required for normal erythropoiesis in red bone marrow. Vitamin B_{12} deficiency leads to a megaloblastic (macroovalocytic) anemia, resulting from increased peripheral red cell breakdown and ineffective erythropoiesis. The patient will require parental vitamin B_{12} supplementation throughout her lifetime to prevent this type of anemia. *(Schrier, 2014)*

9. **(D)** The relationship between the major factors causing resistance to blood flow can be summarized with the Poiseuille equation:

$$\text{Resistance} = \frac{8VL}{\pi r^4}$$

where V is the viscosity of blood; L is the length of a blood vessel; and r is the radius of a blood vessel. When the radius of an arterial blood vessel decreases (as in vasoconstriction), the resistance increases tremendously because the radius is raised to the fourth power. This same effect, in terms of magnitude, would not be achieved with changes to blood viscosity or blood vessel length according to the Poiseuille equation. *(Costanzo, 2014, Ch. 4)*

10. **(B)** The hypoglossal nerve provides motor control of the extrinsic and intrinsic muscles of the tongue. Injury of the hypoglossal nerve (12th cranial nerve) is a recognized complication following soft tissue surgery in the upper and anterior part of the neck. Disorders of the hypoglossal nerve cause weakness and/or wasting (atrophy) of the tongue on the affected side. The tongue will deviate to the affected side upon protrusion because it has lost the strength to resist the push to that side. *(Gelb, 2014)*

11. **(D)** Elevated levels of parathyroid hormone (PTH) raise plasma calcium through its effects on bone (stimulation of bone resorption) and the kidneys (decrease in renal Ca^{+2} excretion). Activation of vitamin D is completed by 1-hydroxylation in the kidneys and is stimulated by parathyroid hormone (PTH). Hence, levels of $1,25\text{-}(OH)_2D_3$ (active vitamin D) rise as PTH increases. PTH also increases renal phosphate excretion, due to the inhibition of phosphate reabsorption in the proximal convoluted tubules. *(Costanzo, 2014, Ch. 9)*

12. **(E)** The middle cerebral arteries supply the following regions:

    - The primary motor cortex (frontal lobe) involved with voluntary control of the muscles of the face and upper extremities
    - The primary somatosensory cortex (parietal lobe) involved with sensation of the face and upper extremities
    - Wernicke's area (temporal lobe) and Broca's area (frontal lobe)

    The patient's symptoms are consistent with stroke to the right middle cerebral artery: contralateral paralysis of the upper extremity and face, contralateral loss of sensation in the upper extremity and face and left hemineglect. *(Ferri, 2015)*

13. **(E)** Blockage of the ureter will cause tubular fluid to collect in the nephrons, leading to an elevation in the hydrostatic pressure within Bowman's spaces (capsules). This particular Starling force opposes filtration, and as a result, the GFR will decrease. Renal blood flow is unaffected by the ureteral stone and will remain the same. The filtration fraction is the ratio of GFR to renal blood flow (RBF). Hence, with a decrease in GFR and no change to the RBF, the filtration fraction decreases. *(Costanzo, 2014, Ch. 6)*

14. (B) The effects of gravity upon standing caused blood to pool in the veins of the patient's lower extremities. This led to a decrease in venous return and ventricular filling. As a result, both stroke volume and mean arterial pressure (MAP) decreased. This triggered the baroreceptor reflex in an attempt to raise the MAP back to normal. As a result of activation of the baroreceptor reflex, the heart rate increased, along with cardiac contractility. Peripheral vasoconstriction also occurred, leading to increased total peripheral resistance (TPR) and MAP. Note that the question asked for the trigger, not the outcomes of the baroreceptor reflex. Answers D and E are outcomes, not triggers. *(Costanzo, 2014, Ch. 4)*

15. (B) Based on the arterial blood gas (ABG), this patient has developed respiratory alkalosis due to the low arterial carbon dioxide causing an elevation in arterial pH. With an alkalosis, buffers are expected to compensate by acting like acids, as the donation of free H^+ is needed to lower the pH toward the normal range (hence, choice A is incorrect). The patient's respiratory alkalosis is due to hyperventilation (not hypoventilation), as reflected by the decreased arterial carbon dioxide (hence, choice C is incorrect). With a pH of 7.52, there is no overproduction of fixed acid, as this would cause metabolic acidosis (hence, choice D is incorrect). Choice E is incorrect as this patient is not suffering from a metabolic alkalosis. If she was, then elevated arterial bicarbonate would be causing the elevated pH; this patient's arterial bicarbonate level is low, not high. Choice B is correct, as the expected compensation for a respiratory alkalosis by the kidneys would be the excretion of bicarbonate in the urine. This would cause the urine pH to become more alkaline. *(Costanzo, 2014, Ch. 7)*

16. (C) A period of prolonged, seated immobility is recognized as one of the major risk factors for developing venous thrombosis. Long-distance air travel and prolonged sitting in relation to work or recreation have been shown to increase the risk of venous thrombosis. With a venous thrombus, there is impedance of blood flow through the affected vein(s), which subsequently causes blood to accumulate in associated capillaries. The raises the hydrostatic pressure in the affected capillaries, causing more fluid to leave and enter into the interstitial spaces, thereby causing edema. *(Costanzo, 2014, Ch. 4)*

17. (A) This patient's signs and symptoms correlate with a suspected case of choledocholithiasis (presence of gallstones within the common bile duct). Jaundice is associated with hyperbilirubinemia, in which the excess bilirubin can deposit in tissues such as the skin, sclera, oral mucosa, and nails. Bilirubin is the waste product generated from the metabolism of hemoglobin. *(Freeman & Arain, 2014)*

18. (A) This case has several clues pointing to a *Candida* infection, including the fact that diabetes mellitus can predispose patients to *Candida* infections and the presence of the white curd-like discharge that is not malodorous. In *Trichomonas vaginalis*, the discharge is malodorous and yellow-green in color. With *Gardnerella*, there is also a malodorous discharge. *Lactobacillus* is the predominant, normal microorganism of the vagina and keeps it slightly acidic to help reduce the growth of potentially harmful organisms. *Staphylococcus epidermidis* is also part of the natural flora of the vagina. *(Sobel, 2014)*

19. (A) Because of their small size, many lung alveoli are prone to collapse. Pulmonary surfactant contains a high concentration of amphipathic phospholipid molecules, which lowers the surface tension of alveoli. According to the law of Laplace, a reduction of surface tension reduces the collapsing pressure on small alveoli and allows them to remain open. Pulmonary surfactant production does not typically begin until the 24th week of gestation; hence, an infant born before this time is at great risk for having collapsed alveoli due to elevated alveolar surface tension. *(Costanzo, 2014, Ch. 5)*

20. (A) If a woman does not become pregnant during her menstrual cycle, there is a lack of human chorionic gonadotropin (hCG) production, as the trophoblast never formed. hCG normally maintains functioning of the corpus luteum and is the signal for the corpus luteum to continue synthesizing progesterone and estradiol, which maintain the endometrial lining. Regression of the corpus luteum and the subsequent loss of progesterone and estradiol cause the endometrial lining to degenerate and menstrual bleeding to occur. *(Costanzo, 2014, Ch. 10)*

21. (C) Purines are normally metabolized into uric acid by the liver and can be found in high amounts in several foods and beverages, including organ meats, seafood, beans, peas, and beer. Higher levels of seafood and beer consumption are associated with an increased risk of gout because of the hyperuricemia that can occur via purine metabolism. *(Becker, 2014)*

22. **(E)** Tumors in the pancreatic head region can often block the flow of bile from the gall bladder and liver to the duodenum, resulting in jaundice and steatorrhea. The bile salts are important for micelle formation within the lumen of the small intestine. Micelles provide a mechanism whereby the hydrophobic products of lipid digestion as well as fat-soluble vitamins (e.g., A, D, E, and K) can be absorbed in the small intestine. *(Mason, 2013)*

23. **(D)** The patient's history, signs, and symptoms are consistent with a diagnosis of Graves' disease. Graves' disease is a form of hyperthyroidism caused by autoantibodies to the thyroid stimulating hormone (TSH) receptor (TSHR-Ab) that activate the receptor, thereby stimulating thyroid hormone synthesis and secretion as well as thyroid growth (causing a diffuse goiter). The elevation in thyroid hormones leads to a decrease in TSH secretion due to negative feedback. *(Davies, 2013; Ross, 2014)*

24. **(D)** Based on the arterial blood gas and history, this patient has developed respiratory acidosis that is related to opiate-induced hypoventilation. The elevation in arterial carbon dioxide (volatile acid) is leading to the formation of higher amounts of free H^+, thereby lowering the arterial pH. The history indicates that this is an acute event, having just occurred over a 20-minute period. Hence, the kidneys have not had sufficient time to compensate for the respiratory acidosis by synthesizing and reabsorbing bicarbonate. This is reflected in the normal arterial bicarbonate level. *(Costanzo, 2014, Ch. 10)*

25. **(C)** Acetylcholinesterase normally degrades acetylcholine within synaptic clefts. Inhibition of this enzyme leads to accumulation of acetylcholine, thereby producing parasympathomimetic effects. These would include bronchoconstriction, increased salivation, increased GI motility, pupil constriction, bradycardia, and hypermotility of bladder smooth muscle. *(Costanzo, 2014, Ch. 2)*

26. **(C)** By definition, residual volume is the volume of air remaining in the lungs after a maximal forced expiration. The residual volume is important physiologically, as it prevents total collapse of the alveoli and minimizes the pressure and energy required to inflate the lungs during inspiration. *(Costanzo, 2014, Ch. 5)*

27. **(A)** The SA node functions as a pacemaker because it exhibits automaticity, which means that it can fire action potentials spontaneously without requiring neural or endocrine input. However, the cells comprising the SA node are not the only myocardial cells that demonstrate automaticity. The heart also has latent pacemakers such as the AV node, bundle of His, and Purkinje fibers. While these tissues can exhibit automaticity and function as a pacemaker, they generally do not because of a physiological concept known as "overdrive suppression." Fundamental to this concept is the fact that the cells that have the fastest rate of phase 4 depolarization are the ones that control the heart rate. The cells of the SA node generate the fastest rate of depolarization and, as a result, the latent pacemakers' ability to spontaneously depolarize is suppressed. *(Costanzo, 2014, Ch. 4)*

28. **(E)** A junctional escape rhythm occurs when there is failure of impulse generation from the SA node. Hence, there are no P waves present on the electrocardiogram (ECG), and the AV node assumes the role of pacemaker. Without atrial depolarization, atrial systole does not occur and ventricular filling only occurs passively. Atrial systole normally represents 15% to 20% of the subsequent stroke volume. *(Costanzo, 2014, Ch. 4)*

29. **(A)** Carbon dioxide is carried in three different forms within the blood: dissolved in plasma, attached to proteins such as hemoglobin and albumin, and as bicarbonate ions. Carbon dioxide is converted into bicarbonate ions because of the activity of carbonic anhydrase, which is present in red blood cells. Approximately 70% of the total carbon dioxide in the blood is carried as bicarbonate ions. *(Costanzo, 2014, Ch. 5)*

30. **(E)** High-density lipoproteins (HDLs) are considered "good" when elevated in the blood because of their ability to lower the risk of coronary heart disease. HDLs accomplish this through a series of biochemical reactions that enable them to target excess cholesterol present in the blood and tissue for biliary excretion by the liver. *(Rosenson, 2014)*

REFERENCES

Becker MA. Clinical manifestations and diagnosis of gout. In: *UpToDate*, 2014.

Bichet DG. Diagnosis of polyuria and diabetes insipidus. In: *UpToDate*, 2013.

Costanzo LS. *Physiology*. 5th ed. Philadelphia, PA: Elsevier Saunders; 2014.

Davies TF. Pathogenesis of Graves' disease. In: *UpToDate*, 2013.

Ferri FF. *Ferri's Clinical Advisor 2015*. Philadelphia, PA: Elsevier Mosby; 2015.

Freeman ML, Arain MA. Choledocholithiasis: clinical manifestations, diagnosis, and management. In: *UpToDate*, 2014.

Gaasch WH. Pathophysiology, clinical features, and evaluation of chronic aortic regurgitation in adults. In: *UpToDate*, 2014.

Gelb D. The detailed neurologic examination in adults. In: *UpToDate*, 2014.

Kelepouris E, Rovin BH. Overview of heavy proteinuria and the nephrotic syndrome. In: *UpToDate*, 2014.

Mann NM, Lafraniere D. Anatomy and etiology of taste and smell disorders. In: *UpToDate*, 2014.

Mason JB. Mechanisms of nutrient absorption and malabsorption. In: *UpToDate*, 2013.

Melmed S. Causes and clinical manifestations of acromegaly. In: *UpToDate*, 2013.

Rosenson RS. Lipoprotein classification, metabolism, and role in atherosclerosis. In: *UpToDate*, 2014.

Ross DS. Diagnosis of hyperthyroidism. In: *UpToDate*, 2014.

Schrier SL. Etiology and clinical manifestations of vitamin B_{12} and folate deficiency. In: *UpToDate*, 2014.

Sobel JD. Candida vulvovaginitis. In: *UpToDate*, 2014.

Index